Bottom Line's Prescription for
NATURAL CURES

With Thousands of Ways to Tap the Astounding Healing Power of Today's Best Natural Remedies

JAMES F. BALCH, MD
MARK STENGLER, ND

Bottom Line Books
www.BottomLineSecrets.com

Bottom Line's Prescription for Natural Cures
With Thousands of Ways to Tap the Astounding Healing Power of Today's Best Natural Remedies
by James F. Balch, MD and Mark Stengler, ND

Published by arrangement with John Wiley & Sons, Inc., Hoboken, New Jersey

Design and production by Navta Associates, Inc.

Exclusive Hardcover Edition published by Bottom Line Books®

Cover Design © Boardroom Inc.

ISBN 0-88723-540-9

Bottom Line Books® publishes the opinions of expert authorities in many fields. The use of a book is not a substitute for health, legal, accounting or other professional services. Consult competent professionals for answers to your specific questions.

Offers, prices, rates, addresses, telephone numbers and Web sites listed in this book are accurate at the time of publication, but they are subject to frequent change.

Bottom Line Books® is a registered trademark of Boardroom® Inc.
281 Tresser Boulevard, Stamford, CT 06901
www.BottomLineSecrets.com

Printed in the United States of America

Contents

Contents

Part Two: The Essentials of Natural Medicine

Part Three: Appendix

Preface

This book was written to provide the public, as well as health practitioners, with the most up-to-date, results-oriented, yet user-friendly, reference book on natural healing available today. It contains information that was published in some of the world's most prestigious medical journals. In addition, it includes invaluable "gems" of clinical advice that you will not likely find in any other book. These tips were either passed on to us by generations of doctors and natural health-care practitioners from around the world or were learned firsthand in our work with thousands of patients.

Prescription for Natural Cures focuses on natural and preventative remedies. It is our belief that the body functions best when we ingest substances that are as close as possible to their natural state. This rule holds true with most foods, herbs, air, and water. While modern pharmaceutical medications can have amazing properties and may be necessary in certain cases, they generally have an inherent potential for causing side effects. Why is this so? Simply put, our genetic code was not designed to be compatible with synthetic, man-made drugs. Does this mean that we do not recommend the use of pharmaceutical medications, surgery, or other conventional therapies? Not at all. As doctors, we are grateful that our medical training has given us a strong background in conventional therapies. For example, Dr. Balch was a skilled urological surgeon before he focused on his new passion for natural healing. We recommend whatever it takes for a patient to get better. Many times, it is a comprehensive protocol of several natural therapies, such as dietary changes, nutritional supplements, exercise, and other natural techniques. In other cases, a patient may require a combination of natural and conventional therapies. This is often seen with cancer, cardiovascular disease, and advanced diabetes, as well as in cases of emergency care.

Where we differ from mainstream doctors is that we believe nonemergency conditions and most chronic health problems should be dealt with by using holistic therapies, whenever possible. They provide a nontoxic way for the body to heal itself, without the risks incurred from the use of suppressive or damaging pharmaceutical agents. By relying on natural therapies as the basis of therapy, we can add conventional treatment if needed, depending on the severity and the response of the patient. Currently, millions of North Americans and countless others around the world are incorporating holistic medicine into their health-care regimens, in an attempt to avoid surgery or stop using pharmaceutical medications. This wise plan may be attainable, but it should be attempted only under the supervision of a qualified doctor. You should not regard the advice in this book as a replacement for proper medical attention.

Let us also focus on the concept of prevention. Remember the last time you had a cold, the flu, or another ailment that you likely could have prevented with rest, sound nutrition, and specific nutrition supplements? The ultimate form of healing is to prevent an illness from occurring in the first place. This requires knowledge about how the body functions at a healthy level. Our book includes this information.

We believe that this book can make a tremendous difference in your health and the health of your loved ones. You now have within reach the powerful and amazing healing tools that were graciously given to us by our Creator.

Acknowledgments

First, I must thank my Lord Jesus Christ, who thirty years ago transformed my mind about healing and wellness. In addition, I thank my wife, Robin Young-Balch, a talented naturopathic doctor, whose research and encouragement spurred us on toward publication of this book. We pray that "the Multitudes" will benefit from the information contained herein.

—James F. Balch, M.D.

I would like to thank the Lord for the blessing of being able to help others with holistic medicine. To my wife, Angela, who is a fine doctor and, more important, an outstanding mother and wife. To my three children, who amaze and inspire me. Also, my thanks to Barb Wallace, for her assistance in the review and the preparation of the manuscript.

—Mark A. Stengler, N.D.

Our thanks to Jeff Herman for representing this book as our agent and to Tom Miller and the staff at John Wiley & Sons for their enthusiasm in publishing *Prescription for Natural Cures*.

—from both authors

How to Use This Book

This book focuses on providing you with results. We have incorporated the best of what science and nature have to offer in the field of natural medicine.

The largest component of the book, Part One, includes entries for health conditions. They are listed in alphabetical order. For easy reference, the exact page number of the condition you are looking for is located in the index at the back of this book. Each condition consists of five main parts, outlined here.

DESCRIPTION OF THE CONDITION

The important features of each condition are described in a thorough, yet easy-to-understand, manner. We provide details on how conventional, as well as holistic, doctors understand and approach these conditions. We mention why researchers believe this disease process is occurring. In many cases, we give our own explanation of why an imbalance or an illness may occur.

SYMPTOMS

A summary of the symptoms helps you to determine whether you have a specific condition. Of course, you should consult a health professional to obtain an accurate diagnosis.

ROOT CAUSES

This section provides a summary of the root causes for a condition or what its initiating factor(s) are. This will help you focus on what is causing your health problem.

TESTING TECHNIQUES

For each condition, we list the most important tests to help determine the root cause of your illness. This section will help you choose the best type of health care. The tests are commonly available through your local medical doctor or natural health-care provider. Please note: not every type of standard conventional test is listed for each condition, because we assume that these are part of your doctor's investigative procedure.

TREATMENT

The Treatment section has a comprehensive description of the following natural methods:

Diet. This section includes foods that are known to prevent or heal the condition. It also describes foods that can cause or worsen an illness.

Detoxification. Detoxification is important for preventing and healing disease. This section gives helpful advice on improving a condition with detoxifying techniques.

Super Seven Prescriptions. One unique aspect of this book, which distinguishes it from other natural healing reference books, is the Super Seven Prescriptions section. Here, we prioritize the top seven prescriptions a person can use for each condition. We chose these prescriptions based on what has worked clinically, is backed by scientific research, and is readily available to the public. You can glance through the top seven prescriptions and get a feel for what most accurately fits your symptom picture. After reviewing the super seven, you can start by using the first choice and see how it affects your condition. Also, you can pick more than one, for an aggressive approach to help prevent or improve a condition.

Studies. For most of the conditions, we provide concise studies demonstrating the scientific validity of the supplements we recommend.

General Recommendations. Since there are so many different choices of nutritional supplements, we also provide a general recommendation section. This includes other fine choices of supplements that are commonly available for each condition.

Homeopathy. Homeopathy is such a distinct field, compared to other nutritional practices, and it often requires more detailed information. We include a section on the most important homeopathic remedies and how to choose one that best fits your profile.

Acupressure. Most conditions have specific acupressure point recommendations that can be incorporated for faster, gentler healing.

Bodywork. Bodywork techniques, such as massage and reflexology, are recommended throughout the book for anyone interested in a comprehensive, self-healing approach.

Aromatherapy. Aromatherapy has had a tremendous surge in popularity in the last decade. Included here are some of the more effective choices for each condition.

Stress Reduction. Research has proved, time and again, that most health conditions can be positively or negatively influenced by how you cope with stress. This section describes practical, well-tested techniques to reduce the effects of stress and improve your health.

Bach Flower Remedies. These popular remedies were once found only in hard-core health food stores. Today they can be purchased in virtually every health food store and a growing number of pharmacies. A summary of the top choices is given for each condition.

Other Recommendations. The field of holistic medicine is vast. The "Other Recommendations" section briefly describes potentially helpful holistic therapies for each condition that were not mentioned in previous sections.

REFERENCES

For the scientifically minded, there is a summarization of the studies that we quoted for each condition.

Part Two, The Essentials of Natural Medicine, gives detailed, user-friendly information on the natural healing tools and methods we recommend throughout the book. It contains helpful advice on the clinical use of Diet and Nutrition, Fasting, Herbal Medicine, Homeopathy, Bach Flower Remedies, Aromatherapy, Traditional Chinese Medicine and Acupressure, Hydrotherapy, Natural Hormones, Bodywork, Exercise and Stress Reduction, and Nutritional Supplements.

Part Three contains a comprehensive glossary of unfamiliar medical terms, as well as a Resource Guide for Holistic Practitioners. This section describes the training and the holistic approach of individual practitioners, as well as contact information for a reliable referral.

PART ONE

Conditions

Abscesses and Boils

An abscess is an accumulation of pus that can occur anywhere in the body, including on the skin and inside of organs and tissues. When an abscess forms around a hair follicle, it is known as a boil. Boils often surface on the buttocks, the underarms, the neck, and the face. They first begin as small, firm, and tender nodules that become red and swollen. Generally, boils do not spread. Within two to four days, a pustule usually forms in the center of the infected area. Then, several days later, it tends to rupture and drain the white or yellow-colored pus. The abscess is called a carbuncle when the skin is red, painful, swollen, and warm, and it forms an elevated lump.

An abscess can occur on anyone at any age. No one is immune to them. They are generally triggered by an impaired immune system, trauma, improper drainage of tissues, bacterial invasion, poor nutrition, and other factors. Skin abscesses tend to develop in places where tight clothing rubs against the skin, as well as around small puncture wounds or cuts. The infected area becomes tender, red, and swollen, and fever may be present.

Delayed or improper treatment can lead to a spreading of the infection. People with a compromised immune system, such as those with HIV/AIDS or diabetes, are more susceptible to a serious infection. Depending on the severity and the location of the infection, antibiotics may be required. In some cases, the abscess will be cut and drained by your doctor. Consult your doctor about any skin abscess that appears on your face, contains red streaks, or is filled with fluids. See your dentist regarding any mouth abscesses. If antibiotics are required, ensure a quicker recovery by simultaneously using natural treatments.

SYMPTOMS

Each of the following symptoms can appear on the face, the chest, or the back.

- Red spots, bumps, or white/yellow pustules, often inflamed and painful
- Swollen, red, and hot area around the lesion
- Fever

Testing Techniques

The following tests will help to assess possible reasons for chronic abscess or boil formation:

Immune system imbalance or disease—blood

Intestinal permeability—urine

Detoxification profile—urine

Vitamin and mineral analysis (especially vitamins C, E)—blood, urine

Digestive function and microbe/parasite/candida testing—stool analysis

Anemia—blood test (CBC, iron, ferritin, % saturation)

Food and environmental allergies/sensitivities—blood, electrodermal

Blood-sugar balance—blood

ROOT CAUSES

- Poor diet and food allergies or sensitivities
- Impaired immune system
- Trauma

- Improper drainage of tissues
- Bacterial invasion, poor nutrition
- Clothing rubbing against the skin
- Puncture wounds or cuts

TREATMENT

Diet

Recommended Food

Dark-green or orange vegetables are especially helpful because they contain beta-carotene, which helps maintain and repair the skin. Eat them raw or lightly cooked to retain their nutrients and fiber.

A quarter of a cup of ground flaxseeds provides helpful essential fatty acids and plenty of fiber for proper elimination. Take with at least 8 ounces of water.

Nuts and seeds, such as almonds, walnuts, and pumpkin seeds, are good sources of skin-healthy vitamin E and essential fatty acids.

Quality protein sources are beans, peas, lentils, eggs, and fresh cold-water fish, such as salmon, mackerel, herring, and sardines. The latter are rich in omega-3 fatty acids.

Meat products should be hormone- and antibiotic-free.

Drink a glass of clean water every two waking hours to flush toxins out of the body and maintain good general health.

If you must use antibiotics, be sure to eat some live unsweetened yogurt every day. The yogurt will replace the "friendly" bacteria in your digestive tract, which are necessary for good health and which antibiotics destroy.

Food to Avoid

Eliminate chips and nachos, colas, sugar, and candy. These products suppress immune function.

Food allergies or sensitivities, such as an allergy to cow's milk, can be a root cause. See the Food Allergies section for more information.

Avoid saturated and hydrogenated fats, which worsen skin inflammation. Stay away from fried foods and solid fats, such as margarine, lard, and vegetable shortening.

Coffee and other caffeinated products may aggravate skin conditions. If they cause problems for you, cut them out and drink herbal teas instead.

People with carbohydrate sensitivity may notice skin improvement by reducing their carbohydrate intake and increasing their protein sources. This is because elevated levels of the blood sugar–regulating hormone insulin increase skin inflammation.

Detoxification

Detoxification helps to cleanse the body of inflammatory poisons. A three-day vegetable juice fast will sweep away toxic buildup. You should drink a variety of juices during your fast, but those made from carrots, apples, and beets with their tops, as well as green drinks (spirulina, wheatgrass, barley grass, chlorella), are especially supportive of a skin cleanse.

℞ Super Seven Prescriptions—Abscesses and Boils

Super Prescription #1   Tea tree (*Melaleuca alternifolia*) **oil**
Apply topically as a cream or 10 drops diluted in a half-ounce of water three times daily. Tea tree oil has antimicrobial effects and helps to draw the pus out.

Super Prescription #2   Colloidal silver
Apply 2 drops four times daily to reduce the infection. Colloidal silver has potent antimicrobial effects.

Super Prescription #3   Echinacea (*Echinacea purpurea*) and **goldenseal** (*Hydrastis canadensis*)
Take 500 mg or 2 to 4 ml of tincture four times daily. Both herbs enhance immune function.

Super Prescription #4   Oregano oil (*Origanum vulgare*)
Take 500 mg in the capsule form four times daily, or take the liquid form as directed on the container. It can be applied directly on the lesions as well. Oregano has powerful antibacterial properties. *Note*: Do not take internally if you are pregnant.

Super Prescription #5   Vitamin C with bioflavonoids
Take 1,000 mg three times daily. Vitamin C supports immune function, and bioflavonoids reduce skin inflammation.

Super Prescription #6   Burdock root (*Arctium lappa*)
Take 3 ml or 500 mg three times daily. Burdock root is used as a skin detoxifier.

Super Prescription #7   Zinc
Take 30 mg twice daily, along with 2 mg of copper. Zinc supports immune function and promotes skin healing.

The antimicrobial activity of oregano oil has been recognized for centuries. A test tube study at the Western University of Australia found that oregano oil had powerful antimicrobial activity against several types of bacteria, including *Staphylococcus aureus,* the bacteria commonly associated with skin infections.

General Recommendations

Super green food supplements, such as chlorella, spirulina, or blends of green foods, support skin healing and detoxification. Take as directed on the container.

Vitamin E is required for a healthy immune system and skin. Take 400 IU of a mixed complex twice daily.

Vitamin A supports immune function. Take 10,000 IU for ten days, and then stop.

Homeopathy

Pick the remedy that best matches your symptoms in this section. For acute abscesses and boils, take a 30C potency four times daily. For chronic abscesses and boils, take a 6x, 12x, 6C, 12C, or 30C twice daily for two weeks to see if there are any positive results. After you notice improvement, stop taking the remedy, unless symptoms return. Consultation with a homeopathic practitioner is advised.

Belladonna (*Atropa belladonna*) is used in the initial stages of an abscess or a boil, where there is a rapid onset characterized by redness, burning, throbbing, and swollen skin. Pus is not usually present. Symptoms are worse from touch or jarring and at midnight. A high fever may also be present.

Hepar Sulphuris is for abscesses that come to a head. The lesion is very sensitive and tender to touch, with a sharp, sticking pain. There may be a cheesy odor with the pus formation. Symptoms are worse in cold air or from cold applications and are better from warmth. This remedy helps to bring the pus out of the abscess or the boil.

Lachesis is used for boils with a purplish or dark-bluish color. Pustules may be bloody and very painful, with a burning sensation. Symptoms are worse at night; with touch, heat, and pressure; and on the left side of the body.

Mercurius Solubilis or Vivus is for burning and stinging pustular discharges. There is often a foul smell and swollen glands. Symptoms are worse at night. Warm applications may make the pain worse.

Silica (*Silicea*) is a great choice for abscesses or boils that do not discharge pus and that fail to heal. It is often used in addition to or following Hepar Sulphuris, to finish the suppuration. Warm compresses feel good on the lesions.

Acupressure

See pages 668–675 for information about pressure points and administering treatment.

- Spleen 10 clears heat from the blood.
- Large Intestine 4 relieves fever and inflammation.

Bodywork

Reflexology

See pages 686–687 for information about reflexology areas and how to work them.

- Work the kidneys and the liver to detoxify the blood.
- If acne is caused by a hormonal imbalance, work the endocrine glands.
- To prevent constipation and speed the elimination of toxins, work the colon.

Hydrotherapy

Alternate a hot and a cold cloth over the affected area to help reduce pain and help expel pus, if the abscess is on the skin: thirty seconds hot, followed by thirty seconds cold, and alternate.

Aromatherapy

Red thyme helps to draw the pus out. Add 1 drop to a hot compress, and apply twice daily to the skin abscess.

Stress Reduction

The effects of stress can worsen skin conditions. Techniques to reduce stress will ultimately help with skin health and appearance. Exercise, prayer, reading, and many other techniques can be used to reduce the effects of stress.

Bach Flower Remedies

Select the appropriate remedy, and place 10 drops under your tongue. Hold the drops in place for thirty seconds, and swallow. Use as often as needed.

Try Crab Apple if your skin is causing feelings of shame about your appearance.

If you've given up hope of finding a cure for your acne, Gorse will renew your spirits.

Larch is helpful for people who lack self-confidence or who are embarrassed because of their skin condition.

Sunlight can inhibit bacterial growth. Get fifteen minutes of sunlight daily, but never allow the skin to burn.

Other Recommendations

Do not squeeze a boil, and keep the area clean.

REFERENCES

Hammer, K. A., C. F. Carson, and T. V. Riley. 1999. Antimicrobial activity of essential oils and other plant extracts. *Journal of Applied Microbiology* 86:985–90.

Acne

The familiar red and white pimples of acne are caused by pores that are blocked and often infected. Although acne is most common in adolescents (more than 80 percent of those between ages twelve and twenty-one are afflicted), it now appears with increasing frequency in adults.

As most people are aware, hormones play a significant role in acne. Normally, the body produces sebum, an oily lubricant, and secretes it through sebaceous glands to the skin. This lubricant is necessary to protect the skin from the elements and to keep it moist. During adolescence and other times of hormonal change, fluctuating hormones change this process and create several conditions that are likely to produce acne. For one, sebum production increases, and the oil, instead of passing harmlessly through the glands, hardens and clogs up the glandular canals. As a result, a red bump—a pimple—appears on the skin. Second, there is also increased production of keratin, a protective protein that covers the skin. Third, the same hormones cause an increase in the number of sebaceous glands, so there are more opportunities for acne to develop.

All of these factors can lead to clogged and infected pores, resulting in increased bacteria and yeast overgrowth on the skin. Overgrowth of these organisms causes skin inflammation. Superficial inflammation results in pustule formation and skin redness. Inflammation that occurs deeper in the skin can result in the formation of nodules and cysts and, possibly, scars.

One must also consider the role of food sensitivities, which can cause or worsen acne. These are discussed further in the foods to avoid section further on. In addition, candida or yeast overgrowth can be an underlying cause of acne. This is most common after chronic antibiotic use, where "friendly bacteria" are destroyed, setting up the overgrowth of candida. Many people are on long-term antibiotic use for the treatment of acne, which sets up not only a further acne problem but potential digestive problems as well. Finally, nutritional deficiencies often need to be addressed to improve acne. Zinc, essential fatty acids, and other nutrients are crucial in preventing acne.

If you suffer from acne, be wary of the usual conventional treatments. Most prescription drugs for acne are either harsh topical lotions, which can cause dryness, redness, scaling, and sun sensitivity, or antibiotics, which disrupt the natural balance of intestinal flora and may give you yeast infections and diarrhea. Instead, try a natural treatment plan for acne that emphasizes dietary changes, detoxification, stress reduction, natural hormone balancing, and identification of possible food allergies.

Surprising Facts about Acne

A key hormone during male adolescence is testosterone. More important, there is greater activity of the enzyme 5-alpha reductase in the skin, which converts testosterone to a metabolite known as DHT (dihydrotestosterone). These hormones, as well as the delicate balance of estrogen and progesterone, along with stress hormones, play a role in female adolescent, as well as in adult female and male, acne.

CAUSES OF ACNE

Hormones can fluctuate at times other than adolescence, most notably during pregnancy, around the time of menses or menopause, and during periods of emotional stress. Oral contraceptives can also affect hormonal production. Acne can appear on babies as well. This is normal and goes away with time.

It would be a mistake, however, to attribute acne solely to fluctuating hormones. The second biggest contributor to acne is poor nutrition. Fat, sugar, and processed foods accelerate skin inflammation and acne. They also contribute to constipation, and thus the body responds by trying to expel the poisons through a different avenue—via the skin.

SYMPTOMS

Each of the following symptoms can appear on the face, the chest, or the back.

- Red spots, bumps, or pustules, sometimes inflamed and painful
- Blackheads
- Whiteheads
- Oily skin

ROOT CAUSES

- Genetics
- Poor diet
- Nutritional deficiencies
- Food sensitivities
- Hormonal fluctuation or imbalance
- Emotional stress
- Poor digestion/toxic body system
- Candida/yeast overgrowth

Testing Techniques

The following tests can be helpful in choosing therapy that will be the most beneficial:

Stool or blood analysis for candida overgrowth

Food allergies/sensitivities (see Food Allergies section)

Saliva hormone analysis for estrogen/progesterone/testosterone balance

Nutritional testing (blood/urine/hair) for nutritional deficiencies

Blood sugar testing

TREATMENT

Diet

Recommended Food

In general, acne sufferers should follow a simple diet of basic, unprocessed foods.

Dark-green or orange vegetables are especially helpful for their beta-carotene, which helps maintain and repair the skin. Eat them raw or lightly cooked to retain their nutrients and fiber.

A quarter cup of ground flaxseeds provides plenty of fiber for proper elimination, as well as helpful essential fatty acids. Take with at least 8 ounces of water.

Nuts and seeds, such as almonds, walnuts, and pumpkin seeds, are good sources of skin-healthy vitamin E and essential fatty acids.

Quality protein sources are beans, peas, lentils, eggs, and fresh cold-water fish such as salmon, mackerel, herring, and sardines. The latter are rich in omega-3 fatty acids.

Meat products should be hormone- and antibiotic-free.

Drink a glass of clean water every two waking hours to flush toxins out of the body and to maintain good general health.

If you must use topical or oral antibiotics for acne, be sure to eat some live unsweetened yogurt every day. Antibiotics destroy the "friendly" bacteria in your digestive tract, which are necessary for good health, and yogurt will replace it.

News about Acne Treatments

- Vitex (chasteberry) and saw palmetto (*Serenoa repens*) alleviate hormone-related acne.
- Homeopathic Silica (*Silicea*) reduces pus formation.
- Reducing simple carbohydrates in the diet decreases skin inflammation.

Food to Avoid

Eliminate junk and processed food, such as chips and nachos, colas, and candy. These products are a large source of toxins in the average diet.

Sugar encourages oil production and provides food for bacteria and yeast. Do not consume foods that contain added sugar. Avoid artificial sugar substitutes like saccharine or aspartame. They have a poisonous effect on the body and also encourage an addiction to sweets.

Adult acne is often an allergic or sensitivity reaction to a certain food or foods. Although any food can conceivably result in an allergic response, by far the most frequent triggers are dairy, wheat, sugar, chocolate, and corn. Try the elimination diet on page 253 to determine whether a food allergy is causing your problem, or see a natural health-care practitioner for testing.

- Saturated and hydrogenated fats are particularly difficult to digest, and they worsen acne. Stay away from fried foods and solid fats, such as margarine, lard, and vegetable shortening.
- An acidic internal environment encourages acne, so avoid alcohol, sugar, chocolate, fried foods, and soda, and limit meat products.
- Coffee and other caffeinated products may aggravate skin conditions. If they cause problems for you, cut them out and drink herbal teas instead.
- People with carbohydrate sensitivity may notice improvement in their skin by reducing their carbohydrate intake and increasing protein sources. This is because elevated levels of the blood sugar–regulating hormone insulin increases skin inflammation.

Detoxification

Detoxification helps cleanse the body of acne-causing poisons. You may find that your acne actually worsens immediately after trying the following therapies because your skin is eliminating toxins at a faster rate than usual. Once the toxins are expelled, your acne should be reduced or even eliminated.

A three-day vegetable juice fast will sweep away toxic build-up. You should drink a variety of juices during your fast, but those made from carrots, apples, and beets with their tops, as well as green drinks (spirulina, wheatgrass, barley grass, chlorella), are especially supportive of an acne cleanse.

Dry brushing removes dead skin and improves circulation. It's also a relaxing way to enhance the effects of a fast. Do not brush areas of the skin where pustules are present.

℞ Super Seven Prescriptions—Acne

Super Prescription #1   Vitex (chasteberry)
Take 160 mg of a standardized Vitex extract (0.6 percent aucubin or 0.5 percent agnuside) or 40 drops of the tincture form daily.

Vitex (chasteberry) is an excellent hormone balancer to reduce acne formation and is effective for men and women. Use this super supplement or a hormone-balancing herbal formula for at least six weeks. If you see improvement, continue with the same dose as long as it remains effective.

Super Prescription #2   Essential fatty acids
Take 1 to 2 tablespoons of flaxseed oil or 3 to 5 grams of fish oil daily.

Essential fatty acids, formulations that contain flaxseeds, fish, or a mixture of omega-3, 6, and 9 fatty acids, are helpful for acne and reduce skin inflammation. Take as directed on container. It may take four to eight weeks for improvements to be noticed.

Super Prescription #3   Zinc
Take 50 mg of zinc twice daily with meals for three months, and then reduce the dosage to 50 mg daily for long-term supplementation. It should be taken in conjunction with copper (3 to 5 mg).

Zinc is one of the best minerals to use for the treatment of acne. It works to reduce the build-up of DHT and promotes skin healing. It may take up to three months for benefits to occur. Do not use zinc sulfate, which is not readily absorbed.

Super Prescription #4   Burdock root (*Arctium lappa*)
Take 300 to 500 mg of the capsule form, 30 drops of tincture, or 1 cup of tea three times daily.

Burdock root works as a blood purifier and a detoxifier, and it improves elimination. It also has hormone-balancing properties. Take it for a minimum of eight weeks.

Super Prescription #5   Tea tree oil (*Melaleuca alternifolia*)
Apply a solution by dabbing it onto blemishes twice daily. It's available in many over-the-counter acne preparations.

A 5 percent solution of tea tree oil in diluted water acts similarly to benzoyl peroxide but without the drying side effects. Since tea tree oil is quite potent, test the solution on a small area of your skin first.

Super Prescription #6   Homeopathy
Use a combination acne formula or one of the following if it matches your symptoms. Use a 6x, 12x, 6C, or a 30C potency for two weeks. If there is improvement, discontinue using it.

Calcarea Sulphurica is for cystic acne or chronic acne where there is a yellow discharge.

Hepar Sulphuris (Hepar sulphuris calcareum) may provide relief if you have several pus-filled spots that are painful when touched, and if your skin lesions feel better with a warm compress.

Ledum palustre is helpful for pustular acne on the nose and the cheeks that feels better with cold applications.

One double-blind study of ninety-one people with moderately severe acne found that 90 mg of zinc significantly improved the acne more than a placebo did.

One study showed that a 5 percent tea tree oil gel extract was comparable to the effects of benzoyl peroxide in the treatment of mild to moderate acne. Tea tree oil users experienced fewer side effects (dryness, burning, redness, and itching).

Pulsatilla (Pulsatilla pratensis) is for acne associated with the hormonal changes of puberty, menstrual onset, or menopause.

Silica (*Silicea*) is for chronic white pustules.

Sulphur is for reddish, inflamed acne pustules that may be itchy or very sore. Heat or washing may cause a worsening of symptoms.

These formulas contain the most common homeopathic medicines for acne and skin health. In rare cases, your acne may initially worsen for a week and then begin to clear up. They are safe to use for all ages. Take as directed on the container.

Super Prescription #7   Vitamin A

Vitamin A is helpful for the skin and has been shown in studies to reduce sebum production and keratin production. Take 5,000 IU to 10,000 IU or higher daily, under the guidance of a doctor.

The problem with vitamin A is that high dosages are needed to be effective for acne, and these may cause side effects. A way around this problem is to use a lower dosage, along with other nutrients that work synergistically for skin health, such as selenium, vitamin E, and zinc. Pregnant women or those trying to conceive should not use more than 5,000 IU daily.

General Recommendations

Saw palmetto (*Serenoa repens*) blocks excessive DHT of the sebaceous glands and is effective for both sexes. Take 160 mg of an 85 to 95 percent liposterolic standardized extract or 30 drops of tincture twice daily.

Dandelion root (*Taraxacum officinale*) supports your liver, which may be overtaxed with toxins. This herb is also a gentle laxative and can facilitate waste removal. Take 300 to 500 mg of the capsule form, 30 drops of tincture, or 1 cup of the tea three times daily.

Milk thistle (*Silybum marianum*) also supports liver detoxification. Find a product that's standardized for 70 to 85 percent silymarin content, and take 200 to 250 mg twice a day.

Passionflower (*Passiflora incarnata*) and hops (*Humulus lupulus*) is used when stress is contributing to your acne. Drink a cup of these calming teas whenever you need to wind down.

Vitamin E-complex enhances the beneficial effects of selenium and vitamin A. Take 400 to 800 IU of mixed vitamin E-complex with tocopherols and tocotrienols.

Selenium, a trace mineral, is helpful in reducing the inflammation of acne. Take 200 mcg daily. Multivitamins contain selenium, and many have a dosage that's close to 200 mcg.

Chromium helps with blood sugar regulation, which can be an important factor with acne. Take 200 to 400 mcg daily.

Vitamin B6 is useful for premenstrual acne. Take a 50 mg B-complex before and during premenstrual flare-ups.

Oregano oil (*Origanum vulgare*) destroys yeast overgrowth associated with acne formation. Take 500 mg twice daily or use a liquid form.

Natural progesterone cream is effective for premenstrual and menopausal acne. To improve premenstrual and premenopausal acne, apply 20 mg once daily for 10 days before your expected menstrual flow. Menopausal women can apply 20 mg one to two times daily for 3 or all weeks of the month.

Colloidal silver has an antimicrobial action. Dab it onto pimples twice daily.

Chamomile (*Matricaria recutita*) has an anti-inflammatory property, as well as a soothing effect on the nervous system.

Super green food supplements, such as chlorella, spirulina, or blends of green foods, support skin healing and detoxification. Take as directed on the container.

Acupressure

See pages 668–675 for information about pressure points and administering treatment.

- Spleen 10 clears heat from the blood.
- Bladder 23 and 47, as well as Stomach 2 and 3, help clear acne.
- Bladder 10 can relieve stress that's related to acne.
- Large Intestine 4 relieves constipation and depression.

Bodywork

Reflexology

See pages 686–675 for information about reflexology areas and how to work them.

- Work the kidneys and the liver to detoxify the blood.
- If acne is caused by a hormonal imbalance, work the endocrine glands.
- To prevent constipation and speed the elimination of toxins, work the colon.

Hydrotherapy

To promote blood circulation and detoxification, soak in a hot tub full of Epsom salts. Rinse well afterward. You can also add any of the oils listed in the Aromatherapy section.

Aromatherapy

Lavender is calming to the emotions and the skin; it also fights bacterial infection. Apply it with a compress or put it in your bath.

Germanium will regulate the production of oil.

Bergamot is both an astringent and an antidepressant. When the skin improves, apply a lotion made with diluted water, lavender, and orange blossom to reduce scarring.

Stress Reduction

The effects of stress can throw the body into a state of imbalance. Stress can affect the skin by altering hormone levels and disrupting digestion and detoxification. People with acne generally feel more self-conscious about their looks. Techniques to reduce stress will ultimately help with skin health and appearance. Exercise, prayer, reading, and many other techniques can be used to reduce the effects of stress.

Bach Flower Remedies

Select the appropriate remedy, and place 10 drops under your tongue. Hold the drops in place for thirty seconds and swallow. Use as often as needed.

Try Crab Apple if acne is causing feelings of shame about your appearance.

If you've given up hope of finding a cure for your acne, Gorse will renew your spirits.

Larch is helpful for people who lack self-confidence or who are embarrassed because of their skin condition.

Sunlight can inhibit bacterial growth. Get fifteen minutes of sunlight, but never allow the skin to burn.

REFERENCES

Bassett, I. B., et al. 1990. A comparative study of tea tree oil versus benzoyl peroxide in the treatment of acne. *Medical Journal of Australia* 153, 455–58.

Hillstrom, L., et al. 1977. Comparison of oral treatment with zinc sulfate and placebo in acne vulgaris. *British Journal of Dermatology* 97:679–84.

Aging

Aging is a natural process and not a disease. It is something we all will experience and, it is hoped, deal with in a positive manner. Ideally, numerous benefits attend old age: wisdom; the pleasure of watching your children, grandchildren, and great-grandchildren flourish; and having time to help others and to enjoy life fully.

But to many people, old age is synonymous with ill health and disability. That's too bad, because most of the diseases we associate with aging—arthritis and other painful conditions, heart disease, diabetes, cancer, digestive problems, frailty, depression, sexual dysfunction, and fatigue—are not an inevitable part of growing older. These "age-related disorders" are mainly caused by lifestyle factors, such as diet, exposure to environmental toxins, lack of exercise, and stress, along with genetic susceptibilities. If you're young or middle-aged, you can prevent many problems by changing your habits now. If you're older and are already experiencing health difficulties, it's not too late to bring balance and harmony to your bodily systems.

Normal aging occurs when old cells start dying at a faster rate than new ones are generated. Since the body's tissues have a smaller supply of cells to draw upon, they begin to degenerate and malfunction. This process happens to everyone; it's simply a natural part of life. It appears that our cells are preprogrammed to have a maximum life span. Yet the key is to prevent premature aging, where one ages faster than one's genetic programming would have ordained. In addition, most people will agree that quality of life is paramount to life span.

In recent years, we have come to understand more about the highly reactive kinds of atoms or molecules called free radicals. In many cases, free radicals assist the body by destroying invaders, producing energy, and helping to carry oxygen through the bloodstream. When they are present in overwhelming numbers, however, they attack healthy cells, sometimes destroying them or mutating their DNA. When cells die before their time or are damaged, the normal aging process is accelerated, and the body becomes vulnerable to life-threatening ailments such as cancer, arteriosclerosis, and many degenerative diseases.

It is becoming more and more difficult to keep the number of free radicals in the body down to a healthy level. Many aspects of modern living, including unwholesome diet and exposure to pollution, tobacco smoke, environmental contaminants, and even the sun, put us in contact with more free radicals than any previous generation ever encountered. Luckily, nature has equipped us with the means to neutralize free radicals in our bodies. Substances called antioxidants accomplish the task, and they're found in many fruits and vegetables and in some herbs. A combination of healthful eating, combined with antioxidant supplements and wise living, can prevent excessive damage from free radicals.

Other major causes of several age-related diseases are diet and nutritional deficiencies. Studies on laboratory mice prove that a reduced-calorie diet significantly extends their lives. Research is starting to show that this is true for humans as well. In addition, diets that are high in fat and sugar lack many essential nutrients, fiber, and antioxidants. Poor diets also contribute to gastrointestinal disorders, which can inhibit the body's ability to absorb important vitamins and minerals. Sometimes, however, a good diet is not enough to keep deficiency at bay. As a result of normal or accelerated aging, older people are often simply less efficient at absorbing nutrients, even if they eat well. If you have reached old age, you will need to redouble your efforts to take in nutrients.

Aging is accelerated by a lack of exercise. If you don't regularly exercise, you increase your risk for almost every kind of disorder, including heart disease, diabetes, arthritis, and osteoporosis.

Hormone balance is a key to healthy aging. This is particularly true of the stress hormones such as cortisol and DHEA. A deficiency or an abnormal elevation of these hormones (particularly cortisol) accelerates aging and immune system breakdown. In reality, all of the hormones are important for healthy aging. Thyroid, estrogen, progesterone, and testosterone, as well as growth hormones, must be kept at balanced levels to slow the aging process. Researchers are finding that growth hormones may play a special role in slowing down the "aging clock."

It is also important to keep blood-sugar levels in the normal range. Elevated levels of glucose lead to a process known as glycosylation. This contributes to a weak immune system and speeds up aging. An example of this process is diabetes.

Finally, the effects of stress appear to play a role in aging. People who experience prolonged periods of intense stress are more likely to develop chronic diseases. One major stressor is loneliness. This has become a big problem with the elderly, who lack companionship and stimulation. Many older people cut back on social obligations, intellectual activities, and sports and exercise. Giving up these essential activities has been linked to a shorter life span and an increased risk of disease. It is up to all of us, whatever our age, to create families and communities in which the elderly are welcome, active members.

SYMPTOMS

- Frequent illness or chronic disease
- Painful conditions and stiffness
- Memory loss or impairment
- Digestive problems
- Weight loss
- Decreased sex drive
- Poor skin and/or muscle tone
- Frailty

ROOT CAUSES

- Free radical damage
- Poor diet and nutritional deficiencies
- Genetics
- Environmental toxins
- Poor digestion and detoxification
- Lack of exercise
- Hormone imbalance
- Elevated blood-sugar levels
- Stress and isolation

Testing Techniques

The following tests can give you an assessment of the degree of your aging:

Oxidative stress analysis—urine or blood testing

Antioxidant testing (urine, blood, or biophoton scanning)

Blood profile for cardiovascular, immune, and blood-sugar markers (glucose and insulin)

Stool analysis

Detoxification profile—urine

Hormone analysis by saliva, urine, or blood (estrogens, progesterone, testosterone, DHEA, cortisol, melatonin, IGF-1, thyroid panel)

TREATMENT

Diet

Recommended Food

Older people often have difficulty absorbing nutrients. When digestive enzymes aren't working at their optimal level, deficiencies, especially in the B-vitamins, can result. To compensate, eat plenty of whole grains and leafy greens, and add brewer's yeast and wheat germ to your meals.

Make sure you get enough fiber. Whole grains, oats, flaxseeds, and raw vegetables can prevent constipation and will reduce toxins in the digestive tract.

Yogurt and other fermented sour products (sauerkraut, kefir) encourage healthful bacteria in the digestive system. These bacteria fight colds and other infections.

Deeply colored fruits and vegetables are packed with antioxidants such as carotenoids, the substances that neutralize free radicals. They can also discourage the build-up of arterial plaque, so it's important to eat several servings with each meal. Remember, "think color!"

Vitamin E and selenium work together to prevent many different diseases. To lower your risk of cancer, heart disease, and arthritis, eat plenty of seeds, nuts, and vegetable oils.

Be sure to incorporate sufficient quality protein into your diet. Beans, soy products, fish, and lean chicken and turkey will give you energy.

Vitamin C helps fight free radical damage, reduces cancer risk, and strengthens the immune system. Good dietary sources of vitamin C include citrus fruits, green leafy vegetables, red peppers, strawberries, tomatoes, asparagus, and avocados.

Garlic and onions also have antioxidant properties and improve circulation, so enjoy them freely.

Whether you're thirsty or not, drink a glass of purified water every two waking hours. Dehydration is linked to kidney malfunction, malabsorption of nutrients, chronic constipation, weight gain, high cholesterol, fatigue, and headaches. It can also cause disorientation and memory loss; many people who are thought to be senile are actually just severely dehydrated.

The skins of red grapes reduce plaque in the walls of arteries. They also have antioxidant properties, so drink a glass of red grape juice or an occasional glass of red wine.

Food to Avoid

Reduce your total caloric intake, while maintaining good nutrition. As you get older, your metabolism slows down, and you require fewer calories to support your activities. Also, studies on laboratory mice have shown that a reduced-calorie diet significantly extended their lives. You can reduce calories by cutting out processed and junk foods, alcohol, sugar, and white flour—but don't skimp on nutritious foods that will keep you healthy.

In addition to the previous suggestions, avoid red meat and processed foods, as well as any food made with additives and preservatives. These foods are all high in free radicals. What's more, they clog up your digestive tract and inhibit proper functioning.

If you have trouble sleeping, don't consume alcohol, caffeine, and simple sugars in the evening. These substances keep you alert. Instead, eat complex carbohydrates, which can promote relaxation and a good night's rest.

Detoxification

Keeping the digestive tract clean is essential for preventing disease, especially if you've spent a lifetime consuming and breathing toxins. Fresh juices and "super green foods," such as chlorella and spirulina, are excellent. Supplements such as milk thistle (*Silybum marianum*) and many of the antioxidants support proper detoxification.

℞ Super Seven Prescriptions—Anti-Aging

Super Prescription #1   Super green food supplement
Take an organic super green food such as chlorella or spirulina or a mixture of these each day. Take as directed on the container.

Super Prescription #2   Green tea
Green tea contains a rich source of antioxidants and substances that assist detoxification. Drink the organic tea regularly (2 cups or more daily), or take 500 to 1,500 mg of the capsule form.

Super Prescription #3   High-potency multivitamin
Take a high-potency multivitamin and mineral formula daily, as it will contain a strong base of the antioxidants and other nutrients that protect against aging.

Super Prescription #4   Essential fatty acids
Take 1 to 2 tablespoons of flaxseed oil or 3 grams of fish oil daily, or a formulation that contains a mixture of omega-3, 6, and 9 fatty acids.

These essential fatty acids are needed for healthy cell functioning and replication, as well as for many other body processes.

Super Prescription #5   Garlic (*Allium sativum*)
Take 1 to 2 capsules of an aged garlic product daily.

Garlic benefits the immune and cardiovascular systems. It also improves detoxification and has antioxidant properties.

Super Prescription #6   Siberian ginseng (*Eleutherococcus Senticosus*)
Take 600 to 900 mg of a standardized product daily. As with most types of ginseng, *Eleutherococcus* works to help the body adapt to mental and physical stress.

Super Prescription #7   Ginkgo biloba
Take 60 to 120 mg twice daily of a standardized product containing 24 percent flavone glycosides and 6 percent terpene lactones.

> This popular herb improves circulation, has potent antioxidant properties, improves memory, and reduces one's tendency to get blood clots.

General Recommendations

Enzymes aid in the digestion of food and are essential for all the metabolic activity in the body. Take 1 to 2 capsules with each meal.

Cordyceps sinensis is a revered fungus used in Chinese medicine as a supplement to combat fatigue and the aging process. Take 2 to 4 capsules daily.

Royal jelly, the substance produced by worker bees as the sole food for their queen, contains a wide range of nutrients. Take as directed on the container.

Alpha lipoic acid is one of the most important antioxidants in the body. Take 50 mg twice daily.

CoQ10 is a potent antioxidant and a nutrient involved in many aspects of cardiovascular function. Take 50 to 300 mg daily.

Reishi extract, revered in Chinese medicine, is made from the "mushroom of immortality." It improves liver and immune system function. Take 2 to 4 capsules daily.

Ashwagandha, known as "Indian ginseng," is a revered herb in Ayurvedic medicine and is used as a tonic for people with chronic disease. Take 1,000 to 3,000 mg daily.

Panax ginseng is revered in Chinese medicine as an antiaging herbal therapy. Take a standardized product containing 4 to 7 percent ginsenosides at 100 to 250 mg twice daily. Do not use if you have high blood pressure.

DHEA is a hormone that research shows is an accurate marker of aging. If your level is low, talk with your doctor about starting at a 15 mg dosage.

Ginger (*Zingiber officinale*) is indeed excellent for aiding the digestion; it also prevents blood clotting and has anti-inflammatory properties. Instead of drinking sugary ginger ale, try ginger tea, made by boiling water over fresh ginger. You can also take 1 to 2 grams of a powdered capsule or a tablet, divided over the course of a day. Or you can use 1 to 3 ml of a ginger tincture three times daily.

A double-blind clinical trial studied the effects of 1,500 mg of *Panax ginseng* on forty-nine elderly people. This herb was found to improve coordination and reaction time, as well as to increase alertness and energy.

Homeopathy

See a homeopathic practitioner who can prescribe a remedy to strengthen your particular state of body and mind.

If you're an older person who has already developed an illness or a painful condition, you will find homeopathic suggestions listed under the specific disorder that's plaguing you.

Acupressure

See pages 668–675 for information about pressure points and administering treatment.

- Stomach 36 is a good point for keeping up health in general. It strengthens the entire body but gives particular support to the immune and digestive systems.

Bodywork

Bodywork is more important than ever in old age. Not only does it increase circulation and reduce aches and pains, it can supply significant emotional benefits to people who are deprived of nurturing physical contact. If you are isolated or depressed, or if your body has become rigid from lack of touch, you might find massage both relaxing and invigorating.

Reflexology

See pages 686–687 for information about reflexology areas and how to work them.

Work the entire foot to provide support for all the systems of the body.

If you want to concentrate on just a few areas, work the kidneys, the liver, and the colon to encourage detoxification.

Hydrotherapy

Hot and cold hydrotherapy will get your circulation going and increase your energy.

Aromatherapy

If you feel tense or irritable or have trouble sleeping, lavender can help you relax. Try it in a bath or as an inhalant, or slip a lavender-filled sachet under your pillow.

If you are depressed, bergamot, clary sage, geranium, or rosemary can be uplifting.

A few drops of jasmine, ylang ylang, sandalwood, or patchouli in a bath will reignite sexual desire.

Stress Reduction

Exercise, prayer, reading, yoga, positive mental imagery, and many other techniques should be used to reduce the effects of stress and aging.

Bach Flower Remedies

You may find the following suggestions useful, but also consult the chart on pages 648–650 to find the appropriate flower remedy for your particular personality and tendencies. Once you've found the right remedy, place 10 drops under your tongue. Hold the drops in place for thirty seconds and swallow. Use as often as needed.

If you have experienced a loss and feel sorrowful and depressed, try Mustard.

Hornbeam will help if you feel too fatigued to participate in everyday activities.

If you are unhappy with present times and tend to dwell on the past as a period of perfect happiness, Honeysuckle will help you cultivate a more positive attitude toward the here and now.

Other Recommendations

- Keep moving. Regular exercise plays a significant role in preventing heart disease, arthritis, osteoporosis, diabetes, and many other disorders. For maximum benefits, your exercise plan should include aerobic exercise (for your heart and lungs), weight lifting (to keep your bones strong), and stretching. It is never too late to start. People who begin exercise and weight-lifting programs as late as their nineties show marked improvement in their general health. If you're older, ill, or overweight, consult with your doctor before beginning an exercise plan.

- If you're having problems digesting your food, your body may not be producing sufficient enzymes. Take an enzyme supplement daily.

REFERENCES

Fulder, S., et al. 1984. A double blind clinical trial of panax ginseng in aged subjects. Presented at the Fourth International Ginseng Symposium, Daejon, Korea.

AIDS and HIV

It is a disturbing and widespread myth that HIV (human immunodeficiency virus) and AIDS, the usually fatal condition believed to be caused by HIV, no longer pose a grave public health threat. The Centers for Disease Control estimates that 5 million Americans are considered to be at high risk for HIV infection. Half of all new cases of HIV occur in people under the age of twenty-five. Although scientists have discovered several treatments that extend the life span of people with the virus, there is still no cure. Even grimmer is the news that AIDS rates, after a short period of decline, are on the rise. Gay men were once thought to be the group most at risk for contracting HIV, but statistics show that heterosexual teenagers, both male and female; Hispanics; blacks; and women are now contracting the disease in rapidly increasing numbers.

HIV is transmitted via vaginal or anal sex or by blood-to-blood contact. It is vitally important for everyone to practice safe sex, preferably in the form of a monogamous relationship with an HIV-free partner, and to abstain from intravenous drug use. Don't rely solely on condoms to protect you, as they sometimes let HIV and other viruses pass through. Intravenous drug users are at a high risk: if you have an addiction, you should seek help, but at the very least you should never share needles with anyone.

The virus may also be passed from mother to child during birth or breastfeeding. It is possible to greatly reduce the chance of transmitting the disease during birth. Pregnant women should be tested for HIV as soon as possible, so that they and their unborn children can receive vital treatment. HIV is sometimes contracted by health-care workers who are stuck with infected needles. Also, be aware that the virus cannot be transmitted through casual contact, such as coughing, sneezing, shaking hands, or dry kissing.

Like all viruses, once HIV has entered the body, it seeks to replicate itself. What makes HIV far deadlier than, say, a cold virus, is that it takes a particularly aggressive tactic within the body: once it invades a cell, it reprograms that cell's genetic material. Normally, a cell will reproduce by dividing and creating a copy of itself. In this way, the body regenerates itself at the most basic level. But when cells that are invaded by HIV divide, they don't create copies of themselves—they create copies of the virus. Those copies then invade other healthy cells, so that, eventually, the virus cells far outnumber the healthy ones. To make matters worse, HIV attacks a particular kind of immune cell, called a Helper T-cell (these lymphocytes have a receptor protein called CD4+ in their outer membrane and so are also referred to as CD4+ lymphocytes). As more and more CD4+ cells are destroyed, the body's ability to fight off infections is dramatically weakened.

Most people do not notice any symptoms when HIV first invades the body. People with HIV will usually go for years without knowing it, unless they are tested for the disease. Before AIDS develops, many will begin to experience symptoms such as night sweats, fatigue, fevers, diarrhea, weight loss, enlarged lymph nodes, thrush, herpes, mouth ulcers, and bleeding gums. Later, as the number of T-cells continues to decrease, their bodies will be highly vulnerable to infection by viruses and bacteria. HIV-positive people might contract a variety of diseases that are otherwise rare, such as Kaposi's sarcoma (a kind of skin cancer characterized by raised purple welts), the Epstein-Barr virus (also known as chronic fatigue syndrome), neurological problems, eye infections (including cytomegalovirus, which can cause blindness), toxoplasmic encephalitis (a brain infection), and systemic candidiasis (yeast infection). Other infections are those we usually consider common, such as pneumonia and various respiratory ailments.

Acquired immunodeficiency virus (AIDS) is the most severe form of HIV infection. A person with HIV infection is considered to have AIDS when at least one complicating illness develops or the person's ability to defend against infection significantly declines, as measured by a low CD4+ lymphocyte count. Since the number of CD4+ lymphocytes in the blood helps to determine the ability of the immune system to protect the body from infections, it is a good measure of the degree of damage done by HIV infection. A healthy person has a CD4+ lymphocyte count of roughly 800 to 1,300 cells per microliter of blood. Typically, 40 to 60 percent of CD4+ lymphocytes are destroyed in the first few months of infection. After about six months, the CD4+ count stops falling so quickly, but it continues to decline. If the CD4+ count falls below about 200 cells per microliter of blood, the immune system is susceptible to severe, life-threatening infections.

It is important to note that while all people with AIDS are HIV-positive, not all people with HIV develop AIDS. Most HIV-positive people develop AIDS within eight to twelve years after first contracting the virus, but some develop it much faster, and many others still remain healthy decades after contracting HIV. It appears that people who are able to ward off full-blown AIDS are those whose immune systems are the strongest. Therefore, complementary therapies for HIV and AIDS work to bolster the ability of the immune system to fight infection.

If you contract HIV, you need to work with a doctor who knows about the latest treatments available for the disease. Although a cure has yet to be found, research is producing new therapies on an almost monthly basis. In addition, you will need medication to combat any infections that might arise.

SYMPTOMS

There are no symptoms during the early stages of HIV, except perhaps a fever when the virus first invades the body. As the virus continues to invade, the following symptoms can occur:

- Night sweats
- Fatigue
- Fevers
- Diarrhea
- Weight loss

- Enlarged lymph nodes
- Thrush (mouth fungus)
- Herpes
- Mouth ulcers
- Bleeding gums

Several conditions are associated with full-blown AIDS. Following are some of the most common:

- Kaposi's sarcoma (a type of skin cancer characterized by raised purple welts)

- Epstein-Barr virus

Neurological problems:

- Eye problems (often related to cytomegalovirus, which can cause blindness)
- Toxoplasmic encephalitis (a brain infection)

- Pneumonia and other respiratory ailments
- Candidiasis
- Salmonella
- Cancer of various organs

Testing Techniques

Diagnosis of HIV is done with the use of the following blood test:

HIV ELISA Test

If this test is positive, it is confirmed with a more accurate test known as Western Blot. Also, the CD4+ count and the viral load are used to monitor progression of the disease.

It is also helpful to have:

Oxidative stress analysis—urine or blood testing

Antioxidant testing (urine, blood, or skin scanning)

Stool analysis

Hormone analysis by saliva, urine, or blood (estrogens, progesterone, testosterone, DHEA, cortisol, melatonin, IGF-1, thyroid panel)

ROOT CAUSES

- Anal or vaginal sex with an infected partner
- Blood-to-blood contact with an infected person (such as from sharing needles for intravenous drug use)
- Transfusions of infected blood (in the United States, blood donations have been screened for HIV since 1985)
- In the womb, at birth, or during breastfeeding

TREATMENT

Diet

To reduce the risk of toxins entering your body, food should be as clean and pure as possible. If you cook meat and poultry at home, reduce your risk of food poisoning by keeping preparation areas sanitary and by cooking at high-enough temperatures. Eat organic food, if it is available. If organic products are not an option, at least wash your food with pure water to get rid of pesticides and other toxins.

Recommended Food

If you have HIV or AIDS, you absolutely must eat well. A good basic diet will include plenty of raw vegetables, seeds, nuts, grains, fresh fruit, and lean protein from quality sources. As the virus continues to invade your body, you may find that you lose your appetite, but try to keep eating healthful meals; an adequate intake of calories is more important now than ever. Protein is particularly important to prevent weight loss and maintain optimal immune function. Try to consume 2.0 grams for every 2.2 pounds of body weight. A high-quality whey protein is helpful in attaining this goal.

Garlic and onions have natural antibiotic effects, so use them often.

To fight HIV or AIDS, include cruciferous vegetables (broccoli, cauliflower, cabbage, brussels sprouts, and others) in your diet.

Drink a glass of clean water every two waking hours. Make sure the water is from a good source, to avoid bacteria and parasite infection.

The "good" bacteria in your digestive tract help fight infection, so maintain their presence by eating yogurt with live cultures, especially *Lactobacillus acidophilus* and *bifidus*. This is especially important if you are taking antibiotics, which kill the good bacteria along with the bad. If you cannot tolerate yogurt, take probiotic capsules.

If you have HIV, it is strongly advised that you invest in a good juicer. Live juices will help your weakened system absorb a maximum amount of nutrients. Drink several glasses daily of a variety of juices, especially those made from cruciferous vegetables, black radishes, cabbage, greens (such as wheatgrass), and carrots.

Food to Avoid

Do not consume raw eggs; unpasteurized milk, cheese, or cider; or rare meat. All of these products can contain harmful bacteria. In people who have compromised immune systems, these bacteria can lead to septicemia, an extremely dangerous and often fatal condition.

Cut out junk food, fried food, sugar, and alcohol, all of which suppress your immune system and tax your entire body.

Find out now if you have any food allergies or sensitivities, because they cause the immune system to attack itself. See the elimination diet on page 253 for further details.

Detoxification

Every month consider doing a juice fast. Juices made from carrots, cabbage, greens, and apples help cleanse the body. Green drinks are another excellent way to purify the blood.

℞ Super Seven Prescriptions—HIV/AIDS

Super Prescription #1   Super green food supplement
Take an organic super green food, such as chlorella or spirulina, or a mixture of super green foods each day. It supplies a host of nutrients and antioxidants. Take as directed on the container.

Super Prescription #2   High-potency multivitamin
Take a high-potency multivitamin and mineral formula daily, as it will contain a strong base of the antioxidants and other nutrients that improve immune function.

Super Prescription #3   Whey protein
Take 25 grams daily or as directed by your doctor. It helps prevent tissue wasting and repairs the digestive tract.

Super Prescription #4   Antioxidant formula
Many studies have shown that people with HIV have a greater need for antioxidants. Take a combination antioxidant formula, as directed on the container.

Super Prescription #5   B-complex
Take a 50 mg complex twice daily. Many people with HIV have deficiencies of the B vitamins, which can impair immune function.

Super Prescription #6   Vitamin C
Take 1,000 to 3,000 mg daily. It supports immune function.

Super Prescription #7   Probiotic
Take a daily probiotic supplement that contains at least 4 billion active organisms. Probiotics are used to replenish healthful bacteria that fight intestinal infection and support immunity.

One clinical trial found that HIV-positive men who took a multivitamin-mineral supplement had a slower onset of AIDS, as compared to men who did not take a supplement.

General Recommendations

DHEA may help prevent the depression and the fatigue associated with an HIV infection. Take 10 to 25 mg or higher, under the supervision of a doctor.

Enzymes aid in the digestion of food and are essential for all the metabolic activity in the body. Take 1 to 2 capsules with each meal.

L-glutathione is one of the most important antioxidants in the body. Take 500 mg twice daily.

CoQ10 is a potent antioxidant and a nutrient involved in energy production and immunity. Take 50 to 300 mg daily.

Reishi (*Ganoderma lucidum*) extract improves liver and immune system function. Take 2 to 4 capsules daily.

Garlic (*Allium sativum*) supports immune function. Take an aged garlic supplement daily.

Milk thistle (*Silybum marianum*) (80 to 85 percent silymarin) supports liver function while you use pharmaceutical medications for HIV/AIDS. Take 250 to 300 mg three times daily.

Aloe (*Aloe vera*) has antiviral effects. Use a food-grade product, and take as directed on the container.

Selenium has antiviral effects. Take a daily dosage of 400 mcg.

Maitake (*Grifola frondosa*) supports immune function and has antiviral properties. Take 1 mg of the MD or D fraction per 2.2 pounds of body weight daily.

Turmeric (*Curcuma longa*) (90 to 95 percent curcumin) is shown in test tube studies to inhibit HIV infection. Take 500 mg three times daily.

Zinc supports immune function. Take a daily total of 30 to 50 mg.

Thymus extract supports healthy immunity. Take as directed on the container.

Homeopathy

HIV and AIDS are complex disorders with many variables. A homeopathic practitioner can suggest a preparation that addresses your individual needs.

Acupressure

See pages 668–675 for information about pressure points and administering treatment.

- Conception Vessel 17 helps the immune system and also eases depression and anxiety.
- To ease digestive problems and improve the absorption of nutrients, try Stomach 36.

Bodywork

Massage

A lymphatic massage, especially with the oils listed in the Aromatherapy section further on, will drain toxins from your body. Massage, in general, can help relieve stress, depression, and fatigue.

Reflexology

See pages 686–687 for information about reflexology areas and how to work them.

Work the liver point to support this critical organ of the immune system.

If you are constipated or experience diarrhea, massage the area corresponding to the colon.

Hydrotherapy

Hot and cold hydrotherapy promotes healing and energy and also combats stress.
See Constitutional Hydrotherapy on pages 676–677.

Aromatherapy

Add juniper to a carrier oil, and use in a lymphatic massage. Juniper helps break down toxins that have built up in fatty deposits.

Several oils have antibacterial properties, especially tea tree and eucalyptus. These oils can be used in any form but are highly recommended for use in lymphatic massage.

To lift your spirits, use lavender or geranium oils in any form.

Stress Reduction

General Stress-Reduction Therapies

A diagnosis of HIV can be devastating. You need someone you can talk to as you work through the initial shock and then face each successive challenge. Although family and friends are always a welcome source of strength, you may also want to recruit the help of a professional who has experience working with people suffering from a difficult illness. A religious adviser, a psychotherapist, or a support group leader can offer you invaluable advice and help.

In a world of expensive and invasive medical treatments, meditation and positive mental imagery can come as a relief. All you need is some private space and a comfortable place to sit. As you grow skilled at meditation, you'll find that you can use its calming techniques whenever necessary, even if you're ill and bedridden.

Bach Flower Remedies

Consult the chart on pages 648–650 to find the appropriate flower remedy for your particular condition. Once you've found the right remedy, place 10 drops under your tongue. Hold the drops in place for thirty seconds and swallow. Use as often as needed.

For fear of the unknown, try Aspen.

For exhaustion and fatigue, Hornbeam or Olive can be useful.

Rescue Remedy is excellent in any stressful crisis.

Other Recommendations

- Get plenty of rest and fresh air.
- Regular exercise will counteract stress and help keep you healthy, but don't overdo it. A daily morning walk is a good idea. Weight lifting helps to maintain muscle mass.
- Try to get early morning sunlight on your skin, but make sure to stay away from harsh or bright sun. People with HIV have a heightened vulnerability to skin cancer.

REFERENCES

Ince, S. 1993. Vitamin supplements may help delay onset of AIDS. *Medical Tribune* 9:18.

Alcoholism. *See* Substance Abuse

Allergies. *See also* Asthma and Food Allergies

An allergic reaction occurs when the immune system misinterprets a normally nontoxic substance, such as grass, pollen, a detergent, or a certain food, as a harmful invader. The immune system then responds to this perceived threat, called an allergen, by releasing substances called histamines. Histamines produce a wide range of bodily reactions, including respiratory and nasal congestion, increased mucus production, skin rashes and welts, and headache. In the case of an actual threat to the body, in the form of, say, a flu virus, these reactions would form an important line of defense against the invader, helping to trap it and expel it, and encouraging you to rest and recover. But during the false alarm of an allergic response, the body overreacts to a harmless agent.

Most allergens are found either in the environment or in food. (For information about allergic reactions to food, see Food Allergies.) Environmental allergens include pollen (reactions to pollen are often called hay fever), mold, animal dander, dust, feathers, insect venom, certain cosmetics and household products, and metals. When the environmental allergens are removed or make their seasonal disappearance, the body returns to normal. If the allergens are not removed, the immune system will continue its artificially high state of alert. In these cases, the allergic response can develop into chronic allergic rhinitis, in which the nasal passages remain persistently inflamed.

Why some people develop allergies to certain substances and others do not remains unclear. It does seem that certain allergic responses, such as hay fever, have a genetic basis. An excess accumulation of mucus in the body, which attracts and stores the irritant, also contributes to or causes allergic responses. In addition, stress and a generally depressed immune system may contribute to the severity of allergies.

A note about allergy tests: many conventional doctors suggest skin or blood tests to determine the source of allergies, but take care. These tests are invasive, expensive, and of questionable reliability. If your doctor recommends one of these tests, question him or her closely about the benefits you should expect.

CAUSES

- Allergies happen when the immune system attacks a harmless substance. Common triggers for allergies include mold; dust; tree, grass, or flower pollen; animal dander; feathers; insect venom, especially from bee stings; metal, particularly nickel; household chemicals; and some cosmetics.
- An excess of mucus, caused by a poor diet
- Stress, which depresses the immune system

SYMPTOMS

Allergic responses can produce any one or a combination of several of the following symptoms:

- Nasal congestion
- Sneezing
- Coughing
- Red, itchy, or watery eyes
- Wheezing
- Sore throat
- Hives, rashes, eczema, or other skin eruptions
- Headache
- Fatigue
- Fluid retention
- Swelling of the throat and the tongue

Caution: If you experience difficulty breathing or develop hives that spread rapidly, *get emergency help at once.* Allergic reactions like these can quickly be fatal. If you know you have severe reactions to certain substances, talk to your doctor about emergency adrenaline kits you can keep on hand.

ROOT CAUSES

- Genetics
- Nutritional deficiencies
- Poor digestion and detoxification
- Limited diet (in cases of food sensitivities, the lack of variety in the diet)

Testing Techniques

Blood IgG4 and IgE food and environmental screen

Electrodermal testing for sensitivities

Muscle testing by a skilled practitioner

TREATMENT

Diet

If you have allergies, dietary therapy should include strategies for mucus reduction, elimination of allergenic pathogens, and general immune support.

Recommended Food

Base your diet on non–mucus-forming foods: whole grains (although gluten sensitivity is common), fresh vegetables and fruits, cold-pressed oils, and raw seeds and nuts. (Many people with environmental allergies also have reactions to nuts, so monitor your reactions carefully.)

To keep your immune system healthy, make sure to get enough lean protein. Seafood and tofu are good sources that don't encourage mucus production.

Drink six to eight 8-ounce glasses of water a day to thin mucus secretions.

Flaxseeds and flaxseed oil can reduce inflammation. Take 2 tablespoons every day.

Food to Avoid

Eliminating foods that cause mucus should be a priority for any allergy sufferer. Mucus-forming foods include all dairy products, fried and processed foods, refined flours, chocolate, and eggs.

The immune response stresses your digestive system, so place as few additional burdens on it as possible. Cut down on bad fats and oils (saturated, hydrogenated, or those containing trans-fatty acids)—as well as the refined flour and the processed foods mentioned earlier—and increase your intake of fiber, especially from raw vegetables.

Many people with environmental allergies also suffer from food allergies. See the Food Allergies section and follow the elimination diet there to ensure that certain foods aren't making your environmental allergies worse.

Wheat is the unsuspected culprit behind many allergies, including those that seem to be triggered by environmental allergens. Try eliminating wheat during the seasons that usually coincide with your allergic responses.

Detoxification

A three-day juice fast to expel mucus is strongly encouraged. During and after the fast, you will feel your congestion begin to clear.

Green drinks are good for flushing out mucus and toxins. Drink one daily, whether you're fasting or not.

℞ Super Seven Prescriptions—Allergies

Super Prescription #1   Homeopathy
Take a combination allergy homeopathic remedy, as directed on the container, or read the description under Homeopathy in this section to pick a single remedy.

Super Prescription #2   Vitamin C
Take 1,000 mg three to five times daily (reduce the dosage if diarrhea occurs). It has a natural antihistamine effect.

Super Prescription #3   Stinging nettles (*Urtica dioica*)
Take 300 to 500 mg daily. Studies show that it is effective for hay fever.

Super Prescription #4   Methylsulfonylmethane (MSM)
Take 3,000 to 5,000 mg daily. It reduces allergic and inflammatory responses.

Super Prescription #5   Quercitin
Take 1,000 mg three times daily. It has a natural antihistamine effect.

Super Prescription #6   Eyebright (*Euphrasia officinalis*)
Take 1 capsule three times daily or apply as a solution to irritated eyes by putting 5 drops of the tincture form in a half ounce of saline. Apply it to the eyes twice daily.

Super Prescription #7   Essential fatty acids
Take 1 to 2 tablespoons of flaxseed oil or 3 grams of fish oil daily. They reduce inflammatory responses associated with allergies.

Study

A randomized, double-blind study involving the use of freeze-dried nettles and people who had hay fever found that after one week of use, 58 percent of participants had a reduction in their sneezing and itching.

Other Recommendations

Thymus extract has been shown to calm the immune response to allergies. Take as directed on the container.

Probiotics reduce the potential for allergies. Take a product containing at least 4 billion organisms of *Lactobacillus acidophilus* and *bifidus*.

Protease enzymes decrease allergic and inflammatory responses. Take 2 capsules twice daily on an empty stomach or as directed on the container.

Digestive enzymes assist in the digestion of food and reduce the likelihood of food sensitivities. Take 1 to 2 capsules with meals.

Betaine hydrochloride assists in the digestion of food and reduces the likelihood of food sensitivities. Take 1 to 2 capsules with meals.

Homeopathy

Pick the remedy that best matches your symptoms. Take 2 pellets of 30C potency twice daily. Should the first three days pass without any sign of improvement, you're probably taking the wrong remedy. Stop using the current one, and switch to something else. When you first notice improvement, stop taking the remedy unless your symptoms begin to return.

Allium Cepa is good for burning, watery eyes and a runny nose. Sneezing is common, and your symptoms feel better in the open air.

Arsenicum Album is for people with burning eyes and a runny nose that doesn't stop, causing the skin under the nose to get red and excoriated. This remedy is effective for the highly sensitive person with many allergies.

Euphrasia is for red, burning, tearing eyes.

Histaminum is for non–life threatening allergy symptoms that come on quickly.

Lycopodium (*Lycopodium clavatum*) is for people who have right-sided nasal and throat symptoms. Bloating after meals is common.

Natrum Muriaticum is for people who sneeze from the sun. They often get cold sores and crave salty foods.

Nux Vomica (*Strychnos nux vomica*) is also for people with diverse allergy symptoms, but those who benefit from this remedy tend to crave sweets, tobacco, and other stimulants. They often wake up sneezing.

Pulsatilla (*Pulsatilla pratensis*) is for people whose allergies are worse in a warm room and who crave the open air. Their nasal passages often get congested at night.

Sabadilla is for people who suffer from many repeated sneezes in a row and a runny nose.

Silica (*Silicea*) will help if your allergies manifest as upper respiratory problems that develop into infections and if you often feel fatigued and low in stamina.

Acupressure

See pages 668–675 for information about pressure points and administering treatment.

- Large intestine 4 relieves headaches and sneezing.
- For fatigue, swollen eyes, and headache, use Bladder 10.
- Triple Warmer 5 fortifies the immune system.
- Stomach 36 is a good all-over toner and promotes balance within the body.

Bodywork

Massage

A percussive massage will help break up mucus. Percussive motions are best used on people who are relatively strong and healthy. If you are frail, thin, or elderly, check with your massage therapist about the suitability of this treatment for you.

A lymphatic drainage massage will carry mucus away from the body.

Almost any massage can help relieve stress, but one that incorporates relaxing essential oils may be the best approach. See the Aromatherapy section for suggested oils.

Reflexology

See pages 686–687 for information about reflexology areas and how to work them.

Working the big toes and the inside of the heels helps abate allergic reactions.

Hydrotherapy

Hot baths induce sweat, which carries toxins out along with it. And if you're congested, a steamy bath feels just plain wonderful. If you want a more powerful release of toxins, add Epsom salts to the water.

A wet compress will help draw out chest congestion. You can add ginger or cayenne for increased strength.

Nasal saline irrigation of both nostrils daily will reduce nasal and sinus symptoms related to allergies.

Aromatherapy

If you suffer from plant allergies, use caution when trying aromatherapy oils.

Several essential oils are excellent at loosening mucus. Try any combination of the following in a steam inhalant or a bath or diffused into the air: eucalyptus, peppermint, lemon balm, and tea tree.

Both lavender and chamomile are good stress relievers, in any form. If you're suffering from allergies, however, they may be of most help when combined with steam, so use them in a steam inhalant or a hot bath.

Bach Flower Remedies

According to Bach remedy philosophy, most allergic conditions are related to some form of emotional intolerance.

If you have little patience for other people, take Beech.

If self-acceptance is the problem, try Rock Water.

Other Recommendations

- Exercise to expel toxins, support the immune system, and reduce stress.
- Don't smoke or expose yourself to secondhand smoke.
- Avoid or reduce exposure to allergy triggers. If you have mold or dust allergies, keep your house extremely clean and dry. A dehumidifier in the basement is a good idea, as are air filters and feather-free pillows and comforters. If you have a wood- or coal-burning fireplace or stove, you may need to find an alternate source of heat. In extreme cases, you may have to rid your home of any item that's likely to collect dust, including upholstered furniture, rugs, and curtains. A HEPA (high-energy particulate air) filter is highly recommended, especially in the bedroom at night.
- Xylitol nasal spray reduces allergy symptoms. Follow directions on the container.
- Consider desensitization treatments from a natural health-care practitioner.

REFERENCES

Mittman, P. 1990. Randomized, double-blind study of freeze-dried Urtica dioica in the treatment of allergic rhinitis. *Planta Medica* 56:44–47.

Alzheimer's Disease

Alzheimer's disease is a progressive brain disorder that begins with memory loss and eventually leads to dementia and death. In the United States, it affects up to 10 percent of people over sixty-five and almost half of those over eighty-five. Scientists predict that in the coming years, these percentages are likely to rise. Such an increase, combined with the rapidly growing size of the older population, could very well result in an epidemic of Alzheimer's cases.

Where Did I Put My Sunglasses?

We all have occasional memory lapses, and many people notice that by late middle age, it's harder to remember details than it used to be. If you've misplaced the remote control again or forgotten to pick up milk at the grocery store—even if you can't remember the names of your new neighbors—you're probably not suffering from Alzheimer's. More likely, you just need to boost your nutritional intake and follow a few other brain-boosting steps. See Memory Problems for further details. And your sunglasses? They're on top of your head.

Alzheimer's disease targets a part of the brain called the hippocampus, which is the seat of memory and intellect. In a person with Alzheimer's, the neurons in the hippocampus become entangled. The resulting formations, often called plaque, result in the loss of brain cells, especially those that make new memories and retrieve old ones. And memory problems characterize the symptoms of Alzheimer's.

In the beginning stages of the disease, people will experience some mild memory problems. They may struggle with complex tasks like planning a party or balancing a checkbook. As the disease progresses, it becomes increasingly difficult to remember events that occurred very recently—say, the day before, or even just a few hours prior to the present time. Memory loss at this point looks more and more like dementia: affected people may not recognize others close to them or be able to recall appropriate words. Eventually, complete dementia sets in. Personal memories disappear and, with them, the ability to recognize beloved people and places. Functional memories also become irretrievable. The person forgets how to perform daily functions, which include getting dressed, brushing the teeth, and using the toilet. Hallucinations or episodes of violence often attend this stage of the disease. At this point, it is rarely possible for a family member or a close friend to look after the sufferer, who needs twenty-four-hour-a-day care.

Many disorders cause symptoms that are quite similar (or even identical) to those of Alzheimer's. Before your doctor makes a diagnosis of Alzheimer's, make sure that he or she rules out the following possibilities:

- Depression
- Anemia
- Heart disease
- Stroke
- Allergies, either food or environmental
- Dehydration
- Hypothyroidism
- Metabolic disorders
- Nutritional deficiencies of vitamins B12 and folic acid
- Alcoholism
- Brain tumor
- Not keeping mentally active (by reading, etc.)
- Head injury
- Drug abuse

In addition, certain pharmaceutical medications, whether alone or in combination, can cause significant memory problems, disorientation, and even dementia. Bring a list of all your current medications, including over-the-counter drugs (better yet, bring all the pill bottles with their labels), to your doctor so that he or she can examine them for potential side effects.

Unfortunately, there is no cure for Alzheimer's, largely because no one is quite sure of the cause. Heredity certainly plays a factor, but as with most inherited diseases, a certain gene probably does not result in Alzheimer's all on its own: it is likely that environmental causes must be present as well. The most promising research into Alzheimer's has discovered that free radicals (the unbalanced molecules that destroy or damage cells of the body) play a significant role in the disorder. Since we know that good nutrition and herbal therapies effectively prevent and fight much free radical damage, it's wise for anyone in the early stages of Alzheimer's (or who has a family tendency toward the disease) to follow the recommendations given here. Environmental toxins seem to be an important factor as well. Although the link between Alzheimer's to toxins like aluminum and mercury has not been firmly established, it is certainly prudent to avoid these poisonous substances as a preventative measure. In addition, stress appears to be a major factor with the development of this disease. Many researchers also feel that prolonged elevation of the stress hormone cortisol is a major causative factor. And finally, elevated levels of the protein metabolism by-product homocysteine is known to contribute to Alzheimer's disease.

Although there is distressingly little that conventional medicine can do for Alzheimer's sufferers, it is very important to see a doctor if you think you may have the disease. One reason is that many elderly people take several different medications at once, and these combinations often result in memory loss, confusion, or even dementia—side effects that can easily be mistaken for those of Alzheimer's. The first step for anyone suffering from memory problems should be a rigorous examination of prescription and other drugs. Furthermore, the symptoms of Alzheimer's mimic those of several other disorders that are quite treatable; many people who believe they have Alzheimer's are actually suffering from depression, hypothyroidism, B12 or folic acid deficiency, or other conditions. Only after your doctor has ruled out all other possibilities will he or she make a diagnosis of Alzheimer's. If your doctor diagnoses you with Alzheimer's after just one or two visits, make an appointment to see someone else—preferably a doctor with a strong background in geriatrics or neurological disorders. If you do have Alzheimer's, it's important to work with a good specialist. Although there's no cure, there are ways to help you improve your health, comfort, and independence.

Natural therapies should be employed to prevent or help slow down the disease and to improve life quality.

In vitro studies at the University of Calgary have shown that mercury vapors cause a degeneration of brain neurons and also cause lesions similar to those found in people with Alzheimer's disease.

SYMPTOMS

Alzheimer's is a progressive disease. Its symptoms are listed here in the order in which they usually occur.

- Memory problems
- Confusion and disorientation
- Mood swings
- Depression
- Paranoia
- Inability to manage basic tasks
- Inappropriate behavior
- Hallucinations and delusions
- Episodes of violence and rage or childlike passivity
- Dementia

ROOT CAUSES

Although researchers are not yet sure what causes Alzheimer's, it is likely that a combination of the following factors plays a significant role in the disease.

- Genetics (including elevated homo-cysteine levels)
- Free radicals
- Nutritional deficiencies (especially of vitamins B1, folic acid, and B12)
- Smoking
- Environmental toxins, especially aluminum and mercury
- Chronically elevated cortisol levels

TREATMENT

Diet

Recommended Food

Eat a wholesome diet of basic, unprocessed foods. Because conventionally grown foods often contain toxins, buy organic whenever possible. If organic food is unavailable or too expensive, wash your food thoroughly before eating.

The antioxidant vitamins A, C, and E will combat damage from free radicals. Fresh fruits and vegetables are among the best sources of antioxidants, so have a couple of servings at every meal. For vitamin E, add wheat germ to salads, cereals, or juices. Nuts and seeds are other good sources of this vital nutrient.

> ### Fish is medicine for the brain.
>
> The *Archives of Neurology* published a study of 815 participants, ages 64 to 94 years. Over a seven-year period, researchers reviewed food frequency questionnaires to quantify fish consumption and dietary intake of the essential fatty acids DHA and EPA. Researchers found that people who ate fish only one to three times a month had a 40 percent lower risk of Alzheimer's than those who never ate fish. Those who consumed fish one time per week had a 60 percent lower risk.

The consumption of fish is very important. Salmon, halibut, cod, sole, and others are healthful sources of DHA, an essential fatty acid involved in brain function and GPA, which reduces inflammation.

A deficiency of the B-complex vitamins can both cause the disease and imitate its symptoms. Brewer's yeast is a potent source of B vitamins, as are wheat germ, eggs, and spirulina.

Use turmeric as a spice when preparing meals.

Many people with Alzheimer's are found to be deficient in zinc. To boost your intake, snack on pumpkin seeds regularly.

To improve circulation, increase energy levels, and detoxify your body, drink a glass of clean water every two waking hours.

Eat plenty of fiber to keep toxins moving through your digestive tract and to prevent them from taking up residence in your body. Whole grains, oats, and raw or lightly cooked vegetables are good sources of fiber that are also nutritionally dense.

If you're older, your digestive system may not be able to absorb nutrients as well as it used to. Fresh fruit and vegetable juices are easily absorbable and packed with the vitamins you need, so have several glasses daily.

Food to Avoid

If you have Alzheimer's or have a family tendency toward the disease, it is imperative that you stay away from all foods containing toxins and additives. Eliminate processed and junk food from your diet. Alcohol and excessive caffeine are also too toxic for you to consume.

This book never recommends drinking tap water, but in your case it is even more important that you avoid it. Tap water is full of environmental contaminants, including those that are linked to Alzheimer's.

Testing Techniques

Conventional testing, such as a CT scan, an MRI, and an electroencephalogram, as well as routine blood work, are standard. Additional helpful testing includes

   Toxic metal testing for elements toxic to brain tissue, such as aluminum, mercury, lead, arsenic, and others. The best test is a toxic element challenge urinalysis. The patient takes a chelating agent such as DMSA or DMPS, which pulls toxic metals out of tissue storage. Urine is then collected, usually for twenty-four hours.

   Oxidative stress analysis—urine or blood testing

   Antioxidant testing (urine, blood, or skin scanning)

   Stool analysis

   Hormone analysis by saliva, urine, or blood (estrogens, progesterone, testosterone, DHEA, cortisol, melatonin, IGF-1, thyroid panel)

It may surprise you to learn that many foods, especially baked goods, contain aluminum. Read all food labels carefully. Don't use self-rising flour, choose nonaluminum baking powder, and avoid pickling salts. You'll also need to avoid food cooked in aluminum pots and pans, as well as beverages that come in aluminum cans.

Sometimes food allergies cause reactions that are similar to the symptoms of Alzheimer's. See the Food Allergies section and the elimination diet discussed there, to determine whether you're allergic to any foods.

Detoxification

A three-day juice fast once a month will help flush toxins out of your body. Support your fast with a wide variety of juices so that you get the nutrition you need.

If you do indeed suffer from heavy-metal poisoning, consider oral or IV chelation therapy to rid your body of these toxins. Make sure you find a qualified, reputable practitioner.

℞ Super Seven Prescriptions—Alzheimer's Disease

Super Prescription #1   Acetyl-L-carnitine
Take 1,000 mg three times daily. It improves brain cell communication and memory.

Super Prescription #2   DHA
Take a fish oil supplement that contains a daily dosage of 1,000 mg of DHA. It supplies essential fatty acids for proper brain function.

Super Prescription #3   Ginkgo biloba (24 percent flavone glycosides)
Take 120 mg two to three times daily. It improves circulation to the brain, improves memory, and has antioxidant benefits.

Super Prescription #4   Club moss (*Huperzia serrata*)
Take a product standardized to contain 0.2 mg of huperizine A daily. This compound has been shown to increase acetylcholine levels in the brain and to improve memory in people with Alzheimer's disease.

DHA is the primary component of the cell membranes of neurons. It also promotes nerve transmission in the central nervous system and protects the mitochondria (energy warehouse of cells). Studies have shown that low levels of serum DHA are a risk factor for Alzheimer's disease.

The herb ginkgo biloba has been shown to be helpful for people with early-stage Alzheimer's disease. It has been approved for the treatment of this disease by the German government. A study done in 1994, involving forty patients who had early-stage Alzheimer's disease, found that 240 mg of ginkgo biloba extract taken daily for three months produced measurable improvements in memory, attention, and mood. In addition, three other double-blind studies have demonstrated that ginkgo is helpful for the early stages of the disease.

S everal clinical trials have found that supplementation of acetyl-L-carnitine delays the progression of Alzheimer's disease, improves memory, and improves overall performance in some people with Alzheimer's disease.

O ne placebo-controlled trial found that 58 percent of people with Alzheimer's disease had significant improvement in memory, as well as in mental and behavioral function, from taking 200 mcg of huperzine A twice a day for eight weeks. This was considered a statistically significant improvement, compared to the 36 percent who responded to placebo.

Super Prescription #5   Phosphatidylserine

Take 300 mg daily. This naturally occurring phospholipid improves brain cell communication and memory and has shown benefits for early-stage Alzheimer's disease.

Super Prescription #6   Vitamin B12

Take 800 to 1,600 micrograms daily. Consider using a sublingual form. Vitamin B12 deficiency mimics the symptoms of Alzheimer's disease.

Super Prescription #7   Vitamin E

Take 2,000 IU daily of a complex with added tocotrienols. Vitamin E is a potent antioxidant that protects against free radical damage. Studies show that it slows the progression of Alzheimer's disease. Do not take this high a dosage if you are on blood-thinning medication.

General Recommendations

Ashwagandha (*Withania somniferum*) is used as a brain tonic in Ayurvedic medicine. It reduces stress hormone levels. Take 100 to 3,000 mg daily.

Panax ginseng improves memory and balances stress hormone levels. Take a standardized product containing 4 to 7 percent ginsenosides at 100 to 250 mg twice daily. Do not use it if you have high blood pressure.

DHEA is an important hormone for cognitive function. If your level is low, talk with your doctor about starting at a 15 mg dosage.

Cordyceps sinensis is used in Chinese medicine for poor memory. Take 2 to 4 capsules daily.

DMAE helps the body produce acetylcholine for memory, and it also has antioxidant properties. Take 600 mg daily.

An antioxidant formula to use should contain a wide range of antioxidants, such as selenium, carotenoids, vitamin C, and others.

Chlorella speeds up the detoxification of toxic metals that may be causing free radical damage. Take as directed on the container.

Phosphatidylcholine increases acetylcholine levels to improve memory. Take 1,000 to 1,500 mg daily.

NADH has been shown to improve mental function in one clinical trial. Take 10 mg daily.

Vitamin B1 has been shown to improve mental function in people with Alzheimer's disease. Take 3 grams daily.

Homeopathy

Although homeopathy cannot cure Alzheimer's, it can reduce or alleviate many of its symptoms. Consult with a licensed homeopath for a constitutional remedy. In the meantime, here are a few temporary suggestions.

Alumina can clear confusion and reduce memory impairment. The person often suffers from constipation. Take 30C daily for three or four days, and see if improvement occurs within a week.

Lycopodium (*Lycopodium clavatum*) can help if you're fearful and have trouble recalling words. Take 30C two times daily for two weeks.

Acupressure

See pages 668–675 for information about pressure points and administering treatment.

- Stomach 36 tones the entire body, while improving the absorption of nutrients into the bloodstream.
- Governing Vessel 24.5 is easy to reach (it's at the center of the forehead, between the eyebrows), and it strengthens both memory and concentration.
- To relieve anxiety or nervous tension, work Pericardium 6.
- Lung 1 will ease depression and encourage deep, slow breathing.

Bodywork

Massage

Lymphatic massage detoxifies the body, while improving circulation (including circulation to the brain). Because it is a gentle therapy, lymphatic massage is ideal for people in the later stages of Alzheimer's, who may be upset by more vigorous manipulation. If your skin is dry, you may want the therapist to use a little lubricating oil during treatment.

Reflexology

See pages 686–687 for information about reflexology areas and how to work them.
  To detoxify cells and tissues, work the area corresponding to the lymph system.
  Encourage blood flow to the brain by working the heart.
  Work the lungs to oxygenate the blood.

Other Bodywork Recommendations

Hot and cold hydrotherapy is invigorating and stimulates blood flow to the brain. Try alternating hot and cold baths for the best effect.

Aromatherapy

Juniper helps break down toxins that reside within fatty deposits. Add it to your bath or use it during a lymphatic massage.

  Black pepper will stimulate digestion, which can improve the absorption of nutrients. Dilute it in some carrier oil, and rub directly onto the abdomen.

  The changing mood states of people with Alzheimer's may sometimes call for relaxing oils; at other times, oils with a stimulating effect are in order. Oils that have relaxing, calming properties include lavender and melissa. To rouse the mind and raise the spirits, try geranium, jasmine, neroli, bergamot, or rose.

Stress Reduction

A diagnosis of Alzheimer's is an extremely stressful event, especially when you are still quite capable and aware of the challenges to come. During these early stages, it's vital that you find stress-reduction techniques that work for you; they will increase the quality—and perhaps even the quantity—of the time you have left.

General Stress-Reduction Therapies

Alzheimer's can make you feel alone, even if you're supported by a loving family. Join a support group of other people who have Alzheimer's, to share your feelings. (You may also want to encourage your loved ones to attend a support group of their own. They're coping with the shock, too.)

  Meditation and prayer will help you manage stress and will also keep your mind and memory functioning at their optimum level for as long as possible.

Bach Flower Remedies

Select the appropriate remedy, and place 10 drops under your tongue. Hold the drops in place for thirty seconds and swallow. Use as often as needed.

Rescue Remedy will help you deal with any crisis calmly, including the initial diagnosis or the difficult times afterward.

If you are so afraid of what the future holds that you tend to cling to the past, take Honeysuckle.

If you usually handle obstacles with aplomb and courage but just can't find the strength to face the challenges posed by your illness, take Oak.

Other Recommendations

- Regular exercise will keep blood flowing to the brain. A daily walk in the morning sunlight can also do wonders for your spirits.
- If you're trying to prevent Alzheimer's, keep yourself active and learning. A lack of mental engagement may be connected to loss of brain function.
- Avoid sources of aluminum and mercury. Some food sources of aluminum were listed earlier, but you must also read the labels on antacids, diarrhea medications, buffered aspirin, deodorants, and douches. You may want to consider having dental fillings composed of a silver-mercury amalgam replaced with a nontoxic substance.
- Simple routines are quite helpful to many people in the early and middle stages of Alzheimer's. Make a schedule for your day, and plan to perform more complicated tasks during the hours when you usually feel your best.
- Although it is very difficult to face the inevitable, many people with Alzheimer's feel much better when they plan ahead. If you work out your legal and financial arrangements now, and discuss your wishes for the future with your family, you may find that you can enjoy a stronger sense of peace and well-being.
- If you are the caregiver of a person who has Alzheimer's, you probably need some help. Contact local support groups to find low-cost assistance with transportation, meals, and even day care for the elderly.

REFERENCES

Bonavita, E. 1986. Study of the efficacy and tolerability of L-acetylcarnitine therapy in the senile brain. *International Journal of Clinical Pharmacology, Therapy, and Toxicology* 24:511–16.

Conquer, J. A., M. C. Tierney, J. Zecevic, W. J. Bettger, and R. H. Fisher. 2000. Fatty acid analysis of blood plasma of patients with Alzheimer's disease, other types of dementia, and cognitive impairment. *Lipids* 35(12):1305–12.

Cucinotta, D., et al. 1988. Multicenter clinical placebo-controlled study with acetyl-L-carnitine (LAC) in the treatment of mildly demented elderly patients. *Journal of Drug Development and Research* 14:213–16.

Hofferberth, B. 1994. The efficacy of EGb 761 in patients with senile dementia of the Alzheimer type: A double-blind, placebo-controlled study on different levels of investigation. *Human Psychopharmacology* 9:215–22.

Kanowski, S., W. Herrmann, K. Stephan, et al. 1996. Proof of efficacy of the *Ginkgo biloba* special extract EGb 761 in outpatients suffering from mild to moderate primary degenerative dementia of the Alzheimer type or multi-infarct dementia. *Pharmacopsychiatry* 29:47–56.

Le Bars, P. L., M. M. Katz, N. Berman, et al. 1997. A placebo-controlled, double-blind, randomized trial of an extract of Ginkgo biloba for dementia. North American EGb Study Group. *Journal of the American Medical Association* 278:1327–32.

Leong, C. C., N. I. Syed, and F. L. Lorscheider. 2001. Retrograde degeneration of neurite membrane structural integrity of nerve growth cones following in vitro exposure to mercury. *Neuroreport* 12(4) (March 26): 733–37.

Maurer, K., R. Ihl, T. Dierks, and L. Frolich. 1997. Clinical efficacy of *Ginkgo biloba* special extract EGb 761 in dementia of the Alzheimer's type. *Journal of Psychiatric Research* 31:645–55.

Morris, M. C., D. A. Evans, J. L. Bienias, C. C. Tangney, D. A. Bennett, R. S. Wilson, N. Aggarwal, and J. Schneider. 2003. Consumption of fish and n-3 fatty acids and risk of incident Alzheimer disease. *Archives of Neurology* 60(7):940–46.

Pettegrew, J. W., W. E. Klunk, K. Panchalingam, et al. 1995. Clinical and neurochemical effects of acetyl-L-carnitine in Alzheimer's disease. *Neurobiological Aging* 16:1–4.

Rai, G., G. Wright, L. Scott, et al. 1990. Double-blind, placebo controlled study of acetyl-L-carnitine in patients with Alzheimer's dementia. *Current Medical Research and Opinion* 11:638–47.

Salvioli, G., and M. Neri. 1994. L-acetylcarnitine treatment of mental decline in the elderly. *Drugs under Experimental and Clinical Research* 20:169–76.

Sano, M., K. Bell, L. Cote, et al. 1992. Double-blind parallel design pilot study of acetyl levocarnitine in patients with Alzheimer's disease. *Archives of Neurology* 49:1137–41.

Xu, S. S., Z. X. Gao, Z. Weng, et al. 1995. Efficacy of tablet huperzine-A on memory, cognition, and behavior in Alzheimer's disease. *Chung Kuo Yao Li Hsueh Pao* 16:391–95.

Anemia

Given the frenetic pace of modern Western life, it can seem almost normal to feel fatigued, weak, or short of breath. But these symptoms are never normal; they always point to a disorder of some kind. For millions of Americans, that disorder is anemia.

Every cell in the human body gets a large portion of its energy from oxygen. In a healthy person, cells receive an adequate supply of oxygen, thanks to a substance called hemoglobin, which transports oxygen through the blood. Without sufficient hemoglobin, the cells don't get enough oxygen; without enough oxygen, the brain, the muscles, and all the other tissues begin to slow down. The anemic person feels weak and tired at first and then may experience several other symptoms, including headaches, difficulty concentrating, and a series of illnesses that are the result of a suppressed immune system.

The body needs iron to produce the necessary amount of hemoglobin, and the vast majority of anemia cases are caused by a deficiency of this mineral. Iron deficiency most often results from a poor diet, especially one that's high in junk food, or from long-term or repeated dieting. There are many other ways a person can end up with a deficiency of iron, however. Blood loss for any reason, including surgery, trauma, gum disease, hemorrhoids, polyps, cancer of the colon, bleeding ulcers, and heavy menstrual periods, can produce an anemic state. So can an increase in the body's need for iron, which usually happens during pregnancy. Iron deficiency can also be caused by an inability to absorb certain nutrients, as can happen with folic acid and vitamin B12. In rarer cases, deficiencies of vitamins A, B2, B6, and C, as well as of copper, may lead to anemia. The elderly often lose their ability to absorb these nutrients, as do people with certain digestive disorders like Crohn's disease or ulcerative colitis. Usually, iron deficiency is caused by a combination of these factors.

In rare cases, anemia is the result of a hereditary blood disorder, in which red blood cells are destroyed prematurely. Thalassemia, sickle-cell disease, and spherocytosis are all very serious and sometimes fatal forms of anemia; people with these diseases must be under lifelong medical care. Anemia can also be caused by an inability to absorb any vitamin B12 at all. This condition can easily be treated with sublingual B12, with regular injections of vitamin B12, or by improving stomach acid levels.

If you suspect that you have anemia, it's likely that you can be cured with simple home treatments and supplementation. It's important, however, that you see a doctor for an official diagnosis. The symptoms of anemia can mimic those of other disorders, so you'll need to get a thorough physical examination. If you are diagnosed with anemia, don't let your doctor stop there. Make sure he or she explains the specific cause of your problem so that you'll know how to address any underlying disorders and prevent a recurrence.

SYMPTOMS

- Fatigue
- Weakness
- Shortness of breath after mild exertion
- Headaches
- Dizziness or fainting
- Difficulty concentrating
- Pale skin, lips, and nail beds
- Cold extremities
- Frequent illnesses
- Cessation of menstruation

ROOT CAUSES

- A poor diet, especially one that's deficient in iron, folic acid, or vitamin B12. This category includes eating disorders, such as anorexia nervosa and bulimia.
- Acute blood loss (most often from menstruation, surgery, or injury)
- Chronic blood loss (commonly from bleeding ulcers, colon disorders, gum disease, or bleeding hemorrhoids)
- Pregnancy
- Inherited blood disorders
- An inability to absorb vitamin B12 or folic acid
- Poor digestion and absorption— particularly, low stomach acid

TREATMENT

Diet

Dietary changes are of utmost importance for the anemic person. If you adhere to the following suggestions for several weeks but still feel tired, consult your doctor. There may be an underlying disorder at work, or you may have something other than anemia.

Recommended Food

Plan your meals so that you get plenty of iron. The best source of this mineral is organic calf's liver; while this book usually discourages the consumption of organ meats, it may be necessary for you to incorporate this one into your diet until your body recovers. Green leafy vegetables (except for spinach—see the note about oxalic acid under Food to Avoid in this section), leeks, cashews, cherries, strawberries, dried fruits, figs, kelp, and eggs are all excellent sources as well. If you're a vegetarian and can't eat calf's liver, include one or two servings of green leafy vegetables at every meal.

Blackstrap molasses is also rich in iron, so take a spoonful of it every day. Blackstrap molasses can usually be found next to the pancake syrup at your grocery store. Make sure to read the label carefully, as you don't want molasses that's been sulfured.

Brewer's yeast is a good source of iron, folic acid, and B12, so add 1 tablespoon to cereals, salads, or juices daily.

Vitamin C will help your body absorb and retain iron. When you're eating foods that are high in iron, have some citrus fruits alongside them or take supplemental vitamin C.

Cook your food in cast-iron pots and pans. The food will absorb some of the mineral from the cookware. This strategy is especially helpful for vegetarians, who have difficulty meeting iron requirements.

If you have a digestive disorder that prevents you from absorbing food properly, juice the vegetables that are suggested here and drink several glasses daily. Juices don't require much digestive work from the stomach and the intestines, and their nutrients are easily passed into the bloodstream.

Testing Techniques

- Blood testing—complete blood count (CBC), ferritin (iron stores), B12, folate
- Comprehensive stool analysis

Food to Avoid

Do not eat spinach, rhubarb, tomatoes, or chocolate. These foods are high in oxalic acid, a substance that inhibits your body's ability to absorb iron.

Sodas, dairy products, coffee, and black tea are other iron-blockers. Eliminate them from your diet.

Iron is removed from your body through the bowels, so eat your fiber or take fiber supplements separately from iron sources. Avoid raw wheat bran entirely: it's a strong laxative that could well deplete an entire day's supply of iron.

Avoid cow's milk, which may cause hidden bleeding in the intestinal tract. This is particularly true with children.

Many young women—and, increasingly, men—become anemic as a result of following fad diets. If you truly need to lose weight, don't starve yourself; instead, restrict your consumption of fats and sugars, while eating lots of foods with high nutritional density, such as vegetables, fruits, soy products, and whole grains. For further weight-loss suggestions, see Obesity.

℞ Super Seven Prescriptions—Anemia

Super Prescription #1   Iron
Take 50 to 100 mg of a well-absorbed form of iron, such as iron citrate, gluconate, glycinate, or fumarate, one to two times daily. Also, labels that state iron chelate

are generally well absorbed. Avoid the use of iron sulfate (ferrous sulfate), which is poorly absorbed and can cause digestive upset. *Note:* Supplement iron only if you have iron-deficiency anemia.

Super Prescription #2   B12

Take 1,000 to 2,000 mcg of B12 daily, preferably in the methylcobalamin form. Sublingual is very absorbable, or your doctor may use the injection form to start. *Note:* Supplement this higher dose of B12 if your doctor has diagnosed a B12 deficiency.

Super Prescription #3   Folic acid

Take 800 to 1,200 mcg of folic acid daily. Sublingual is very absorbable, or your doctor may use the injection form to start. *Note:* Supplement this higher dose of folic acid if your doctor has diagnosed a folic acid deficiency.

Super Prescription #4   Homeopathic Ferrum phosphoricum

Take 5 pellets of the 3x or 6x potency three times daily. This homeopathic remedy improves iron utilization in the cells.

Super Prescription #5   Spirulina

Take 2,000 mg daily, as it has been shown to help improve anemia by stimulating the bone marrow production of red blood cells.

Super Prescription #6   Yellow dock (*Rumex crispus*)

Take 1 capsule or 20 drops of the tincture form with each meal. It contains iron and improves iron absorption.

Super Prescription #7   Vitamin C

Take 250 to 500 mg with each dose of iron. It provides an acidic environment for enhanced iron absorption.

Phycocyanin, a phytonutrient found in spirulina, has been shown in animal studies to stimulate the bone marrow to produce blood cells more effectively. Spirulina is considered a rich source of vitamins, minerals, and amino acids.

General Recommendations

Gentian root (*Gentiana lutea*) increases stomach acid for improved absorption. Take a 300 mg capsule or 20 drops of tincture at the beginning of each meal.

Betaine hydrochloride increases stomach acid. Take 1 to 3 capsules with each meal.

Several herbs leach iron from the soil as they grow. When you consume them, you get the benefit of their mineral density. Some of the best herbs for anemia treatment include dandelion (*Taraxacum officinale*), pau d'arco (*Tabebuia avellanedae*), and nettle leaf (*Urtica dioica*). There are several commercial preparations available that combine these herbs into one "blood-building" formula; take as directed on the product label. If you wish to buy and take the herbs separately, here are the recommended dosages:

Dandelion (*Taraxacum officinale*), in addition to having a high iron content, cleanses the blood and detoxifies the liver. Choose a product made from dandelion root, and take 3 to 5 grams or 5 to 10 cc daily.

Pau d'arco (*Tabebuia avellanedae*) can be used as a tea; drink several cups a day. Take 100 mg or 0.5 to 1.0 cc three times daily.

Nettle leaves (*Urtica dioica*) are used for anemia because they have a rich nutritional content. Take 300 mg two or three times daily, or use 2 to 4 cc of a tincture three times daily.

Ashwagandha (*Withania somniferum*) has been shown in human studies to increase red blood cell count. Take 2,000 to 3,000 mg daily.

Dong quai is a traditional Chinese blood builder. Take 500 mg twice daily for one month.

Homeopathy

Select the appropriate remedy from the following list, and take 30C two times daily for two or three weeks.

Calcarea Phosphorica is for anemia in school children or chronic anemia in adults.

China Officinalis will improve anemic conditions that are a result of blood loss or illness.

Natrum Muriaticum is for anemia that's accompanied by headaches and constipation.

Acupressure

See pages 668–675 for information about pressure points and administering treatment.

- Improve your strength and energy, along with your ability to absorb nutrients from food, by working Stomach 36.
- For tension, work Lung 1 and Pericardium 6.
- If you have a headache, use Large Intestine 4.

Bodywork

Massage

While massage won't address any of the causes of anemia, it's an effective way to improve your circulation and increase your energy level. A full-body massage is probably the best choice, but there are easy home-care techniques you can use to relieve headaches or to warm up cold extremities.

Reflexology

See pages 686–687 for information about reflexology areas and how to work them.

Work the spleen to encourage the manufacture and the recycling of hemoglobin.

To aid circulation, blood formation, and detoxification, stimulate the liver.

Aromatherapy

Eucalyptus, ginger, black pepper, and rosemary all improve poor circulation. Add any of these oils—or if you prefer, a combination of them—to a bath. You can also dilute them in a carrier oil and use in a massage.

For an uplifting effect, try geranium or jasmine oils. Use them in any preparation you like, but for a long-lasting effect, you might like to add a few drops to a diffuser and let the scent envelop your room or office.

Bach Flower Remedies

Select the appropriate remedy, and place 10 drops under your tongue. Hold the drops in place for thirty seconds and swallow. Use as often as needed.

Olive is a potent way to address the prolonged fatigue that accompanies anemia.

Clematis is for people who feel dreamy and unable to concentrate. It is also good for people who feel a constant, almost overpowering urge to sleep.

If anemia has drained you of the hope that you'll ever feel better, take Gorse. It will help you regain the more balanced outlook that's often necessary for healing.

REFERENCES

Chamorro, G., M. Salazar, K. G. Araujo, C. P. dos Santos, G. Ceballos, and L. F. Castillo. 2002. Update on the pharmacology of spirulina (*Arthrospira*), an unconventional food. *Archives Latinoamericanos de Nutricion* 52(3):232–40.

Zhang, C., et al. 1994. The effects of polysaccharide and phycocyanin from spirulina platensis variety on peripheral blood and hematopoietic system of bone marrow in mice. Second Asia Pacific Conference on Alga Biotechnology, April 25–27, p. 58.

Angina. *See* Cardiovascular Disease

Anorexia Nervosa. *See* Eating Disorders

Anxiety

Anxiety is a tool of the human body that is meant to be a healthy response to stresses in life or even to a dangerous situation. When we are afraid, our metabolism speeds up, our muscles tighten, and our adrenal glands produce extra quantities of adrenaline (a hormone that makes our hearts beat faster).

Anxiety becomes a troublesome response only when we can't burn up the nervous energy it creates. When a meeting, a deadline, or a family problem sets us on edge, our bodies signal "danger"—but physical action is rarely appropriate. Instead, we endure the unpleasant sensation of a rapid heartbeat and tensed muscles, often while having to smile at the opponent who sits across the desk or the dinner table. We are all able to handle occasional bouts of unreleased anxiety, but if the anxiety doesn't go away, or if it recurs frequently, it can lead to serious health problems. People who are exposed to prolonged anxiety—those who are going through a divorce, for example, or who are subject to intense pressures at work—often suffer from high blood pressure, insomnia, digestive problems, skin disorders, mood swings, depression, and many other conditions. The effects of anxiety can also make any existing health problems much worse.

Sometimes people feel the symptoms of anxiety even when they're not facing a serious challenge or danger. Anxiety disorder is the name given to an excessive amount of worry that lasts longer than six months. What's excessive? Any nervous response that's out of proportion to its cause. A new job or a serious illness should naturally produce more anxiety than, say, planning a party. And if people cannot pinpoint the source of anxiety, or if it constantly changes, there's a good chance that they suffer from anxiety disorder.

People with anxiety disorders are vulnerable to the same health problems as anyone else with prolonged anxiety. They may also experience extreme states of nervousness and worry, called panic attacks. During a panic attack, the heart pounds and breathing becomes rapid or difficult. Sufferers may break into a cold sweat, experience tingling in the extremities, or feel dizzy and weak. Although panic attacks rarely last long—they can take anywhere from a few seconds to half an hour—they are quite frightening. People may feel certain that they are having a heart attack or a stroke or may simply feel overwhelmed by intense terror.

If you suffer from prolonged anxiety, whether as a result of an anxiety disorder or from a major unresolved source of tension, you can take certain steps to ease your symptoms. Bodywork and stress-reduction techniques will give you immediate relief but can also help you work on the root of your problem. Dietary changes and herbal therapies can have a calming, stabilizing effect on your mood.

As you employ these complementary healing strategies, it's also important to rule out any underlying physical causes. Disorders like low blood sugar, thyroid problems, heart problems (mitral valve prolapse), and clinical depression can lead to the symptoms of anxiety, as can nutritional deficiencies. Certain substances can also create anxiety or make it worse. Caffeine is perhaps the most notorious tension-inducing chemical, but sugar and other food allergens, nicotine, alcohol, environmental toxins and allergens, and other causes can all be just as potent.

SYMPTOMS

- Restlessness and tension
- Trembling
- Heart palpitations
- Dry mouth
- Sweaty palms
- Diarrhea
- Lump in the throat
- Mood swings
- High blood pressure
- Dizziness

- Sleep disturbances
- Appetite disorders
- Fatigue
- Impotence
- Chest pains
- Hyperventilation
- Headache
- Backache
- Muscle tension and/or spasms
- Panic attacks

ROOT CAUSES

- Stress
- Caffeine
- Sugar
- Nicotine
- Alcohol and street drugs
- Prescription medications
- Disturbed sleep
- Food allergies

- Environmental toxins
- Poor nutrition
- Thyroid problems
- Mitral valve prolapse
- Low blood sugar
- Depression
- Adrenal disorders

Testing Techniques

The following tests can give you an assessment of possible metabolic reasons for your anxiety:

Hormone analysis by saliva, urine, or blood (estrogens, progesterone, DHEA, cortisol, thyroid panel). DHEA and cortisol are of particular importance.

Fasting blood sugar

Food allergy/sensitivity testing

TREATMENT

Diet

Some foods can create anxiety, and others soothe it. If you're a victim of prolonged or frequent tension, a good diet can significantly—and sometimes completely—alleviate your symptoms.

Recommended Food

An anxiety-healing diet starts with a good base of nutrients. Plan well-rounded meals of basic, clean foods. To keep your blood-sugar levels stable, eat smaller meals throughout the day, rather than three large ones.

Complex carbohydrates contain serotonin, a neurotransmitter that has a calming effect on the brain. Have some whole grains, like brown rice or oats, at every meal.

Make sure you get enough B-vitamins by increasing your intake of brewer's yeast, brown rice, and leafy green vegetables.

If you have a bowel disorder, fibrous foods will help regulate your digestive tract. The whole grains and vegetables that were suggested earlier are an excellent source of fiber. For further suggestions, see the entry that addresses your particular problem.

Calcium and magnesium calm the body. Good sources include sea vegetables, green leafy vegetables (except spinach), soybeans, nuts, molasses, salmon, oysters, sardines (with the bones), broccoli, and unsweetened cultured yogurt.

Food to Avoid

Caffeine and alcohol cause anxiety or the symptoms of anxiety. Wean yourself off black tea, coffee, and alcohol, even if they seem to comfort you when you're stressed. Ultimately, these substances just put a further strain on your system.

Refined sugars are another enemy of anxious people. Whole fruits and naturally sweet products are fine in moderation, but candy, cake, cookies, refined flour products, and soft drinks will cause your blood sugar to spike and then plummet. The resulting low levels of blood sugar produce feelings of irritability, tension, and depression.

A response to food allergies can lead to trembling, dry mouth, heart palpitations, misbehaving bowels, and other symptoms that mimic anxiety. See Food Allergies to learn more, and use the elimination diet presented there to identify any problematic foods.

If you suffer from anxiety, chances are that you're short on B vitamins. Since refined flour and processed foods deplete your body of this nutrient, cut them out of your diet.

Detoxification

Stress can be a result of toxins, and stress itself is poisonous to your entire system. Consider doing a three-day supervised juice fast. Be sure most of your juices are made from vegetables, as too many fruit juices can give you unwanted sugar shock. A fast is also an ideal time to rest up and enjoy various types of therapy, like a massage or a hot bath, that combine detoxification with relaxation.

℞ Super Seven Prescriptions—Anxiety

Super Prescription #1   Homeopathy
Take a combination anxiety homeopathic remedy, as directed on the container, or read the descriptions further on in the Homeopathy and Bach Flower sections to pick a single remedy.

Super Prescription #2   5-hydroxytryptophan (5-HTP)

Take 50 to 100 mg two to three times daily. Note that 5-HTP increases serotonin levels, which have a calming effect on the mind. *Note:* Do not take in conjunction with a pharmaceutical antidepressant or an antianxiety medication.

Super Prescription #3   Kava (*Piper methysticum*)

Take 200 to 250 mg two to three times daily of a product standardized to 30 percent kava lactones. Kava (*Piper methysticum*) can significantly relieve a panic attack, as well as the symptoms of generalized anxiety. If you're using a pharmaceutical tranquilizer, you should talk to your doctor about making the switch. Do not, under any circumstances, take kava at the same time you're taking a medication for anxiety, depression, or Parkinson's disease. Do not use kava while consuming alcohol or if you have elevated liver enzymes. This supplement should be used with a doctor's supervision.

Super Prescription #4   Calcium and magnesium

Take a combination of 500 mg of calcium and 250 mg of magnesium twice daily. These minerals help calm the nervous system.

Super Prescription #5   Passionflower (*Passiflora incarnata*)

Take 250 mg or 0.5 ml two to three times daily. Passionflower relaxes the nerves and is gentle enough to use during the day.

Super Prescription #6   B-complex

Take a 50 mg complex one to two times daily. B vitamins help combat the effects of stress and will balance your brain chemicals. Vitamin B6 is especially important.

Super Prescription #7   GABA

Take 500 mg two to three times daily between meals. This amino acid has a calming effect.

Double-blind studies have shown that kava *(Piper methysticum)* is effective in helping people with mild to moderate anxiety. One trial found that kava also reduced anxiety symptoms in menopausal women.

General Recommendations

Valerian (*Valeriana officinalis*) is a strong nerve relaxer and is especially helpful for insomnia caused by anxiety. Take 300 mg or 0.5 to 1.0 ml two to three times daily.

Saint-John's-wort (*Hypericum perforatum*) can lift anxiety that's accompanied by depression. Take 300 mg three times daily. If you're on medication for depression or anxiety, talk to your doctor before switching to an herbal preparation.

Ashwagandha (*Withania somniferum*) helps balance stress hormone levels and reduce tension. Take 2,000 to 3,000 mg daily.

Chromium balances blood-sugar levels. Take 200 mcg two to three times daily.

Inositol has been shown in studies to be helpful for panic attacks. Take 4 grams three times daily.

Chamomile (*Matricaria recutita*) and oatstraw (*Avena sativa*) are great herbal nerve relaxers. They can be taken as a tea or in supplement form.

Homeopathy

Pick the remedy that best matches your symptoms. Take 2 pellets of 30C potency twice daily to prevent or reduce anxiety. Should the first three days pass without any sign of improvement, you're probably taking the wrong remedy. Stop using the current one, and switch to something else. After you first notice improvement, stop taking the remedy, unless symptoms begin to return. For acute anxiety or a panic attack, take a 30C potency every fifteen minutes for up to 6 doses. After improvement is noticed, stop taking the remedy, unless symptoms return.

Aconitum Napellus is for acute panic attacks, especially those that make you feel as if you might die. You may experience shortness of breath, a sensation of impending doom, and heart palpitations.

Arsenicum Album is for anxiety and insecurity that are accompanied by a fast heartbeat, chills, and a disturbed appetite. People who benefit from this remedy are often obsessively tidy and organized.

Calcarea Carbonica is for symptoms of anxiety and a feeling of being overwhelmed. You are generally chilly and tire easily.

Gelsemium (*Gelsemium sempervirens*) is effective for acute anxiety from stage fright or from being in crowds. Trembling and diarrhea often accompany anxiety.

Ignatia (*Ignatia amara*) is for when you feel moody, weepy, and brooding and may feel a lump in your throat. It is excellent for anxiety that results from an emotional trauma.

Kali Phosphoricum is for generalized anxiety, poor memory, and fatigue. Take a 6x potency three times daily.

Lycopodium (*Lycopodium clavatum*) will ease stage fright or social anxiety due to low confidence. You often crave sweets and have a digestive upset, such as gas and bloating.

Acupressure

See pages 668–675 for information about pressure points and administering treatment.

- For quick relief of anxiety, work Lung 1. A detailed method for working this point can be found on page 670.
- Pericardium 6 is another good point for nervous tension. Because it's located on the wrist, you can easily work this point whenever you need quick relief—at the office, in meetings, or on a bus.
- For fear, work Bladder 23.
- For anxiety that leads to depression, work Conception Vessel 17.

Bodywork

Massage

A regular full-body massage is a great way to relieve the tension that collects in your muscles. If you don't have the time or the money for a professional treatment, you or a loved one can easily perform some spot techniques at home. A neck, a shoulder, or a foot rub can help you unwind. Use any of the essential oils recommended under Aromatherapy in this section for an even more relaxing effect.

Reflexology

See pages 686–687 for information about reflexology areas and how to work them.

Work the areas corresponding to the diaphragm, all the glands, the heart, and the solar plexus.

Hydrotherapy

If you suffer from insomnia, it's important to draw blood away from your head before bedtime. Take a ten-minute hot foot bath to encourage the blood to move down and out toward your limbs.

Aromatherapy

Many essential oils have relaxing properties, but lavender, melissa, jasmine, and ylang ylang are among the best for anxiety. Use them in a bath or a massage, or add some to a room diffuser for extended relief.

During a panic attack, inhale frankincense to encourage deep breathing.

If you have diarrhea, use chamomile, peppermint, lavender, and melissa to soothe gastric cramps. Add a few drops to a massage oil, and rub gently onto your abdomen.

Bergamot will restore a lost appetite. Try some in a room diffuser, or simply inhale deeply over the bottle.

Stress Reduction

If you suffer from anxiety, it's wise to have a repertoire of stress-reduction techniques you can call upon. Any of the techniques discussed in the Exercise and Stress Reduction chapter can help, but following are some specific suggestions.

General Stress-Reduction Therapies

Use prayer to alleviate and prevent anxiety. The Bible contains many scriptures that address anxiety.

It is also prudent to seek help from a counselor who specializes in anxiety disorder.

Positive mental imagery and meditation are useful. Whenever you feel your mind racing ahead to upcoming deadlines or unpleasant situations, try to bring it back to an awareness of the present. Focus for a moment on something beautiful: the sound of a bird, the color of the sky, the steam drifting up from your cup of tea.

Many people with anxiety have cold hands and feet, because the panic response pulls blood away from the extremities. Thermal biofeedback can help you use this symptom to your advantage. During a thermal biofeedback session, you'll be asked to try to warm your hands. As you learn this technique, you'll actually learn to control the nervous-system arousal mechanism that is set off by anxiety. Soon you'll be able to ward off a panic attack just by mentally warming your hands.

If you suffer from severe anxiety, consider EEG biofeedback. This form of biofeedback can be expensive, but it does have an excellent track record of helping people calm their brainwaves.

Don't let stress management itself become a source of stress. You're not a failure if you have a panic attack or an episode of anxiety; no one can manage anxiety perfectly. Just keep practicing tension-relieving techniques daily, and try to accept whatever comes your way as best you can.

Bach Flower Remedies

If none of the remedies suggested here applied to you, consult the chart on pages 648–650 to find one that suits your personality. Once you've found the appropriate remedy, place 10 drops of it under your tongue. Hold the drops in place for thirty seconds and swallow. Use as often as needed.

If you are prone to acute anxiety, keep a bottle of Rescue Remedy on hand. When a panic attack strikes, it will restore your peace of mind.

Rock Rose is one of the primary components of Rescue Remedy and is extremely helpful in a physical or emotional emergency. If a bad shock or a fright leaves you feeling helpless or blank, Rock Rose will help you return to a calmer state.

Aspen is for people who are gripped by fears they can't name. Their anxiety may come on suddenly and may produce intense feelings of dread.

For people who are all too able to name the fears that provoke their anxiety, Mimulus can help. This remedy is especially good for people who tend to keep these fears to themselves.

If your anxiety is brought on by excessive concern for others, Red Chestnut will help you put things in perspective.

Other Recommendations

- Exercise is still one of the best anxiety-relievers. A daily walk is enough for many people, although most methods of exercise will help reduce the effects of stress and anxiety.
- Acupuncture is helpful in controlling anxiety for some people.

REFERENCES

Lehmann, E. E., J. Kinzler, and J. Friedmann. 1996. Efficacy of a special kava (*Piper methysticum*) extract in patients with states of anxiety, tension and excitedness of non-mental origin. A double-blind placebo-controlled study of four weeks treatment. *Phytomedicine* 3:113–19.

Volz, H. P., and M. Kieser. 1997. Kava (*Piper methysticum*)—Kava (*Piper methysticum*) extract WS 1490 versus placebo in anxiety disorders. A randomized placebo-controlled 25-week outpatient trial. *Pharmacopsychiatry* 30:1–5.

Warnecke, G. 1991. Psychosomatic dysfunctions in the female climacteric. Clinical effectiveness and tolerance of kava (*Piper methysticum*) extract WS 1490. *Fortschritte de medizin* 119–22 [in German].

Arteriosclerosis. *See* Cardiovascular Disease

Arthritis

Arthritis is a degenerative joint disease that causes swelling and pain that can range from mild to excruciating. Although more than two hundred diseases are classified under the name "arthritis," most arthritic conditions fall into one of two categories: osteoarthritis and rheumatoid arthritis.

Osteoarthritis is by far the more common, afflicting 40 million Americans and 80 percent of people over fifty. The pain and the inflammation occur when the cartilage that protects the bones from rubbing against each other wears down. Not surprisingly, the disease usually appears in joints that do most of the body's hard work: the knees, the hips, the spine, and the hands. Although injury or the normal wear and tear of life often bring on cartilage damage, it can be made much worse by food allergies, poor diet, and mineral deposits in the joints. For some people, the effects of mental and emotional stress aggravate arthritis pain. Changes in the weather—usually, rain and falling barometric pressure—often cause arthritis flare-ups

Rheumatoid arthritis (RA) is quite another story. Most experts believe it is caused by an inappropriate immune reaction, in which white blood cells attack the cartilage in the joints; it can go on to destroy the bones themselves and even the muscles and the skin. It is often exceedingly painful and can cripple its sufferers. While osteoarthritis affects men and women equally, RA appears three times more frequently in women. It affects only 2 to 3 percent of the population and can occur at any age, even in childhood. The course of the disease is difficult to predict. It may disappear a few months after its appearance, or it may grow progressively worse. Experts disagree over the causes of RA, but it seems clear that genes, food allergies, bacterial or viral infection, stress, excess acid in the body, and the presence of certain antibodies in the blood all play a role. Many of the complementary therapies used for osteoarthritis are also effective in reducing the pain and slowing the spread of rheumatoid arthritis.

Underlying factors for both of these conditions may include poor digestive function (intestinal permeability), hormone imbalance, nutritional deficiencies, food allergies, and lifestyle factors.

SYMPTOMS OF OSTEOARTHRITIS

Symptoms usually come on gradually, progressing as follows:

- Morning stiffness
- Painful, swollen joints
- Restricted range of motion
- Deformity of joints (in some cases)

SYMPTOMS OF RHEUMATOID ARTHRITIS

- Inflammation, pain, tenderness, and discoloration in the joints, usually the shoulders, the elbows, the wrists, the fingers, the ankles, or the toes
- Morning stiffness
- Lumps under the skin at the site of damaged joints
- Deformity of joints in long-term cases
- Fatigue, weight loss, weakness, and occasionally fever.
- Chronic infections

ROOT CAUSES OF OSTEOARTHRITIS

- Fractures or other injuries, even those that occurred early in life
- Food allergies
- A diet high in fats, animal products, and other foods that promote an internal acidic environment
- Excess of body fat, which places extra stress on joints
- Emotional stress
- Poor digestion heath (increased intestinal permeability, bacteria imbalance)
- Hormone imbalance
- Biomechanical imbalance (e.g., poor posture and abnormal foot arch)

ROOT CAUSES OF RHEUMATOID ARTHRITIS

No one is exactly sure what causes RA. It is likely multifactorial.

- Autoimmune malfunction (presence in the blood of the rheumatoid factor [RF], a set of antibodies in
- the blood that leads to an attack on the body's joint tissue)

Canadian researchers examined the association between synthetic hormone replacement and a new diagnosis of arthritis. It was discovered that women who use synthetic hormones for five years or longer were twice as likely as nonusers to develop osteoarthritis. A separate study examining synthetic estrogen replacement therapy and arthritis found a 96 percent increased risk among women who used it from four to ten years.

- Infection (mycoplasma, bacterial, or viral)
- Overgrowth of harmful bacteria in the gastrointestinal tract (dysbiosis)
- Food allergies
- Toxic metal accumulation
- Emotional stress

Testing Techniques

The following tests can give you an assessment of possible metabolic reasons for arthritis:

Hormone analysis by saliva, urine, or blood (estrogens, progesterone, DHEA, cortisol, IGF-1, thyroid panel).

Fasting insulin levels—blood

Food allergy/sensitivity testing (including screening for celiac disease or gluten intolerance)

Intestinal permeability—urine test

Stool analysis—bacteria balance, parasites, candida, food breakdown

Vitamin and mineral analysis—blood or urine

Toxic metal test—hair analysis or urine

TREATMENT

Diet

An effective diet will go a long way toward controlling arthritis for many people.

Recommended Food

Flaxseeds and cold-water fish are high in essential fatty acids and have anti-inflammatory properties. Salmon and mackerel are good examples.

Eat lots of fiber in the form of raw vegetables and whole grains. It will help sweep away mineral and acid build-up and keep your digestive system free of harmful bacteria. Cruciferous vegetables such as broccoli and cauliflower also have anti-inflammatory properties.

Foods high in sulfur will help repair cartilage and bone. Try eating some asparagus, cabbage, garlic, or onion every day.

To keep cartilage lubricated and healthy, drink a glass of clean water every two waking hours. Dehydration has been linked to arthritis pain.

Raw pineapple, whether whole or juiced, has an enzyme called bromelain, which has been shown to reduce inflammation.

Food to Avoid

Too much acid in the body causes inflammation, which leads to pain. Avoid acid-promoting foods such as red meat, eggs, saturated fats, oils, fried foods, sugar, dairy products, refined carbohydrates, foods high in gluten (such as breads, pasta, and pastries), alcohol, and caffeine. Although this list is long, allergy sufferers who eliminate these foods often experience great relief. Food allergy or sensitivity testing helps to narrow down the group of offending foods (see the Food Allergies chapter).

Animal products generally worsen inflammation in the joints. Avoid all eggs, dairy, and meat, with the exception of fish, which contains anti-inflammatory oils.

Use the list on page 252 to determine whether you have food allergies. Allergies cause inflammation, and for people with RA, they also do further damage to the immune system and may increase the intestinal tract's vulnerability to bacteria.

The nightshade vegetables—tomatoes, potatoes, eggplant, and peppers—contain a substance called solanine, which can trigger allergic responses and pain in some allergy sufferers. Eliminate these foods from your diet for a period of six weeks to see if there is improvement.

Detoxification

A vegetable juice or water fast is helpful to reduce joint pain. Work with a nutrition-oriented doctor.

Lemon and grapefruit juices are especially supportive of an arthritis fast.

Mix 1 teaspoon of apple cider vinegar and 1 teaspoon of honey into a glass of clean water, and drink it every day of your fast. This concoction will help alkalinize your body.

Green drinks are excellent for detoxification.

℞ Super Seven Prescriptions—Arthritis

Super Prescription #1 Glucosamine sulfate
Take 1,500 mg daily. Many formulas combine it with 600 to 1,200 mg of chondroitin sulfate, a related compound that also reduces joint pain and rebuilds cartilage. Benefits are usually noticed within four to eight weeks.
Note: Glucosamine and chondroitin sulfate are specific remedies only for osteoarthritis.

Super Prescription #2 Methylsulfonylmethane (MSM)
Take 2,000 to 8,000 mg daily. MSM has natural anti-inflammatory benefits and contains the mineral sulfur, an integral component of cartilage. Reduce the dosage if diarrhea occurs.

Super Prescription #3 Fish oil
Take a daily dosage of at least 1.8 mg of DHA and 1.2 mg of EPA. Fish oil contains a direct source of the omega-3 fatty acids that reduce joint inflammation and promote joint lubrication. This makes it a better choice than flaxseed oil, although flaxseeds are an option for vegetarians. Improvement may take up to twelve weeks of use.

Super Prescription #4 High-potency multivitamin
Take a formula that is rich in a blend of antioxidants, which will prevent joint tissue destruction. Take as directed on the container.

Super Prescription #5 Betaine HCL or bitter herb digestion formula
Take betaine HCL or a bitter herb digestion formula. These supplements increase stomach acid and improve digestion. Take as directed on the container with each meal.

Super Prescription #6 Bromelain
Take 500 mg three times daily between meals. Look for products standardized to 2,000 M.C.U. (milk-clotting units) per 1,000 mg or 1,200 G.D.U. (gelatin-dissolving units) per 1,000 mg. Bromelain has a natural anti-inflammatory effect. Protease enzyme products also have this benefit.

Many studies have confirmed the efficacy of glucosamine sulfate for relieving osteo-arthritis symptoms. A three-year, double-blind, placebo-controlled trial involving 212 people with knee osteoarthritis found that 1,500 mg of glucosamine sulfate taken daily significantly reduced symptoms. In addition, diagnostic images found that people supplementing glucosamine had no significant joint space loss, while those on placebo had joint deterioration.

> **Super Prescription #7   Cayenne** (*Capsicum annuum*) **cream**
> Apply the cream to the affected area two to four times daily for symptomatic relief. Choose a cream standardized to between 0.025 and 0.075 percent capsaicin. Capsaicin depletes the nerves of substance P, a neurotransmitter that transmits pain messages.

General Recommendations

Many excellent herbs reduce inflammation. Devil's claw root (*Harpagophytum procumbens*), alfalfa (*Medicago sativa*), and yucca root (*Yucca schidigera*) capsules are among the best. Give these herbs at least two months to take effect. Recommended dosages are as follows:

Devil's claw (*Harpagophytum procumbens*) should not be taken if you have a history of gallstones, heartburn, or ulcers. Take 1,500 to 2,500 mg of the standardized powdered herb in capsule or tablet form daily, or use 1 to 2 ml of a tincture three times a day.

White willow (*Salix alba*) products that are standardized to contain 240 mg of salicin daily or 5 ml of the tincture form should be taken three times daily.

Alfalfa (*Medicago sativa*) comes in the form of capsules or tablets made from dried alfalfa leaves. Take 500 to 1,000 mg daily, or take 1 to 2 ml of a tincture three times daily.

Yucca root (*Yucca schidigera*) in the capsule form is taken in 1,000-mg doses twice daily.

Ginger (*Zingiber officinale*) is a popular choice for relief of both inflammation and pain. Pour boiling water over the grated root and drink the tea, or try adding ginger fresh to your meals. If you want something stronger, take 1 to 2 grams of dried powder in a capsule two or three times daily, or use 1 to 2 ml of a tincture three times daily.

Boswellia (*Boswellia serrata*) is taken in doses of 1,200 to 1,500 mg of standardized extract, containing 60 to 65 percent boswellic acids, two to three times daily.

Plant sterols and sterolin is more specifically used for rheumatoid arthritis, to calm down an overactive immune system. Take as directed on the container, between meals, three times daily.

DHEA: If your levels are low, work with a holistic doctor and start with 10 to 25 mg daily.

SAMe (S-adenosylmethionine) is an excellent supplement to reduce the symptoms of osteoarthritis. Take 600 to 1,200 mg for two months and then 400 to 800 mg as a maintenance dosage.

Evening primrose oil, black currant, or borage oil contain the essential fatty acid GLA, which reduces joint inflammation. Take up to 2.8 grams of GLA daily.

Cetyl myristoleate (CMO) is shown in preliminary studies to be helpful for arthritis. Take 540 mg daily.

Vitamin E is preferably taken via a vitamin E-complex with additional tocotrienols. If you are on blood-thinning medication, use a lower amount under your doctor's supervision. Take 800 to 1,200 IU daily.

Vitamin C: Take 1,000 two to three times daily.

Boron: Take 1 mg per day.

Niacinamide: Take 500 mg four times daily.

Plant enzymes: Take as directed on the container to improve food absorption.

Chlorella or spirulina are super green foods high in antioxidants and aid detoxification. Take as directed on the container.

DMSO (dimethyl sulfoxide) is a topical substance used for pain relief. Work with a doctor to use this substance.

Protease enzymes reduce inflammation. Take 1 to 2 capsules twice daily between meals.

Homeopathy

Pick the remedy that best matches your symptoms. Take 2 pellets of 30C potency twice daily. Should five days pass without any sign of improvement, you're probably taking the wrong remedy. Stop using the current one, and switch to something else. After you first notice improvement, stop taking the remedy, unless symptoms begin to return.

Apis (*Apis mellifica*) is for joints that are swollen and hot and having stinging pain that feels better with cool applications. It is more commonly used with rheumatoid arthritis.

Arnica (*Arnica montana*) is for bruising pain, especially for osteoarthritis arising from injuries.

Belladonna (*Atropa belladonna*) works on joints that are hot, red, and burning and that feel worse with motion. Pain and swelling may come on suddenly.

Bryonia (*Bryonia alba*) is for stitching pains and swollen, hot joints that are worse with any movement. People who benefit from Bryonia tend to be irritable from the pain.

Calcarea Carbonica is for joint pains made worse from dampness and coldness. The person usually is overweight and chilly.

Calcarea Fluorica is for arthritis with enlarged joints or bone spurs, as well as for hypermobile joints.

Calcarea Phosphorica is for joint and bone pains that are made worse from cold and drafts of cold air. It's useful for arthritis that occurs from bone spurs, especially in the neck region.

Dulcamara is for arthritis that flares up from cold, damp weather.

Pulsatilla (*Pulsatilla pratensis*) is helpful if your pain wanders from joint to joint and if your symptoms improve in fresh, cool air or with cool applications.

Rhus Toxicodendron relieves arthritis that is worse in the cold and the damp or during long periods of inactivity. Stiffness is the main symptom, which improves with some movement and warmth.

Sulphur is for arthritis characterized by burning pains. Symptoms are better with cold applications.

Acupressure

Acupressure can be quite helpful in reducing or even eliminating arthritis pain. Because the suggested points may be very tender, be sure to press them firmly instead of massaging them. You may need to work the appropriate points two or three times a day for up to six months before you see complete results; afterward, reduce your practice to once daily. For more information about pressure points and administering treatment, see pages 668–675.

- To relieve arthritis in the hands, the wrists, the elbows, the shoulders, or the neck, use Large Intestine 4.
- Large Intestine 11 reduces pain and swelling in the elbow and the shoulder.
- For ankle pain, try Spleen 5 and Kidney 3.
- Stomach 36 supports the entire body, including the joints. In addition, it promotes the sense of well-being that arthritis sufferers sometimes lack.

Bodywork

Massage

A light drainage massage of the areas surrounding an arthritic joint will reduce the build-up of lymphatic fluid.

Stress and tension can trigger painful episodes, especially for sufferers of RA. Regular massage will relax the body and the mind. It will also loosen muscles that have tightened in reaction to pain.

Reflexology

See pages 686–687 for information about reflexology areas and how to work them.

Massage of the entire foot is best for relief of arthritis pain, with special attention to the region that corresponds to the painful area (i.e., shoulder, hands, or back).

Hydrotherapy

Soak in a hot bath with Epsom salts or mineral salts for at least twenty minutes. You'll eliminate toxins through sweat, and the salts will help replenish the body's mineral stores. Constitutional hydrotherapy is excellent (see the Hydrotherapy section for directions).

Aromatherapy

A number of different oils will reduce stress, so you should try several to see which ones work best for you. Some good choices are chamomile, jasmine, lavender, and rose.

To assist in cleansing the joints of mineral and acid deposits, use juniper or lemon balm in a hot bath.

Chamomile, lavender, and rosemary all have anti-inflammatory properties. Use them in a bath, or combine them with a base oil and apply gently to the painful area. Lavender is an especially good choice for people with rheumatic pain.

Black pepper, ginger, and eucalyptus all stimulate blood flow around the joints and are invigorating in a bath.

Stress Reduction

Many doctors and other experts have noted that emotional stress and an inability to accept criticism seem to appear frequently in arthritis sufferers. In addition, arthritis itself can cause great tension, both muscular and emotional, and even depression.

General Stress-Reduction Therapies

Yoga works wonders for some people, as may tai chi or Pilates. Take a class with a qualified instructor, preferably one who has experience with arthritic clients.

Thermal biofeedback has produced good results for many arthritis sufferers. It teaches you to open up your blood vessels and stimulates warmth and nourishment to your hands and joints.

Bach Flower Remedies

Consult the chart on pages 648–650 if the following suggestions do not apply to your particular needs. Once you have selected the right remedy, place 10 drops under your tongue. Hold them in place for thirty seconds and swallow. Use as often as needed.

If you are inflexible and critical of yourself and others, try Rock Water.

To relieve fatigue and exhaustion brought on by pain, use Hornbeam or Olive.

If you are sensitive to weather changes, use a combination of Aspen, Olive, Elm, and Holly.

Other Recommendations

- Vitamin D from sunshine is crucial to bone health. Don't let arthritis pain keep you from getting out in the early morning sun every day.
- Arthritis sufferers often cut back on activity, but studies show that moderate exercise actually reduces pain and swelling. While you must avoid joint-pounding workouts like jogging or tennis, low- or no-impact exercises like swimming, aqua-aerobics, cycling, and walking are excellent choices.

REFERENCES

Reginster, J. Y., et al. 2001. Long-term effects of glucosamine sulphate on osteoarthritis progression: A randomised, placebo-controlled clinical trial. *Lancet* 357:251–56.

Sahyoun, N. R., et al. 1999. Estrogen replacement therapy and incidence of self reported physician diagnosed arthritis. *Preventive Medicine* 28(5):458–64.

Wilkins, K. 1999. Hormone replacement therapy and incident arthritis. *Health Reports* 11(2):49–57.

Asthma

Asthma is a serious respiratory disease that literally leaves its victims breathless. People with asthma usually have a combination of problems in the lungs: bronchial muscle spasms, swelling of the mucus linings, and increased mucus production. When a susceptible person is exposed to a trigger, such as environmental irritants, allergens, heavy exertion, or even anxiety, the passages inflame further and block air from flowing freely, resulting in an asthma attack. In a severe attack, a person who doesn't receive emergency medical care can suffocate.

In America, the number of people with asthma has increased by one-third in the last decade, probably because of pollution, the effects of emotional stress, and a Western diet that's high in additives, meat products, and fats, all of which can cause inflammation and excess mucus production. Alarmingly, the incidence of asthma continues to rise among children. It is most common in children under the age of ten.

Diet, nutritional supplements, bodywork, and other therapies can go a long way toward preventing and relieving asthma, but if you suffer from this potentially life-threatening disease, you also need to be under the care of a good doctor.

SYMPTOMS

- Difficulty breathing
- Wheezing
- Coughing
- Tightness in the chest
- Loss of sleep due to coughing and blocked airways
- Increased heart rate
- Constriction of the muscles in the bronchial airways
- Inflammation of the mucus linings
- Increased mucus flow

ROOT CAUSES

Triggers that bring on an attack vary from person to person but most often include

- Allergies, either environmental or food
- Pollution and irritants
- Infections (colds, flu, or other respiratory infections)

- Cold air
- Heavy physical exertion
- Poor digestive function
- Hormone imbalance
- Emotional stress

Important: If you experience a severe asthma attack, *get emergency help at once.* Have someone call an ambulance or drive you to the hospital, where you will receive medication to open your air passages.

TREATMENT

Diet

While it may take some discipline, following an antiasthma diet will reduce inflammation and the clogging of air passages. If you have trouble getting started, try the detoxifying fast recommended further on. It will help break your addiction to unwholesome food and will allow you to "hear" clearly what your body needs.

Note: Check with a pediatrician or a holistic doctor before eliminating any food group from a child's diet.

Recommended Food

Eat a simple, light diet, based on foods that don't promote mucus production: raw vegetables and fruits, seeds, whole grains, lean poultry, and fresh fish.

Carotenoids are antioxidants that have natural antioxidant and anti-inflammatory benefits. They are found in dark-green leafy vegetables and deep-yellow and orange vegetables.

Studies show that children who eat fish more than once a week have one-third the risk of developing asthma.

Garlic and onions have anti-inflammatory properties and are a savory addition to vegetable dishes.

A glass of clean water every two waking hours will help keep your system clean. Water is especially helpful after an asthma attack to break up mucus.

Ground flaxseeds are an excellent source of anti-inflammatory omega-3 fatty acids. For children over five years of age, use 1 to 2 teaspoons, and for adults, the dosage is 1 to 2 tablespoons daily.

Food to Avoid

It is most important to discover whether certain foods provoke allergic reactions. See the Food Allergies entry, especially the elimination diet on page 253.

Even if you don't have an allergy to dairy products, eliminate them from your diet. They encourage the production of mucus that plugs your airways. For the same reason, stay away from sugar, junk food, and fried and refined foods.

Do not eat foods that contain additives or preservatives. This means avoiding processed foods, dried or smoked foods, and salad bars, which are often sprayed with preservatives, such as tartrazine (yellow dye number 5), red dye, sulfites (as found in dried fruits), benzoates, and monosodium glutamate (MSG).

Never eat frozen or extremely cold foods, which can cause the muscles in your airways to tighten.

Keep pressure off your diaphragm by eating small meals and by avoiding foods that cause gas, such as beans and cruciferous vegetables (broccoli, cauliflower, and brussels sprouts are the most common offenders).

Detoxification

Every three months, consider doing a three-day vegetable cleansing juice fast to expel mucus. Also, daily consumption of super green foods, such as chlorella and/or spirulina, is recommended.

Testing Techniques

The following tests can give you an assessment of possible metabolic reasons for your asthma:

Food allergy/sensitivity testing—blood, electrodermal testing (see Food Allergies for more details)

Vitamin and mineral analysis—blood

Candida and flora balance—stool analysis

Toxic metals—hair or urine analysis

Intestinal permeability—urine

Stress hormones DHEA and cortisol—saliva or urine

℞ Super Seven Prescriptions—Asthma

Super Prescription #1   Homeopathy
Read the description under Homeopathy in this section, and pick the single remedy that best matches your symptoms. If possible, work with a practitioner who is well trained in homeopathy.

Super Prescription #2   Essential fatty acids
Take 1 to 2 tablespoons of flaxseed oil or 4 to 8 grams of fish oil daily. Essential fatty acid formulations that contain flaxseed oil, fish oil, or a mixture of omega-3, 6, and 9 fatty acids are helpful for preventing asthma. Take as directed on the container. It may take four to eight weeks for you to notice an improvement.

Super Prescription #3   Magnesium
Take 250 mg two to four times daily. Reduce the dosage if loose stools occur. Magnesium relaxes the bronchial tubes and improves lung function. Nutrition-oriented doctors may also use magnesium intravenously for acute asthma.

Super Prescription #4   Vitamin C
Take 1,000 mg two to four times daily. Reduce the dosage if loose stools occur. Vitamin C lessens spasms of the bronchial passages and has antiallergy benefits. Use a nonacidic product, such as calcium ascorbate.

Super Prescription #5   Astragalus (*Astragalus membranaceus*)
Take 500 to 1,000 mg twice daily. Astragalus is used to strengthen the lungs and to prevent respiratory infections that can trigger asthma. Do not use if you have a fever.

> **Super Prescription #6   Antioxidant formula**
> Take as directed on the container. Antioxidants decrease inflammatory responses of the airways.
>
> **Super Prescription #7   Enzymes**
> Take a full-spectrum enzyme product with each meal to improve the absorption of nutrients and decrease reactions to foods.

General Recommendations

Vitamin B12 reduces the reaction to sulfites that causes asthma symptoms in some people, especially in children. Take 1,500 mcg orally or 400 mcg sublingually. The injectable form is also used by nutrition-oriented doctors.

Vitamin B6 has been found to be low in people who have asthma. In addition, asthma medications may lower B6 levels in the body. Take 100 to 200 mg daily.

N-acetylcysteine is a good antioxidant that also liquefies mucus in the bronchial tubes and the sinuses. Take 500 mg two to three times daily.

Lycopene is an antioxidant that has been shown to reduce exercise-induced asthma. Take 30 mg daily of a natural Lycopene complex.

Betaine HCL is helpful for some people with asthma. This supplement increases stomach acid levels, which tend to be low in people with asthma. Take as directed on the container, with meals, or as directed by a doctor.

Ginkgo biloba has anti-inflammatory and antioxidant benefits for the lungs. A study using ginkgo extract found that it decreased asthma symptoms. Take 120 to 240 mg daily of an extract containing 24 percent flavone glycosides.

Quercitin is useful for its anti-inflammatory and anti-allergy benefits. Take 1,000 mg three times daily.

Mullein (*Verbascum thapsus*), licorice, and marshmallow (*Althea officinalis*) root have historically been used in the herbal treatment of asthma. Choose formulas that contain a combination of these herbs, and use as directed on the container.

Cordyceps is a medicinal mushroom used in Chinese medicine to reduce bronchial secretions, improve lung function, and energize the body. Take 800 mg twice daily of a standardized product.

Adrenal-support formulas are helpful in the prevention of asthma. They include herbs such as *Panax ginseng,* American ginseng, adrenal glandular, and pantothenic acid (vitamin B5). Take as directed by a nutrition-oriented doctor.

Homeopathy

Many homeopathic remedies exist for asthma. The following suggestions are for use until you can consult with a qualified homeopath to find the remedy appropriate for your constitution. During an asthma attack, take 30C every ten or fifteen minutes until the symptoms subside. Long-term use of the proper homeopathic remedy can reduce your susceptibility to asthmatic attacks.

Aconitum Napellus is for attacks that start suddenly, especially after exposure to cold air, and that cause a great deal of fear or anxiety.

Arsenicum Album is for people with asthma who feel anxious, restless, and worse in the cold air and between midnight and 2 A.M. They feel better sitting up and when sipping warm drinks. This remedy is used for chronic and acute asthma.

Carbo Vegetabilis is for people who feel chilly and faint, yet better when being fanned or near a window. They may have a sensation of fullness in the upper abdomen

A double-blind trial found that more than half of people with exercise-induced asthma had significantly fewer asthma symptoms after taking 30 mg of lycopene per day for one week, compared to when they took a placebo.

and the chest and may feel relief from burping. They feel worse from talking, eating, or lying down.

Ipecacuanha is helpful when a lot of mucus formation causes coughing, gagging, and vomiting.

Kali Carbonicum is for asthma that is worse between 2 A.M. to 4 A.M. The person is usually chilly. Sitting up and leaning forward help to relieve symptoms.

Lachesis is for a feeling of constriction in the throat and the chest. Symptoms are better with fresh air. The person cannot stand any touching or pressure on the throat or the chest and tends to feel warm.

Medorrhinum is for chronic asthma, where the person is prone to reoccurring respiratory tract infections, is usually very warm, and craves citrus fruit, especially oranges.

Natrum Sulphuricum is for asthma that comes on or is worse in cold, damp weather. Symptoms are often worse from 4 A.M. to 5 A.M.

Nux Vomica (*Strychnos nux vomica*) is for a constricted feeling in the chest and fullness in the stomach or stomach upset. Asthma symptoms are often worse upon awakening in the morning. Overindulging in food, especially alcohol, spicy foods, or sweets, can bring on symptoms. The person feels chilly and irritable.

Pulsatilla (*Pulsatilla pratensis*) is for asthma symptoms that are worse in the evening; in hot, stuffy rooms; or after eating fatty foods. The person often coughs up yellowish mucus, which may also cause gagging. The person desires fresh air and to be comforted by someone.

Acupressure

Acupressure is highly effective at increasing lung capacity and relaxing the muscles of the airways. Massage these points daily for best results. For more information about pressure points and administering treatment, see pages 668–675.

- Lung 1, 7, and 9 relieve congestion and coughing due to asthma.
- Conception Vessel 17 relieves tension in the chest.

Bodywork

Massage

A back massage will relax your bronchial muscles. A professional treatment is always nice, but you can ask a loved one to rub your back, if you like. And children enjoy receiving back massages from their parents, especially just before they go to bed.

To break up congestion, get a cupping massage on your back or chest.

Any kind of massage, especially with a calming essential oil, will dispel stress and anxiety.

Other Bodywork Recommendations

Osteopathic, acupuncture, and chiropractic treatments are useful for long-term treatment. Craniosacral therapy should also be highly considered, especially for children.

Reflexology

See pages 686–687 for information about reflexology areas and how to work them.

Massage the points that correspond to the lungs, the diaphragm, and the adrenal glands.

Hydrotherapy

Hot baths and saunas are relaxing ways to sweat out toxins and mucus. Do not take a sauna if you have hypertensive cardiovascular disease.

Aromatherapy

Test separate oils for an allergic response before using any in a combination.

- Many oils open airways and loosen congestion. Try eucalyptus, lavender, tea tree, or a combination of these in a steam inhalation or a bath.
- Frankincense encourages deep, relaxed breathing. Do not use frankincense in a steam, as it can inflame the mucus membranes.
- Mix lavender oil in a base, and rub it directly on your chest to ease breathing and loosen congestion.

Stress Reduction

Anxiety can trigger an asthma attack, so keeping stress levels down is not a luxury, it is a necessity. Children in particular often feel helpless and fearful as a result of asthma; teaching them to manage stress can help them live normal lives that are not dictated by their disease.

General Stress-Reduction Therapies

Yoga and deep breathing will help train asthma sufferers to take deep, regular, and calm breaths.

EEG biofeedback can teach you to control your brainwaves, and children, who love working with computers and machinery, respond especially well to this therapy.

Bach Flower Remedies

Consult the chart on pages 648–650 to find the right flower remedy for your particular condition. Once you've found the right remedy, place 10 drops of it under your tongue. Hold them in place for thirty seconds and swallow. Use as often as needed.

Take Rescue Remedy if you feel a crisis coming on. It is in no way, however, adequate treatment for a full-blown asthma attack.

Other Recommendations

- Mild to moderate exercise will increase your ability to take in oxygen, so get in a daily walk or other activity. Cold air can trigger an attack, though, so either wear a mask over your face and mouth during the cold months or exercise indoors.
- Perform deep breathing exercises every day.
- Use a HEPA (high energy particulate air) filter to clean the air in your room and home.
- Have the air vents in your house professionally cleaned each year.
- Wash all bedding in hot water one to two times weekly to remove dust and dust mites, which can trigger asthma. Use allergy-proof coverings for the bed mattress, the pillow covers, and the box spring.
- Vacuum twice weekly with a HEPA filter vacuum. Consider removing carpets and rugs, especially in the bedroom, and replace with nontoxic wooden or laminate flooring.
- Avoid all sources of smoke.

REFERENCES

Guinot, P., C. Brambilla, J. Dunchier, et al. 1987. Effect of BN 52063, a specific PAF-ascether antagonist, on bronchial provocation test to allergens in asthmatic patients—a preliminary study. *Prostaglandins* 34:723–31.

Neuman, I., H. Nahum, and A. Ben-Amotz. 2000. Reduction of exercise-induced asthma oxidative stress by lycopene, a natural antioxidant. *Allergy* 55:1184–89.

Athlete's Foot

Athlete's foot, also known as tinea pedis, is a persistent and annoying fungal infection of the foot. It commonly occurs between the toes and the toenails but can also occur on other areas of the foot. The skin between the toes can appear red, cracked, and scaly. Sores and blisters can form on the soles of the feet and between the toes. The infected areas may burn or itch.

Moisture and warmth provide an environment for this fungus to thrive. Public or private showers, locker rooms, gym floors, and hotel bathrooms are common places for a child to contract this fungus. People with sweaty feet are more susceptible to getting athlete's foot. Some have a natural resistance to athlete's foot, while others must be more careful with hygiene. Changing into clean socks reduces the risk of reinfection.

We find that in many cases of chronic athlete's foot, there is an underlying systemic problem with candidiasis. For more effective therapy in these cases, it is important to have a systemic treatment to eradicate the fungus. See the Candidiasis section for detailed information.

Most cases of athlete's foot can be treated at home. However, complications can arise when a bacterial infection sets in, along with the existing fungal infection. If your athlete's foot does not improve with natural treatment or gets worse, see a doctor for evaluation.

SYMPTOMS

- Burning, itching, and cracking between the toes and on other places of the foot
- Patches of dry skin
- Yellowish-brown toenails

ROOT CAUSES

- Prolonged or frequent use of antibiotics or corticosteroids, leading to a depletion of good bacteria that normally keep fungus in check
- Poor digestion and elimination
- Depressed immune system (e.g., diabetes)
- A high-sugar diet
- Poor hygiene (feet in a damp environment)

Testing Techniques

The following tests help assess possible metabolic reasons for candidiasis:

Candida levels—stool, blood (antibodies), or urine (yeast metabolites)

Intestinal permeability—urine test

TREATMENT

Diet

Recommended Food

For high-density nutrition and immune support, base your meals around fresh vegetables, whole grains, and quality sources of lean protein, such as beans, lentils, fish, and organic poultry.

For severe toenail fungal infections, you can try the following home therapy. Make sure the nails are trimmed as short as possible. Please note that this therapy cannot be used if you have cuts or openings in the skin.

1. In a bucket, dilute 1 cup of bleach in 10 cups of water.

2. Dip the affected foot in the bucket for five seconds. Remove and towel dry.

3. Repeat this procedure every other day for four weeks. Make a new mixture each time.

You should notice that the skin dries out and flakes off. This is normal. You can apply tea tree (*Melaleuca alternifolia*) oil and calendula (*Calendula officinalis*) between treatments for better results.

To replace friendly bacteria, eat unsweetened yogurt daily. Make sure the brand you're using has live yogurt cultures. Sauerkraut and miso are other examples of foods that contain friendly bacteria.

Vegetable and green drinks will improve your resistance.

Drink 8 glasses of pure water a day to help flush out yeast toxins.

Consume 1 to 2 tablespoons of ground flaxseeds daily. Flaxseeds have antifungal properties.

Food to Avoid

Fungus feeds on sugar and yeast, so reduce or eliminate obvious sugars in the diet, such as refined foods, which are likely to be loaded with sugars.

Avoid or reduce the use of fruits and fruit juices during the initial phase (first month) of treatment. It is especially important to avoid these foods between meals.

Detoxification

Consume foods such as garlic, onions, chlorella, spirulina, wheatgrass, and others known to support detoxification.

℞ Super Seven Prescriptions—Athlete's Foot

Super Prescription #1   Tea tree (*Melaleuca alternifolia*) oil
Apply tea tree oil liquid directly to the fungal infection. For toenail fungus, trim the nails, wash the feet with soap (tea tree oil soap is a good choice), and apply as far under the nail as possible. Repeat daily for six to eight weeks or until the infection is cleared.

Super Prescription #2   Oregano oil (*Origanum vulgare*)
Take a 500 mg capsule or the liquid form (as directed on the container) orally, three times daily with meals. The tincture variety can also be applied topically. Oregano oil (*Origanum vulgare*) has a powerful antifungal effect, internally and externally.

Super Prescription #3   Garlic (*Allium sativum*)
Take 500 to 1,000 mg of garlic twice daily. Garlic fights fungal infections and also boosts immune strength.

Super Prescription #4   Grapefruit seed extract
Take 200 mg two to three times daily. Practitioners rely on this herb for its antifungal properties.

Super Prescription #5   Caprylic acid
Take 1,000 mg three times daily. This type of fatty acid has been shown in studies to have antifungal properties.

Super Prescription #6   Echinacea (*Echinacea purpurea*) and **goldenseal** (*Hydrastis canadensis*)
Take 500 mg or 2 to 4 ml of tincture three times daily. Both herbs enhance immune function. Echinacea has been shown to have antifungal effects.

Super Prescription #7   Probiotic
Take a product containing 4 billion active organisms, twice daily, thirty minutes after a meal. It supplies friendly bacteria such as *Lactobacillus acidophilus* and *bifidus,* which fight fungus and prevent its overgrowth.

General Recommendations

Calendula (*Calendula officinalis*) tincture or gel can be applied to the affected area in-between treatments of tea tree (*Melaleuca alternifolia*) oil. This herb has an antiseptic effect and promotes skin healing.

Thuja (*Thuja occidentalis*) oil has potent antifungal effects. Apply 2 drops to the affected area twice daily.

Pau d'arco (*Tabebuia avellanedae*) has strong antibacterial and antifungal properties. Drink several cups every day.

Wormwood (*Artemisia absinthium*), Oregon grape (*Berberis aquifolium*), and rosemary (*Rosmarinus officinalis*) all have antifungal properties. Take as part of a candida formula.

A high-potency multivitamin provides the many nutrients needed to support immune function. Take as directed on the container.

Vitamin C is used to enhance immune function. Take 1,000 mg two to three times daily.

One double-blind study reported in the *Australian Journal of Dermatology* looked at the effect of tea tree oil on people with a diagnosis of athlete's foot (tinea pedis). Patients applied the solution twice daily to affected areas for 4 weeks and were reviewed after 2 and 4 weeks of treatment. Fungal cure was assessed by a culture of the skin and was found to be 64 percent in those applying a 50 percent tea tree oil, compared to 31 percent in the placebo group.

Homeopathy

Pick the remedy that best matches your symptoms in this section. Take a 6x, 12x, 6C, 12C, or 30C potency twice daily for two weeks to see if there are any positive improvements. After you notice improvement, stop taking the remedy, unless symptoms return. Consultation with a homeopathic practitioner is advised.

Graphites is helpful when there is cracked skin that oozes a thick, yellow fluid.

Silica (*Silicea*) is a good choice when there is profuse foot sweating and an offensive smell that excoriates feet.

Sulphur is the best choice for chronic athlete's foot when there is intense itching and burning of feet.

Thuja (*Thuja occidentalis*) is used when you have long-standing fungal infections of the skin that do not respond to other remedies.

Other Recommendations

- Expose your feet to the open air. Wear sandals or porous slippers around the home or outside (if the climate permits).

- Use cotton socks. If your feet perspire a lot, change socks twice daily.
- Wear waterproof slippers or sandals in locker rooms and showers.
- Make sure your feet are washed with soap daily.

REFERENCES

Satchell, A. C., A. Saurajen, C. Bell, and R. S. Barnetson. 2002. Treatment of inter-digital tinea pedis with 25% and 50% tea tree oil solution: A randomized, placebo-controlled, blinded study. *Australian Journal of Dermatology* 43(3):175–78.

Attention Deficit Hyperactivity Disorder

Attention deficit hyperactivity disorder (ADHD) is defined as age-inappropriate impulsiveness, lack of concentration, and sometimes-excessive physical activity. This condition is associated with learning difficulties and a lack of social skills. Because there is no laboratory or physical test that diagnoses ADHD, its diagnosis is based on a clinical history of symptoms and behavior. Since it is a subjective diagnosis, it brings up controversy as to whether the behavior is actually normal in many cases, especially for younger boys. There are three subtypes of ADHD, one of which mainly involves an attention problem and not a hyperactivity issue. Between 30 and 40 percent of children with ADHD have learning disabilities, although in many cases these children are quite bright. ADHD often goes undiagnosed, if not caught at an early age, and it affects many adults who may not be aware of their condition.

Many parents instinctively believe that the problem is connected to their children's diet. They know that children can respond negatively to sugar or other foods, and they wonder if their child is simply suffering from an extreme version of this reaction. In most cases, these parents are absolutely correct. In the last few decades, sugars, preservatives, and colorings have been added to our food at an increasing rate. Too many children consume nothing but convenience foods, like hot dogs, fried chicken fingers, and highly sweetened fruit drinks and sodas. Since children's small bodies are especially vulnerable to additives in these foods, it is not surprising that many of them have a toxic response. For some, the response takes the form of traditional allergies—say, a runny nose or hives. For others, however, the poisons surface as extreme behavior problems.

Unfortunately, Western doctors have been trained to discount the importance of diet in hyperactive kids. Instead of nutritional therapy, they will often suggest medication to suppress the symptoms of ADHD: it is estimated that more than two million children take drugs like Ritalin on a daily basis. While medications may be necessary in a few cases, parents should cultivate a healthy wariness of giving them to their children. The long-term effects of ADHD medications are not yet well known, and there are signs that the drugs can retard growth and lead to substance abuse or emotional problems later in life. Teens who take Ritalin may be tempted to mix it with alcohol, marijuana, or other recreational drugs, creating a dangerous brew with unknown consequences. And as with many conventional prescription drugs, the most compelling argument against ADHD drugs is that they fail to address the cause of the problem. Without the underlying cause being treated, children may have to take Ritalin well into their twenties.

There are many underlying reasons why a child may have attention or behavior problems. Studies show that frequent ear infections and the regular use of antibiotics, as well as premature birth and family history, are associated with a greater likelihood of developing this disorder. Holistically speaking, causative factors include food additives and food allergies, environmental allergens, and heavy metal toxicity (such as lead, mercury, and aluminum). A poorly functioning digestive system and increased intestinal permeability lead to an increase in metabolic toxins that disrupt brain chemistry. Nutritional deficiencies of essential fatty acids, B vitamins, magnesium and other minerals, and iron appear to play a role. Finally, do not underestimate the role of emotional stress and its relationship to ADHD. The breakdown of the family unit in our culture places abnormal stresses on a child, which can result in attention and behavior changes.

If your child has ADHD, try the home-care suggestions here for at least a month and optimally for three months. Some children settle down to a normal level of activity after just a few days without troublesome foods; others will need three or four weeks before the toxins are out of their bodies. Buying and preparing natural foods can be a challenge for busy parents, but your perseverance will be rewarded with a healthier child and a stronger family. Nutritional supplements can work extremely well for most children to correct underlying biochemical imbalances.

SYMPTOMS

- Inability to sit still
- Mood swings
- Restlessness
- Short attention span
- Inability to concentrate
- Frequent tantrums
- Poor coordination and motor skills
- Impaired memory
- Failure to complete age-appropriate tasks
- Impulsiveness
- Speech or learning disorders

ROOT CAUSES

- A diet that's high in sugar and additives
- Food allergies/sensitivities
- Hypoglycemia
- Nutritional deficiencies
- Poor digestion and absorption
- Heavy metal poisoning
- Emotional stresses

Testing Techniques

The following tests can give you an assessment of possible metabolic reasons for ADHD:

Food allergy/sensitivity testing—blood, electrodermal testing (see the Food Allergies section for more details)

Vitamin and mineral analysis—blood

Candida and flora balance—stool analysis

Toxic metals—hair or urine analysis

Intestinal permeability—urine

Blood-sugar levels—fasting blood test

Essential fatty-acid levels—fasting blood test

Amino acid levels—urine or fasting blood test

TREATMENT

Diet

Nutritional therapy should be an important component of the treatment of ADHD. The strategies described here will improve behavior and promote age-appropriate concentration and stability, and they will also help keep your child free of many other diet-related disorders. The same general recommendations hold true for adults with this condition.

Recommended Food

The best way to ensure that your child eats an additive-free diet is to buy only fresh foods and prepare them yourself. You don't need to prepare special meals for your child; instead, feed your entire family a whole-foods diet. Younger children will usually eat what everyone else is eating, especially if you can reserve a small portion for them before you season the meal to the taste of adult palates.

B vitamins are healing to stressed-out nerves. Good sources include brown rice, brewer's yeast (which you can add to smoothies and yogurt), and leafy green vegetables.

Many children with ADHD suffer from an excess of copper or lead. Food that's high in vitamin C will encourage the release of these toxins from the body, so feed your child citrus fruits for dessert.

Iron deficiency is linked to short attention spans and memory problems. If a blood test finds an iron deficiency, a daily tablespoon of unsulfured blackstrap molasses is a naturally sweet way to give your child an adequate amount of this mineral.

Tryptophan encourages the production of serotonin, a chemical that produces a sense of calm. Incorporate soy products, live unsweetened yogurt, whole grains, and organic turkey and chicken into meals and snacks. If your child has trouble sleeping, be sure to include some of these foods at dinner, and try a snack of turkey or chicken on whole-grain crackers before bedtime.

Healthful Bean Dip

Let your kids dip to their hearts' content.

Ingredients

Black beans, cooked

Juice of 1 lime

1 teaspoon cumin

¼ cup fresh cilantro leaves

½ clove of minced garlic (optional)

Combine the previous ingredients (leave out the garlic, if you like) in a food processor, and whirl until the consistency is smooth. For a fancy presentation and added nutrition, garnish with chopped tomato.

Anyone with food sensitivities should drink lots of clean water. Children over ten years of age should have a glass every two waking hours; children ten and under should drink half this amount.

Make sure to keep blood-sugar levels balanced by avoiding simple sugars and refined carbohydrates and providing adequate protein with meals (nuts, legumes, lean poultry, and fish). Also, as much as possible include vegetables with meals, as they slow down blood sugar release. Eating smaller, more frequent meals and snacks (every two to three hours) works well. Make sure that breakfast is not skipped, as it sets the biochemical balance for the rest of the day.

Regularly serve brain-healthy foods that are rich in essential fatty acids. Examples include fish (trout, salmon, halibut), nuts (walnuts, almonds), and ground flaxseeds (1 to 2 teaspoons for children and 1 to 2 tablespoons for adults).

Food to Avoid

If your child suffers from ADHD, it's likely that he or she is allergic to at least one food product, if not several. Read the Food Allergies section in this book, and follow the elimination diet and testing techniques to determine which foods may be causing behavior problems. You may already suspect that a certain food is a trigger for your child, and you should target that product right away. You should also closely examine your child's consumption of the following, all of which are common allergens: wheat, dairy, corn, chocolate, peanuts, citrus, soy, food coloring, and preservatives.

- Do not feed your child anything with artificial colors, flavors, or preservatives. This means you'll have to eliminate fast food, as well as all junk and processed food. If you must buy canned or frozen products, read the labels carefully. Even items advertised as "all natural" may contain small amounts of additives.
- Sugar is famous for making children hyper, and, in fact, excess sucrose often leads to hypoglycemia, a factor in ADHD. Obviously, candy, sodas, and sweets are out of the question, but so are most store-bought fruit juices, which usually contain added sugar, and products made with white flour. If your child has been eating large quantities of refined sugar, you may see a dramatic difference in his or her behavior within just a few days of eliminating it.

Detoxification

Teenagers may want to try a short juice fast to cleanse their bodies of toxins and prepare themselves for their new diets. Don't force a teen to fast, however, as you may set the stage for a future eating disorder. Never put a child on a fasting program.

For preadolescent children and teens who don't want to go without solid food, try to increase the amount of raw fruits and vegetables in the diet, so that your child is eating 50 to 75 percent raw foods for several days. This will help move toxins through the body at an accelerated rate. Kids who usually balk at vegetable dishes are often happy to eat a platter of raw crudités served with yogurt or a homemade bean dip.

℞ Super Seven Prescriptions—ADHD

Super Prescription #1   Essential fatty acids
Take a product that contains a daily dosage of 500 to 1,000 mg of DHA. Also, take 100 mg of GLA, which is found in evening primrose oil, black currant, or borage oil. Products are available that have a combination of these essential fatty acids.

Super Prescription #2   Homeopathy
Pick the remedy that best matches your symptoms. Take a 6x, 12x, 6C, or 30C potency twice daily for two weeks to see if there are any positive improvements. After you notice improvement, stop taking the remedy, unless symptoms return. Consultation with a homeopathic practitioner is advised.

Super Prescription #3   Phosphatidylserine
Take 300 to 500 mg daily for three months. A maintenance dosage of 100 to 300 mg may be effective for some kids and adults. Phosphatidylserine is a naturally occurring substance found in high concentrations in brain cells; it helps brain cells function properly.

Super Prescription #4   Calcium and magnesium complex
Take a combination of these two minerals, at a dosage of 500 mg of calcium and 250 mg of magnesium twice daily. These two minerals relax the nervous system.

Super Prescription #5   Probiotic
Take a probiotic to maintain good bacteria levels in the digestive tract. Take as directed on the container.

A study involving 21 cases of youths ages 4 to 19 with ADHD found that daily supplementation of phosphatidylserine at dosages between 200 and 300 mg daily for 4 months benefited greater than 90 percent of cases. Attention and learning were the symptoms most improved.

Super Prescription #6   Vitamin B6

Give 100 mg daily for children five years or older. B6 is involved in the formation of serotonin, a neurotransmitter that has a calming effect. High doses of this vitamin are best used under the guidance of a nutrition-oriented doctor, along with a B-complex for balance.

Super Prescription #7   High-potency multivitamin

Take as directed on the container. It provides a base of nutrients required for brain function.

REFERENCES

Schoenthaler, S. J., I. D. Bier, K. Young, D. Nichols, and S. Jansenns. 2000. The effect of vitamin-mineral supplementation on the intelligence of American schoolchildren: A randomized, double-blind placebo-controlled trial. *Journal of Alternative and Complementary Medicine* 6(1):19–29.

General Recommendations

Western Herbal

Ginkgo biloba brings oxygen and nutrients to the brain. Look for a product standardized to 24 percent flavone glycosides. People who are 16 and older should take 60 to 120 mg twice a day. Give 30 to 60 mg twice a day to children ages 10 through 15. Those under 10 should be given 15 to 30 mg twice daily.

GABA is an amino acid that has a calming effect on the mind. Give 250 mg two to three times daily between meals.

Zinc deficiency can contribute to ADHD symptoms. Children ages 2 and older should get a daily total of 10 to 15 mg, along with 2 mg of copper.

B-complex vitamins supply all the B vitamins involved with brain function. Give a 50 mg B-complex daily.

Passionflower (*Passiflora incarnata*) can be effective in calming children with ADHD. Those 16 years of age and older should take 100 to 200 mg twice a day. Children ages 10 through 15 should take 50 to 100 mg twice daily. Children under 10 should be given 25 to 50 mg twice daily.

If your child is depressed, Saint-John's-wort (*Hypericum perforatum*) may help. Children ages 10 through 15 should take 50 to 150 mg twice a day. Children under 10 should take 25 to 75 mg twice a day. Adolescents and young adults who are 16 and older can take 100 to 300 mg twice a day.

Homeopathy

Pick the remedy that best matches your symptoms. Take a 6x, 12x, 6C, or 30C potency twice daily for two weeks to see if there are any positive results. After you notice improvement, stop taking the remedy, unless symptoms return. Consultation with a homeopathic practitioner is advised.

Anacardium Orientale is for children who tend to be cruel to animals and people. There is low self-esteem, and they are antisocial and absentminded. They often curse and swear.

Hyoscyamus Niger is for children who are very impulsive and violent, especially toward younger siblings. They are very talkative and sexually precocious.

Medorrhinum is for children who have major temper tantrums and are violent toward other kids. They have a hard time concentrating, are very warm, and crave oranges and ice.

Stramonium is for children who have many fears, such as of the dark or of animals. They have fits of anger and rage and destroy things. Night terrors are common.

Sulphur is for children who are curious, stubborn, and hyperactive. They are very warm, sweat easily, have a great thirst for cold drinks, and crave spicy foods.

Tarentula Hispanica is for children who are extremely hurried and restless. They are mischievous, destructive, and impulsive. They love music and dancing.

Tuberculinum is for children who are very stubborn, demanding, and impatient and get bored easily. They often have violent tempers and may hit other people and animals. They crave milk and smoked meats and are prone to respiratory infections.

Acupressure

Even young children can be taught acupressure techniques to practice when they feel upset. In fact, by teaching them to identify disquieting emotions and to take time out for a calming acupressure session, you'll give them a valuable life skill. For information about pressure points and administering treatment, see pages 668–675.

- Lung 1 releases tension and helps restore normal, deep breathing.
- If your child's hyperactivity seems to be triggered by frustration, teach him or her to press Conception Vessel 12 while slowly repeating the point's descriptive name, Center of Power.

Bodywork

Massage

Young children—if you can persuade them to remain still long enough—enjoy soothing massages from their parents. Teenagers may prefer to have an appointment with a massage therapist; you can also show them the self-care techniques listed in the Bodywork chapter of this book.

Reflexology

See pages 686–687 for information about reflexology areas and how to work them.

Work the areas corresponding to the diaphragm and the solar plexus to encourage a sense of peace and stillness.

Other Bodywork Recommendations

Craniosacral therapy by a qualified practitioner is highly recommended to balance out the nervous system for people with ADHD.

Aromatherapy

Aromatherapy makes a relaxing complement to the other treatments suggested here. Use chamomile, lavender, or sandalwood to encourage serenity; try them in a bath or a massage, or add a few drops to diffuser and let the pleasing scent waft through an entire room. These applications are especially helpful just before bedtime.

Stress Reduction

General Stress-Reduction Therapies

Although biofeedback may seem like the stress-reduction technique that's least likely to work for children, it is actually highly effective for kids with ADHD, many of whom enjoy the interaction with machines and computers. Of all the biofeedback techniques, EEG seems to work best for hyperactivity.

Consider signing up for a parent-and-child yoga class. Children usually have fun making the animal poses, and you'll both enjoy the lifelong health benefits of this ancient discipline.

Bach Flower Remedies

Select the appropriate remedy and place 5 drops of the liquid under your child's tongue. For children over fifteen, you can use 10 drops. Hold the drops in place for thirty seconds and swallow. Use as often as needed.

Rescue Remedy will help soothe a child in an emotional crisis.

Impatiens is for children who move, talk, and think quickly and who are angered by people who don't keep up with them.

Children who are plagued by recurring destructive impulses should take Cherry Plum.

Crab Apple will help children who are ashamed of their hyperactive behavior.

Other Recommendations

- Encourage your child to play or exercise outside in the fresh air. Limit exposure to sedentary, passive activities, like watching television or playing video games.
- Consider buying an air filter to purify your household of environmental allergens.
- Work with a counselor to help your child with behavior modification and learning styles. Every child is different and requires an individualized approach. Emotional counseling may be necessary for healing, especially in cases of broken families or abuse.

REFERENCES

Kidd, P. 2000. Attention deficit/hyperactivity disorder (ADHD) in children: Rationale for its integrative management. *Alternative Medicine Review* 5(5):402–28.

Back Pain

If you're an American, you have an 80 percent chance of experiencing back pain at some point in your adult life. Back pain is one of the most common reasons for emergency room visits; in fact, it is the fourth most common ailment in our country.

A few years ago, it was generally believed that back pain was caused by the degeneration of one or more discs, the "shock absorbers" of the spine. This results in an impingement and possible damage to the nerves that exit the spinal column. Today we know that almost all adults over forty have some disc deterioration; moreover, many people with degenerated discs don't feel any pain at all. While disc problems can be one cause of back pain, a more common cause is strained muscles. Stress, bad posture, and long periods of inactivity all weaken the back, making it vulnerable to pain from injury or exercise. When the back is very weak, even minor actions like twisting or coughing can trigger severe pain. Chronic back pain is frequently caused by muscular imbalance in the back, poor flexibility, spinal misalignment, and ligament or tendon injuries.

Although many cases of back pain have their roots in the muscles, other conditions can cause or contribute to pain. Pregnancy and obesity, which place stress on the muscles, are two common factors, as are arthritis, osteoporosis, and disorders of the kidney, the bladder, the pelvis, and the prostate. Constipation and other digestive disorders can also refer pain to the back area.

Proper lifting techniques are very important to prevent strain and injury of the back. This is especially true for people who have had previous back injuries.

Back pain does not automatically mean surgery and a lifetime of agony. It is now considered highly preventable and treatable with exercise, stretching, bodywork, supplements, and stress management. However, if you have pain that lasts for several weeks or extremely acute pain, contact your doctor so that he or she can check for underlying disorders that may be causing your pain. For example, certain kinds of back pain can signal a stroke, osteoporosis, or other serious medical conditions like cancer. If the pain radiates down your leg or is accompanied by numbness or loss of muscular, bowel, or bladder control, get medical help immediately.

SYMPTOMS

- Any kind of pain—sharp, lancing, dull, aching, gradual, sudden—usually in the lower or middle back
- Pain can radiate to the hips or the neck

ROOT CAUSES

- Inactivity, especially when punctuated by sudden exercise
- Poor posture and spinal misalignment
- Muscle strength and flexibility imbalances
- Sleeping on a poorly made mattress
- High heels
- Obesity
- Pregnancy
- Disorders of the kidney, the bladder, the prostate, or the pelvic region
- Arthritis
- Osteoporosis
- Emotional stress
- Premenstrual syndrome (PMS)
- Nutritional deficiencies
- Constipation
- Smoking

TREATMENT

Diet

Constipation, extra weight, and toxic build-up can aggravate back pain. Diet and detoxification therapies will help keep your body free of these stressors.

Recommended Food

Eat small, light meals. Heavy eating puts a burden on your digestive tract and weakens the back.

Constipation makes back pain worse, so eat plenty of fiber, preferably in the form of vegetables.

Dehydration aggravates back pain. Drink a glass of clean water every two waking hours. If you have an episode of back pain, drink a few glasses as soon as the pain starts.

Keep your bones well fed. Get protein from fish, soy products, and beans; for calcium, eat your leafy greens, sea vegetables, nuts and seeds, and tofu.

Consume foods that are rich in essential fatty acids (salmon, mackerel, almonds, walnuts, and ground flaxseeds).

Food to Avoid

Stay away from products that are high in saturated fat and sugar, especially if you are overweight. Extra pounds on the waist and the hips means a heavier load on the back.

Avoid caffeine and alcohol products, which are known to worsen inflammation.

Detoxification

A three-day juice fast will speed the removal of waste. If you're overweight and are starting a diet to reduce strain on your back, a juice fast may be a good way to break food addictions.

If you are chronically constipated, take 1 to 2 tablespoons of ground flaxseeds daily, along with 12 ounces of water.

℞ Super Seven Prescriptions—Back Pain

Super Prescription #1   Methylsulfonylmethane (MSM)
Take 3,000 to 8,000 mg daily in divided doses. Reduce the dosage if diarrhea occurs. MSM alleviates muscle spasms and has natural anti-inflammatory effects.

Super Prescription #2   Calcium and magnesium
Twice daily, take a complex of these two minerals that contains 500 mg of calcium and 250 mg of magnesium. These minerals alleviate muscle spasms.

Super Prescription #3   Homeopathy
Pick the remedy that best matches your symptoms under Homeopathy in this section. For acute back pain, take a 30C potency four times daily. For chronic back pain, take twice daily for two weeks to see if there are any positive improvements. After you notice improvement, stop taking the remedy, unless symptoms return. Consultation with a homeopathic practitioner is advised.

Super Prescription #4   Bromelain
Take 500 mg three times daily between meals. Look for products standardized to 2,000 M.C.U. (milk-clotting units) per 1,000 mg or 1,200 G.D.U. (gelatin-dissolving units) per 1,000 mg. Bromelain has a natural anti-inflammatory effect. Protease enzyme products also have this benefit.

Super Prescription #5   White willow (*Salix alba*)
Take a product standardized to contain 240 mg of salicin daily or 5 ml of the tincture form three times daily. This herb reduces pain.

Super Prescription #6   Glucosamine sulfate
Take 1,500 mg daily. It's useful for back pain that is caused by osteoarthritis.

Super Prescription #7   Cayenne (*Capsicum annuum*) **cream**
Apply the cream to the affected area two to four times daily for symptomatic relief. Choose a cream standardized to 0.025 to 0.075 percent capsaicin. Capsaicin depletes the nerves of substance P, a neurotransmitter that transmits pain messages.

General Recommendations

Vitamin C reduces inflammation and strengthens connective tissue. Take 1,000 mg three times daily.

Pine bark or grape seed extract reduces inflammation. Take 100 mg three times daily.

Ginger (*Zingiber officinale*) is a popular choice for relief of both inflammation and pain. Pour boiling water over the grated root and drink the tea, or try adding ginger fresh to your meals. If you want something stronger, take 1 to 2 grams of dried powder in capsule form, two or three times daily, or use 1 to 2 ml of a tincture three times daily.

Boswellia (*Boswellia serrata*): Take 1,200 to 1,500 mg of a standardized extract containing 60 to 65 percent boswellic acids two to three times daily.

DMSO (dimethyl sulfoxide) is a topical pain-relieving substance. Work with your doctor to use DMSO.

Many excellent herbs reduce inflammation. Devil's claw root (*Harpagophytum procumbens*), alfalfa (*Medicago sativa*), and yucca root (*Yucca schidigera*) capsules are among the best. Give these herbs at least two months to take effect. Recommended dosages are as follows:

Devil's claw should not be used if you have a history of gallstones, heartburn, or ulcers. Take 1,500 to 2,500 mg of the standardized powdered herb in capsule or tablet form daily, or use 1 to 2 ml of a tincture three times a day.

Arnica (*Arnica montana*) oil reduces pain and spasm. Rub this oil over the affected area twice daily.

Saint-John's-wort oil (*Hypericum oil*) reduces nerve pain. Rub over the affected area twice daily.

D-L phenylalanine is an amino acid used to reduce pain. Take 500 mg three times daily on an empty stomach.

Vitamins B1, B6, and B12 have been shown to reduce the amount of medication needed for back pain. Take 50 mg of B1 and B6 and 400 mcg of B12 three times daily. Also, when using these individual B vitamins long term, make sure to also supplement a 50 mg B-complex for a balance of all the B vitamins.

Protease enzymes reduce inflammation. Take 1 to 2 capsules twice daily between meals or as directed on the container.

Homeopathy

Pick the remedy that best matches your symptoms in this section. For acute back pain, take a 30C potency four times daily. For chronic back pain, take twice daily for two weeks to see if there are any positive improvements. After you notice results, stop taking the remedy, unless symptoms return. Consultation with a homeopathic practitioner is advised.

Aesculus is for lower back or sacral pain that is worse when you are sitting. The pain often radiates into the right hip.

Arnica (*Arnica montana*) is for an injury that leaves your back feeling bruised and sore and is helpful if you have difficulty moving around.

Bryonia (*Bryonia alba*) is for lower back pain and stiffness that feel worse with any movement and in cold, dry weather, and that feels better when the area is rubbed.

Calcarea Carbonica is for chronic lower back pain and weakness in overweight individuals who also are chilly. Symptoms are worse in the cold and in dampness.

Cimicifuga Racemosa is for a stiff and aching neck and back. Muscles feel bruised, but feel better with warmth. Also, it is used for menstrual cramps with lower back pain radiating to the thighs.

Ignatia (*Ignatia amara*) is for back spasms and cramping as the result of emotional stress.

Magnesia Phosphorica is for a muscle spasm in the back that feels better from warmth.

Nux Vomica (*Strychnos nux vomica*) is for back spasms and cramping, especially in the lower back. The person may also have constipation and feel chilly and irritable. The symptoms are worse from cold and feel better with warmth.

Rhus Toxicodendron is for a stiff lower back that is worse in the cold and the damp and feels better with movement. It is specific for a sprained back muscle or ligaments.

Ruta Graveolens is for pain near the neck or for lower back pain. The area of the injury feels lame, and the pain is worse at night. This remedy is useful for back sprains and strains.

Acupressure

Acupressure relieves back pain by stimulating blood flow, unblocking energy, and strengthening the internal organs. Some of the following points may be quite tender; if so, use a very light, continuous touch, instead of heavy pressure. In cases of severe pain or true disc damage, always consult a doctor before working these points. For more information about pressure points and administering treatment, see pages 668–675.

- For lower back pain, work Bladder 25, 31, and 40.
- Bladder 20 is the point for pain in the middle back.
- Upper back pain can be eased by using Gallbladder 20 and Governing Vessel 14.
- For back pain accompanied or caused by tension, use Bladder 48.
- If you have arthritis as well as back pain, Bladder 54 is a good choice.

Bodywork

Complementary therapy for back pain should usually include some kind of bodywork. You may want to try several of the following methods until you find the combination that works best for you. For a thorough evaluation, check with an osteopathic doctor, a naturopathic doctor, a chiropractor, or a medical doctor. Then a course of treatment can be recommended.

Massage

Most people know instinctively that massage will relieve their back pain and tension, but many are held back by their inability to travel to a massage therapist or by fear of making the pain worse. Massage is so effective, it's worth taking extra steps to overcome any obstacles to treatment. Check around to find a licensed, experienced professional who knows how to work with different kinds of back pain. He or she may also be willing to come to your house if you're immobilized.

Reflexology

See pages 686–687 for information about reflexology areas and how to work them.

Work the spine, the hips, and the tailbone area, all of which exist at the base of the heel.

Hydrotherapy

Hot water therapies are popular ways to treat backache and release stress. Although their relief is usually temporary, they feel wonderfully soothing and can get you mobile enough to receive other therapies.

To release spasms and tension, soak in a warm bath (90 to 100 degrees F). For an extra soothing effect, add any of the essential oils recommended under Aromatherapy in this section, or try a little mustard or ginger.

A hot water bottle is an old-fashioned remedy for back spasms, and it still works.

Constitutional hydrotherapy is helpful. See the Hydrotherapy section for directions.

Other Bodywork Recommendations

For chronic or severe pain, a visit to a chiropractor or an osteopath is highly recommended. He or she will correct postural problems and manipulate your spine so that your body is balanced and aligned.

Pay attention to your posture. Stand up straight, with your pelvis tucked in. When seated, keep your back erect and your feet flat on the floor. If you have serious back problems, try postural methods such as Hellerwork or the Alexander technique, which seek to retrain the body so that it moves naturally, correctly, and painlessly. Contact a specialist for instruction.

Throw out your high heels. Most footwear companies now make beautiful shoes that aren't hard on your feet and back.

If you feel stiffness and pain in the middle of the night and in the morning, but not during the rest of the day, your mattress may be the culprit. Find one that's firm and

The following exercise will often relieve lower back pain:

1. Take your shoes off and stand against a wall so that your heels touch it.
2. Now adjust your posture so that your buttocks and shoulders also touch the wall.
3. Imagine that you are straightening the curvature of your spine, and try to make your entire back press flat against the wall. Take the stretch as far as you comfortably can, and hold it for twenty to thirty seconds.

supportive. In addition, you should sleep on your side, with your knees bent. Placing a pillow between your knees may make you more comfortable.

Unless your health-care provider recommends this, it is best to avoid bed rest with a back injury. Studies show that it often slows down recovery.

Aromatherapy

- A massage with ginger, black pepper, or peppermint oils will help warm up muscles and dissolve cramps.
- To help relieve stress, try some of the many oils that have relaxing properties. Add geranium, jasmine, or lavender to a hot bath, or if you suffer from chronic tension, use a diffuser or a candle to release the scent throughout a room for long periods of time (just make sure you don't leave the flame unattended).
- If you tend to breathe shallowly in a crisis, use frankincense to encourage deep, relaxing breaths. Hold the vial directly under your nose and inhale.

Stress Reduction

General Stress-Reduction Therapies

Many people with back problems find that yoga eases their pain. Yoga releases emotional stress, as well as the physical tension that often deposits itself in the back; it also strengthens the spine and improves all-over flexibility. If you have or have had severe pain, take a class with an instructor who knows how to handle your condition.

If you have severe or chronic back pain, look into biofeedback. EMG biofeedback will help you identify just when you tense up your back muscles and will show you how to release them.

Many of the techniques mentioned throughout this section, such as massage, hot baths, and herbal treatments, treat stress as well as pain. Keep them in mind, and employ the ones you like best on a regular basis.

Bach Flower Remedies

Consult the chart on pages 648–650 to find the appropriate flower remedy for your individual personality. Following are some suggestions. Once you've selected the remedy that's right for you, place 10 drops of it under your tongue. Hold the drops in place for thirty seconds and swallow. Use as often as needed.

If you suffer from recurring attacks of pain, keep some Rescue Remedy on hand. Try taking it when you feel a strong emotional or physical crisis coming on, as it may prevent your back from seizing up.

Beech is for hard-driving perfectionists who are highly critical of others.

If you are a quick, efficient thinker who is irritated by slower people, Impatiens will help. It is especially effective when a deadline or a high-pressure event draws near.

If you deny yourself pleasures because of your single-minded pursuit of a goal, take Rock Water.

Other Recommendations

Regular exercise is the best way to prevent and treat back pain. While acute attacks may keep you in bed for a day or two, you should plan to get moving again as soon as possible. Gentle, nonjarring exercises such as walking, swimming, and cycling (with your back straight), are excellent choices. Whatever you do, do it consistently. Inactivity on the weekdays, punctuated by rigorous workouts on Saturday or Sunday, will only set your back up for injury.

REFERENCES

Bruggemann, G., C. O. Koehler, and E. M. Koch. 1990. Results of a double-blind study of diclofenac + vitamin B1, B6, B12 versus diclofenac in patients with acute pain of the lumbar vertebrae. A multicenter study. *Klin Wochenschr* 68:116–20 [in German].

Kuhlwein, A., H. J. Meyer, and C. O. Koehler. 1990. Reduced diclofenac administration by B vitamins: Results of a randomized double-blind study with reduced daily doses of diclofenac (75 mg diclofenac versus 75 mg diclofenac plus B vitamins) in acute lumbar vertebral syndromes. *Klin Wochenschr* 68:107–15 [in German].

Schwieger, G., H. Karl, and E. Schonhaber. 1990. Relapse prevention of painful vertebral syndromes in follow-up treatment with a combination of vitamins B1, B6, and B12. *Annals of the New York Academy of Science* 585:54–62.

Bad Breath (Halitosis)

If you've ever eaten garlic or onions—or stood next to someone who has—you know that certain foods reliably produce a sour or strong odor on the breath. These foods, usually ones that are pungent or spicy, contain foul-smelling sulfur compounds that are released not just into the mouth but into the bloodstream and the lungs as well. Even if you brush and gargle, you'll continue to exhale the sulfur with every breath until the food is fully metabolized, a process that can take up to twenty-four hours. This kind of food-induced bad breath can sometimes be socially troubling (especially if your companions have not eaten the same sulfur-producing food that you have), but it is in no way a health threat. If you enjoy eating spicy, strong food, complementary medicine offers some effective ways to mask the temporarily offensive result.

Persistent bad breath, on the other hand, is medically known as halitosis and is a symptom of an underlying problem. Many cases are warning signs of insufficient oral hygiene. If you do not clean your teeth after eating, bacteria will feed on the food particles left in your mouth and emit sulfur as a digestive by-product. Eventually, these bacteria will cause tooth decay and gum disease, disorders that, in turn, lead to even worse-smelling breath.

If regular brushing and flossing don't improve chronic bad breath, it's quite possible that you are suffering from a toxic body system. An improper diet and a poorly functioning digestive system can lead to the accumulation of toxins, which is reflected in bad breath. If you are constipated (as are many people who follow poor diets) and cannot eliminate the poisons via your bowels, the body may try to expel some of them every time you breathe out. A cleansing program, followed by dietary changes, should help get rid of the toxins and, with them, the cause of bad breath.

Also, undetected infections of the throat such as tonsillitis, as well as sinusitis can be the underlying cause of foul breath. These conditions may be the result of food or environmental allergens causing mucus formation and postnasal drip. Along these lines are chronic root canal infections, as well as teeth and mercury fillings that are decaying. The repeated use of antibiotics can wipe out the good flora in your mouth, which leads to the overgrowth of bad bacteria that cause bad breath.

Smoking is another obvious method of poisoning your body, and the best way to clear up the breath it causes is to give up the habit.

In rare cases, halitosis is a symptom of a serious disease. If the suggestions listed here don't improve your breath, consult a holistic dentist first and then a doctor, if necessary. It is possible that you have a dental disorder or even a disease of the kidneys or the liver. Take chronic bad breath seriously, but do exercise some common sense. Our society places an unnaturally high priority on eliminating body odors, and many dentists have noted that otherwise healthy patients can become convinced their breath is offensive, when in fact it is perfectly normal. If your close friends and health professionals assure you that your breath is fine, it's probably wisest to trust them.

SYMPTOMS

- Unpleasant odor on the breath

ROOT CAUSES

- Pungent or spicy foods
- Inadequate dental hygiene
- Poor diet
- Constipation
- Smoking
- Tooth decay
- Gum disease
- Chronic infection in the mouth
- (especially root canals), throat, or sinuses
- Decaying mercury fillings
- Flora imbalance in the mouth and the respiratory tract
- Liver failure
- Kidney disease
- Diabetes

TREATMENT

Diet

Recommended Food

Base your meals on healthful sources of fiber. Whole grains, raw or lightly cooked fruits and vegetables, beans, and raw nuts and seeds will all improve your digestive system's ability to process food and expel toxins.

Drink a glass of clean water every two waking hours. You'll keep your digestive system regular and help eliminate poisons.

If you go to a diner or an old-fashioned restaurant, you may notice that a sprig of parsley accompanies your meal. The parsley is meant to be more than a garnish; it's a traditional breath freshener that really works. Parsley is high in chlorophyll, an agent that neutralizes odor in the bloodstream and the lungs. Other good sources of chlorophyll include green vegetables, watercress, and alfalfa. If you know you're going to eat a type of food that causes bad breath, you may want to incorporate some of these greens into your meal.

Vitamins A and C are necessary for good dental health. For vitamin A, consume green or orange vegetables like carrots, kale, squash, sweet potatoes, and spinach. Eat citrus fruits for vitamin C.

Cultured products, especially live unsweetened yogurt, will encourage healthy bacteria to grow in the intestines and will improve digestion.

Food to Avoid

- Avoid foods that take a long time to travel through the digestive system. Red meat, fried food, and processed food all linger in the system and cause both constipation and halitosis.

- Mucus slows waste matter in its passage through the intestines. Cut down on mucus-forming foods like dairy products, refined flours, chocolate, and bananas.
- Avoid foods that are high in refined sugar, which leads to tooth decay. Be especially wary of sticky treats like caramels or hard candies, which can lodge themselves between your teeth and attract oral bacteria.
- Foods that are most likely to cause temporary bad breath include garlic, onions, strong cheese, cured meats, and anchovies. If the resulting odor bothers you, limit or stop your consumption of these items.

Detoxification

To get rid of undigested food, go on a three-day juice fast. Emphasize green drinks during your fast, and go easy on juices made with sweet fruits. If you're constipated, add 1 tablespoon of ground flaxseeds to your drinks for fiber.

℞ Super Seven Prescriptions—Bad Breath

Super Prescription #1   Chlorophyll
Take a teaspoonful of liquid chlorophyll after meals. Chlorella, alfalfa, and spirulina are also rich sources. Take as directed on the container.

Super Prescription #2   Xylitol
Use 4 to 12 grams of xylitol in natural gums, mints, toothpastes, or as a mouth rinse. This natural sweetener prevents the bacteria that cause bad breath from sticking to the mucosa of your mouth and teeth.

Super Prescription #3   Parsley
Take 5 drops of a liquid parsley extract after each meal to freshen your breath.

Super Prescription #4   Probiotic
Take a product containing at least 4 billion organisms. Mix it into water, swish it in your mouth, and swallow. It contains friendly bacteria that prevent the build-up of bacteria that cause bad breath, and it improves digestive function and elimination.

Super Prescription #5   Enzymes
Take a full-range enzyme with each meal to enhance the breakdown and the absorption of food.

Super Prescription #6   Bitter herbs
Take a digestion formula that contains bitter herbs, such as gentian, to improve overall digestive function. Take as directed on the container at beginning of each meal.

Super Prescription #7   Milk thistle (*Silybum marianum*)
If you are frequently constipated, you probably need to detoxify your liver. Cleanse it with milk thistle (*Silybum marianum*) extract. Choose a product standardized to 70 to 80 percent silymarin, and take 200 to 250 mg twice a day.

General Recommendations

Coenzyme Q10 is for people with active gum disease. Take 200 mg daily.

Cooled rosemary and peppermint tea makes a highly effective mouthwash.

Homeopathy

Pick the remedy that best matches your symptoms. Take a 6x, 12x, 6C, or 30C potency twice daily for two weeks to see if there are any positive results. After you notice improvement, stop taking the remedy, unless symptoms return.

Mercurius Solubilis is for offensive breath caused by tooth decay and accompanied by a yellow coating on the tongue and excessive salivation.

Nux Vomica (*Strychnos nux vomica*) is helpful if you have bad breath after drinking alcohol or have a history of constipation and/or heartburn.

Pulsatilla (*Pulsatilla pratensis*) is for sour breath caused by eating too much fatty food.

Acupressure

See pages 668–675 for information about pressure points and administering treatment.

- You can reduce the frequency of constipation by strengthening your colon. Use Large Intestine 11 to achieve this goal.
- Stomach 36 tones your digestive system.

Aromatherapy

Essential oils are much more effective than commercial mouthwashes are at eliminating oral bacteria and neutralizing bad breath. To make your own mouthwash, add a few drops of peppermint or eucalyptus oil to clean water.

Other Recommendations

- Brush after every meal, and floss your teeth before you go to bed. Many people who are assiduous brushers neglect flossing, but this step is vital to keep food particles out of the spaces between the teeth.
- Avoid toothpastes that are full of chemicals and artificial sweeteners. Natural toothpaste is now available at many drugstores, as well as at health food stores. You can also make your own with baking soda and hydrogen peroxide. Just before you brush, combine the two ingredients until they form a paste with a consistency that's to your liking. You should make a fresh mixture each time you brush your teeth.
- Commercial mouthwashes are just as bad as most toothpastes. They irritate the soft tissues of the mouth and can actually encourage bacterial growth. Instead, use a homemade mouthwash of water and essential oils, as previously recommended.
- Even if you keep your teeth scrupulously clean, see your holistic dentist for regular check-ups. He or she can remove plaque and other buildup that you may not be able to reach and will also check for any early signs of decay.

Bee Stings

When a bumblebee or a honeybee attacks, it leaves its stinger and attached venom sac in the skin. In most cases, the sting creates only slight pain, swelling, and irritation. It is more of a nuisance than a concern. However, look for signs of an allergic reaction, such as swollen eyelids or hands, difficulty breathing or wheezing, dizziness, fainting, nausea, vomiting, and the appearance of a hive-like rash. For these symptoms, go immediately to the emergency room or your doctor's office. The bee sting can be fatal in people who are allergic to its venom.

Other insects, including fire ants, paper wasps, hornets and yellow jackets, are capable of stinging, but they do not leave stingers in their victims.

Tips for Avoiding a Bee Sting

1. Wear light-colored, smooth-finished clothing.
2. Avoid perfumed soaps, shampoos, and deodorants. Don't wear cologne or perfume. Avoid bananas and banana-scented toiletries.
3. Wear clean clothing and bathe daily. Sweat angers bees.
4. Cover the body as much as possible with clothing.
5. Avoid flowering plants.
6. Check for new nests during the warmer hours of the day during July, August, and September. Bees are very active then.
7. Keep outside areas clean. Social wasps thrive in places where humans discard food, so clean up picnic tables, grills, and other outdoor eating areas.
8. If a single stinging insect is flying around, remain still or lie face down on the ground. The face is the most likely place for a bee or a wasp to sting. Swinging or swatting at an insect may cause it to sting.
9. If you are attacked by several stinging insects at the same time, run to get away from them. Bees release a chemical when they sting. This alerts other bees to the intruder. More bees often follow. Go indoors. Outdoors, a shaded area is better than an open area to get away from the insects.
10. If a bee comes inside your vehicle, stop the car slowly, and open all the windows.

What to Do If Someone Is Stung

1. Have someone stay with the victim to be sure that the person does not have an allergic reaction.
2. Wash the site with soap and water.
3. The stinger can be removed by wiping a four-inch gauze pad over the area or by scraping a fingernail or a credit card over the area. Never squeeze the stinger or use tweezers. It will cause more venom to go into the skin and will injure the muscle.
4. Apply ice to reduce the swelling.
5. Do not scratch the sting. This will cause the site to swell and itch more and will increase the chance of infection.
6. If the victim is having a severe allergic reaction, seek emergency medical attention.
7. Epinephrine is given by injection to stop allergic reactions.

TREATMENT

Diet

Recommended Food

Consume foods rich in omega-3 fatty acids that promote skin healing and reduce inflammation, such as fish (salmon, cod, mackerel). Ground flaxseeds, avocados, and wheat germ are also recommended.

Eat green, orange, and yellow vegetables at every meal. These foods are packed with vitamins A and C, which will speed your skin's recovery from the inflammation.

Food to Avoid

Sugar worsens the inflammatory response. Stay away from refined sugar products, including cookies, cakes, sweet baked goods, and sodas, and eat naturally occurring sugars, such as those found in fruit, in moderation.

℞ Super Seven Prescriptions—Bee Stings

Please note that these therapies do not replace conventional therapy for people who are having a severe allergic reaction to a bee sting.

Super Prescription #1   Homeopathic Apis (*Apis mellifica*)
Take a 30C potency every thirty minutes to reduce swelling and pain. The stinging or burning pain, along with great swelling, is reduced with cold applications.

Super Prescription #2   Homeopathic Carbolic Acid (Carbolicum Acidum)
Take a 30C potency every five minutes to reduce severe reactions to a bee sting, while waiting to get conventional therapy with an epinephrine injection.

Super Prescription #3   Homeopathic Ledum (Ledum Palustre)
Take a 30C potency every thirty minutes to reduce swelling and pain. The person has a bruising pain that feels better with cold applications.

Super Prescription #4   Vitamin C with bioflavonoids
Take 1,000 mg three times daily to reduce swelling and inflammation. *Note:* Reduce the dosage if loose stools occur.

Super Prescription #5   Super green food supplement
Take a super green food product, such as spirulina, chlorella, or a combination of greens, to reduce the inflammatory response. Take as directed on the container.

Super Prescription #6   Bach Flower Rescue Remedy
This decreases anxiety and emotional upset. Take 10 drops four times daily.

Super Prescription #7   Quercitin
Take 500 mg three times daily. This flavonoid reduces inflammation of the skin.

Bladder Infection (Cystitis)

The uncomfortable and irritating symptoms of a bladder infection send American women to their doctors 6 to 9 million times every year. Most of these women will be treated with a course of antibiotics, a strategy that kills the current infection but that leaves the bladder vulnerable to a future bacterial invasion. As a result, most of the women who see a doctor about a bladder infection will return; 10 to 20 percent of all women experience a bladder infection at least once over a twelve-month period.

When the bladder is infected, usually by bacteria, its interior walls become inflamed. This inflammation, medically known as cystitis, leads to a frequent and urgent need to urinate, although the urine produced may be scanty, and the bladder may not feel completely empty. There is usually pain or burning upon urination, and there may be cramping in the abdomen or the lower back, and fever.

Women suffer from bladder infections far more frequently than men do, mainly because of the female anatomy. In women, the urethra—the tube that conducts urine away from the bladder and out of the body—is very short, and its opening is in close proximity to both the anus and the vagina. It's relatively easy for vaginal or intestinal bacteria to travel to the opening to the urethra, make their way up the tube, and infect the bladder. Although bacteria are the cause of most infections, several other conditions put women at risk for this disorder. Frequent use of antibiotics is one of the most prevalent, since these medications destroy the "good" bacteria needed to fight infections. Anything else that weakens the immune system, such as stress or a poor diet, increases the likelihood of an infection. Pregnancy, sexual intercourse, and injury to the area are associated with a higher risk. Hormone imbalances can also contribute to an increased susceptibility. Menopause is a time when many women first start to experience bladder infections.

Most bladder infections respond well to home care that treats the symptoms, while strengthening the immune system. You should still consult a doctor, however, as there is a possibility that the infection can spread to the kidneys. Your physician should monitor your progress and make sure the infection isn't traveling upward. And if you have recurring infections, your doctor should examine you for a structural abnormality in the urethra or the bladder that prevents urine from flowing properly. Should your doctor want to prescribe antibiotics, explain to him or her your desire for more conservative treatment and ask whether antibiotics are really necessary. (In some cases, they're needed to prevent a kidney infection.) If you are a man with a bladder infection, you may have a more serious condition. For more information, see the sections on prostate problems in this book.

SYMPTOMS

- Pain or burning upon urination
- Frequent need to urinate
- Scanty flow or dribbling
- Cramps in abdomen or lower back
- Nausea or vomiting
- Fever

ROOT CAUSES

- Vaginal or intestinal bacteria, usually *E. coli*
- Frequent use of antibiotics
- Stress
- Poor diet and food allergies
- Pregnancy
- Sexual intercourse
- Injury
- Use of a diaphragm for contraception
- Structural abnormality
- Hormonal imbalance

TREATMENT

Diet

Recommended Food

Make sure that you're getting all the nutrients you need. Plan well-rounded, wholesome meals, made with basic foods that you prepare yourself.

One of the best strategies for fighting a bladder infection is to increase your urine output. Drink as much clean water as you can stand. Try for one 6- to 8-ounce glass every waking hour.

Cranberry juice has long been a folk remedy for bladder infections, and now science helps us understand why: it appears that cranberry juice keeps bacteria from clinging to the linings of the bladder and the urethra. You can find unsweetened cranberry juice at most health food stores and many supermarkets. Drink several glasses of it a day.

Natural diuretics will help flush out the infection. Eat plenty of watermelon, celery, or parsley, or use them to make fresh juices.

Add some garlic to clear soups or other meals. It's a potent infection-fighter.

If you must take antibiotics, eat a cup of unsweetened live yogurt or another cultured product every day. These foods help return "good" bacteria to your body.

Food to Avoid

Sugar depresses the immune system and encourages the growth of bacteria.

Avoid all refined sugars (including those in alcohol) while you're battling the infection, and restrict them once you've recovered.

During the course of the infection, stay away from salty, spicy, processed, or refined foods, as well as caffeine. All of these substances will further aggravate the problem.

Food allergies can cause recurring bladder infections. See the Food Allergies section and the accompanying elimination diet to determine whether a food is at the heart of your problem.

Many women who are frequent consumers of sodas (both sugary and diet) experience recurring bladder infections. Sodas, whether made from natural or artificial sweeteners, are never a good idea; if you are troubled by bladder infections, you now have another compelling reason to avoid sodas.

Detoxification

A three-day juice fast is a strong weapon against recurring infections. Concentrate on vegetable juices, rather than on fruit juices, at this time, since you want to avoid too much sugar. When you drink fruit juice, dilute it with clean water.

℞ Super Seven Prescriptions—Bladder Infection

Super Prescription #1   Uva ursi
Take a standardized capsule containing 250 mg of arbutin or 5 ml of the tincture form four times daily. Arbutin is a constituent in uva ursi that is converted in the body to a chemical called hydroquinone, which destroys bacteria.

Super Prescription #2   D-mannose
Take 500 mg four times daily. This substance prevents bacteria from being able to attach to the urinary tract and the bladder wall.

Super Prescription #3   Homeopathy
Pick the remedy that best matches your symptoms under Homeopathy in this section. For acute bladder infection, take a 30C potency four times daily. After you notice improvement, stop taking the remedy, unless symptoms return. Consultation with a homeopathic practitioner is advised.

Super Prescription #4   Echinacea (*Echinacea purpurea*) and **goldenseal** (*Hydrastis canadensis*)
Take 500 mg of the capsule form or 4 ml of the tincture four times daily. These herbs enhance immune function to combat infection.

Super Prescription #5   Cranberry (*Vaccinium macrocarpon*) **extract**
Take 400 to 500 mg twice daily of cranberry extract capsules. Cranberry prevents bacteria from adhering to the bladder wall. This herb is best used for the prevention of urinary tract infections but can also be used as part of a comprehensive protocol for acute infection.

Super Prescription #6   Horsetail (*Equisetum arvense*)
Take 500 mg of the capsule or 2 ml of the tincture four times daily. This herb has a long history of use for urinary tract infections.

Super Prescription #7   Vitamin C
Take 1,000 mg four to five times daily. Vitamin C enhances immune function, inhibits the growth of *E. coli,* and makes the urine more acidic so that bacteria cannot grow as easily.

General Recommendations

Oregano oil (*Origanum vulgare*) has powerful antibacterial and antiviral effects. Take 500 mg of the capsule form four times daily or as directed on the container.

Vitamin A enhances immune function. Take 25,000 to 50,000 IU daily for one week. Do not use if you are pregnant.

Probiotic contains friendly bacteria that prevent the overgrowth of harmful bacteria. It is especially important to take if you are using antibiotics. Take it at a separate time during the day, and continue use for two months. Take a product containing at least 4 billion organisms daily.

Homeopathy

Pick the remedy that best matches your symptoms in this section. For acute bladder infection, take a 30C potency four to six times daily. After you notice improvement, stop taking the remedy, unless symptoms return. Consultation with a homeopathic practitioner is advised.

Aconitum Napellus is helpful for the very first two hours of a bladder infection. Urination feels hot, and the person feels anxious. A fever comes on quickly.

Apis (*Apis mellifica*) is good for sharp, stinging pains that feel better with cold compresses or cool drinks and feel worse with warm applications (such as a warm bath). There are often only small amounts of urine passed.

Belladonna (*Atropa belladonna*) is for burning in the urethra, with a feeling of great urgency and with bladder spasm. A high fever comes on quickly.

Cantharis is the homeopathic remedy of choice for bladder infections. Use it if you have a strong urge but produce very little urine. You may have burning and cutting

A study reported in the *Journal of the American Medical Association* found that regular consumption of cranberry juice (10 ounces a day) significantly reduced the amount of bacteria and pus in the urine of elderly women. Another study found that cranberry capsule extract (400 mg twice daily) for three months significantly reduced the recurrence of urinary tract infections in women ages eighteen to forty-five who had a history of reoccurring infections.

pain upon urination, as well as cramps in your abdomen and lower back. Small tinges of blood may be present.

Mercurius Corrosivus is helpful when blood and pus are in the urine. The person feels great burning pains and spasm in the bladder.

Nux Vomica (*Strychnos nux vomica*) helps when there is a constant urge to urinate, with only small amounts being passed. The person feels chilly and irritable. Symptoms are better with warmth (a warm bath).

Sarsaparilla can be taken when there is burning pain at the end of urination. The person seems to urinate only when standing and not sitting.

Staphysagria is for the burning pains of a bladder infection that come on after sexual intercourse. It is also used for bladder infections that result from the use of a catheter.

Bodywork

Reflexology

Reflexology is helpful to prevent bladder infections, and you should see improvement after two or three treatments. For information about reflexology areas and how to work them, see pages 686–687.

Work the areas corresponding to the bladder, the kidneys, and the ureters.

Hydrotherapy

A hot sitz bath is a comforting and powerful therapy for bladder infections. Take it once or twice a day until you are healed. Add vinegar or garlic oil for an even stronger effect.

Constitutional hydrotherapy can also be used for an acute bladder infection.

Aromatherapy

- Bergamot, chamomile, and lavender all have gentle antiseptic qualities. Use them in a sitz bath. If you prefer, a regular hot bath is still an effective delivery system for these oils.
- Tea tree oil (*Melaleuca alternifolia*) is a potent infection-fighter that also stimulates the immune system. It can be irritating to some people, so add just a few drops to a bath for your first use. If you do not have a reaction, you can add a few more.
- If you need to relieve stress, several oils can help you. See page 658 for information on oils. Here are some good ones to get you started: lavender, jasmine, rose, geranium, and bergamot.

Stress Reduction

General Stress-Reduction Therapies

Stress depletes the immune system and leaves you vulnerable to recurring infections. If you need to reduce the level of stress in your life, experiment with the different techniques described in the Exercise and Stress Reduction chapter until you find the ones that are best for you.

Bach Flower Remedies

The chart on pages 648–650 will help you determine the flower remedy best suited to your personality. Select the appropriate remedy, and place 10 drops under your tongue. Hold the drops in place for thirty seconds and swallow. Use as often as needed.

Crab Apple is a good choice if bladder infections make you feel impure or unclean.

Other Recommendations

- Always empty your bladder when you feel the need. Delaying urination sets the stage for an infection.
- Empty your bladder prior to and, if possible, after sexual intercourse to reduce the likelihood of infection. It's a good idea for women to drink a big glass of water before and after intercourse.
- After swimming, immediately change out of your wet bathing suit and into dry clothes. Damp conditions are a breeding ground for bacteria.
- If you're prone to bladder infections, wear cotton underwear that lets the genital area breathe.
- After going to the toilet, always wipe from front to back. This reduces the chances that intestinal bacteria will travel to the urethra.
- Avoid products that may irritate the urethra or the vagina. Do not use powders, sanitary napkins, or tampons that are scented.
- A hot compress is very soothing to an irritated urinary tract. Lie down somewhere comfortable, and place the compress on your lower abdomen.
- For bladder infections that occur around menses or that began with menopausal changes, hormone balancing is likely the issue. See the chapters that correspond to your situation, such as PMS and Menopause.

REFERENCES

Avorn, J., M. Monane, J. H. Gurwitz, et al. 1994. Reduction of bacteriuria and pyuria after ingestion of cranberry juice. *Journal of the American Medical Association* 271:751–54.

Walker, E. B., D. P. Barney, J. N. Mickelsen, et al. 1997. Cranberry concentrate: UTI prophylaxis. *Journal of Family Practice* 45:167–68 [letter].

Blood Pressure, High

As blood circulates through the body, it presses against the walls of the arteries. The force of this action is called blood pressure. When the pressure is too high, the arterial walls become distorted—they may narrow or thicken—and an extra burden of stress is placed on the heart.

Blood pressure may temporarily rise from exercise, stress, and emotions ranging from joy to anger. Usually, the pressure returns to normal once the situation has passed. In many people, however, blood pressure is high all the time. More than 50 million Americans have high blood pressure (also known as hypertension), including almost half of those over the age of sixty-five. The disorder can lead to very serious conditions, including stroke, heart disease, diabetes, eye damage, and kidney problems, so it is considered one of the country's leading health problems.

Sometimes there are symptoms of high blood pressure. You may have unexplained headaches, nosebleeds, or spells of dizziness or sweating. But most of the time high blood pressure is completely asymptomatic, so it's vital that you have it checked regularly. The disorder can strike anyone at any age, but it is most common among the elderly, African Americans, and people of all races living in the southeastern United States. If you fall into any of these risk categories, or if you have a family history of hypertension, you should be doubly sure to have routine checks and to take preventative measures.

About 90 percent of all cases of high blood pressure are called primary or essential hypertension, meaning that there is no underlying disease and no obvious cause. Most likely, a cluster of lifestyle factors is to blame: diet, lack of exercise, stress, and smoking have all been linked to an increase in blood pressure. If another disease or condition, such as cardiovascular disease or kidney, adrenal, or thyroid disorders causes the problem, it is called secondary hypertension. A very small percentage of people suffer from malignant hypertension, in which blood pressure can suddenly soar to extremely dangerous levels.

Essential hypertension can often be controlled with home treatment, but if you have any kind of high blood pressure, you must be under the care of a doctor. Talk to him or her about the strategies you want to employ for wellness.

SYMPTOMS

High blood pressure does not usually produce symptoms. If, however, you experience any of the following, see a doctor:

- Recurring headaches
- Dizziness
- Unexplained sweating
- Nosebleeds
- Visual disturbances
- Shortness of breath
- Flushed cheeks
- Ringing in the ears

ROOT CAUSES

- A diet that's high in fat, sugar, and/or salt
- Use of alcohol or caffeine and other stimulants
- Smoking
- Obesity
- Inactivity
- Pregnancy or birth-control pills
- Underlying medical disorders
- Heavy-metal poisoning

Testing Techniques

The following tests help assess possible metabolic reasons for high blood pressure:

Vitamin and mineral analysis—blood or urine

Food allergy testing—blood or electrodermal

Toxic metals (lead, cadmium, etc.)—hair or urine

TREATMENT

Diet

The Western diet has a lot to do with hypertension. Following the suggestions here will make a real difference in your blood pressure and your overall wellness.

When you have your blood pressure checked, the doctor or the nurse usually tells you the two numbers of your reading and whether you have cause for concern. But most health-care professionals don't take the time to explain exactly what those numbers mean. Since this is one of the most important medical tests people receive on a regular basis, here's a quick analysis.

The first number is called the systolic pressure. It is measured when the heart beats and indicates the highest amount of pressure against the arterial walls. Between heartbeats, the heart is at rest and pressure drops to its lowest level. This low reading is called the diastolic pressure.

Sample blood pressure reading of 120/80

systolic pressure = 120

diastolic pressure = 80

Blood pressure varies with age and fluctuates many times over the course of a day; it often rises in a doctor's office, when many people feel nervous or tense. Blood pressure should be taken when you are calm and unstressed, and it is best to average a total of three readings, taken on different days. The consensus is that for most healthy adults, 120/80 is normal.

Readings are broken down into several categories:

Normal: 110–130/70–85

High normal: 130–139/85–89

Mild hypertension: 140–159/90–99

Moderate hypertension: 160–179/100–109

Severe hypertension: 180 or higher/110 or higher

Recommended Food

A diet high in fiber is an excellent way to control or reverse high blood pressure. Your meals should be based around fresh, raw vegetables; soy products; whole grains, like oats; beans; nuts; and seeds.

Dehydration increases the risk of hypertension, so drink a glass of clean water every two waking hours.

As you lower your intake of salt, you must also increase your consumption of potassium. A combination of excess sodium and a deficiency in potassium has been found in many people with hypertension. Good sources of potassium include apples, asparagus, cabbage, oranges, tomatoes, bananas, kelp (*Ascophyllum nodosum*), and alfalfa.

Apples are superfoods for people with high blood pressure. Not only do they have high levels of potassium, they're also a good source of pectin, which is an excellent type of soluble fiber.

Onions, garlic, and parsley have been shown to bring down blood pressure. They also add flavor to vegetarian meals, so take advantage of their healing properties daily.

Celery has been shown in animal studies to reduce blood pressure. Consume up to four stalks a day.

Food to Avoid

People with high blood pressure generally benefit from restricting their intake of salt. Salt contains sodium, which causes water retention and increases the pressure inside the arteries. It is not enough to simply stop using table salt; you must also cut out all processed and packaged foods, as well as smoked meats and cheeses, as they are loaded with sodium.

Avoid the use of the herbs ephedra (*Ma huang*), Chinese ginseng (*Panax ginseng*), and large amounts of licorice (*Glycyrrhiza glabra*), as they may increase blood pressure.

- Saturated, hydrogenated, and partially hydrogenated fats cause high blood pressure and place a terrible burden on your arteries and heart. Eliminate animal products, margarine, butter, shortening, and refined vegetable oils.
- Sugar is linked to hypertension. If you do not eat packaged or processed foods, you will eliminate the largest sources of added sugar from your diet, but you should also avoid sugary baked goods and limit your intake of foods that are sweetened naturally.
- Overindulgence in caffeine is a cause of high blood pressure. Cut back on your intake of coffee, colas, chocolate, and caffeinated teas.
- Allow yourself no more than one alcoholic beverage a day.

Detoxification

Do a one- to three-day juice fast every month. Drink a wide variety of juices to support your fast, including those made from apples, bok choy, carrots, onions, leafy greens, apricots, cranberries, cantaloupe, papayas, and red grapes.

℞ Super Seven Prescriptions—High Blood Pressure

Super Prescription #1   Hawthorn (*Crataegus oxycanthae*)
Take 250 mg of a standardized extract three times daily. This herb dilates the artery walls and decreases blood pressure.

Super Prescription #2   Calcium and **magnesium**
These minerals have been shown in studies to lower blood pressure. Take a combination of 500 mg of calcium and 250 mg of magnesium twice daily.

Super Prescription #3   Coenzyme Q10
Studies show that this nutrient reduces blood pressure. Take 100 mg two to three times daily.

Super Prescription #4   Garlic (*Allium sativum*)
Several studies confirm garlic's ability to lower blood pressure. Take 600 mg twice daily of an aged garlic extract.

Super Prescription #5   Fish oil
Fish oil reduces blood pressure when taken on a long-term basis. Take 3,000 mg three times daily.

Super Prescription #6   Potassium
This mineral has been shown in repeated studies to lower blood pressure. Take as part of a salt-substitute product. Otherwise, use up to 2,000 mg under the supervision of a doctor. Do not use if you are taking a potassium-sparing diuretic medication or have kidney disease or serious heart disease.

Super Prescription #7   Vitamin C
Vitamin C has mild blood-lowering effects and helps the body detoxify toxic metals, such as lead, which contribute to high blood pressure. Take 1,000 to 2,000 mg daily.

A randomized, double-blind, placebo-controlled study of seventy-four people with type 2 diabetes found that 100 mg of coenzyme Q10 taken twice daily significantly lowered blood pressure over a period of twelve weeks. Other studies have also found CoQ10 blood pressure–lowering benefits.

General Recommendations

Passionflower (*Passiflora incarnata*) relaxes the nerves and is helpful for blood pressure that increases with stress. Take 250 mg or 0.5 ml two to three times daily.

Valerian (*Valeriana officinalis*) is a strong nerve relaxer and may indirectly lower blood pressure. Take 300 mg or 0.5 to 1.0 ml two to three times daily.

Chamomile (*Matricaria recutita*) and oatstraw (*Avena sativa*) are great herbal nerve relaxers. They can be taken as a tea throughout the day.

Taurine is an amino acid shown in research to lower blood pressure in humans and animals. Take up to 6 grams daily between meals.

Reishi (*Ganoderma lucidum*) extract should be taken in 500-mg doses three times daily for a blood pressure–lowering effect.

Dandelion leaf (*Taraxacum officinale*) acts as a gentle, natural diuretic to lower blood pressure. Take 300 mg of the capsule form or 2 ml three times daily.

Homeopathy

Argentum Nitricum is for elevated blood pressure that occurs with anxiety. Symptoms often come on from a stressful event or "stage fright." The person is usually very warm and has strong salt and sweet cravings.

Belladonna (*Atropa belladonna*) is for high blood pressure that comes on suddenly. The person has a flushed face and dilated pupils and feels a great deal of heat, although the hands and the feet are cold. Pounding headaches may occur, and the person is sensitive to light.

Glonoinum may be helpful for high blood pressure that's accompanied by a bursting headache and a flushed face. The person is worse from the heat and sun exposure or from consuming alcohol.

Lachesis is for a person who is very intense, who feels suspiciousness and jealousy, and who is very talkative. The person feels warm and is intolerant of anything touching the neck.

Natrum Muriaticum is for high blood pressure that begins after an emotional upset. The person desires to be alone and often experiences headaches, heart palpitations, and insomnia. There is a strong craving for salt, a great thirst, and an aversion to being in the sun.

Nux Vomica (*Strychnos nux vomica*) is for high blood pressure that occurs from the effects of stress. The person feels irritable and impatient and has a strong desire for stimulants such as coffee, as well as alcohol. The person is usually chilly and is prone to constipation.

Acupressure

See pages 668–675 for information about pressure points and administering treatment.

- Bladder 38 simultaneously lowers blood pressure and relieves nervous tension.
- If you tend to get heart palpitations when you're agitated, take some time out of a tense situation to work Pericardium 6. This spot is located at your wrist, so it's easy to use even in a public place like the office.
- People who feel chest tension when they're upset or worried should use Conception Vessel 17.
- Encourage circulation to your heart and chest by working Heart 3 and 7.

Bodywork

Massage

Massage can be of great help to people with high blood pressure. It regulates the body's rhythms, improves circulation, and promotes relaxation, so make a regular appointment with a good therapist, if possible.

If stress makes your chest feel tight and full, try a neck massage to relieve tension and steady your heartbeat. You can do this yourself or have a loved one do it for you.

Reflexology

See pages 686–687 for information about reflexology areas and how to work them.

Work the areas corresponding to the thyroid, the kidneys, the solar plexus, and the pituitary and adrenal glands.

Hydrotherapy

Do not use saunas. The hot steam can make your blood pressure rise to dangerous levels.

Other Bodywork Recommendations

Acupuncture is helpful for high blood pressure, especially when the underlying cause is stress.

Osteopathic and craniosacral therapy can help normalize circulation.

Aromatherapy

Take advantage of the soothing effects of essential oils. Many oils will help you relax, but lavender, marjoram, and ylang ylang are those most often used to calm the body and bring down blood pressure. You can use them in any preparation that suits you.

When used in a massage, juniper oil will help break down fatty deposits in your arteries and elsewhere in your body.

Stress Reduction

General Stress-Reduction Therapies

Meditation is a cheap, portable technique that you can use anywhere for a calming effect. You can practice meditation on a regular basis in a quiet room at home. If you feel your blood pressure rise while sitting at a stoplight, during a meeting, or while waiting up for your teenager to come home, you can easily spend a few moments paying attention to your breath. Meditative breathing won't stop the stress, but it can help you take a few steps back and view the problem with detachment.

Stress can make your body constrict its blood vessels, making it harder for blood to get through and thus raising your blood pressure. Biofeedback, however, can help you identify when you constrict your blood vessels, and it can train you to relax them.

Bach Flower Remedies

Select the appropriate remedy, and place 10 drops under your tongue. Hold the drops in place for thirty seconds and swallow. Use as often as needed.

When you feel panicked, upset, angry, or stressed in any way, take Rescue Remedy to help yourself calm down.

If you tend to cover up insecurity with aggressive, irritable behavior, Holly will help you feel more patient and gentle.

Rock Water is for people who work very hard and blame themselves for every problem.

Oak will help people who—whether for reasons of duty, responsibility, self-sacrifice, or ambition—refuse to give up or yield. Those who will benefit from Oak tend to place themselves in high-pressure, strenuous situations.

Take Aspen if you have general anxiety or vague, unnamed fears.

Other Recommendations

- If you are obese, you must lose weight. The dietary suggestions in this section will help you take off the pounds safely, but if you'd like to learn more, see Obesity. Do not rely on stimulant diet products; they may contain additives that could make your condition worse.
- Moderate exercise is a reliable way to reduce blood pressure, but consult with your doctor before starting an exercise program. As a person with hypertension, you may have special needs that should be addressed.
- Do not smoke or expose yourself to secondhand smoke.
- If testing shows that you have high toxic metal levels (such as lead, cadmium, and mercury), work with a doctor who is knowledgeable in chelation therapy.

REFERENCES

Digiesi, V., F. Cantini, and B. Brodbeck. 1990. Effect of coenzyme Q10 on essential arterial hypertension. Current Therapeutic Research 47:841–45.

Hodgson, J. M., G. F. Watts, D. A. Playford, V. Burke, and K. D. Croft. 2002. Coenzyme Q10 improves blood pressure and glycaemic control: A controlled trial in subjects with type 2 diabetes. European Journal of Clinical Nutrition 56(11):1137–42.

Singh, R. B., M. A. Niaz, S. S. Rastogi, et al. 1999. Effect of hydrosoluble coenzyme Q10 on blood pressures and insulin resistance in hypertensive patients with coronary artery disease. *Journal of Human Hypertension* 13:203–8.

Bone Fractures

A bad fall, a hard blow, an automobile collision, a sports injury, or an underlying medical condition such as osteoporosis can result in a broken bone.

When a bone breaks, it triggers not only pain, swelling, bruising, and immobility but also trauma and shock throughout the entire body. Fractures located near joints are sometimes misidentified as simply bad sprains.

There are varying degrees of fractures. Here are definitions and causes for the main types of fractures:

1. *Partial* (incomplete): The break across the bone is incomplete.
2. *Complete:* The bone is broken in two pieces.
3. *Closed* (simple): The broken bone does not protrude through the skin.
4. *Open* (compound): The broken bone protrudes through the skin.
5. *Comminuted:* The bone is splintered at the broken area and many smaller fragments of bone are found between the two main pieces.
6. *Greenstick:* This occurs only in children and is defined by having one side of the bone break and the other side just bend, often seen on the radius (forearm bone).
7. *Spiral:* A breaking force twisted the bone apart.
8. *Transverse:* This occurs at right angles to the bone.
9. *Impacted:* One fragment is forcibly driven into the other.
10. *Colles':* This is a fracture of the distal end of the radius (wrist), and the fragment is displaced posteriorly (behind).
11. *Pott's:* This is a fracture of the distal (lower portion of leg) end of the fibula, with serious injury of the distal tibia articulation.

12. *Nondisplaced:* The correct anatomical alignment of the bone is maintained.
13. *Displaced:* The correct anatomical alignment of the bone is not maintained.
14. *Stress:* This is a partial fracture, resulting from the inability of the bone to withstand repeated stresses (such as doing aerobics on hard surfaces or running long distances for prolonged periods of time). Almost one-fourth of stress fractures occur in the fibula.
15. *Pathologic:* This fracture is a result of normal stress on a weakened bone. It occurs in such diseases as osteoporosis, neoplasia, osteomyelitis, and osteomalacia.

If you have had an accident where you may have broken a bone, it is important to get immediate medical attention. For a more serious injury and if you have someone to help you, try to stay immobilized until medical personnel assess and move you. Otherwise, if you must move, it is important to have the fracture site immobilized with splinting materials. Even magazines or a towel can be used.

Once your fracture has been assessed and immobilized by medical personnel, it is very helpful to utilize the natural therapies in this chapter. They can help to speed healing of the fracture and can reduce pain and swelling. Remember, our bones are living tissues that have the ability to repair themselves when damaged. They must be given the correct nutrients to do so. Many vitamins and minerals are required for healthy bones. Calcium is the obvious one, but magnesium; boron; silicon; strontium; vitamins D, C, and K; and others play important roles in bone metabolism.

SYMPTOMS

- Bone pain
- Swelling
- Bleeding

ROOT CAUSES

- Fall or injury
- Osteoporosis

TREATMENT

Diet

Recommended Food

Eat foods that are high in calcium and the other nutrients needed for calcium's assimilation. Sea vegetables, green leafy vegetables (except spinach), soybeans, nuts, molasses, salmon, oysters, sardines (with the bones), broccoli, and unsweetened cultured yogurt are all good sources.

Green vegetables, such as collard greens, kale, romaine lettuce, and others, are important for their vitamin K content, which helps with bone formation.

Fermented soy products, such as tofu and miso, are good for the bones.

Essential fatty acids found in walnuts, almonds, flaxseeds, and fish are important for healthy bones.

Food to Avoid

Eliminate sugar, refined grains, and soda pop drinks from your diet, as they contribute to bone loss.

Testing Techniques

The following tests help assess possible reasons for people whose bones fracture easily:

Hormone testing (thyroid, DHEA, cortisol, testosterone, IGF-1, estrogen, progesterone)—saliva, blood, or urine

Intestinal permeability—urine

Vitamin and mineral analysis (especially magnesium, calcium, vitamin K, vitamin D)—blood, hair

Toxic metals—urine or hair

Digestive function and microbe/parasite/candida testing—stool analysis

Food and environmental allergies/sensitivities—blood, electrodermal

Bone resorption (pyridinium and deoxypyridinium)—urine

High salt intake is linked to bone loss. Do not eat processed foods, which are usually loaded with salt, and never add conventional table salt to your meals.

Moderate your use of caffeine and alcohol, as they contribute to bone loss.

℞ Super Seven Prescriptions—Bone Fracture

Super Prescription #1   Homeopathic Symphytum (*Symphytum officinale*)
Take a 30C potency four times daily for two weeks. Symphytum is a specific remedy for healing bones and reducing fracture pain more quickly. Make sure to use Symphytum only after the fracture has been set, as it rapidly speeds knitting of the bone.

Super Prescription #2   Calcium
Take 500 to 600 mg twice daily in divided doses of well-absorbed calcium complexes, such as citrate, citrate-malate, chelate, or hydroxyappatite. Calcium is the main mineral that bone is composed of.

Super Prescription #3   Magnesium
Take 250 to 350 mg twice daily in divided doses. Magnesium is required for proper calcium metabolism and bone formation. Some researchers feel that it is as important as calcium. *Note:* Reduce the dosage if loose stools occur.

Super Prescription #4   Vitamin D
Take 800 IU daily for one month and then 400 IU daily. This vitamin improves intestinal calcium absorption and reduces the urinary excretion of calcium.

Super Prescription #5   Vitamin K
Take 5 mg daily for one month and then 100 to 500 mcg daily to finish bone healing. Vitamin K is needed to form the protein osteocalcin, a substance that attracts calcium into the bone matrix. Low levels of vitamin K are associated with osteoporosis and fractures. *Note:* Do not use if you are taking blood-thinning medications.

Super Prescription #6   High-potency multivitamin
This provides a base of the nutrients required for healthy bones. Take as directed on the container.

A study in the *American Journal of Clinical Nutrition* reported that a low intake of vitamin K was associated with an increased risk of hip fracture. The data from the study came from the review of the diets of over 72,000 women. Studies have also shown that vitamin K supplementation improves bone density.

> **Super Prescription #7   Essential fatty acids**
>
> Take 4 grams of fish oil daily, along with 3,000 mg of evening primrose oil. Studies show that these essential fatty acids improve calcium absorption and deposition into the bone.

General Recommendations

Boron is a mineral that activates vitamin D for effective calcium metabolism. Take 3 to 5 mg daily.

Vitamin C is used to manufacture collagen, an important component of bones. Take 500 to 1,000 mg twice daily.

Silicon is a mineral that is involved in calcification and making collagen. Take 50 to 200 mg daily.

Zinc is required for enzymatic reactions that build bone. Take a daily total of 30 mg, along with 2 to 3 mg of copper.

Manganese helps with bone calcification. Take 15 to 30 mg daily.

A greens formula that contains super green foods, such as chlorella, spirulina, and others, has an alkalinizing effect and is rich in minerals. Take as directed on the container.

Soy protein powder has been shown to protect against bone loss. Take 40 grams daily; this amount contains 90 mg of isoflavones.

Strontium is a nutrient that was shown to be helpful in increasing bone density when combined with calcium. Take 340 to 680 mg daily.

Homeopathy

Pick the remedy that best matches your symptoms in this section. For acute fracture pain, take a 30C potency four times daily. For chronic fracture pain, take a 6x, 12x, 6C, 12C, or 30C potency twice daily for two weeks to see if there are any positive results. After you notice improvement, stop taking the remedy, unless symptoms return. Consultation with a homeopathic practitioner is advised.

Aconitum Napellus is used when people are in shock from a trauma. They are restless and fearful. Aconitum will help calm them down as you seek medical attention.

Arnica (*Arnica montana*) is the first remedy to give immediately after a fracture has occurred. This will help reduce pain, shock, and swelling. Give the highest potency available. Most health food stores carry a 30C potency; take it four times daily for two days.

Bryonia (*Bryonia alba*) is to be given during the first week of a fracture, when the slightest movement aggravates the pain. The person exhibits great irritability from the pain. Bryonia can be alternated with homeopathic Symphytum (*Symphytum officinale*).

Calcarea Carbonica is a remedy for people with signs of calcium imbalance, such as a slow-healing fracture, osteoporosis, aching bones, muscle cramps, and swollen joints. People requiring this remedy are generally chilly and flabby and feel worse in the cold and the dampness. They are easily fatigued and get overwhelmed. There is a craving for sweets, milk, and eggs.

Calcarea Phosphorica is a good remedy for fractures that are slow to heal. This remedy stimulates bone building.

Hypericum (*Hypericum perforatum*) is for crushing injuries that result in nerve damage. There are sharp, shooting pains. It is especially good for fractures of the coccyx (tailbone).

Phosphorus is a remedy for weak bones or fractures that heal slowly. People requiring this remedy tend to be tall and thin. There is a strong craving for ice-cold drinks. The person tends to be very social and suggestible.

Silica (*Silicea*) is for people who have poor bone density and tend to be very thin. People who need this remedy are often nervous, easily fatigued, and chilly and have low resistance to infection.

Symphytum (*Symphytum officinale*) is a specific remedy for healing and reducing fracture pain more quickly. Make sure to use it after a bone has been set.

Acupressure

See pages 668–675 for information about pressure points and administering treatment.

- To increase your ability to absorb nutrients (including calcium), work Stomach 36. With regular practice, your digestion will improve, and you'll find that you have more energy than before.
- If you have pain, work Large Intestine 4. Do not use this point if you are pregnant.

Bodywork

Massage

Massage is a good wellness measure after the fracture has been set, to encourage blood flow and healing.

Acupuncture

Acupuncture is recommended to help relieve the pain and the swelling from a fracture.

Magnet Therapy

Magnets can be used by a knowledgeable practitioner to reduce fracture pain and stimulate healing.

Reflexology

See pages 686–687 for information about reflexology areas and how to work them. Work the areas corresponding to the area of injury.

Aromatherapy

Black pepper and rosemary both have warming qualities that soothe aching bones and joints. Use them in a massage, a lotion, or a bath.

Hydrotherapy

Alternate hot and cold towels over the opposite body part affected. For example, if the left arm is broken, alternate a hot towel (two minutes) with a cold towel (two minutes) over the right arm, repeat three times, and perform twice daily. There is a reflex action whereby circulation will be increased in the opposite body part, which increases nutrition to the healing bone.

Bach Flower Remedies

Rescue Remedy is a good choice for the shock and the emotional stress brought on by a fracture. Take 10 drops twice daily.

Other Recommendations

- Start doing a regular weight-bearing exercise once you have been instructed to by your doctor, as it stimulates bone healing.
- Don't smoke or expose yourself to secondhand smoke. Smoking makes bones brittle and weak.

REFERENCES

Feskanich, D., P. Weber, W. C. Willett, H. Rockett, S. L. Booth, and G. A. Colditz. 1999. Vitamin K intake and hip fractures in women: A prospective study. *American Journal of Clinical Nutrition* 69(1):74–79.

Bronchitis

Acute bronchitis is the deep, wet, or dry cough that comes on and lingers after an infection, such as a cold, sinusitis, or the flu. The cough, which may start out dry and then turn productive, is the body's way of expelling infected mucus (phlegm) from the lungs. An episode of bronchitis may last for one to two weeks, and because a virus usually causes it, antibiotics may not be helpful. The best treatment is usually rest, combined with immune-enhancing natural therapies, as well as symptomatic therapy to calm the cough and promote removal of the mucus.

Chronic bronchitis develops in the continual presence of irritants, usually tobacco smoke, but also environmental allergies and damp, foggy weather; it sometimes results from food allergies. It often begins as a protracted case of acute bronchitis that returns every few months and, if the irritants are not removed, will develop into a constant cough, often accompanied by breathlessness and sometimes wheezing. The weakened condition of the lungs leaves the body vulnerable to infections like acute bronchitis, pneumonia, and emphysema. In its advanced stage, even minor colds can grow into deadly diseases. The best treatment is to eliminate the irritants that caused the condition. This is accomplished by identifying the offending allergens and removing them or reducing your body's sensitivity to them.

SYMPTOMS

Acute bronchitis

- A cough that may start out dry but that turns deep and productive, with thick clear or yellow mucus
- Usually follows a viral infection

Chronic bronchitis

- Long bouts of acute bronchitis that recur frequently
- A persistent, constant cough that's worse upon waking
- Breathlessness
- Wheezing

ROOT CAUSES

Acute bronchitis

- Food or environmental allergens, causing excess mucus in the lungs
- Viral infection

Chronic bronchitis

- Smoking or exposure to second-hand smoke
- Food allergies
- Environmental irritants (especially dust, pollen, animal dander, or mold)
- Cold, damp, foggy weather

TREATMENT

Diet

Recommended Food

To thin mucus secretions, drink a glass of clean water every two waking hours.

Homemade chicken soup also thins mucus. Add garlic or ginger for flavor and immune support.

To reduce phlegm, have some hot barley soup.

Onions are an old folk remedy and have anti-inflammatory properties, so eat them often.

If you have bacterial bronchitis and are taking antibiotics, consume nondairy sour products, such as kefir or sauerkraut, daily to replenish disease-fighting bacteria.

Food to Avoid

Eliminate foods that encourage mucus production: dairy products, chocolate, and bananas, as well as processed, refined, fried, and junk foods. Avoid simple sugars, as they suppress immune function.

Detoxification

Fast on water, soup, juice, and herbal tea for a few days to let your body turn its full attention to fighting the infection. Fasting will also speed the elimination of mucus, especially when expectorant herbal teas are part of the regimen. (See the herbal recommendations further on.)

℞ Super Seven Prescriptions—Bronchitis

Super Prescription #1   N-acetylcysteine (NAC)
NAC reduces the viscosity of phlegm so that it is easier to expectorate. It's useful for acute and chronic bronchitis (especially for smokers and people with asthma or emphysema). Take 300 to 500 mg twice daily.

Super Prescription #2   Homeopathy
Use a combination cough remedy, as directed on the container, or pick the remedy that best matches your symptoms under Homeopathy in this section. For acute

bronchitis, take a 30C potency four times daily. For chronic bronchitis, take twice daily for two weeks to see if there are any positive improvements. After you notice improvement, stop taking the remedy, unless symptoms return. Consultation with a homeopathic practitioner is advised.

Super Prescription #3   Vitamin C

Take 500 to 1,000 mg three times daily. It enhances immune function for acute bronchitis and has anti-allergy benefits for chronic bronchitis. Vitamin C is particularly important for smokers.

Super Prescription #4   Echinacea (*Echinacea purpurea*) and goldenseal (*Hydrastis canadensis*)

Take 500 mg or 2 ml of this combination four times daily for acute bronchitis with a wet cough. Both herbs enhance immune function, and goldenseal works to dry up mucus.

Super Prescription #5   Mullein (*Verbascum thapsus*)

Take 500 mg of the capsule or 2 ml of the tincture four times daily. This herb promotes the discharge of mucus and has soothing/anti-inflammatory effects for the respiratory tract.

Super Prescription #6   Astragalus (*Astragalus membranaceus*)

Astragalus is an excellent treatment for chronic, as well as acute, bronchitis. It strengthens weak lungs and increases the body's general resistance to infection. Take 500 to 1,000 mg or 3.5 ml of a tincture two or three times daily. Do not take astragalus if you have a fever.

Super Prescription #7   Colloidal silver

Take one-half to 1 teaspoon, or as directed on the container, three times daily for five days. It has an antimicrobial effect, especially for bacteria.

Testing Techniques

The following test helps assess possible metabolic reasons for chronic bronchitis:

Food and environmental allergy testing—blood or electrodermal

---

General Recommendations

Garlic (*Allium sativum*) has antimicrobial effects. Take 300 to 600 mg of garlic extract twice daily.

Licorice (*Glycyrrhiza glabra*) reduces coughing, enhances immune function, and soothes the respiratory tract. Use caution when supplementing licorice if you have high blood pressure. It's best used short term under the guidance of a holistic doctor. Take 500 mg of the capsule or 1 ml of the tincture four times daily.

Bromelain has a natural anti-inflammatory effect and enhances the effectiveness of some antibiotics. Take 500 mg three times daily between meals or along with antibiotic therapy. Look for products standardized to 2,000 M.C.U. (milk-clotting units) per 1,000 mg or 1,200 G.D.U. (gelatin-dissolving units) per 1,000 mg.

Vitamin A enhances immune function. Take 25,000 to 50,000 IU daily for five days.

Ivy leaf (*Hedera helix*) may be helpful for chronic bronchitis for both children and adults. Take as directed on the container.

Other useful herbs that can be found in respiratory formulas include horehound, pleurisy root, plantain, marshmallow, ginger, peppermint, and cherry bark.

Homeopathy

Antimonium Tartaricum is for a congested, wet cough that produces a rattling noise in the chest. The person has trouble expectorating and may find it hard to breathe at times. The person feels better in a cool room and with the windows open.

Arsenicum Album is for a cough with a burning pain that feels better from taking sips of warm drinks. The person feels anxious and restless and may be very fatigued. Symptoms are worse from 12 A.M. to 2 A.M.

Bryonia (*Bryonia alba*) will treat a dry cough that causes stitching pain in the throat or the chest and that is worse at night. Movement of any type feels worse. The person has a great thirst and prefers to be left alone.

Coccus Cacti is for a cough that produces stringy mucus. The person feels like constantly clearing the throat. Coughing often leads to vomiting.

Drosera is for a dry, barking cough that may end in gagging. The cough is worse when lying down and is also worse after midnight.

Hepar Sulphuris (*Hepar sulphuris calcareum*) is for a rattling, barking cough that comes on after exposure to dry, cold air. The person coughs when uncovered and feels chilly and irritable. There is often yellowish mucus.

Kali Bichromium is for a hoarse cough that produces thick, stringy, yellow mucus. The cough is worse from eating and drinking.

Phosphorous is for a dry, tickling cough that is worse in the cold air, with talking or laughing, and when lying on the left side. The person may have a burning sensation in the chest and feels better with cold drinks.

Pulsatilla (*Pulsatilla pratensis*) will clear up a cough with yellow or green phlegm that is looser in the morning and drier at night. The person has a low thirst and feels better near an open window. The cough is worse when the person lies down.

Rumex Crispus is for a dry cough that begins as soon as a person lies down. The person feels a tickling sensation in the throat that leads to a cough. The cough is worse in cold air.

Silica (*Silicea*) is for someone who seems to have bronchitis all winter long. The person has weak immunity and low stamina and feels chilly. Coughing up mucus takes a lot of effort.

Spongia Tosta helps when one has a dry, barking cough that is better after ingesting warm foods or liquids.

Sulphur is for bronchitis with burning pains that are better after having cold drinks. The person feels warm and desires a cool room. Sulphur is often used after a long bout of bronchitis, for complete recovery.

Acupressure

See pages 668–675 for information about pressure points and administering treatment.

- To relieve chest congestion, massage Kidney 27, Conception Vessel 22, and Lung 1 and 7.
- If you have difficulty breathing and need to calm your emotions, use Bladder 38.

Bodywork

Massage

A back massage will break up excess phlegm. If you have chronic bronchitis, you might want to schedule regular sessions with a professional massage therapist. If you're generally a strong and healthy person, ask your therapist to use percussive motions, which are highly effective at releasing phlegm. People who suffer from an occasional bout of acute bronchitis might prefer to rely on a loved one to perform this task each evening.

Hydrotherapy

Sit in a hot, steamy bath or a sauna to thin mucus secretions and sweat out toxins. If you have hypertension, do not use saunas.

Constitutional hydrotherapy works well for acute and chronic bronchitis. Follow the directions for treatment on pages 676–677.

Aromatherapy

Add eucalyptus, peppermint, lemon balm, or tree tea oil to a hot bath or a steam inhalation to drain congestion. You can also add any of these oils to a base oil and rub it directly onto your chest.

Stress Reduction

General Stress-Reduction Therapies

Stress can weaken your immune system, leaving your lungs open to infection. If you're vulnerable to frequent bouts of bronchitis, or if you suffer from chronic bronchitis, experiment with the techniques in the Exercise and Stress Reduction chapter until you find ones you like. Practice them on a daily basis, or more often as needed.

Bach Flower Remedies

Select the remedy that meets your needs, and place 10 drops of the liquid under your tongue. Hold the drops in place for thirty seconds and swallow. Use as often as needed.

Take Clematis if you tend to give in whenever you feel a respiratory infection coming on.

Red Chestnut is for people who worry a great deal about their loved ones, even to the extent of neglecting themselves.

Other Recommendations

- Rest, preferably in bed, while the illness is at its worst. When you feel better, move around to keep the infection from settling into your lungs, but continue to rest after periods of activity.
- Don't take a cough suppressant. The lungs need to expel phlegm to get healthy, and suppressants keep them from doing so. Consistent use of suppressants can lead to worse cases of acute bronchitis or even to chronic bronchitis or pneumonia.
- Encourage expectoration by applying warm compresses to your chest.
- Don't smoke or expose yourself to secondhand smoke.

- If you have chronic bronchitis and live in a damp, cold climate, you may have to move to another location that's dry and warm. You should have your doctor consider mold allergies as a possible cause of chronic bronchitis.
- People with chronic bronchitis need to keep their lungs as elastic and strong as possible. Exercise, breath deeply, and, if you enjoy music, take up a wind instrument.

Bruises

A bruise is an injury caused by a blow or a bump that does not cut the skin but breaks blood vessels underneath the skin. Blood seeps out of these vessels, producing the tell-tale black-and-blue discoloration, as well as swelling and soreness.

The deeper the bruise, or contusion, the longer it will take to heal. Leg bruises, for instance, can linger for up to four weeks because leg vessels have greater blood pressure than arm vessels.

Bruises also change in color, first starting off red, then becoming blackish-blue, and finally turning yellowish-green. The final color is a sign that the body has worked to remove the dead cells and tissues and replace them with healthy, new cells to restore color to the skin.

Falls, sprains, pinches, and suction can cause bruises. These are occupational hazards for active children who love to run, jump, bike, climb, or skate. People who are anemic or obese tend to bruise easily. Nutritional deficiencies of vitamin C, iron, vitamin K, bioflavonoids, and other nutrients can contribute to easy bruising. Sometimes, unexplained bruising can be a clue that a person's blood vessel walls are brittle or that a child has insufficient blood-clotting factors. Bruising can also signal the onset of serious illnesses such as leukemia or hemophilia.

Parents should have their child's bruise examined by a doctor if

- The bruise is located on the head or the eye areas.
- Bruising seems to show up without any apparent cause.
- A minor bump or blow creates a large bruise.
- Bruises are located in unusual places, such as the back, the calves, or the backs of the arms.
- Your child has difficulty talking, walking, or seeing, or appears drowsy and dizzy.

People of all ages should see a doctor if a fever accompanies the bruising or for bruises that do not heal.

Medications such as aspirin and other blood thinners like Coumadin can cause bruising. Check with your doctor if you use one or more of these medications to see if it is related to your bruising.

If your doctor has determined that your bruising occurs as the result of anemia, see the Anemia section for more information.

SYMPTOMS

- Red, black and blue, or yellowish skin discoloration

ROOT CAUSES

- Trauma to soft tissues
- Anemia
- Clotting disorders or other underlying medical conditions

Testing Techniques

The following tests help assess possible reasons for chronic bruising:

Immune system imbalance or disease—blood

Hormone testing (thyroid)—saliva, blood, or urine

Intestinal permeability—urine

Vitamin and mineral analysis (especially iron, B12, folic acid, vitamin C, and vitamin K)—blood

Digestive function and microbe/parasite/candida testing—stool analysis

Anemia—blood test (CBC, iron, ferritin, % saturation)

Food and environmental allergies/sensitivities—blood, electrodermal

TREATMENT

Diet

Recommended Food

Dark-green leafy vegetables provide many minerals that help heal bruising, such as vitamin C and vitamin K.

Citrus fruits, bell peppers, and other brightly colored vegetables and fruits provide bioflavonoids that help heal bruises.

Fish such as salmon, nuts like walnuts, and seeds such as flaxseeds provide essential fatty acids that are necessary for tissue repair.

Brussels sprouts, broccoli, potatoes, and many citrus fruits are good sources of vitamin C.

Food to Avoid

Reduce or eliminate sugars, as they interrupt the healing of tissue.

Avoid saturated, hydrogenated, and trans-fatty acids found in meat and packaged, processed foods, as they interfere with the healing of cells.

In one early clinical trial, 74 boxers who regularly suffered bruising on the face, the lips, the ears, the chest, and the arms were given bromelain. When bromelain was given 4 times a day, all signs of bruising disappeared by the fourth day among 58 of the boxers. In contrast, those in a control group receiving a placebo required 7 to 14 days before the bruises healed.

℞ Super Seven Prescriptions—Bruises

Super Prescription #1   Homeopathic Arnica (*Arnica montana*)
Take a 30C potency four times daily for five days. Arnica is a specific remedy for healing bruises and soft tissue injuries.

Super Prescription #2   Bromelain
Take 500 mg three times daily between meals. Look for products standardized to 2,000 M.C.U. (milk-clotting units) per 1,000 mg or 1,200 G.D.U. (gelatin-dissolving units) per 1,000 mg. Bromelain has a natural anti-inflammatory effect. Protease enzyme products also have this benefit.

Super Prescription #3   Vitamin C
Take 500 to 1,000 mg three times daily. Vitamin C is used to manufacture collagen, the protein that holds blood vessels and connective tissue together. Vitamin C also improves wound healing.

Super Prescription #4   Bioflavonoids

Take a 500 mg complex three times daily. Bioflavonoids such as rutin and hesperedin act similarly to vitamin C and improve vitamin C's therapeutic effect.

Super Prescription #5   Arnica oil (*Arnica montana*)

Apply arnica oil topically over the area of the bruise twice daily. This herb in oil form has anti-inflammatory benefits. Do not use on broken skin.

Super Prescription #6   Vitamin K

Take 2 mg daily for two weeks for an acute bruise and 500 mcg daily to prevent bruising. Vitamin K is involved with the blood-clotting process. *Note:* Do not use if you are taking blood-thinning medications.

Super Prescription #7   High-potency multivitamin

This provides a base of the nutrients required for healthy blood vessels. Take as directed on the container.

General Recommendations

Essential fatty acids, as found in fish oil or flaxseed oil, are required for tissue healing. Take 3 grams of fish oil daily or 1 tablespoon of flaxseed oil. A greens formula that contains super green foods, such as chlorella, spirulina, and others, has an alkalinizing effect and is rich in minerals such as vitamins K and C, which promote healing of the soft tissue. Take as directed on the container.

Maritime pine bark or grape seed extract are rich sources of proanthocyandins, which promote tissue healing. Take 50 mg twice daily.

Homeopathy

Pick the remedy that best matches your symptoms in this section. For acute bruises, take a 30C potency four times daily. For chronic bruising, take a 6x, 12x, 6C, 12C, or 30C twice daily for two weeks to see if there are any positive results. After you notice improvement, stop taking the remedy, unless symptoms return. Consultation with a homeopathic practitioner is advised.

Arnica (*Arnica montana*) is for any injury to the soft tissues and will treat or prevent bruising. Arnica is generally the first remedy to use for bruising. It's also used for early-stage sprains and strains that result in bruising. The injury feels bruised and sore. Symptoms are worse from touch and motion and feel better with a cold compress and in the open air.

Bellis Perennis is for bruising of the deep and internal tissues, especially of the abdomen, the back, and the breasts. It is also used for bruises that do not respond to Arnica. Swelling and tumors may occur at the site of the injury. Symptoms are worse from cold bathing and touch. Improvements are noted from movement and rubbing the injury.

Ferrum Phosphoricum is the indicated remedy when bruising occurs as the result of anemia.

Hamamelis is a good choice when there is intense soreness associated with a bruise; it is especially good for injuries to the veins and for black eyes. One's symptoms are worse with pressure and cold applications.

Ledum (*Ledum palustre*) should be used for bruises that are a result of puncture wounds. It is also used for bruising that results from sprains and strains, such as a sprained ankle. Symptoms feel better with cold applications.

Ruta (*Ruta graveolens*) is useful for bruising of bone coverings, such as the shinbone, or from a cartilage or joint injury.

Sulphuricum Acidum is for large, red or black-blue, itchy bruises that do not heal, especially after using Arnica. The person feels weak from the injury.

Bodywork

Aromatherapy

Add 2 drops of lavender oil to a carrier oil, and rub over the bruise twice daily.

Hydrotherapy

Ice the bruise for the first twenty-four hours, then alternate hot (one minute) and cold cloths (one minute) over the affected area and repeat four times. Perform twice daily. This improves circulation to the injury site and speeds up healing.

REFERENCES

Blonstein, J. L. 1960. Control of swelling in boxing injuries. *Practitioner* 185:78.

Bulimia. *See* Eating Disorders

Burns (including Sunburn)

Few injuries are more frightening or painful than a serious burn. The skin may be burned from heat, steam, scalding liquids, the sun, chemicals, or electricity. Treatment is based on the type of burn, the severity of the burn, the location of the burn, and the source of the burn. Severe burns can destroy all skin layers and damage the underlying muscle and fat.

Heat burns can be caused by wet heat, such as scalding hot water, or dry heat, caused by a flame. These burns are classified by degree. A first-degree burn affects only the skin surface and is considered the most minor of all burns. The skin is usually red and slightly swollen. A second-degree burn affects the skin surface and the layer just beneath the skin surface. Blisters and swelling may occur. A third-degree burn, the most serious, results in white or blackened skin layers, is extremely painful, and involves all layers of the skin.

Chemical burns are caused by caustic substances that can be either acidic or alkaline. If the source of the burn is acidic, use water to wash the chemical off the wound. If the source of the burning agent is alkaline, it is vital not to wet the wound because that can cause further burning. Symptoms of chemical burns include redness of the skin, blistering, swelling, and peeling.

Electrical burns are caused by electric shock. It is important to realize that the body is electrically charged and that the heart functions on tiny pulses of electricity. Electrical burns have the potential to disrupt the heartbeat and cause cardiac and respiratory arrest. Be aware that severe electrical burns quite often do not display much damage on the surface layer of skin. The real damage is deeper in the layers underneath.

Consult your doctor about your burn under the following circumstances:

- All electrical burns
- Any burn located on the face, the mouth, the hands, or the genitals
- Any burn that covers more than 10 percent of the body or completely encircles an arm or a leg
- Any burn that blisters or turns the skin white
- Any burn that remains red or oozes longer than twenty-four hours and intensifies in pain

Natural therapies can be very effective in relieving the pain of minor burns and, to some degree, major burns (along with pain medicines). They are even more effective in promoting faster skin healing and may help in the prevention of secondary skin infections.

SYMPTOMS

- Burning sensation and damage of the skin

ROOT CAUSES

- Heat, chemicals, or electricity

TREATMENT

Diet

Recommended Food

Drink electrolyte drinks and plenty of water to replace lost fluids.

Citrus fruits, bell peppers, and other brightly colored vegetables and fruits provide bioflavonoids that help heal the skin.

Fish such as salmon, nuts like walnuts, and seeds such as flaxseeds provide essential fatty acids that are necessary for tissue repair.

Brussels sprouts, broccoli, potatoes, and many citrus fruits are good sources of vitamin C, which helps heal the skin.

Food to Avoid

Reduce or eliminate sugars, as they interrupt the healing of tissue.

℞ Super Seven Prescriptions—Burns

Super Prescription #1   Homeopathic Cantharis (*Cantharis vesicator*)
Take a 30C potency four to six times daily for acute burns, including sunburns. This remedy prevents or reduces blistering and burn pain.

Super Prescription #2   Aloe vera
Choose an aloe gel product (80 percent or higher) and apply to the burned area twice daily. Aloe has a soothing effect and may stimulate skin healing.

Super Prescription #3   L-glutamine
Take 500 to 1,000 mg three times daily on an empty stomach or in the intravenous form given by your doctor. L-glutamine is required for tissue healing and to prevent secondary infection that often occurs with burns.

Super Prescription #4   Zinc
Take 30 mg twice daily, along with 2 mg of copper. Zinc promotes skin healing.

L-glutamine is proving to be a valuable supplement for burns. It is currently used orally and in intravenous methods to increase body levels of this healing nutrient. One study of people with burns serious enough to require hospitalization found that oral glutamine supplementation resulted in a shorter hospital stay.

> **Super Prescription #5   Calendula** (*Calendula officinalis*)
> This herb can be used topically in the liquid or gel form to help heal burns. Apply twice daily.
>
> **Super Prescription #6   Mixed carotenoids**
> Take 25,000 IU of a mixed carotenoid complex daily to protect against sunburns. Carotenoids help to absorb the UV rays of the sun.
>
> **Super Prescription #7   Antioxidant complex**
> Take a complex composed of antioxidants such as vitamins E, C, selenium, and others, which will neutralize free radical damage as the result of burns, including sunburns.

General Recommendations

Topical creams that contain vitamins C and E, CoQ10, and carotenoids may be helpful in preventing sunburns. Apply as directed on the container.

Vitamin C promotes skin healing. Take 1,000 mg three times daily. Reduce the dosage if loose stools occur.

Vitamin E is a good antioxidant that helps with tissue healing. Take 400 IU daily. Vitamin E gel, cream, or oil can be applied topically for burn healing.

Propolis is a bee product that speeds healing of a burn and prevents secondary infections. It's available as a spray, a salve, or a tincture.

Manuka honey, applied to burns, helps to speed healing and prevent infection. This is commonly done in countries such as New Zealand.

Colloidal silver is used topically to prevent secondary skin infections.

Homeopathy

Pick the remedy that best matches your symptoms in this section. For acute burns, take a 30C potency four times daily. For chronic burn pain, take a 6x, 12x, 6C, 12C, or 30C potency twice daily for two weeks to see if there are any positive results. After you notice improvement, stop taking the remedy, unless symptoms return. Consultation with a homeopathic practitioner is advised.

Apis (*Apis mellifica*) is for burns characterized by stinging, burning pains that feel better from cool applications and worse from warmth. The skin is hot, dry, and puffy and may have small vesicles.

Arsenicum Album is for people with burning skin pain that are worse from cold and better from warm applications. They are restless, anxious, and weak. It is also for severe burns that turn blue or black.

Cantharis (*Cantharis vesicator*) is for intense scalding burns or sunburns. This remedy is used for any burn but particularly for second- or third-degree burns. Cold water gives relief to the pain.

Causticum is indicated for severe burns, especially caustic chemical burns, and for old burns that do not heal. Symptoms are worse from dry, cold drafts and better from warmth or damp weather.

Hypericum (*Hypericum perforatum*) is a remedy for burns that affect the nerves and cause a sharp, radiating nerve pain.

Phosphorous is a specific remedy for electrical shocks and burns.

Rhus Toxicodendron is a good choice when the skin has itching, burning vesicles. The person is restless. Symptoms feel better from applying hot water to the burn and feel worse in cold air.

Urtica Urens is a good remedy to use if Cantharis (*Cantharis vesicator*) is not helpful. The person experiences scalding, burning pain, and fluid-filled blisters. It is mainly used for first- and second-degree burns.

Bodywork

Electrical acupuncture has been shown to reduce the pain associated with burns. See a qualified practitioner for treatment.

Other Bodywork Recommendations

Magnet therapy can be effective in reducing pain and stimulating skin healing. Use under the guidance of a knowledgeable practitioner.

REFERENCES

Zhou, Y., Y. Sun, Z. Jiang, G. He, and N. Yang. 2002. [The effects of glutamine dipeptide on the improvement of endotoxemia in severely burned patients.] *Zhonghua Shao Shang Za Zhi* 18(6):343–45.

Cancer

Almost all the cells in our bodies must be replaced on a regular basis. Some cells, like those that make up the intestinal lining, die out quickly and are replaced every few days. In other parts of the body, the cells live for years before they divide and form new ones. Under special circumstances, such as an injury or an illness, healthy new cells may grow more quickly than usual to replace those that are damaged. When the area is healed, the cell growth slows back down to its normal rate.

Normally, the genes that control the growth of cells automatically know when to start and stop the replication process. But when those genes are mutated—perhaps because of an inherited flaw, or more commonly, because of dietary and environmental factors—cells may begin to multiply and divide at an unusually fast rate. Eventually, these cells form a lump. Sometimes lumps are benign (meaning that they are noncancerous and relatively harmless), as in the case of warts or uterine fibroids. Other growths, however, are malignant. They pull nutrients away from the healthy tissues that surround them, and they interfere with the body's normal functions, to a potentially life-threatening extent. If a tumor continues to grow, its cells may spread via the blood vessels or the lymphatic system to other parts of the body, where they form new tumors. Once this process, called metastasis, is underway, there is a risk of dying from the complications that can occur. Although many cancers can be treated successfully when caught early, the sad fact remains that they are the second-leading cause of death in the United States. Every minute, another person dies of some form of the disease.

The word *cancer* refers to the process of uncontrolled cell division, but, technically, it is not, in itself, the name of a specific disorder. Instead, *cancer* is an umbrella term that refers to more than one hundred different kinds of diseases, which are generally named according to the area where a tumor first appears. In men, prostate cancer is most common; in women, breast cancer is most frequent. But both of these cancers can be highly treatable when caught early. Lung cancer is common and one of the deadliest. Cancer also tends to strike the skin, the urinary tract, the colorectal region, and the female reproductive organs, although it can attack anywhere. It's beyond the scope of this book to discuss each individual type of cancer, but the suggestions here apply to anyone who is fighting off a tumor, wants to keep a cancer in remission, or hopes to avoid developing cancer in the first place. We also have recommendations on what to take if you are undergoing chemotherapy and/or radiation, to reduce side effects and optimize immune function, as well as outcome.

Scientists break cancers down into four very broad categories, and if you're trying to communicate with your doctor or keep up with medical literature, it's helpful to understand the difference among them. Carcinomas affect soft tissues in organs and glands, like the skin, the breasts, the lungs, and the pancreas. Sarcomas, which are quite rare, occur in solid tissues, especially bone, muscle, and cartilage. Lymphomas appear in the lymphatic system. Leukemias are cancers of the tissues that form blood; these cancers are unusual, in that they don't form hard tumors.

As with so many other chronic and deadly diseases, researchers have not been able to pinpoint the cause of uncontrolled, cancerous cell growth, despite decades of hard work and billions of dollars in funding. It's likely that there isn't just one cause. We know, for example, that faulty genes play a role in some cancers—but most people with genetic flaws aren't doomed to develop cancer; they simply have a greater chance of doing so. Although a family history of cancer carries with it increased risk, most cancer researchers agree that as a sole cause, genetics is relatively insignificant, accounting for only 5 to 15 percent of cancers. It appears that most cancers are caused by largely controllable factors, such as nutrition, lifestyle, and environmental factors. One of the criticisms of conventional medicine in preventing and treating cancer is that diet, lifestyle, stress, and the ability to rid the body of environmental toxins rarely are addressed in a comprehensive fashion. Yet these factors are both most influential and most controllable in the prevention of cancer, and they play important roles in the recovery from cancer. To reduce the risk of developing cancer, we all need to reduce free-radical formation in the body, limit exposure to dietary and environmental sources of free radicals, and increase our intake of antioxidant nutrients.

We also know that environmental carcinogens like cigarette smoke, man-made food, and pollution can have a devastating effect on the body. These toxins encourage the formation of free radicals, and many experts now believe that these unbalanced molecules contribute to uncontrolled cell growth. People with strong immune systems and high levels of antioxidants—the substances that neutralize free radicals—are in a much better position to stave off tumor growth. But again, not everyone exposed to high levels of carcinogens or with a weakened immune system will necessarily suffer from cancer. An increasing amount of research is demonstrating how the effects of stress may be the root cause for some people. In all probability, a combination of several factors leads to this group of diseases.

Since we can't control the genes we inherit (not yet, anyway), it's wise for people who are battling cancer or who want to prevent it to turn their attention to things we can control. First things first: Early detection is the key to successful treatment, so have regular checkups and cancer screenings, as are appropriate for your age, sex, and medical history. Learn the warning signs of cancer, and contact a doctor immediately if one shows up on your body. Aside from these common-sense strategies, you must do everything you can to support your immune system and increase your intake of antioxidants, while minimizing your exposure to environmental toxins. You should also

Toxins That Cause Cell DNA Damage

- Pesticides and herbicides
- Toxic metals
- Tobacco
- Alcohol
- Metabolites of poor digestion and elimination
- Radiation

cleanse your body by drinking lots of clean water and eating plenty of fiber. Periodic fasts will further detoxify your system. Your liver is one of the most crucial organs for cancer defense; under normal conditions, it filters out toxins and helps them pass out of the body. But when unhealthful food, pollution, or other carcinogens overtax

Recommended Screening Tests for Cancer

Regular screening tests can help you and your doctor detect any cancerous growths at the earliest possible stage. When cancer is caught early, your chances of healing rise dramatically. Early detection also gives you a broader range of treatment options, along with more time to consider the ones that are right for you.

Breast exams and mammograms: Every woman should practice a monthly self-examination of her breasts. If you find any kind of change—a lump, dimpling of the skin, a swelling, an unexplained discharge from the nipples, or a rash—contact your doctor. In addition to self-exams, women should get a yearly breast examination by a health-care professional. And women over forty should receive mammograms as directed by their doctors.

Colon and rectal exams: If you're fifty or older, your doctor should give you a digital rectal exam (DRE) every year. Because the first sign of colorectal cancer is blood in the stool, you should also have an annual stool test for occult, or hidden, blood.

Oral exams: Be sure that your dentist examines your entire mouth during your twice-yearly visits. He or she should perform a manual, as well as a visual, inspection of your oral cavity and your neck.

Pap tests: All women over the age of eighteen, as well as younger women who are sexually active, should have annual Pap tests to screen for cervical cancer. The Pap test can detect precancerous cervical changes; with a relatively simple outpatient procedure, your doctor can stop cancer before it starts. If you've had three negative Pap tests in a row and have never had a positive result, your doctor may allow you to reduce the frequency of the exams.

Prostate exams and PSA tests: If you're a man age forty years or older, your doctor should perform manual prostate exams at your yearly checkup. Starting at age fifty, you should also have a prostate-specific antigen (PSA) blood test. Men who have a family history of prostate cancer should begin PSA tests a little earlier, at age forty-five.

Pelvic exams: In addition to Pap tests, women should have yearly pelvic exams to check for ovarian cancer. A doctor will feel your ovaries and uterus to make sure they're healthy.

Skin exams: Everyone, even people who have avoided the sun, should have a skin exam during his or her yearly physical. It's also wise to perform a self-exam once every month. Use a full-length mirror, as well as a hand mirror, to check places that are hard to see, like your back, as well as the backs of your knees and your upper thighs. If you detect any changes, give your doctor a call.

Testicular exams: Men should have their testes examined during their annual check-up. While self-exams are generally not necessary, you should be alert to any changes in your testicles. If you find a lump or any other change, call your doctor.

it, some of those toxins are reabsorbed into the body, where they may encourage cancerous growths. Good nutrition and a detoxification plan will support your liver, but you'll also want to give it a boost with cleansing herbs. And because stress can produce free radicals and lower immunity, it's also important to find measures that release tension and get your stress levels under control.

As most of us know, the conventional measures for treating cancer—chemotherapy, radiation, and surgical removal of the tumor or the affected organ—are extremely harsh and sometimes even life-threatening. There are also highly promising reports of dietary and supplementation therapies that have caused cancer remission in some people, but as yet, we have few studies that can actually prove their effectiveness. Talk to your doctor, do some research, and weigh the pro's and cons of the different treatments available for your type of cancer. If you choose to undergo chemotherapy or other conventional treatments, try to find a doctor who is sympathetic to your desire to incorporate natural strategies into your healing process. Dietary changes, herbs, and other natural treatments can significantly reduce your discomfort and boost your ability to fight the disease.

ROOT CAUSES

There is no single cause of cancer, but the factors that are tied to a greater likelihood of developing cancer are listed as follows:

- Genetic flaws
- Environmental toxins, including pollution, toxic metals, and radiation
- A poor diet, especially one high in fat, additives, pesticides, and improperly prepared meats
- A toxic liver
- Viruses and other stealth infections
- A weakened immune system
- Stress
- Poor digestion and detoxification
- Lack of exercise
- Nutritional deficiencies
- Certain medical therapies (such as synthetic hormone replacement related to breast cancer)

Testing Techniques

The following tests help assess possible reasons for cancer:

Immune system imbalance or disease—blood

Genetic defects—blood, saliva

Hormone testing (thyroid, DHEA, cortisol, testosterone, IGF-1, estrogen, progesterone)—saliva, blood, or urine

Intestinal permeability—urine

Detoxification profile—urine

Oxidative stress—urine or blood

Vitamin and mineral analysis (especially magnesium, B12, iron, and CoQ10)—blood

Digestive function and microbe/parasite/candida testing—stool analysis

Food and environmental allergies/sensitivities—blood, electrodermal

Blood-sugar and insulin balance—blood

SYMPTOMS

Cancers often grow for years, even decades, before they manifest in symptoms. Nevertheless, there are some early warning signs you should watch for. If you experience any of the following symptoms, don't panic. Most likely, you don't have cancer: the symptoms of cancerous growths are similar or identical to the symptoms of many other illnesses, often ones that are much less frightening. Nevertheless, you should see your doctor right away for an accurate diagnosis. If you do have a cancerous growth, the sooner you start treatment, the better your chances of sending the disease into permanent remission.

- A mole, a wart, or a blemish that changes in diameter, shape, color, or thickness
- A sore that doesn't heal within three weeks
- A lump or a swelling under the skin
- Thickening of the skin on any part of your body
- Chronic indigestion or difficulty swallowing
- A change in bowel or bladder habits
- Blood in the urine or the stool
- Rectal bleeding
- An unexplained vaginal discharge or bleeding between periods
- Recurring headaches
- An unexplained loss of weight or appetite
- An unexplained pain, especially in the bones
- A persistent low-grade fever
- Recurrent infections
- Hoarseness that lingers for more than a week
- A persistent cough or a cough that brings up blood
- Persistent fatigue, nausea, or vomiting

TREATMENT

Diet

Dietary therapies for cancer seek to return your body to its natural state of balance and health. Focus on a diet of whole foods, as outlined in this chapter, which optimize immune function and detoxification.

Recommended Food

Wherever possible, eat clean, live foods. Look for food that's organically grown. If you're eating poultry, check the label to be sure the animal was not raised on antibiotics or other unnatural substances. When buying fish, ask whether the product comes from a clean water source.

When the liver processes toxins, cancer-promoting free radicals are produced in high quantities. Of all the antioxidants, glutathione is the best at counteracting the free radicals created during this process. Asparagus, avocados, broccoli, brussels sprouts, cabbage, and walnuts are all excellent sources of glutathione. Make it a priority to put one or more of these foods on your menu every day.

Eat as many raw vegetables and fruits as possible, especially those that have deep, rich colors. These foods are high in fiber, which helps flush toxins from your system, and they're potent sources of antioxidants. When you eat them raw, you will also retain their natural enzymes, which help you digest food and absorb the maximum amount of nutrients into your bloodstream.

For even more fiber, eat plenty of whole grains, including oats and brown rice.

Eat wheat germ, nuts, and seeds for their vitamin E content. Vitamin E is another powerful antioxidant.

Garlic, onions, and legumes will help keep your liver functioning at optimum capacity.

Fermented soy products, such as tofu, tempeh, and miso, appear to have anticancer properties, based on population studies. Consume these products three to four times weekly, unless you are sensitive to soy products. (But don't take isoflavone extracts. Their effects on the body are still unknown.)

If you're battling cancer, you don't need to be told how important it is to keep up your strength and energy. Eat lean protein from beans, eggs, tofu, poultry, or fish. People undergoing conventional cancer therapy require increased protein intake to prevent tissue wasting.

Studies in Japan show that in areas where people drink green tea, there are significantly lower rates of stomach, esophageal, and liver cancer. It also acts as a mild stimulant of the immune system.

Tomatoes are high in lycopene, a substance that's been shown to prevent and even help counteract prostate cancer. Cooked tomatoes are higher in lycopene than raw ones are.

Make sure to drink plenty of clean water to promote healthy detoxification. Fresh juicing with vegetable and fruit juices is highly advised. Try to consume 8 to 10 ounces a day of a variety of juices.

For extra fiber and cancer-fighting phytonutrients known as lignans, take 4 tablespoons of ground flaxseeds daily with 10 ounces of water.

Food to Avoid

Do not eat foods that don't come from nature. Processed food, junk food, and anything containing chemicals, additives, or dyes should be banished from your menu.

Make every effort to avoid foods that have been sprayed, waxed, or otherwise treated. If you absolutely cannot avoid eating these foods, at least be sure to remove their peels, skins, or outer layers and to wash the food thoroughly in clean water before eating.

While there's no evidence that refined sugar directly causes cancer, we do know that too much of it significantly depresses your immune system. A weak immune system may leave you vulnerable to cancer, and it can also sap your ability to handle aggressive cancer treatment. Do not eat products containing refined sugar. This includes sodas, candy, cakes, and cookies, as well as store-bought juices and many processed foods. You should also restrict your intake of natural sugars. Go easy on homemade fruit juices and baked goods sweetened with molasses or honey.

Saturated, hydrogenated, and partially hydrogenated fats are linked to most degenerative disorders, and cancer is no exception. High consumption of these "bad" fats (as opposed to the "good" essential fatty acids found in cold-pressed oils and some fish) has been strongly linked to several types of cancer, including breast, prostate, and colorectal cancers. Avoid red meat, butter, margarine, shortening, and products made with these foods. Especially carcinogenic are meats that have been grilled, charcoal-broiled, cured, or smoked. If you're trying to prevent cancer and want to enjoy red meat as an occasional treat, it would be wise to stay away from meats prepared in any of these manners, including hot dogs, cold cuts, and luncheon meats, as well as most types of bacon, ham, and sausage.

Be wary of alcohol. Heavy use is linked to mouth and throat cancers and possibly to cancer of the stomach, the colon, and the rectum. If you're a healthy person trying to avoid cancer, limit yourself to a glass or two of wine per week. If you have cancer, it's best to avoid alcohol entirely, as it depletes much-needed nutrients from your body.

Detoxification

If you've been diagnosed with cancer, make regular detoxification a priority. Do a 3-day juice fast once every month; once every 6 months, do a longer fast—for 5 or 7 days. People who are in an advanced stage of cancer should use common sense: although it's normal to have some bodily response like headaches or nausea while fasting, you should stop if those responses become severe or unbearable. Instead, simply add juices to your normal good diet.

None of us can completely avoid exposure to toxins, no matter how well we eat or change our lifestyle habits, so a person hoping to avoid cancer would do well to practice regular short fasts. You do not need to undertake the longer fasts recommended for a person diagnosed with cancer. Try doing a three-day juice fast once a month, or fast one day out of every week. These should be done under medical supervision.

Coriolus enhances a disease-free period after colon cancer surgery. A 10-year, randomized, double-blind trial was performed by administering coriolus (PSK) to 56 patients and a placebo to another group of 55 patients after surgical operations on their colorectal cancers. The rate of patients in remission (or disease-free) was significantly higher (more than doubled) in the PSK group than in the placebo group. Researchers also found that the white blood cells for the PSK group showed "remarkable enhancement in their activities."

Maitake Cancer Study

A total of 33 cancer patients in stages II, III, and IV, ages 33 to 68, participated in this trial. Data was collected under the cooperation of their medical doctors in Japan. Patients were given either MD fraction with tablets only, or MD fraction and tablets in addition to chemotherapy. Cancer regression or significant symptom improvement was observed in 11 out of 16 breast cancer patients, 7 out of 12 liver cancer patients, and 5 out of 8 lung cancer patients.

℞ Super Seven Prescriptions—Cancer

Super Prescription #1   Coriolus versicolor (*Trametes versicolor*)
Take 1,000 mg three times daily of the PSP or PSK standardized extracts on an empty stomach. Coriolus contains polysaccharides that have been shown to enhance immune function. It is mainly used for esophageal, lung, stomach, and colon cancer. *Note:* It can be safely used in conjunction with conventional treatment (surgery, chemotherapy, and radiation).

Super Prescription #2   Maitake (*Grifola frondosa*l)
Take 0.5 to 1 mg of the standardized MD or D fraction per kg of body weight per day in divided doses on an empty stomach. Maitake enhances immune cells that fight cancer. It was found to be most effective for breast, prostate, liver, and lung cancers. *Note:* It can be safely used in conjunction with conventional treatment (surgery, chemotherapy, and radiation).

Super Prescription #3   Proteolytic enzymes
Take a complex of proteolytic enzymes (dependent on the dose of the formula, take as directed on the container) three times daily between meals. Proteolytic enzymes have been

Coriolus Alleviates Side Effects of Chemotherapy and Radiation

A study at the University of Shanghai examined whether coriolus polysaccharides (PSP) could lessen the side effects of chemotherapy or radiation. In this study, 650 people with cancer who were undergoing chemotherapy and radiation were given either PSP or a placebo, and their side effects were assessed. Researchers used twenty different criteria to assess adverse reactions and determined that people receiving PSP had markedly fewer side effects than did those receiving placebo.

shown to have numerous anticancer effects. *Note:* They can be safely used in conjunction with conventional treatment (surgery—except not three days before or after surgery—chemotherapy, and radiation).

Super Prescription #4 Astragalus (*Astragalus membranaceus*)
Take 1,000 mg or 4 ml of the tincture three times daily. Astragalus enhances natural killer and other immune cells that fight cancer. *Note:* It can be safely used in conjunction with conventional treatment (surgery, chemotherapy, and radiation).

Super Prescription #5 Vitamin C
Take 5,000 to 10,000 mg or higher in divided doses. One technique is to build up to as high a dose as you can tolerate. When diarrhea occurs, cut back on the dosage. *Note:* Vitamin C can be administered in very therapeutic levels by a doctor who was trained in intravenous therapy.

Super Prescription #6 Curcumin
Take 400 mg of curcumin extract three times daily on an empty stomach. This extract from turmeric has many different anticancer effects. *Note:* It can be safely used in conjunction with conventional treatment (surgery, chemotherapy, and radiation).

Super Prescription #7 Essiac
Essiac is a combination of detoxifying herbs derived from an ancient Indian healing formula, and it has attained a reputation for great success in treating cancers of all kinds. When buying Essiac—many brands use the name—look for the following set of herbs: sheep sorrel, burdock root (*Articum lappa*), slippery elm (*Ulmus fulva*), rhubarb root, watercress, blessed thistle (*Cnicus benedictus*), red clover (*Trifolium pratense*), and kelp (*Ascophyllum nodosum*). Essiac is most potent as a tincture or a tea; take as directed on the package label.

℞ Super Seven Prescriptions—Cancer Prevention

Super Prescription #1 Green tea (*Camella sinensis*)
Drink three cups of organic green tea daily. *Note:* If you are sensitive to caffeine, there are many brands that have removed the caffeine. Or, take 1,500 mg daily of the capsule form standardized to contain at least 80 to 90 percent polyphenols and 35 to 55 percent epigallocatechin-3 gallate (EGCG).

Super Prescription #2 Super green food blend
Use a formula that contains a blend of super green foods, such as chlorella, spirulina, wheatgrass, and other green foods. They contain an array of phytonutrients and antioxidants that promote healthy cells in the body. Take as directed on the container.

Super Prescription #3 High-potency multivitamin
Take a high-potency multivitamin and mineral formula, as directed on the container. It provides a base of nutrients and antioxidants for immune health.

Super Prescription #4 Probiotic
Take a product containing at least 4 billion organisms of the friendly bacteria per daily dose. These good bacteria support immune function, digestion, and detoxification of carcinogenic matter.

Super Prescription #5 Indole-3-carbinol
Take 400 mg daily to support detoxification, particularly of cancerous hormone metabolites.

In a study at the University of Texas Medical Center in Houston, researchers found that astragalus restored or enhanced the function of white blood cells that were taken from people with cancer. Interestingly, some of the damaged cells were so much improved that they became more active than normal cells taken from people who were cancer free. This herb is also used to support bone marrow function for patients undergoing chemotherapy.

In one small human study, MCP was shown to decrease PSA levels (a marker for prostate cancer) in four out of seven men with prostate cancer.

Super Prescription #6   D-glucarate

Take 400 mg daily to support detoxification of carcinogens and cancerous hormone metabolites.

Super Prescription #7   Fish oil

Take a daily dosage of 1,000 mg of combined DHA and EPA daily. These essential fatty acids support healthy cell structure.

General Recommendations

Modified citrus pectin (MCP), studies suggest, reduces the risk of prostate cancer metastasis. Take 10 mg of the powder form three times daily.

IP6 (inositol hexaphosphate) has been shown in studies to be an effective immune booster. Take 4 to 8 grams of IP6. *Note:* It can be safely used in conjunction with conventional treatment (surgery, chemotherapy, and radiation).

Quercitin is a type of flavonoid that has been shown to inhibit tumor formation in test tube studies. Take 400 mg three times daily on an empty stomach.

Fish oil is an important supplement, especially in preventing cachexia (tissue wasting). Take a product that contains a daily combined total dosage of 1,500 to 2,000 of DHA and EPA.

Whey protein provides valuable protein to support the immune system. It also increases the levels of the important antioxidant glutathione. Take 25 grams twice daily as part of a protein shake or a smoothie.

A greens drink containing super green foods, such as chlorella, spirulina, wheat grass, and others, supports detoxification. Take daily, as directed on the container.

Probiotic supplements are important for optimal immune function and for digestion and detoxification. Take a product containing a daily total of at least 4 billion active organisms.

Colostrum is a good supplement to support the immune system. Take 500 mg three times daily.

Melatonin has been shown in several studies to be helpful as an adjunctive therapy for certain types of cancers. It activates immune cells and improves the action of chemotherapy drugs and radiation. Take 20 mg or more under the direction and the guidance of a doctor.

Milk thistle (*Silybum marianum*) will protect your liver during chemotherapy and radiation treatments. Find a product standardized for 70 to 80 percent silymarin content, and take 150 to 200 mg twice a day.

A high-potency multivitamin and mineral formula provides a base of nutrients for immune support. Take as directed on the container.

A substance called carnosol, which is found in rosemary, has been found to inhibit cancer in laboratory animals. Take 2 to 3 grams twice a day, or use 2 to 3 cc of a tincture three times daily.

If you are undergoing radiation treatment or chemotherapy, drink fennel tea to reduce the side effects.

Garlic (*Allium sativum*) strengthens the immune system. Take 300 to 450 mg twice a day.

Cat's claw (*Una de bato*) stimulates the activity of white blood cells. Take 500 mg or 1 to 2 cc twice a day.

In this study, researchers examined the association between consumption of green tea prior to clinical cancer onset among 472 patients with stages I, II, and III breast cancer. Consumption of green tea was closely associated with decreased numbers of axillary lymph node metastases among premenopausal patients with stages I and II breast cancer. They also found that increased consumption of green tea was correlated with decreased recurrence of stages I and II breast cancer.

The researchers concluded, "Our results indicate that increased consumption of green tea prior to clinical cancer onset is significantly associated with improved prognosis of stage I and II breast cancer."

Pau d'arco (*Tabebuia avellanedae*) is another highly potent immune-system enhancer. Take 100 mg or 0.5 to 1.0 ml three times daily.

Take 300 mg of echinacea (*Echinacea purpurea*) three times a day for its immune-boosting properties.

If cancer treatment is making you nauseated, drink peppermint or ginger tea to soothe your stomach.

Homeopathy

Homeopathic treatment can be helpful for someone with cancer but requires a skilled homeopathic practitioner. The following remedies can be used safely to reduce the side effects of chemotherapy and radiation. Pick the remedy that best matches your symptoms in this section. For acute symptoms, take a 30C potency four times daily. After you notice improvement, stop taking the remedy, unless symptoms return.

Cadmium Sulphuratum is used to prevent and treat fatigue, vomiting, and loss of hair.

Ipecacuanha (*Cephaelis ipecacuanha*) is for persistent nausea and vomiting, when vomiting does not provide any relief from symptoms.

Nux Vomica is for symptoms of heartburn, reflux, constipation, and nausea. The person feels irritable and chilly.

Traditional Chinese Medicine

Many Chinese patent herbal remedies can strengthen your immune system and help you fight infection while undergoing conventional treatment. Consult a TCM practitioner for a combination that meets your individual needs.

Acupressure

See pages 668–675 for information about acupressure points and administering treatment.

- Liver 4 is the point for general pain relief.
- Stomach 36 is a good addition to a healthful eating plan, as it improves your body's ability to digest food and absorb nutrients.

Bodywork

Massage

Massage won't cure cancer—and you should run from anyone who claims it can—but in the midst of conventional treatments, the compassionate touch of a massage therapist can be quite welcoming. Depending upon your individual need, you can ask for a relaxing massage or an invigorating one. Or you may prefer to opt for a lymphatic massage, which breaks up toxins and carries them away from the body. A note of caution is in order, however: Do not allow the area where a tumor is located to be massaged.

Reflexology

See pages 686–687 for information about reflexology areas and how to work them.

When time permits, work the whole foot to stimulate all areas of your body's defense and promote a general sense of well-being.

If you have a limited amount of time, focus on the region or the regions where the growth is located. You should also work the liver and the colon to facilitate detoxification.

Hydrotherapy

Many cancer patients have responded well to fever therapy, which stimulates the body's immune response in the same way that a fever does. It also pulls toxins from the body and expels them as you sweat. At the very least, hydrotherapy will help fight bacteria or viruses that may be trying to take advantage of your body's weakened state. Saunas also can be used. We recommend constitutional hydrotherapy, which you can do at home. See the Hydrotherapy chapter for directions.

Aromatherapy

Juniper breaks down toxins that are hiding in fatty deposits. To bolster the detoxifying effects of a lymphatic massage, ask your massage therapist to use an oil mixed with a little juniper. You can also add a few drops of juniper to your bath.

If you are fatigued, use rose, geranium, or jasmine for an energy lift. You can employ these oils in almost any preparation, but for all-day relief, you may want to place a few drops in a diffuser and let the scent waft throughout your room.

Lavender and melissa are calming when you feel anxious and stressed.

Warming oils like black pepper, rosemary, and ginger can help relieve pain. Add them to a bath, a compress, or a lotion.

Tea tree oil (*Melaleuca alternifolia*) is antibacterial, antifungal, and antiviral. When treatment has left you vulnerable to infection or if you're exposed to a contagious illness like the flu, take a hot bath and run a few drops of tea tree oil under the tap. (Add just 2 or 3 drops for your first use, as this oil can be irritating to some people.)

If cancer treatment leaves you feeling queasy or downright sick, you can use peppermint or ginger oils to calm your stomach. If your nausea is unpredictable, try carrying a vial around with you; place the vial under your nose and inhale deeply as needed. You can also make a lotion or a cream with either oil and rub it into your skin. The scent will stay with you and reduce your chances of feeling ill.

Stress Reduction

General Stress-Reduction Therapies

Stress is a carcinogen, just like radiation and pesticides. Reducing stress has an inhibiting effect on tumor growth; it will also improve the quality of your life during treatment. Support groups are an excellent way to handle stress and reduce tension. One famous study of breast-cancer patients showed that women who discussed their problems in support groups lived a full two years longer than women who did not. It's a good idea to supplement weekly sessions with a daily stress-reducing exercise, like meditation, yoga, or deep breathing.

Cancer also causes stress. In order to keep yourself in peak fighting condition, do everything you can to avoid tense situations, even those that you usually accept as a normal part of a full life. This is the time to unload a demanding project at work or to avoid your personal stress triggers, like crowded roads or difficult relatives.

Bach Flower Remedies

Select the appropriate remedy, and place 10 drops under your tongue. Hold the drops in place for thirty seconds and swallow. Use as often as needed.

Rescue Remedy comes to your aid in emotional or physical crises. It soothes your body and mind and allows you to turn your focus away from panic and back to healing.

Other Recommendations

- One of the most avoidable—but most prevalent—carcinogens is cigarette smoke. Everyone knows it causes lung cancer, but the free radicals produced by inhaling smoke may contribute to many other forms of the disease. Do not smoke, not even socially, and do not expose yourself to secondhand smoke.
- As much as possible, avoid radiation. Do not sit or stand close to television sets or microwave ovens (a distance of about eight feet is preferable). If you work on a computer, invest in a radiation screen. And limit X-rays to those that are absolutely necessary for your health.
- You must also avoid harsh chemicals. A good rule of thumb is to stay away from any substance that releases fumes: Nail polish remover, hair spray, gasoline, household cleaners, and dry-cleaning solvent are all dangerous.
- Establish a healthy relationship with the sun. You need about fifteen minutes of sunshine a day to keep your body in proper working order, but sunburn and prolonged exposure can result in skin cancer. (The sun is, after all, a source of radiation.) Try to get your daily dose of sunlight in the early morning hours, when the rays are weak; if you must go out in broad daylight, wear protective clothing and use sunscreen.
- Radon is a radioactive gas that is strongly linked to lung cancer. It's usually found in the soil, but it may seep out, contaminating the air in your house and the water you drink. Radon cannot be detected with the senses, so you should buy a radon test kit and use it in your home. Should you have a radon problem, you can insulate your home by sealing up leaks.
- A sexually transmitted organism called human papilloma virus is a leading cause of cervical cancer, so do not engage in sexual intercourse with people whose sexual histories you do not know. Don't rely on condoms to protect you, as the virus can pass through them.

REFERENCES

Mavlit, G., Y. Ishii, Y. Patt, et al. 1979. Local xenogenic graft-vs-host reaction: A practical assessment of T-cell function among cancer patients. Journal of Immunology 123(5):2185–88.

Nakachi, K., K. Suemasu, K. Suga, T. Takeo, K. Imai, and Y. Higashi. 1998. Influence of drinking green tea on breast cancer malignancy among Japanese patients. *Japanese Journal of Cancer Research* 89(3):254–61.

Nanba, H. October 1999. Presented at the 3rd International Conference on Mushroom Biology and Mushroom Products in Sydney, Australia.

Strum, S., et al. 1999. Modified citrus pectin slows PSA doubling time: A pilot clinical trial. Presentation: International Conference on Diet and Prevention of Cancer, Ampere, Finland. May 28–June 2.

Sun, Z., et al. 1999. The ameliorative effect of PSP on the toxic and side reaction of chemo and radiotherapy of cancers. In *Advanced Research* in PSP, ed. Q. Yang. Hong Kong: Hong Kong Association for Health Care Ltd.

Torisu, M., Y. Hayashi, T. Ishimitsu, T. Fujimura, K. Iwasaki, M. Katano, H. Yamamoto, Y. Kimura, M. Takesue, M. Kondo, et al. 1990. Significant prolongation of disease-free period gained by oral polysaccharide K (PSK) administration after curative surgical operation of colorectal cancer. Cancer Immunology and Immunotherapy 31(5):261–68.

Candidiasis (Thrush and Yeast Infection)

Candida albicans is one of the many types of fungi that live and grow inside most human bodies. Normally, candida causes no harm; our bodies are equipped with probiotic (or "friendly") bacteria and immune cells that keep it under control. However, some medications, high-sugar diets, allergies, and other factors can all cause the friendly bacteria to die, leaving candida free to grow unchecked in parts or all of the body.

The medical name for this overgrowth is candidiasis, but most people know the condition as either thrush or as a yeast infection. Thrush is marked by soft white patches in the oral cavity, around the anus, or on the skin. It most often appears in babies and in the elderly, but people with seriously compromised immune systems—such as those who have AIDS or who are undergoing chemotherapy—are also quite vulnerable. Many conventional doctors do not believe that such a condition exists except in cases of a seriously compromised immune system such as AIDS. Our view is different, and we find that many people with chronic fatigue and other chronic health conditions have problems with yeast overgrowth.

A vaginal yeast infection, by far the more common manifestation of candidiasis, causes burning, itching, and soreness in the vagina, along with a thick, sticky discharge. It's often the result of antibiotic use, poor diet, hormone imbalance, or a combination of these causes.

Sometimes the fungus spreads throughout the entire body in a condition known as systemic candidiasis. This disorder can produce any of a wide variety of symptoms and is often at the root of a persistent, mysterious illness. If you feel sick but are told by doctors that nothing is wrong, there's a good chance that you're actually suffering from systemic candidiasis. For people with dramatically weakened immune systems, systemic candidiasis is a grave threat, as the fungus can actually poison the blood.

Complementary treatments, which emphasize therapies that reduce the levels of candida to normal levels, are the best ways to resolve this condition. Depending on the person, several steps are often required for success in treating candida overgrowth. This requires treating the underlying cause(s). One of the obvious steps is to eliminate or cut down on simple sugars, alcohol, and so on, which feed yeast. Also, direct therapy that destroys candida works to assist the body in getting candida levels down to a controllable level. Examples include oregano oil and garlic. However, many chronic cases require a change in the biological terrain. By this, we mean the state and the health of the digestive tract, the organs of detoxification and elimination, the immune system, and hormone balance. In particular, one often needs to improve digestion and elimination. The by-products of poor digestion can form metabolites that can promote candida growth. Leaky gut syndrome, as the result of intestinal permeability, is often a root problem of chronic candida. It is also imperative to promote the growth of the friendly flora that inhabit the digestive tract and many other areas of the body. These good bacteria are an essential component of the immune system's presence that keeps yeast levels in check. Also, keep in mind that chronic stress can alter flora balance and can suppress immune function. And finally, hormone balance is important, especially for women. The use of the birth control pill or other forms of synthetic hormones may set the stage for candida overgrowth.

In a small percentage of cases, antifungal medications may be required. They, of course, should be used sparingly and with close supervision. They are not a magic bullet, and the root causes described in this chapter must still be addressed for long-term success.

SYMPTOMS OF THRUSH

- White patches on the inside of the mouth
- Inflamed, red patches on the skin
- Bad breath
- Heavily coated tongue
- Dry mouth

SYMPTOMS OF YEAST INFECTION

- Vaginal itching, pain, and burning
- Thick yellow discharge
- Burning during urination

SYMPTOMS OF SYSTEMATIC CANDIDIASIS

The list of symptoms that systematic candidiasis can cause is too long to print here, but following are some of the most common:

- Persistent fatigue
- Constipation
- Diarrhea
- Colitis
- Abdominal pain
- Rectal itching
- Kidney and bladder infections
- Muscle pain
- Arthritis
- Canker sores
- Congestion
- Cough
- Headaches
- Numbness or tingling in the limbs
- Poor memory and concentration
- Mood problems (depression, anxiety)
- Chronic skin rashes
- Genital or toenail fungus
- Allergies

ROOT CAUSES

- Prolonged or frequent use of antibiotics or corticosteroids, leading to a depletion of good bacteria
- Poor digestion and elimination
- A depressed immune system
- A high-sugar diet
- Allergies
- Stress
- Hormonal changes and birth-control pills
- Aging

Testing Techniques

The following tests help assess possible metabolic reasons for candidiasis:

Candida levels—stool, blood (antibodies), or urine (yeast metabolites)

Intestinal permeability—urine test

TREATMENT

Diet

Recommended Food

For high-density nutrition and immune support, base your meals around fresh vegetables, whole grains, and quality sources of lean protein, such as beans, lentils, fish, and organic poultry.

To replace friendly bacteria, eat unsweetened yogurt daily. Make sure the brand you're using has live yogurt cultures. Sauerkraut and miso are other examples of foods that contain friendly bacteria.

Despite its name, brewer's yeast does not encourage *Candida albicans;* in fact, it enhances your immune system, so add some to your salads and other dishes. Vegetable and green drinks will improve your resistance. Drink 8 glasses of pure water a day to help flush yeast toxins out.

Consume 1 to 2 tablespoons of ground flaxseeds daily. Flaxseeds have antifungal properties.

Food to Avoid

The fungus that causes candidiasis feeds on sugar and yeast, so you must absolutely avoid all foods (especially alcohol) containing these substances during the initial phase of treatment.

Many people with candidiasis also have undiagnosed allergies. See the Food Allergies entry on pages 251–256 to determine whether you're one of them.

During the course of your infection, avoid foods with mold (aged cheese, nuts, and nut butters)

Avoid refined foods that are likely to be loaded with sugars.

Avoid or reduce the use of fruits and fruit juices during the initial phase (first month) of treatment. It is especially important to avoid these foods between meals.

Detoxification

Consume foods such as garlic, onions, chlorella, spirulina, wheatgrass, and others that are known to support detoxification.

R̥ Super Seven Prescriptions—Candidiasis

Super Prescription #1   Oregano (*Origanum vulgare*) oil
Take a 300 to 500 mg capsule or the liquid form (as directed on the container) three times daily with meals (to avoid digestive upset).

Super Prescription #2   Probiotic
Take a product containing 4 billion active organisms twice daily, thirty minutes after a meal. It supplies friendly bacteria, such as acidophilus and bifidus, which fight candida and prevent its overgrowth.

Super Prescription #3   Garlic (*Allium sativum*)
Take 500 to 1,000 mg of aged garlic twice daily. Garlic fights fungal infections and also boosts immune strength.

Super Prescription #4   Grapefruit seed extract
Take 200 mg two to three times daily. Practitioners rely on this herb for its anti-candida properties.

Bacteria Basics

Many cultured and sour products contain the friendly bacteria that will prevent candidiasis and many other infections. Yogurt can be an especially good source, but you need to shop carefully—many mass-produced yogurt products just don't have enough of the bacteria you need. When you're reading labels, look for one or more of these Latin names:

Lactobacillus acidophilus

Bifidobacterium bifidum

Lactobacillus bulgaricus

Strepococcus thermophilus

When buying yogurt, be sure the label or the container lists yogurt cultures that are "live," "living," or "active." And since sugar encourages the growth of *Candida albicans,* buy unsweetened yogurt only.

A study compared the anti-candida effect of oregano oil to that of caprylic acid. Researchers found that oregano oil is over one hundred times more potent than caprylic acid against candida.

> **Super Prescription #5   Caprylic acid**
> Take 1,000 mg three times daily. This type of fatty acid has been shown in studies to have antifungal properties.
>
> **Super Prescription #6   Gentian root** (*Gentiana lutea*)
> Take 250 mg or 0.5 to 1.0 ml at the beginning of each meal. It improves stomach acid levels and overall digestive function. It's often used with other bitter herbals.
>
> **Super Prescription #7   Echinacea** (*Echinacea purpurea*) and **goldenseal** (*Hydrastis canadensis*) combination
> Take 500 mg or 2 to 4 ml of tincture three times daily. Both herbs enhance immune function. Echinacea has been shown to have antiyeast effects.

General Recommendations

Pau d'arco (*Tabebuia avellanedae*) has strong antibacterial and antifungal properties. No matter what kind of candida infection you have, drink several cups of this tea every day.

Peppermint (*Mentha piperita*) oil relieves intestinal cramping often associated with candida. Studies also show that it has antifungal properties. Take 1 to 2 enteric-coated capsules or 0.2 ml of peppermint oil two to three times daily.

Wormwood (*Artemisia absinthium*), Oregon grape (*Berberis aquifolium*), and rosemary (*Rosmarinus officinalis*) all have antifungal properties. Take as part of a candida formula.

Tea tree oil (*Melaleuca alternifolia*) is mainly used topically for skin-related yeast infections. The tincture form can also be mixed in water (5 to 15 drops) and swished in the mouth for treating thrush.

A high-potency multivitamin provides the many nutrients used to support detoxification.

Vitamin C is used to enhance immune function. Take 1,000 mg two to three times daily.

Milk thistle (*Silybum marianum*), Reishi (*Ganoderma lucidum*), and dandelion (*Taraxacum officinale*) are herbs used individually or in formulas to support liver and kidney detoxification while you undergo an anticandida program. Generally, you take 1 to 2 capsules with each meal or as directed on the container.

Betaine HCL, taken with meals, improves stomach acid levels and absorption. Take 1 to 2 capsules with meals.

Enzymes also support digestion when taken with meals. Protease enzymes, taken between meals, may have antifungal effects and reduce inflammation.

Homeopathy

See a qualified homeopathic practitioner for an individually prescribed remedy. For specific problems related to candida, see the corresponding sections in this book, such as AIDS, Constipation, Diarrhea, Fatigue, Headache, Indigestion, and so on. Otherwise, try the following recommendation:

Candida Albicans 6x, 12x, or 30x. This is a homeopathic preparation of candida that can be used to stimulate the immune system to target candida organisms. Take 2 pellets three times daily.

Acupressure

See pages 668–675 for information about acupressure points and administering treatment.

- Spleen 6 and 10 detoxify the blood.
- If candidiasis is accompanied by nervousness and stress, massage Large Intestine 4 and Liver 3.

Bodywork

Massage

Any massage, especially with one of the following relaxing oils, is wonderful for reducing stress. If you have a yeast infection and prefer to remain clothed, try a shoulder, a head, or a foot rub. Lymphatic massage is particularly good to support detoxification for people undergoing treatment for chronic candida.

Reflexology

See pages 686–687 for information about reflexology areas and how to work them.

Work the areas that correspond to the location of your symptoms. For thrush, massage the head region. For a yeast infection, concentrate on the pelvic area. If you have systematic candidiasis, work the entire foot or the hand.

Aromatherapy

- To relax and reduce stress, try any of the following in a bath, in steam inhalation, or in a diffuser: chamomile, jasmine, lavender, or rose.
- Tea tree oil, peppermint, and myrrh all have a natural antifungal action. Use any one of them in a massage, a bath, or a compress. Tea tree oil can sometimes be irritating, so if you're adding it to a bath or a compress, use just a few drops.

Stress Reduction

General Stress-Reduction Therapies

High levels of stress have been implicated in candida infections. If you're prone to candidiasis, any stress-reduction technique is likely to help. Exercise, yoga, and prayer are very good.

Bach Flower Remedies

Consult the Bach Flower Remedy chart on pages 648–650 to find the best remedy for your personal situation. Following are some suggestions to get you started. Once you've selected the right remedy, place 10 drops of the liquid under your tongue. Hold the drops in place for thirty seconds and swallow. Use as often as needed.

If you are nervous or tense, and if you have a hard time sitting still, take Impatiens.

If a lack of self-confidence causes you anxiety in work or social situations, try Larch.

Rock Water is helpful if a perfectionist nature makes you hard on yourself and those around you.

Other Recommendations

- Whether you have thrush, a yeast infection, or systemic candidiasis, change your toothbrush monthly to avoid reinfecting yourself.
- For a yeast infection, wear cotton underwear and loose clothes to keep the area dry.
- If you have a yeast infection, you can apply live yogurt locally to replace pro- biotic bacteria. Spoon the yogurt onto a towel or a sanitary pad, or douche with yogurt and distilled water.
- Be aware that sexual intercourse can spread candida. Partners should both be treated if vaginitis is a chronic problem.

REFERENCES

Stiles, J. C. 1995. The inhibition of Candida albicans by oregano. *Journal of Applied Nutrition* 47:96–102.

Cardiovascular Disease

Numerous disorders fall under the broad category of heart and vascular disease. Here, discussion is restricted to arteriosclerosis, angina, and heart attack. For related sub- jects, see High Blood Pressure and Stroke.

Arteries transport blood from the heart and deliver it to other parts of the body. Arteriosclerosis occurs when the inside of the artery wall thickens, leaving a narrower passageway for the blood to travel through. This disorder is often called hardening of the arteries. Arteriosclerosis can affect the coronary arteries—the arteries that lead to the heart—and is usually caused by a buildup of fatty deposits within the arterial walls. This buildup is often the result of a poor diet, one that's high in bad fats and low in fiber. Most people who have arteriosclerosis are not aware of it, as it does not trigger symptoms in the body until later in the disease.

Unfortunately, when arteriosclerosis is left untreated, it just gets worse. Without treatment, the arteries will eventually become so constricted that adequate supplies of oxygenated blood can't reach the heart muscle. This oxygen deprivation may result in the chest pain known as angina. Angina is often a precursor to a heart attack.

In some ways, people with angina are lucky. Their pain usually leads to a diagno- sis of cardiovascular disease, and they can then take several steps to slow or reverse their condition before it results in a trip to the emergency room or even death. But for many, a heart attack is the first outward sign of trouble; 25 percent of people who suf- fer heart attacks have never felt any previous symptoms. A heart attack—or myocar- dial infarction, as it's called by doctors—is brought on when blood flow to a section of the heart muscle is completely cut off, either because a clot has backed up behind a thickened artery, or because the artery itself has become so narrow that no blood at all can pass through. If you ever suspect that you are having a heart attack, you must receive emergency medical care at once. Instead of having someone drive you to a hospital (unless you are really close), call for an ambulance. Life-saving treatment for heart attacks requires special medical techniques and tools, and the sooner profession- als arrive with their equipment, the greater your chances of survival.

Heart disease is so prevalent now, most people are surprised to hear that it was actually quite rare until the turn of the twentieth century. Our modern diet and way of life are at the root of most heart problems, and the best way to prevent or reverse heart disease is to change our habits. Because heart disease is caused by a variety of factors, it is best to include several kinds of therapies in your treatment or prevention plan. Eat well, exercise, manage stress, and identify and treat genetic susceptibilities that are known to bring on cardiovascular disease.

In recent years, researchers have found that chronic inflammation in the blood vessels is a central factor in the development of heart disease. This chronic inflammation leads to arterial wall damage and the resulting plaque formation. Although cholesterol levels have some importance, it appears that this substance is not the "villain" that it was once thought to be. While diet and lifestyle factors are root causes of chronic inflammation, there are also genetic reasons beyond inheriting a disposition to high cholesterol levels. They includes one's levels of homocysteine and lipoprotein(a) and other heredity factors. Fortunately, these genetic susceptibilities can be reduced through natural therapies. Stealth or hidden infections in the body are also suspected of increasing the inflammatory response. Therefore, it is imperative you are tested for these newer, more predictive markers of heart disease.

Finally, the impact of stress and negative emotions cannot be underrated as a cause of heart disease. This chapter will explore the mental/emotional connection to heart disease, in addition to the physical causes.

> ### Homocysteine
>
> One theory regarding the origins of arteriosclerosis has to do with a substance called homocysteine. Homocysteine is a toxic substance created in your body at too high a level. It is a by-product of protein metabolism when you ingest foods like meat or dairy products; luckily, most people who eat these foods in moderation are usually able to convert homocysteine into a chemical called methionine, which is harmless. But a significant percentage (approximately 10 to 20 percent) of us are born with genetic flaws that make it impossible for us to neutralize homocysteine in this manner, and this substance stays around, inflaming the blood vessels and contributing to arteriosclerosis. A simple blood test will show if you have an elevated level. B vitamins, such as B12, folic acid, and B6, can bring it down to normal levels.

SYMPTOMS OF ARTERIOSCLEROSIS

There are usually no overt symptoms until later in the disease. See your doctor if you experience any of the following:

- Dizziness
- Fainting
- Leg pain that starts after walking a short distance and that goes away with rest

SYMPTOMS OF ANGINA

- Mild to severe chest pain. Often, it feels like the heart is being squeezed.
- There is tightness in the chest.
- Pain may feel worse after exercise or a heavy meal and better when resting.

SYMPTOMS OF HEART ATTACK

If you have any of the following symptoms, call 911 immediately. Even if the symptoms pass, you need emergency medical attention.

- The classical symptoms are crushing or tight pain in the chest, which may extend to the arms, the back, the shoulders, the neck, or the jaw. The pain may be intense and severe, or it could be so mild that you might mistake it for indigestion.
- Women sometimes have heart attack symptoms that are different from the previous ones. The pain may begin in the stomach or the jaw or with stabbing pains between the breasts. The symptoms in general may be more vague than for men.
- Other possible symptoms include profuse sweating, a drop in blood pressure, difficulty swallowing, dizziness or faintness, ringing in the ears, or, more rarely, nausea and vomiting.

ROOT CAUSES

- Poor diet, especially one that's high in saturated fat and low in fiber and antioxidants
- Genetics
- Smoking
- High blood pressure
- Stress, depression, and anxiety
- Obesity
- Inactivity
- Diabetes and syndrome X
- Stealth infections
- Excess of toxic metals

Testing Techniques

The following tests help assess possible metabolic reasons for cardiovascular disease. We have included the historic markers, as well as a description of the new predictive blood markers, of cardiovascular risk.

Blood tests

Historic

Total cholesterol

Normal range is 165–200 mg/dL.

LDL cholesterol

Normal range is below 130 mg/dL.

HDL cholesterol

Normal range is 50 mg/dL or higher.

Triglycerides

Normal range is less than 150 mg/dL.

New Markers
C-reactive protein is a marker of inflammation in the body, including in the blood vessel walls. It is considered the best predictor of heart disease.

Normal range is less than 32 mg/dL.

Homocysteine—Buildup of this toxic metabolite increases plaque formation in the artery walls. Genetics, low thyroid, B vitamin deficiencies, and a high animal protein diet increase the level.

Normal range is less than 10 micro mol/L.

Lipoprotein(a) is a more specific cholesterol marker and a stronger risk factor than is LDL cholesterol.

Normal range is less than 32 mg/dL.

Fibrinogen plays an important role in blood clotting. Elevated levels increase the risk of stroke and coronary artery disease.

Apolipoprotein B is a type of lipid that binds to LDL cholesterol and accelerates plaque formation.

Normal range is 55–125 mg/dL.

Apolipoprotein A-1 is found in HDL cholesterol and provides a protective effect against heart disease.

Normal range is 125–215 mg/dL.

Apolipoprotein B and the apolipoprotein ratio are overall predictors of heart disease risk.

Normal range is 0.30–0.90.

Normal range is between 180 and 300 mg/dL.

Glucose—Diabetes predisposes one to early heart disease.

Normal range is between 80 and 110 mg/dL.

Insulin—Elevation of this hormone is seen with syndrome X, a condition characterized by rising blood-sugar and insulin levels. Spiked insulin levels increase arterial inflammation, as well as triglyceride, cholesterol, and blood pressure levels. They also contribute to weight gain.

Normal range is between 4 and 15 micro mol (fasting).

Iron—Excessive iron in the body produces free radicals and oxidative damage.

Normal range is less than 150 mg/dL.

TREATMENT

The following therapies are recommended as ongoing support for your heart. They are not treatments for a heart attack. If you suspect that you're having a heart attack, get emergency medical help immediately.

Diet

When most people think of diets to prevent or reverse heart disease, they think of reducing cholesterol and fat. In reality, many other factors must be taken into account, such as an adequate intake of "good" fats, fiber, and antioxidants. A heart-healthy diet, in fact, is much like the basic wholesome eating plan this book suggests for almost everyone.

Recommended Food

A whole-foods, plant-based diet (with the addition of fish) has been shown to sweep away arterial plaque. Your meals should emphasize vegetables, fruits, and whole grains, with soy products, beans, and fish for protein. People who require a higher-protein diet can add more lean poultry to their menu.

Highly reactive molecules known as free radicals are closely linked to heart disease. Foods that contain antioxidants will help prevent damage caused by free radicals, so eat a wide variety of fruits and vegetables every day.

Essential fatty acids are "good" fats that actually protect the heart and help the rest of the body function smoothly. Essential fatty acids are found in cold-water fish like halibut, salmon, and mackerel; raw nuts (excluding peanuts); olive oil; and flaxseeds.

Eat lots of fiber. A whole-foods diet will automatically increase your fiber intake, but if you need more, include oat bran or flaxseeds with your meals.

Garlic and onions reduce levels of bad cholesterol and lower the blood pressure. They make excellent additions to low-fat meals, like vegetable stir-fries, clear soups, and bean dishes.

The skins of red or purple grapes help clear the arteries of plaque. Have a glass of purple grape juice daily.

Potassium or magnesium are heart-protective minerals. Good sources include green vegetables, whole grains, wheat germ, soybeans, garlic, legumes, bok choy, and potatoes. Sea salt, listed previously, is another good choice.

Follow the Mediterranean diet: the consumption of plant foods; olive oil; and low to moderate amounts of fish, poultry, meat, dairy, eggs, and wine. Researchers believe that the consumption of fish is one of the keys to this heart-healthy diet, which results in a lower incidence of obesity, heart disease, and diabetes.

> A four-year study published in the *Journal of the American Heart Association* found that people following the Mediterranean diet could reduce their risk of a heart attack by as much as 70 percent.

Food to Avoid

If you have heart disease, you must eliminate or drastically reduce your consumption of harmful fats (saturated fat, trans-fatty acids, or hydrogenated fats). Common sources of saturated fat or cholesterol include meat, poultry, dairy products, butter, eggs, palm oil, and coconut oil. Don't forget that many foods are made with these ingredients. Sweet baked goods, for instance, are likely to contain eggs and butter, as well as other fats and oils.

Don't make the mistake of substituting margarine or vegetable shortening for butter. These products are made with oils that have been artificially processed under high heat. This processing creates mutated molecules, called trans-fatty acids, that are most likely even worse for your heart and cholesterol levels than saturated fats are.

People who cut down on fat sometimes end up gorging themselves on non- and low-fat processed foods, especially packaged cookies and other sweets. Avoid this trap. These foods have little or no nutritional content, and they rely on sugar to make up for the presence of fat. Excess sugar is tied to a number of health problems, and when used as a replacement for starch, it reduces the level of good, heart-protecting cholesterol.

Avoid simple sugars. Simple sugars cause elevated levels of cholesterol, triglycerides, C-reactive protein, insulin, and other markers that contribute to cardiovascular damage.

Radically reduce your consumption of sodium. Packaged and processed foods are by far the highest source of sodium in the Western diet, so stay away from them. A high sodium intake, combined with a low potassium intake, increases your likelihood of having high blood pressure.

Detoxification

The buildup of heavy metals in the arteries can also cause damage and diminished blood flow. If you have heart disease, consider chelation therapy, either oral or intravenous, to encourage the excretion of these toxic substances.

℞ Super Seven Prescriptions—Cardiovascular Disease

Super Prescription #1   High-potency multivitamin
Take as directed on the container. It provides a base of the many nutrients and antioxidants that promote cardiovascular health. The formula should contain 400 IU of natural vitamin E (d'alpha tocopherol).

Super Prescription #2   Garlic (*Allium sativum*)
Take 300 to 500 mg of aged garlic twice daily. It reduces cholesterol and homocysteine, has a natural blood-thinning effect, and has antioxidant properties.

Super Prescription #3   Coenzyme Q10
Take 100 to 300 mg daily. This nutrient is used by the heart cells to pump efficiently and with regular rhythm. Studies show that it lowers blood pressure and helps improve angina, mitral valve prolapse, and congestive heart failure. It also prevents the oxidation of LDL cholesterol.

Super Prescription #4   Fish oil
Take a daily dosage of a fish oil product containing at least 480 mg of EPA and 360 mg of DHA daily. Fish oil reduces inflammation in the arteries, lowers cholesterol/triglycerides, and is a natural blood thinner.

Super Prescription #5   Policosanol
Take 10 to 20 mg each evening. This supplement reduces LDL cholesterol and lipoprotein(a), improves HDL cholesterol, and helps angina.

Super Prescription #6   Hawthorn (*Crataegus oxycantha*)
Take 500 to 900 mg daily. It improves circulation to the heart and reduces blood pressure.

Super Prescription #7   Magnesium
Take 500 mg daily. The heart, to produce energy for contraction and regular rhythm, uses this mineral. It also relaxes the blood vessel walls, for improved circulation and reduced blood pressure.

> ### Study
> Researchers at UCLA Medical Center completed a one-year, double-blind, randomized clinical study with people taking aged garlic extract. Researchers found that people taking aged garlic extract had significantly less coronary plaque formation than did those in the placebo group. Also, the group supplementing the garlic tended to have lower blood homocysteine and cholesterol levels.

> ### Study
> A review published in the *American Heart Journal* found that Policosanol lowered total cholesterol by 17 to 21 percent, as well as raised the good HDL cholesterol by 8 to 15 percent. It also reported that Policosanol was found to be equally as effective in lowering total or LDL cholesterol as the statin drugs Simvastatin or Pravastatin.

General Recommendations

Antioxidant formula contains a wide spectrum of antioxidants that prevent the oxidative damage of cholesterol. Take as directed on the container.

Ginkgo biloba improves blood flow, has antioxidant benefits, and has blood-thinning properties. Select an extract made with 24 percent ginkgo flavone glycosides and take 80 to 120 mg twice a day.

L-carnitine is a nutrient that lowers triglyceride levels and improves heart contraction. Take 500 to 2,000 mg daily.

Vitamin E has well-researched cardioprotective properties as an antioxidant and a blood thinner. Take 400 to 800 IU of a vitamin E-complex containing tocotrienols and tocopherols. If you are on blood-thinning medication, take E-complex under the guidance of a doctor at a lower dosage.

Vitamin C prevents cholesterol oxidation and mildly lowers blood pressure. Take up to 3,000 mg daily.

Cayenne (*Capsicum frutescens*) extract reduces cholesterol levels and improves circulation. Take 500 mg two to three times daily.

Green tea reduces cholesterol oxidation. Take 250 to 500 mg of a standardized extract two to three times daily.

New Risk Markers and Their Supplement Solutions

If testing shows that your levels of these markers are elevated, the following supplements can be helpful:

C-reactive protein

Vitamin C: 1,000 to 3,000 mg daily

Vitamin E: 400 to 800 IU daily

Fish oil: 5,000 mg daily

Gamma linoleic acid (GLA): 250 to 500 mg daily

Bromelain: 500 mg three times daily, between meals

Lipoprotein(a)

Niacin (flush free): 1,500 mg twice daily

Coenzyme Q10: 100 to 300 mg daily

Policosanol: 10 to 20 mg daily

Fish oil: 5,000 mg daily

Homocysteine

Vitamin B12: 800 to 2,000 mcg daily

Folic acid: 1 to 10 mg daily

Vitamin B6: 20 to 100 mg daily

Trimethylglycine (TMG): 500 to 1,000 mg daily

S-Adenosylmethionine (SAMe): 400 mg daily

Fibrinogen

Fish oil: 5,000 mg daily

Vitamin E: 400 to 800 IU daily

Bromelain: 500 mg three times daily between meals

Garlic (*Allium sativum*): 350 to 500 mg twice daily

Homeopathy

If you have cardiovascular disease, see a licensed homeopath for a constitutional remedy. If any of the following remedies seem appropriate for you, try them, but only on a temporary or emergency basis. After that, see a homeopath for further help.

Homeopathy may help you recover from a heart attack. Once you've received emergency help and are under a doctor's care, consult with a naturopathic or homeopathic practitioner.

If you have symptoms of a heart attack, call 911 and follow their instructions. While you are waiting for the ambulance to arrive, you can take a 30C potency every two or three minutes.

Aconitum Napellus is for numbness and pain in the left arm. The person feels very fearful and anxious.

Arnica (*Arnica montana*) is helpful when you have the sensation that your heart is being squeezed or you feel a bruising pain.

Cactus (*Cereus grandiflorus*) can also ease the pain of angina. Take it if you feel as if a band is tightening around your chest.

Acupressure

See pages 668–675 for information about acupressure points and administering treatment.

- If you have a heart attack, first call an ambulance. While you are waiting, you can squeeze the tips of the little fingers. This action may reduce the severity of the attack.
- To stimulate circulation around the heart and the chest, use Heart 3 and 7.
- Governing Vessel 24.5 produces a general sense of calm and well-being.
- Conception Vessel 17 relaxes chest tension caused by nerves or sadness.
- Pericardium 3 eases chest pain and anxiety.
- If your anxiety causes heart palpitations, massage Pericardium 6.

Bodywork

Massage

A full-body massage improves circulation, steadies the body's rhythms, and relieves stress. As such, it is a valuable addition to heart disease treatment.

If tension causes pressure in your chest, a neck massage may calm you down and regulate your pulse. You can easily give yourself a simple neck rub by learning a few techniques.

Chiropractic or osteopathic treatment can be helpful for improved circulation.

Reflexology

See pages 686–687 for information about reflexology areas and how to work them.

To strengthen a weakened heart, massage the chest and lung area.

Working the sigmoid colon will prevent gas from backing up and causing pain in the chest.

Aromatherapy

Many oils stimulate relaxation. Try several until you find a few that you like, then alternate them to preserve their effectiveness. Some good oils to start with are lavender and jasmine. A diffuser that releases scent into a room will allow you to benefit from an oil's relaxing qualities all day long.

Add juniper to a massage oil. It will encourage the breakdown of fatty deposits and other toxins.

Stress Reduction

General Stress-Reduction Therapies

Conventional medicine is finally beginning to accept that stress is a primary factor in heart disease. If you have heart disease, you must take several steps to reduce the amount of stress in your life. Dr. Dean Ornish has produced remarkable results by putting his patients on a program of yoga and daily meditation. He's found that even the most resistant of patients have eventually come to enjoy and look forward to these relaxing sessions.

Consider joining a support group for people with heart disease. Again, Dr. Ornish's work shows that when people can talk out their worries and frustrations with others who share some of their experiences, stress levels decline dramatically, along with the risk of a heart attack (or a repeat heart attack).

Bach Flower Remedies

Consult the chart on pages 648–650 to find the appropriate flower remedy for your particular kind of stress. Following are a few suggestions. Once you've selected the remedy that meets your needs, place 10 drops of the liquid under your tongue. Hold the drops in place for thirty seconds and swallow. Use as often as needed.

Sweet Chestnut is helpful for people suffering from great anguish, whether mental or physical, and who feel that hope has run out.

People who use aggression to cover up feelings of insecurity will benefit from Holly.

If you work hard and deny yourself pleasures, try Rock Water.

Perfectionists who are rarely satisfied and who tend to blame themselves, even for others' mistakes, should take Pine.

If you are easily irritated and have little patience for others' slowness, Impatiens will help.

Aspen is for unexplained sudden fears.

Other Recommendations

- Quit smoking, and eliminate your exposure to secondhand smoke. Tobacco smoke is known to weaken artery walls and is one of the leading causes of heart disease.
- Exercise is a crucial component of heart fitness, but you don't need to force yourself into a punishing regimen. Just enjoy a brisk thirty-minute walk daily; move quickly enough that you're breathing hard but not so fast that you can't carry on a conversation. If you have heart disease, see a doctor before beginning any exercise program.
- If you're a heart-disease patient and have been told to lose weight, the dietary suggestions given here should help you take off the pounds safely. People who are very heavy will find additional suggestions under the heading Obesity.
- Women who smoke or who are over thirty-five should not take oral contraceptives or synthetic hormone replacements. This is particularly true if they are over thirty-five and smoke.
- If you suffer from depression, you are at a significantly greater risk of developing heart disease. See the Depression section for more information.

REFERENCES

Budoff, M., et al. 2003. Anti-atherosclerotic effect of aged garlic (Kyolic) in the bypass surgery patients analyzed by computed tomography. *FASEB Journal*. April 15, 2003, San Diego.

De Longeril, M., et al. 1999. Circulation. *Journal of the American Heart Association* 99:733–85.

Gouni-Berthold, I., and H. K. Berthold. 2002. Policosanol: Clinical pharmacology and therapeutic significance of a new lipid-lowering agent. *American Heart Journal* 143(2):356–65.

Carpal Tunnel Syndrome (CTS)

The carpal tunnel is a very small opening just below the base of the wrist, between the arm and the hand. It allows the median nerve to pass from the bones and the muscles of the forearm to the palm, the thumb, and the fingers. Because the opening is so small, it is vulnerable to pressure and swelling. Inflammation from overuse, hormonal changes, or arthritis causes the pain and the numbness of carpal tunnel syndrome (CTS). CTS may begin as a mild tingling that's worse in the morning or the evening and can progress to a crippling, excruciating pain.

CTS has always afflicted people who consistently use their hands in a repetitive motion: Knitters, musicians, writers, grocery clerks, and assembly-line workers have traditionally suffered from the effects of CTS. But in the last decade, as work has increasingly centered on the personal computer, CTS has reached near-epidemic proportions. At least 10 percent of people who work at computers have CTS, and that number is projected to rise.

The best way to treat CTS is to prevent it from happening. If you work at a computer, use a wrist rest to relieve pressure on the carpal tunnel, and take a break every hour to rotate your hands. If you think you may already have CTS, see your doctor for a test called an electromyograph. If the test proves that you do have CTS, complementary therapies can help relieve your pain. Treatments include removing the source of pain when possible, improving circulation, and reducing swelling. Since a vitamin B6 deficiency has been linked to CTS, complementary treatment also encourages the consumption of that nutrient. Specific treatments from a chiropractor, an acupuncturist, or an osteopath can be very effective in addressing the underlying structural cause of carpal tunnel syndrome. Surgery for this condition should be avoided, if at all possible, because of its high failure rate.

In a preliminary trial, people with CTS (some of whom had previously undergone surgery) received either acupuncture or electroacupuncture (acupuncture with electrical stimulation). Researchers found that 83 percent of the participants experienced complete relief that lasted two to eight years after follow-up.

SYMPTOMS

Symptoms can occur in one or both hands.

- Numbness, tingling, or pain in the thumb and the first three fingers
- Pain is worse at night and/or in the morning.
- Weakness of the thumb and the first three fingers
- Inability to make a fist
- Pain may radiate to the forearm or the shoulder.

ROOT CAUSES

- Continuous use of the fingers and the hand
- Constant vibration of the fingers and the hand (as in holding a jack-hammer for long periods of time)
- Pregnancy or other hormonal changes that cause fluid retention
- Inflammatory arthritis in the wrist
- Bone spurs in the wrist
- Vitamin B6 deficiency

Testing Techniques

The following test helps to assess possible metabolic reasons for carpal tunnel syndrome:

Vitamin B6—blood test

TREATMENT

CTS is often brought on or made worse by pregnancy. If you're pregnant or nursing, check with your doctor before taking any herbs or supplements or making radical changes to your diet.

Diet

Recommended Food

If you're overweight, there's a good chance you will find relief from the pain of CTS by following a wholesome diet based on whole grains, fresh fruits and vegetables, and lean protein (especially beans and soy). This eating plan will help you lose weight safely and will take pressure off the carpal tunnel.

Drink a glass of clean water every two waking hours to combat fluid retention.

A deficiency of vitamin B6 may be a cause of CTS, so consume plenty of beans, brewer's yeast, and wheat germ. Green leafy vegetables are good sources of B6 as well.

Green drinks are also good for reducing inflammation.

Food to Avoid

Fluid retention puts pressure on the carpal tunnel, so eliminate sources of sodium from your diet.

Avoid saturated fat, which slows circulation.

℞ Super Seven Prescriptions—Carpal Tunnel Syndrome

Super Prescription #1   Vitamin B6
Take 100 mg three times daily. Studies show that this vitamin reduces the nerve inflammation that is found with carpal tunnel syndrome. Also, take a B-complex to prevent an imbalance of the other B vitamins.

Super Prescription #2   Bromelain
Take 500 mg three times daily between meals. Look for products standardized to 2,000 M.C.U. (milk-clotting units) per 1,000 mg or 1,200 G.D.U. (gelatin-dissolving units) per 1,000 mg. Bromelain has a natural anti-inflammatory effect. Protease enzyme products also have this benefit.

Super Prescription #3   Boswellia (*Boswellia serrata*)
Take 1,200 to 1,500 mg of a standardized extract containing 60 to 65 percent boswellic acids, two to three times daily. It acts as a natural anti-inflammatory.

Super Prescription #4   Calcium and magnesium
Take a complex containing 500 mg of calcium and 250 mg of magnesium twice daily. This reduces muscle tightness and nerve irritation.

Super Prescription #5   White willow (*Salix alba*)
Take a product standardized to contain 240 mg of salicin daily or 5 ml of the tincture form three times daily. This herbal extract reduces pain and inflammation.

Super Prescription #6   Homeopathy
Pick the remedy that best matches your symptoms in the Homeopathy section. For acute wrist pain, take a 30C potency four times daily. For chronic wrist pain, take twice daily for two weeks to see if there are any positive improvements. After you notice improvement, stop taking the remedy, unless symptoms return. Consultation with a homeopathic practitioner is advised.

Super Prescription #7   Ginkgo biloba
Take 120 mg twice daily of a product standardized to 24 percent flavone glycosides. Gingko improves circulation.

General Recommendations

Dandelion leaf (*Taraxacum officinale*) is a natural diuretic that is considered to be safe during pregnancy. Take 300 mg or 2 ml three times daily. It should be used under the supervision of a doctor, though.

DMSO (dimethyl sulfoxide) is a topical pain reliever. Work with a doctor to use this substance.

Arnica (*Arnica montana*) and hypericum (Saint-John's-wort) oil can be rubbed over the affected area to reduce pain and swelling.

Homeopathy

Arnica (*Arnica montana*) is for deep pain that feels bruised. It is best used for the first two days after an injury.

Causticum is a remedy for recurring or long-lasting carpal tunnel syndrome. The wrist area feels bruised, with burning or drawing pains. There is often stiffness and contracture of the wrist and the forearm. Symptoms are better with warm applications.

Hypericum (*Hypericum perforatum*) is for shooting nerve pains that extend from the wrist.

Rhus Toxicodendron is for achy pain that improves with movement and dry warmth and is worse with inactivity and windy, rainy weather.

Ruta (*Ruta graveolens*) is for stiff, bruised pain and aching of the wrist. The wrist feels lame and weak from overuse.

Acupressure

See pages 668–675 for information about acupressure points and administering treatment.

- The best points for easing wrist pain are Pericardium 6 and 7 and Triple Warmer 5. You can easily practice this short acupressure routine while at your desk or when you're taking a break from work.

Work Those Wrists!

Your wrists, like the rest of the body, need exercise to stay strong and supple. Practice the following recommended exercises at the beginning of every workday, and take breaks every few hours to go through the routine again. It's also a good idea to use these exercises as a warm-up for yoga, tennis, rock climbing, and other hand-intensive sports.

- Begin by shaking out your wrists for about ten seconds.

- Gently rotate your wrists clockwise through their full range of motion. Do this five times, and then repeat, this time going counter-clockwise.

- Hold your arm straight out in front of you, palm facing outward, and use the opposite hand to gently pull back your fingertips. Hold for a few seconds and then release. Repeat with the other arm.

Bodywork

Reflexology

See pages 686–687 for information about reflexology areas and how to work them.

Work the areas corresponding to the lymph system, the kidneys, and the adrenals to reduce swelling and inflammation. This gentle therapy is especially good for pregnant women.

Hydrotherapy

Contrast hydrotherapy will improve blood flow and provide pain relief. Submerge your hand and wrist in hot water for a couple of minutes; then immerse them in cold water for about thirty seconds. Repeat the sequence several times.

Other Bodywork Recommendations

You may want to look into magnet therapy, which many pain sufferers claim to be quite effective. Although the benefits of magnets are not proven, it is thought that they relieve pain by stimulating blood flow.

An experienced chiropractor or osteopath, especially one who specializes in sports therapy, can perform adjustments of the wrist, the arm, the shoulder, and the neck. Make sure to find a qualified practitioner.

Other Recommendations

- Use a cold compress to reduce swelling.
- Cigar and cigarette smoke disturbs the circulation. If you smoke, quit. If you're exposed to secondhand smoke, remove yourself from the smoky environment as much as possible.
- Pregnant women whose CTS is brought on by edema will find that their symptoms disappear after their babies are born.
- If your CTS has been caused by overuse of the wrist and the fingers, stop all repetitive hand motions for a few days. When you return to your work, you'll need to alternate repetitive tasks with other activities. Take a break every hour to rest and to rotate your wrists, and try to keep your work environment warm and dry, as cool, humid conditions can aggravate CTS.
- If you work on a computer, make sure your screen is two feet away from your body and slightly below your line of vision. Also, use a wrist rest. Most employers are now aware of CTS and will provide ergonomic workspace if you ask for it.

REFERENCES

Chen, G. S. 1990. The effect of acupuncture treatment on carpal tunnel syndrome. *American Journal of Acupuncture* 18:5–9.

Cataracts

Cataracts are the leading cause of vision loss in the United States and worldwide. Because they develop gradually, and because most of us tend to associate some vision disturbances with "normal" aging, most cases go undetected until it is too late to stop the damage. This is a shame, because when cataracts are caught in their early stages, it is possible to halt or even reverse their progression. If your eyes are healthy, you can also take steps that may help prevent cataracts altogether.

Cataracts are cloudy or opaque spots that develop on the usually translucent lens of the eye. When these spots first appear, you may not notice any difference in your vision.

Over a period of years, however, the cataract spreads across the lens. You may notice that it's harder to make out details or that colors look different. Night driving becomes more challenging. If you've been farsighted for most of your life, a cataract may actually improve your vision—for a short while. As the cataract continues to grow, it will become more difficult to see medium-sized and larger objects. In the worst-case scenario, cataracts can leave a person completely blind. In fact, 40,000 Americans go blind every year as a result of cataracts.

Most cases fall under the category that doctors call "senile cataracts." These are lens spots that commonly accompany old age, although they are by no means an inevitable part of growing older. We now know that senile cataracts are caused by damage from free radicals, the unbalanced, destructive molecules that destroy cells in the body. While the production of free radicals does naturally increase somewhat with aging, most of these dangerous agents are caused by lifestyle choices. Excess sun exposure, poor diet, and smoking are all primary causes of free radicals. Changing these habits can prevent and sometimes stop cataracts, as can taking steps to supply your body with antioxidants, the substances that fight free radicals.

In some instances, cataracts are inherited or caused by a preexisting disorder. Cataracts that begin in youth or middle age are extremely rare and are usually related to an inherited condition. In addition, people with diabetes and Down's syndrome have a higher risk of developing cataracts than the rest of the population does.

Poor digestive function can be at the root of cataracts. Low stomach acid can lead to malabsorption of nutrients from foods and can create more free radicals. In addition, toxic metals such as cadmium, mercury, and others accelerate free radical damage of the lens. Elevated blood sugar levels, as is seen with diabetes, is a major risk factor for developing cataracts.

If at any stage of your life you experience vision changes, it's important to consult a doctor or an optometrist as soon as possible. For many eye disorders, an early diagnosis can mean effective treatment. Nutritional therapy is important in the prevention and the treatment of cataracts.

SYMPTOMS

Symptoms are painless and usually progress in the following order:

- Blurring of details
- Temporary improvement of farsightedness
- Changes in color perception
- Difficulty driving at night
- Blurring of larger objects
- Darkening of vision
- Blindness

ROOT CAUSES

- Exposure to ultraviolet or infrared light
- Poor diet, especially one low in antioxidants
- Obesity
- Poor digestion
- Smoking
- Radiation

- Heavy metal poisoning
- Mineral deficiencies
- Injury to the eye
- Long-term use of steroids
- Diabetes
- Down's syndrome
- Heredity
- Pharmaceutical medications

TREATMENT

Diet

A diet to prevent or reverse cataracts can require some dedication at first. Once you've established healthful eating habits, however, you'll not only improve your eye health, you'll reduce your risk of developing almost every other disease we commonly associate with aging.

Recommended Food

Build your diet around deeply colored fruits and vegetables, which are the best sources of antioxidants, the substances that fight free radical damage. Of the antioxidants, the carotenoids are most important for eye problems. Good sources of carotenoids are dark-green leafy vegetables, bell peppers, yellow squash, carrots, tomatoes, celery, oranges, red grapes, mangoes, and melons.

Consume spinach and kale, as these foods are high in the carotenoids lutein and zeaxanthin. These carotenoids have been reported to lower the risk of developing cataracts.

Egg yolks are also rich in carotenoids.

Vitamin C and bioflavonoids work in combination to fight free radical damage. In addition, they improve the tissues and the capillaries of the eye. Good sources of bioflavonoids include berries, cherries, tomatoes, and plums; for vitamin C, eat plenty of citrus fruits.

> ### Study
>
> People who consume small amounts of fruits and vegetables and those with low blood levels of antioxidants have been reported to be at high risk for cataracts.

Food to Avoid

Banish from your diet all fried foods, as well as those that contain saturated, hydrogenated, or partially hydrogenated fats or oils. Refined and processed foods, including white flour, are also out of the question. All of these foods are high in free radicals, the atoms that destroy your body's cells—and your eyesight.

Alcohol puts a heavy burden on the liver and impairs its ability to detoxify your blood, so avoid it.

Some eye doctors have noted a link between cataracts and an inability to digest milk sugars properly. While no one has proven a connection between dairy and eye disorders, it seems prudent for people with cataracts to eliminate milk products from their diet.

Detoxification

As we age, our organs of detoxification lose some of their potency. Support your body's ability to purge itself of free radicals by undertaking a three-day juice fast once a month.

Heavy metal poisoning may cause or contribute to cataracts by preventing antioxidants from doing their job. Consider getting a hair or urine analysis to find out if you have metal poisoning; if you do, be sure to fast regularly, and be sure to look into chelation therapy.

Testing Techniques

The following tests help assess possible metabolic reasons for cataracts:

Vitamin and mineral analysis—blood

Intestinal permeability—urine

Digestion—stool analysis

Toxic (heavy) metal toxicity—urine or hair

Antioxidant scan—skin

℞ Super Seven Prescriptions—Cataract

Super Prescription #1   High-potency multivitamin
This provides a base of nutrients that will neutralize free radicals.

Super Prescription #2   Vitamin C
Vitamin C is one of the main antioxidants that protects the eye lens. Take 1,000 mg two to three times daily.

Super Prescription #3   Gentian root (*Gentiana lutea*) or **betaine HCL**
Gentian root and other bitter herbs improve stomach acid and overall digestive function. Take 250 mg or 0.5 to 1.0 ml with meals. Betaine HCL increases stomach acid levels for improved absorption. Take 1 to 2 capsules with meals.

Super Prescription #4   Bilberry (*Vaccinium myrtillus*)
Take 160 mg two to three times daily of a 25 percent anthocyanosides extract. Phytochemicals in bilberry protect the lens from free radical damage.

Super Prescription #5   B complex
Take a 50 mg complex daily. Vitamins B2 and B3 have been shown to have a protective effect against cataracts.

Super Prescription #6   Vitamin E
This potent antioxidant protects against free radical damage. Take 400 IU of a vitamin E complex with tocotrienols and tocopherols.

Super Prescription #7   Mixed carotenoid complex
Take 25,000 IU one to two times daily. It provides lutein, zeaxthanin, beta carotene, and other carotenoids that protect the lens.

Population studies show that people who take multivitamins or supplements containing vitamins C or E for more than ten years have up to a 60 percent lower risk of forming cataracts.

General Recommendations

Ginkgo biloba has a well-deserved reputation as a free-radical scavenger. It also offers general support and protection to the eyes. Choose an extract standardized to 24 percent flavone glycosides, and take 120 mg twice a day.

Alpha lipoic acid is an important antioxidant. Take 100 mg twice daily.

N-acetylcysteine increases glutathione levels, an important antioxidant for the eyes. Take 500 mg twice daily.

Bioflavonoid complex provides additional protection for the lens. Take with your vitamin C formula or separately at a dose of 500 mg twice daily. *Note:* A separate antioxidant formula can also be used to provide a broad base of antioxidants.

Grape seed or pine bark extract are both potent antioxidants that improve the micro-circulation of the eye. Take 50 mg three times daily.

Homeopathy

Many homeopathic practitioners have reported good success in slowing cataract development. The following suggestions are meant to help you get started, but it is strongly advised that you see a professional for a constitutional treatment. For temporary treatment, choose the appropriate following remedy and take 6C two or three times a day for one month. If you see improvement, take a rest from the remedy for a week, and then keep taking it in a cycle of one month on, one month off.

If a doctor or an optometrist has told you that you have cataracts in the very early stages, take Calcarea. By the time you experience symptoms, you'll need to move on to a different remedy.

Phosphorus is the remedy if you feel that there's a veil over your eyes.

If you have dimmed vision, with hot, red eyes, take Ruta Graveolens.

At the very first sign of impaired vision, take Silica (*Silicea*).

Acupressure

See pages 668–675 for information about pressure points and administering treatment.

- To improve circulation to your head and to deliver oxygen and nutrients to your eyes, work Large Intestine 3 and 4.

Bodywork

Reflexology

See pages 686–687 for information about reflexology areas and how to work them.
Work the eye/ear region and the neck.
To encourage detoxification, stimulate the liver, the kidneys, and the colon.

Stress Reduction

Although stress is not a direct cause of cataracts, unresolved tension and anxiety inhibit the body's ability to neutralize and eliminate free radicals. Review the stress-reduction techniques in the Exercise and Stress Reduction chapter and find one or two that you'd like to practice on a regular basis.

Other Recommendations

- Smoking is a leading cause of free radical damage and a factor in almost every disease we associate with "natural" aging. If you smoke, stop. And if you don't smoke, you still need to make a conscious effort to avoid secondhand smoke.
- Wear sunglasses that protect against both UVA and UVB rays. Try to avoid excursions that take place in the glare of the full sun.
- Consider the use of intravenous vitamin and mineral therapy. This provides a more aggressive treatment for cataracts.
- For many people with cataracts, surgery is a real option. If the cataract is caught early enough, a doctor can remove the entire lens and replace it with a

plastic one. The operation is not painful, and it has a high rate of success. As always, it's best to try to avoid invasive procedures by employing complementary healing strategies, but if you experience significant loss of vision, surgery may be the only way to restore sight. Talk to your doctor about your options.

REFERENCES

Jacques, P. F., and L. T. Chylack Jr. 1991. Epidemiologic evidence of a role for the antioxidant vitamins and carotenoids in cataract prevention. *American Journal of Clinical Nutrition* 53:352S–55S.

Knekt, P., M. Heliovaara, A. Rissanen, et al. 1992. Serum antioxidant vitamins and risk of cataract. *British Medical Journal* 305:1392–94.

Mares-Perlman, J. A., et al. 2000. Vitamin supplement use and incident cataracts in a population-based study. *Archives of Ophthalmology* 118:1556–63.

Cholesterol, High

High levels of cholesterol in the blood are one of the many risk factors for serious future health problems (see the Cardiovascular Disease section for information on other risk markers). Too much cholesterol can increase the chances of developing heart disease (including possibly fatal heart attacks) and stroke. By inhibiting circulation, too much of this substance can also cause gallstones, impotence, high blood pressure, and loss of mental acuity.

Cholesterol isn't all bad, however. Your body requires it in moderation for the proper function of cells, nerves, and hormones. It is an essential component of every cell in your body, and life without it would be impossible. To distribute cholesterol throughout the body, substances called lipoproteins transport it in the blood. One class of lipoproteins, called low-density lipoproteins, or LDLs for short, carries cholesterol from the liver, where it is produced, to the cells that need it. Then another kind of lipoprotein, called high-density lipoproteins, or HDLs, picks up the excess cholesterol from the cells and takes it back to the liver, where it is broken down and excreted from the body or reprocessed.

Under normal conditions, the lipoproteins keep cholesterol levels in balance. But this carefully calibrated system can be overtaxed when the body creates more cholesterol than HDL can sweep away. After the cells take what they need, the existing HDLs remove what they can, and the extra cholesterol simply remains in the blood. Then if cholesterol becomes oxidized (especially LDL cholesterol) and attaches to the artery walls, it sets the stage for inflammation of the arteries. This chronic inflammation contributes to further buildup and deposition of cholesterol and plaque on the interior walls of the arteries. We call this buildup, which narrows the arteries and limits the amount of blood that can pass through them, arteriosclerosis or hardening of the arteries. Arteriosclerosis is the first stage of heart disease; when left untreated, it will lead to a heart attack or stroke. For more information about arteriosclerosis, see Cardiovascular Disease.

Normal Cholesterol Levels

Total cholesterol: 165–200 mg/dL.

LDL cholesterol: below 130 mg/dL.

HDL cholesterol: 50 mg/dL or higher.

Total cholesterol/HDL ratio: less than 3.7

LDL/HDL ratio: less than 3.0

Note: The relative amount of total cholesterol to HDL, and the ratio of LDL to HDL is considered more important than total cholesterol.

Getting More Specific with Cholesterol

Apolipoprotein B (apoB) is a cholesterol particle that is believed to promote heart disease by affecting how cholesterol is transported into the arteries and the tissues. ApoB is found in low density lipoprotein (LDL) and other potentially harmful cholesterols, such as very low density lipoproteins (VLDL). Conversely, apolipoprotein A (apoA-1) is found in HDL cholesterol and provides a protective effect against heart disease.

A large study known as the AMORIS (Apolipoprotein-related Mortality Risk) measured the levels of apoA-1 and apoB, as well as other lipids, in more than 175,000 men and women in Sweden. Researchers found that people at greatest risk of dying from a heart attack tended to have the highest ratios of apoB to apoA01. In this study, these newer markers were more predictive of a heart attack than were the typical total, HDL, and LDL cholesterol and triglycerides. Men with the highest apoB/apoA-1 ratio had almost four times the risk of a fatal heart attack, compared to those with the lowest ratios; and in women the relative risk was threefold. ApoB appears to be an important marker for people with normal to low LDL cholesterol, as well as for those with diabetes and insulin resistance.

ApoB reference range: 55–125 mg/dL

Apo A-1 reference range: 125–215 mg/dL

ApoB/ApoA-1 ratio reference range: 0.30–0.90

Elevated cholesterol levels are often caused by the standard Western diet, which relies heavily on animal products, saturated fats, and refined carbohydrates. It can also be caused by heredity conditions or preexisting diseases like diabetes and insulin resistance, or syndrome X. Although, in these cases, diet usually plays a role as well. It stands to reason, then, that high cholesterol can often be treated with dietary changes and exercise. Specific supplements discussed in this section are also excellent non-pharmacological ways to normalize cholesterol levels. Stress reduction has a beneficial effect as well. It is strongly suggested that you employ these natural strategies before trying any of the cholesterol-lowering medications on the market. These drugs, while effective at reducing cholesterol, are potentially toxic to the liver and may cause nutritional deficiencies. While they may be necessary in some cases, many doctors prescribe them as a matter of routine—often because they're afraid that their patients won't make the lifestyle changes that can lower cholesterol naturally. If your doctor wants to prescribe a cholesterol-lowering agent for you, explain to him or her that you're willing to embark on a new regimen in the hopes of avoiding a lifelong dependency on drugs. Whatever your decision, be sure that it is based on your physician's and your analysis of your individual situation.

SYMPTOMS

Often, there are no symptoms of high cholesterol, so it's important to have your doctor perform a blood analysis regularly. One sign of high cholesterol can be a buildup of cholesterol rings on the skin under the eyes. Make an appointment if cholesterol or heart problems run in your family, or if you experience any of the following:

- Dizziness
- Mental confusion or dullness
- Circulatory problems
- Difficulty breathing after minor exertion

ROOT CAUSES

- Poor diet, especially one high in cholesterol, saturated fats, and refined carbohydrates
- Inactivity

- Hereditary tendency to high cholesterol
- Diabetes, insulin resistance
- Hypothyroidism
- Stress

Testing Techniques

Total cholesterol, HDL, LDL, VLDL, Apolipoprotein B, Apolipoprotein A-1—all are blood tests

See the Cardiovascular Disease section for a review of all cardiovascular markers that should be tested.

Oxidative damage—blood or urine

TREATMENT

Diet

Just as a poor diet is a primary cause of high cholesterol, dietary changes are one of the best ways to treat it. One major key to balancing cholesterol levels is to consume a diet that's high in fiber. This means increasing the amount of vegetables, fruits, nuts, seeds, and whole grains in the diet. Soluble fiber is a great choice. This type of fiber does not dissolve in water and binds cholesterol as it passes through the digestive tract. Oat bran is a great example of soluble fiber, and more than twenty studies show that it reduces total and LDL cholesterol when consumed on a daily basis. One bowl of oatmeal can lower cholesterol levels between 8 and 23 percent in just three weeks. Pectin, found in the skin of apples, is also effective, as is ground flaxseeds.

The reduction of fats in the diet, especially the harmful fats described in the sidebar, is important as well. In addition, eating less sugar products and refined carbohydrates can make all the difference in the world for some people's cholesterol levels. Finally, many people with diabetes and insulin resistance find that cutting down on simple carbohydrates and increasing the consumption of protein foods can dramatically reduce cholesterol levels.

Recommended Food

Soluble fiber can dramatically decrease cholesterol levels (along with your risk of developing many other diseases). Oats, brown rice, beans, and fruits are all good sources; have some at every meal. For breakfast, you might like to have a bowl of hot oatmeal, flavored with soy milk, bananas, and a little molasses, and an orange or a half grapefruit on the side.

The molecules in cholesterol are highly vulnerable to damage by free radicals. Reduce your risk of developing heart disease and other serious degenerative illness by increasing your consumption of deeply colored fruits and vegetables. Eat a wide variety for the broadest protection, and try for at least five raw or lightly cooked servings every day.

Not all fats are forbidden to people with elevated cholesterol. Essential fatty acids actually have a heart-protecting effect, so be sure to incorporate cold-water fish like salmon or mackerel into your meals several times a week. Flaxseeds are another good source of EFAs; you can sprinkle them over salads or use the oil as a dressing.

Olive oil increases levels of HDL (the "good cholesterol). The uses for this fruity oil are numerous: it can enrich pasta sauces, or you can add a little to a skillet and sauté your favorite vegetables.

Garlic and onions are savory complements to vegetarian meals—and they help lower LDL cholesterol while raising HDL.

Add spices to your meals, such as cayenne, basil, rosemary, and oregano. These spices are rich in antioxidants to prevent cholesterol oxidation.

Nuts, such as walnuts, have been shown to reduce cholesterol and trigylceride levels. Eat a handful daily.

Food to Avoid

Fats that are saturated, hydrogenated, or partially hydrogenated tend to increase cholesterol levels. By avoiding foods that contain the bad fats, you can decrease cholesterol and improve your cardiovascular health. Fried foods, sweet baked goods, and most crackers are all dangerously full of fats. Even margarine and vegetable shortening—

Hydrogenated and Partially Hydrogenated Fats

Hydrogenation is a process that turns vegetable and seed oils into soft or solid fats that, unlike the oils in their natural state, can be used as table spreads and that hold up when used in cooking or baking. During hydrogenation, the oil's carbon molecules are saturated with hydrogenation and exposed to extremely high heat. The oil is kept in the heat until it reaches the desired consistency. Shortening, for example, remains in the heat until it is completely solid; it is said to be a hydrogenated fat. Margarine, on the other hand, is removed from the heat before the oil completely hardens, just as it reaches a soft, "spreadable" consistency. Products like margarine are called partially hydrogenated oils.

It's ironic and unfortunate that margarine and even vegetable shortening are touted as heart-healthful products. For years, doctors have told us to replace butter with margarine, and most brands of shortening loudly proclaim that they have less saturated fat than butter does. But as you have probably heard, researchers have discovered that the hydrogenated process produces altered molecules called trans-fatty acids. These substances appear to pack a double whammy: not only do they raise LDL, they lower HDL and cause free radical damage. Not even butter does that kind of damage to your arteries. Scientists still have to perform more studies before they can pronounce their findings conclusive, but no matter what the ultimate results are, the fact remains: it's never a good idea to eat processed and chemically altered foods, even those that are claimed to be good for you.

This news is not a reason to eat all the butter and saturated fat you like. It's far wiser to cut down on three kinds of fats: saturated, hydrogenated, and partially hydrogenated. Instead, eat cold-water fish and sauté your vegetables and dress your salads with oils like olive, canola, and flaxseed. These foods fill you up, while raising your "good" cholesterol levels. Remember, though, that they're still fats. Enjoy them in moderation.

items that cholesterol patients often use as substitutes for butter and lard—are high in partially hydrogenated fats, which are even deadlier than the saturated kind.

Sugar and alcohol stimulate the liver to produce more cholesterol. Avoid alcoholic beverages and all sources of refined sugar, including sodas, candy, and low-fat baked goods.

An excess consumption of caffeine has been linked to high cholesterol. You don't need to cut out your coffee or black tea completely—just keep your intake down to a cup or two a day. Green tea is a much better choice, as it is rich in antioxidants that have been shown to prevent cholesterol oxidation.

Detoxification

Most people who have high cholesterol levels have been eating toxic foods. Detoxify your body (especially your liver) with a one- to three-day vegetable juice fast. As mentioned earlier, you may also find that a juice fast is an excellent way to break old eating habits.

℞ Super Seven Prescriptions—High Cholesterol

Super Prescription #1   Policosanol
Take 10 to 20 mg each evening. Numerous studies show that policosanol reduces total and LDL cholesterol, lipoprotein(a), and increases the good HDL cholesterol.

Super Prescription #2   Red yeast rice (*Monascus purpureus*)
Take 1,200 mg twice daily. This extract has been shown to reduce cholesterol levels and increase HDL. The type of product used in successful studies contained 10 to 13.5 mg of monacolins per day. *Note:* Take 100 mg of CoQ10 daily when using this product.

Super Prescription #3   Garlic (*Allium sativum*)
Take 300 to 500 mg twice of aged garlic daily. It reduces cholesterol levels and increases HDL cholesterol.

Super Prescription #4   Niacin (inositol hexaniacinate, or IP6)
Take 1,500 to 3,000 mg daily of the no-flush form (inositol hexaniacinate). It reduces cholesterol levels and increases HDL cholesterol.

Super Prescription #5   Fish oil
Take a daily dosage of a fish oil product containing at least 480 mg of EPA and 360 mg of DHA. Fish oil reduces inflammation in the arteries and lowers cholesterol and triglyceride levels.

Super Prescription #6   Guggul (*Commiphora mukul*)
Take a daily total of 1,500 mg standardized to 5 percent guggulsterone (equivalent to 75 mg of guggulsterones). This Ayurvedic herb reduces cholesterol levels and increases HDL.

Super Prescription #7   Antioxidant formula
Take a complex of antioxidants or a multivitamin, as directed on container. Several of the antioxidants prevent cholesterol oxidation.

A twelve-week study demonstrated that 1,500 mg of guggulipid reduced total cholesterol by an average of 22 percent and triglycerides by 25 percent. A different study of 233 people with elevated cholesterol levels showed that Guggul worked better than the cholesterol-lowering drug clofibrate. Only people who took Guggul had improvements in HDL cholesterol.

General Recommendations

Pantetheine is a metabolite of vitamin B5 that has been shown in studies to reduce total and LDL cholesterol, as well as to increase HDL. It can be particularly effective for people with diabetes. Take 600 to 900 mg daily.

Numerous studies have shown that vitamin C reduces the risk of dying from heart disease. One of the mechanisms, in addition to its ability to prevent cholesterol oxidation, is that it is involved in the formation of bile salts. Bile is produced by the liver and released by the gallbladder to digest fats. Cholesterol is converted into bile salts and eliminated through the digestive tract. Vitamin C enhances this process by improving bile salt formation and thus cholesterol elimination.

Soy protein has been shown in studies to reduce total and LDL cholesterol and to increase HDL. Take 25 to 50 grams daily.

Reishi (*Ganoderma lucidum*) is a mushroom extract that reduces cholesterol. Take 800 mg two to three times daily.

Vitamin E prevents LDL oxidation. Take 400 to 800 IU of a mixed blend daily.

Vitamin C reduces total cholesterol and LDL levels and acts to prevent their oxidation.

Chromium reduces total cholesterol and increases HDL levels. Take 200 to 400 mcg daily.

Green tea contains potent antioxidants known as polyphenols that reduce cholesterol oxidation. It has also been shown to reduce total cholesterol levels, while increasing good HDL cholesterol.

Cholesterol Drugs and CoQ10

The cholesterol-lowering drugs known as "statins" are among the most widely prescribed drugs today. These "statin" drugs work by inhibiting the liver enzyme HMG CoA reductase, which acts to help the liver synthesize cholesterol. This same enzyme is also involved in the synthesis of CoQ10, a vital nutrient that's required for proper heart function. A 1993 study in the *Journal of Clinical Pharmacology* found that the use of statin drugs reduced CoQ10 levels by an average of 40 percent after three months of use. Other studies have also found CoQ10 depletion effects. In one study, 100 mg per day of supplemental CoQ10 reversed this effect.

Homeopathy

If you have cardiovascular disease, see a licensed homeopath for a constitutional remedy.

Acupressure

See pages 668–675 for information about acupressure points and administering treatment.

- Keep blood flowing to your heart and chest by working Heart 3 and 7.
- If you can feel your chest tense up when you're under pressure, take some time out to work Conception Vessel 17.
- Pericardium 3 is another point for anxiety and chest pain.
- Should tension and anxiety bring on heart palpitations, work Pericardium 6.

Bodywork

Massage

If you have high cholesterol, your blood may not be able to travel through your body, especially to your extremities, as quickly as it used to. Massage can't directly lower your cholesterol levels, but it can greatly improve your circulation, as well as strengthen your heart and reduce stress. For maximum circulatory and heart benefits, a full-body massage is recommended.

Reflexology

See pages 686-687 for information about reflexology areas and how to work them.

Work the areas corresponding to the heart, the chest, the adrenals, the liver, and the thyroid.

Aromatherapy

Juniper oil will help release toxic buildup in your body. Add some to a bath, or combine it with a carrier oil and use it in a massage.

No essential oil can lower your cholesterol, but several have soothing properties that can help you relax and reduce stress. You can experiment with any of the relaxing oils mentioned on page 658, but you might like to start with lavender, marjoram, or ylang ylang. You can use any of these oils in a bath or a massage or add them to a diffuser and let the scent linger in your room or office throughout the day.

Stress Reduction

General Stress-Reduction Therapies

Persistent, unresolved stress has been linked to high cholesterol problems, as well as to heart disease and stroke. Stress reduction should be part of a comprehensive approach to preventing heart disease.

Other Recommendations

- Know your cholesterol and cardiovascular risk marker levels—all of them. Get regular checkups, and find a doctor who is willing to explain the numbers to you.
- Smoking is the number-one risk factor in heart disease. If you smoke and have high cholesterol, you're in grave danger of having a heart attack. People who smoke must quit immediately; even if you've never picked up the habit but are exposed to secondhand smoke, you must find a cleaner environment in which to live or work.
- Exercise lowers LDL levels, while raising those of HDL. Find an activity you enjoy, and pursue it regularly. A brisk thirty-minute walk every day does wonders for almost everyone.
- If you have diabetes or hypothyroidism, work with a doctor to keep your disease in check and to devise an individual plan for controlling your cholesterol.
- Many cholesterol patients are told to lose weight. The dietary suggestions here will help most people take off excess pounds, but if you're more than twenty pounds overweight, you may need additional help. See Obesity for further suggestions.

REFERENCES

Bargossi, A. M., M. Battino, A. Gaddi, et al. 1994. Exogenous CoQ10 preserves plasma ubiquinone levels in patients treated with 3-hydroxy-3-methylglutaryl coenzyme A reductase inhibitors. International Journal of Clinical and Laboratory Research 24:171–76.

Folkers, K., et al. 1990. Lovastatin decreases coenzyme Q levels in humans. *Proceedings of the National Academy of Sciences of the United States of America* 87(22):8931–34.

Ghirlanda, G., A. Oradei, A. Manto, S. Lippa, L. Uccioli, S. Caputo, A.V. Greco, and G. P. Littarru. 1993. Evidence of plasma CoQ10-lowering effect by HMG-CoA reductase inhibitors: A double-blind, placebo-controlled study. *Journal of Clinical Pharmacology* 33(3):226–29.

Kishi, T., H. Kishi, and K. Folkers. 1977. Inhibition of cardiac CoQ10 enzymes by clinically used drugs and possible prevention. In *Biomedical and Clinical Aspects of Coenzyme Q, Vol. I.* Ed. K. Folkers and Y. Yamamura. Amsterdam: Elsevier/North Holland Biomedical Press, pp. 47–62.

Mortensen, S. A., et al. 1997. Dose-related decrease of serum coenzyme Q10 during treatment with HMG-CoA reductase inhibitors. *Molecular Aspects of Medicine* 18(Suppl.):S137–S144.

Niyanand, S., et al. 1989. Clinical trials with guggulipid: A new hypolipidemic agent. *Journal of the Association of Physicians of India* 37(5):323–28.

Srinivasan, S. R., and G. S. Berenson. 2001. Apolipoproteins B and A1 as predictors of risk of coronary artery disease [commentary]. *Lancet* 358:2012–13.

Walldius, G., I. Jungner, I. Holme, A. H. Aastveit, W. Kolar, and E. Steiner. 2001. High apolipoprotein B, low apolipoprotein AI, and improvement in the prediction of fatal myocardial infarction (AMORIS study): A prospective study. Lancet 358:2026–33.

Chronic Fatigue Syndrome (CFS)

Chronic fatigue syndrome is one of the most mysterious and controversial maladies of our time. Even now, more than fifteen years after the disease was recognized and named, doctors argue about its origin or origins: Is it caused by a viral infection? Blood pressure abnormalities? Chronic infection? Food allergies? Chemical sensitivities? Some doctors wonder if the symptoms of CFS are indeed real.

Despite the doubts of a few doctors, chronic fatigue syndrome most definitely is real. And as its victims well know, it can also be horribly debilitating. Its predominant symptom is persistent, overwhelming fatigue that dramatically reduces its sufferers' ability to participate in the regular activities of life. Along with the fatigue are problems with memory and concentration. It is also usually accompanied by several out of a long list of symptoms, including but not limited to headaches, insomnia, sore throat, and muscle and joint pain. These problems can come and go over a period of years. If you have deep fatigue for more than two weeks, or if for any reason you suspect that you have CFS, do not make a diagnosis on your own. See a doctor so that he or she can rule out other possible disorders. Once other disorders have been ruled out, your best chances of recovery are, in our opinion, from the use of natural therapies.

CFS is probably caused by a combination of factors and often results in a depressed immune system. Of course, the key to treatment is to find out and treat the reason(s) for the immune system imbalance, which can be related to many factors. For example, chronic infections are thought to play a role for some people, such as the viruses Epstein-Barr (EBV), cytomegalovirus (CMV), and human herpes virus (HHV-6).

Other infections, such as mycoplasma and chlamydia, are also suspect. The overgrowth of yeast (*Candida albicans*) seems to be a common problem for people with this condition, and health practitioners frequently find parasite infection to be present.

One common finding in people with this condition is hormone imbalance. The most common one is adrenal gland insufficiency, also referred to as "adrenal burnout." The adrenal glands, located on top of both kidneys, produce the stress hormones cortisol and DHEA. These hormones are commonly depleted in people with chronic fatigue, and we find that restoring the levels to normal is generally quite helpful. The same can be said of many of the hormones in the body. Low thyroid function can be a core problem and will result in suboptimal energy production within the cells. In addition, deficiencies in testosterone or growth hormone and deficiencies or imbalances of estrogen and progesterone are common. Underlying much of the hormone imbalance can be hypothalamic dysfunction. This refers to an imbalance of the hormonal and the neural messages from the brain to the adrenal and the thyroid glands and other hormonal organs of the body.

Poor digestion and impaired detoxification also need to be considered as root causes of chronic fatigue. Malabsorption of foods and nutrients contributes to nutritional deficiencies. Environmental toxins, such as mercury and others, inhibit enzyme functions that are required for energy production.

An unhealthful diet can set the stage for chronic fatigue. A high amount of refined carbohydrates contributes to blood sugar problems, yeast overgrowth, increased demand on the adrenal glands, and chronic inflammation, and immune suppression can set in. In addition, a diet of processed foods is deficient of nutrients required for energy production and a healthy immune system.

Also of prime importance are the effects of chronic stress on the body. People who do not deal with mental, emotional, and spiritual stresses effectively are more likely to suffer fatigue. As well, unresolved problems with anxiety and depression contribute to fatigue.

Movement and exercise are fundamental keys to health. Too little exercise contributes to fatigue, while, at the opposite end of the spectrum, overtraining and overexertion lead to breakdown of the organs involved with energy production.

A final area worth mentioning is sleep. This is your body's way of recovering and regenerating. Adequate sleep is essential. If you suffer from a sleep problem, seek medical help and focus on natural ways to alleviate it. See the Insomnia section.

A good complementary care regimen will address the whole body—and therefore many of the possible causes. If you have CFS, it's important to find the treatments that give you the most relief; what works for one person might not be right for another.

SYMPTOMS

Constant, disabling fatigue is the primary symptom, but CFS usually incorporates several of the following:

- Low-grade fever
- Headache
- Sleep disturbances
- Depression and anxiety
- Difficulty concentrating
- Temporary loss of memory
- Muscle and joint pain
- Weakness
- Exhaustion after even mild exercise
- Loss of appetite
- Upper respiratory tract infections
- Sore throat
- Intestinal problems
- Sore or swollen lymph nodes

ROOT CAUSES

- Chronic infection (often viral)
- Immune system damage
- Low blood pressure
- Nutritional deficiencies
- Intestinal permeability
- Impaired detoxification
- Parasites and dysbiosis
- Food allergies
- Chemical sensitivities
- Neurological malfunction
- Chronic candidiasis
- Hypoglycemia
- Hypothyroidism
- Poor adrenal function
- Sleep disorders (such as apnea)
- Hormone deficiencies
- Environmental toxins (e.g., toxic metals)
- Unresolved stress
- Side effects of pharmaceutical medications

In a randomized, double-blind study in the *Journal of Chronic Fatigue*, researchers found that people who received an integrated treatment approach, based on each individual's symptoms and laboratory analysis, had significantly greater benefits than did people receiving a placebo. Long-term follow up found that the active group had increasing improvement.

TREATMENT

Diet

Recommended Food

Your diet should be dense with nutrients and strong in immune-building foods. Sea vegetables and whole grains are high in minerals that your body may lack; cultured foods with probiotics will fight infection, especially candidiasis; cruciferous vegetables are high in nutrients and fiber; and nuts, seeds, and cold-water fish contain lots of essential fatty acids, which support immune function.

Drink a glass of clean water every two waking hours to flush out toxins and encourage good general health.

Intestinal pain is an unpleasant symptom of CFS. Keep your digestive tract working efficiently by eating foods that are high in fiber, especially cruciferous vegetables.

Food to Avoid

People with CFS usually have severely depleted immune systems. Keep as much stress off the body as possible by avoiding caffeine, alcohol, junk and processed food, and refined sugars. In addition to taxing the immune system, some of these items aggravate conditions that may cause CFS. Caffeine depresses the adrenal glands, excess sugar consumption can lead to hypoglycemia, and junk and processed foods contain additives that stimulate chemical sensitivities.

CFS is often accompanied by food allergies; in fact, allergies may cause some cases of CFS. See the Food Allergies section and the accompanying elimination diet to help you determine which foods, if any, trigger an allergic response for you.

Be wary of wheat. Fatigue is a common symptom of wheat or gluten allergy or intolerance. Talk with your nutrition-oriented doctor about testing for a reaction to this food. Or, avoid gluten products for two to four weeks, and see if you notice an improvement.

Detoxification

Do a one- to three-day juice fast once a month to remove toxins. Green drinks are especially helpful; they speed the elimination of poisons, stimulate red blood cell production, and boost your energy.

Whiteout

When eliminating processed foods, a good rule of thumb is to watch out for the "whites." White flour, white sugar, and salt are all hallmarks of artificial or junk food products.

Testing Techniques

The following tests help assess possible metabolic reasons for chronic fatigue syndrome:

Immune system imbalance or disease—blood

Low blood pressure

Hormone testing (thyroid, DHEA, cortisol, testosterone, IGF-1, estrogen, progesterone)—saliva, blood, or urine

Intestinal permeability—urine

Detoxification profile—urine

Vitamin and mineral analysis (especially magnesium, B12, iron, and CoQ10)—blood

Digestive function and microbe/parasite/candida testing—stool analysis

Anemia—blood test (CBC, iron, ferritin, % saturation)

Food and environmental allergies/sensitivities—blood, electrodermal

Blood sugar balance—blood

Sleep disorder—sleep study

Heart function—EKG

Toxic metals—urine or hair analysis

℞ Super Seven Prescriptions—Chronic Fatigue

Super Prescription #1   B-complex
Take a 50 mg B-complex twice daily. B vitamins are involved with energy production.

Super Prescription #2   Magnesium
Take 250 mg two to three times daily. Magnesium is crucial for energy production within the cells. Reduce the dosage if diarrhea occurs.

Super Prescription #3   Vitamin B12
Take 200 to 400 mcg of the sublingual form daily or 1 cc (1,000 to 2,000 mcg) of the injectable form 1 to 2 times weekly from your doctor.

Super Prescription #4   Cordyceps sinensis
Take 800 mg twice daily of a standardized product. It supports adrenal gland function.

Super Prescription #5   DHEA
Take 5 to 25 mg daily under a doctor's supervision if testing shows that your levels are low. This adrenal hormone helps with energy production and the effects of stress.

Super Prescription #6   CoQ10
Take 100 mg two to three times daily. It is utilized within cells to produce energy.

Super Prescription #7   NADH
Take 10 mg on an empty stomach each morning.

One double-blind study looked at the effect of using 10 mg of NADH or a placebo each day for four weeks on people with chronic fatigue syndrome. Thirty-one percent of those receiving NADH reported an improvement in fatigue, a decrease in other symptoms, and improved overall quality of life, in contrast to 8 percent of those in the placebo group.

General Recommendations

Vitamin C is used by the adrenal glands to manufacture stress hormones, and it also supports immune function.

A probiotic supplies the good bacteria needed for proper digestion, detoxification, and immunity. Take a product that contains at least 4 billion organisms daily.

Essential fatty acids are important for healthy cell and brain function. Take 1 to 2 tablespoons of flaxseed oil or 3 to 5 grams of fish oil daily.

L-carnitine is used by the cells for energy production. Take 500 mg three times daily.

Panax ginseng is a strong adrenal gland tonic. Take 100 mg two to three times daily of a product standardized to between 4 and 7 percent ginsenosides.

Eleutherococcus (Siberian) ginseng is good for energy production. Take 600 to 900 mg of a standardized product daily.

Reishi (*Ganoderma lucidum*) is an adaptogen that can help with energy and mental function. Take 800 mg of a standardized product twice daily.

Ginkgo biloba is a popular herb that improves circulation, which is good for people with low blood pressure, and improves memory. Take 60 to 120 mg twice daily of a standardized product containing 24 percent flavone glycosides and 6 percent terpene lactones.

Saint-John's-wort (*Hypericum perforatum*) can be helpful when depression accompanies fatigue. Take 300 mg three times daily of a 0.3 percent hypericin extract. Do not combine with pharmaceutical antidepressants.

5-HTP is for insomnia and depression related to the fatigue. Take 100 mg two to three times daily. For insomnia, take 100 mg a half hour before bedtime on an empty stomach. Do not combine with pharmaceutical antidepressants.

Olive leaf (*Olea europa*) is for antiviral support. Take 500 mg three times daily.

Phosphatidylserine is a naturally occurring phospholipid that improves memory and increases cortisol levels. Take 300 mg daily.

Ashwagandha, known as "Indian Ginseng," is a revered herb in Ayurvedic medicine and is used as a tonic for fatigue and anxiety. Take 1,000 to 3,000 mg daily.

Enzyme complex can be taken with meals to improve digestion and absorption.

Oregano (*Origanum vulgare*) oil is for chronic infections. Take 500 mg of the capsule form four times daily or as directed on the container.

Malic acid is used by cells for energy production. Take 500 mg two to three times daily.

Licorice (*Glycyrrhiza glabra*) works to increase the levels of cortisol in the body. Take 1,000 mg two to three times daily. Blood pressure should be monitored, because in some individuals it may elevate blood pressure.

Note: The use of low doses of cortisol can be effective for people with chronic fatigue syndrome and diagnosed cortisol deficiency. Consult with your local holistic doctor for its proper use.

Homeopathy

Arsenicum Album is helpful for feelings of exhaustion, combined with anxiety and depression. The person is usually chilly, feels worse from cold food or cold environments, and often has trouble sleeping between the hours of midnight and 2 A.M.

Calcarea Carbonica is for a person with fatigue and anxiety, who tends to take on too much. He or she also suffers from swollen glands, joint pain, headache, intestinal distress, constipation, and food allergies. The person tends to be chilly, yet sweats easily.

Gelsemium (*Gelsemium sempervirens*) is for fatigue that includes drowsiness, weakness, and a bruising pain in the muscles.

Kali Phosphoricum is for a feeling of fatigue and mental weariness.

Phosphoric Acid is for extreme fatigue, where the person has an unusually strong craving for carbonated drinks. Fatigue may come on after episodes of emotional grief.

Silica (*Silicea*) is for bouts of fatigue and poor stamina. The person gets sick easily and is usually thin and chilly. Constipation is often present.

Acupressure

See pages 668–675 for information about acupressure points and administering treatment.

- Stomach 36 is an important point for CFS, because it helps your digestive system absorb nutrients.
- Gallbladder 21 stimulates circulation. It also alleviates anxiety, irritability, and headaches.
- Pericardium 6 is good for indigestion, sleeplessness, and nervous tension.
- Bladder 23 and 47 support the nervous system and are especially good for fatigue, weakness, and confusion. Do not press on these points if you have severe back pain.
- Lung 3 helps tiredness, head pain, confusion, and lightheadedness.
- Triple Warmer 5 soothes joint pain.

Bodywork

Bodywork is a good way to address the many causes and symptoms of CFS. Include at least one bodywork strategy in your treatment program.

Massage

In general, massage improves the systems weakened by CFS: immune, muscular, circulatory, digestive, and limbic. Almost any kind of massage will make you feel better, but if you're seeing a professional, you may want to ask for a lymphatic drainage massage to stimulate your immune response. Any of the essential oils listed in this section under Aromatherapy will compound the beneficial effects of massage.

You can practice gentle self-massage of your gums, tongue, and lower abdomen to strengthen your digestive system.

Chiropractic and osteopathic treatments are also helpful for proper nerve and energy flow.

Acupuncture can be very effective for fatigue. Consult with a qualified practitioner.

Reflexology

See pages 686–687 for information about reflexology areas and how to work them.

Since CFS is a systemic disorder, it's best to massage the entire foot. If you want to focus on specific symptoms, here are some suggestions.

For fatigue, work the adrenals, the diaphragm, the spine, and all the glands.

Work the endocrine glands, the solar plexus, the pancreas, and the head in case of depression.

If your doctor suspects that hypoglycemia is a cause of your CFS, massaging the pancreas area can help (although it's not a substitute for other treatment).

The liver, the gallbladder, and the stomach will ease indigestion.

Hydrotherapy

Constitutional hydrotherapy renews the nervous system. See pages 676–677 for more information.

Aromatherapy

Many oils may reduce your levels of tension and depression. Several suggestions are listed here, but you may want to refer to page 658 and try others that seem best suited to your particular needs. All of the oils mentioned here can be used as inhalants (with steam or without), in baths or diffusers, or as part of a massage.

To stimulate your muscular and nervous systems, use lavender, peppermint, or rosemary.

Geranium, bergamot, and neroli combat fatigue related to depression.

Tea tree oil fights bacteria, viruses, and fungi. Because it strengthens the immune system, it's an especially good complement to a lymphatic massage.

For general relaxation and calming benefits, try rose, jasmine, lavender, or bergamot in any preparation you like. If you need all-day stress relief, consider using a diffuser that allows the scent to fill your home or office.

Stress Reduction

CFS sufferers can grow weary of well-meaning friends and family members who suggest that their problem is "all in your head." But don't let exasperation regarding this popular misconception prevent you from seeking relief from depression, tension, and anxiety—all of which are linked in some way to CFS, as either a cause or a symptom. Experiment with several stress-reduction techniques, and practice them daily.

General Stress-Reduction Therapies

If you're ready for a gentle workout, take a yoga class. Yoga relieves joint and muscle pain, and several of the poses help strengthen the digestive muscles.

If you suffer from anxiety, consider EEG biofeedback to teach you to control your brainwaves.

Bach Flower Remedies

Consult the chart on pages 648–650 to find the appropriate flower remedy for your particular condition. Once you've select the right remedy, place 10 drops of the liquid under your tongue. Hold the drops in place for thirty seconds and swallow. Use as often as needed.

If you are burned out and exhausted at the thought of any activity, whether mental or physical, take Hornbeam.

Olive is the remedy for people who have little interest in anything or anyone.

Mustard is for sadness and depression without an obvious cause.

If you despair of ever feeling better again, try Gorse.

Other Recommendations

- Take a walk every day in the early morning sunlight. You'll stimulate your immune system, get vitamin D, and ward off the depression and the anxiety that often attend CFS.

- Don't try to do too much. Listen to your body; when it tells you to get rest, do so.
- Don't smoke or expose yourself to secondhand smoke. You'll wreak havoc on your immune system.
- Breathe slowly and deeply to encourage relaxation and to diminish stress.
- Try to keep an optimistic outlook, and focus on a positive outcome.
- Go to bed by 9 P.M. and take a thirty-minute nap after lunch each day.

REFERENCES

Forsyth, L. M., H. G. Preuss, A. L. MacDowell, L. Chiazze Jr., G. D. Birkmayer, and J. A. Bellanti. 1999. Therapeutic effects of oral NADH on the symptoms of patients with chronic fatigue syndrome. Annals of Allergy, Asthma & Immunology 82(2):185–91.

Teitelbaum, J., et al. 2001. Effective treatment of chronic fatigue syndrome and fibromyalgia—A randomized, double-blind, placebo-controlled, intent to treat study. Journal of Chronic Fatigue Syndrome 8(2).

Common Cold

Colds are caused by any of more than two hundred viruses that infect the upper respiratory tract. Colds are spread through the air, such as by sneezing or coughing, or by contact with a contaminated object. In response to an invasion by a cold virus, the membranes that line the nose and the throat become swollen and start producing additional mucus. The result is congestion, sneezing, coughing, sore throat, and a general feeling of malaise—all of which are your body's way of expelling the virus and getting you to slow down and rest. Although colds can come on at any time of the year, they are most common during late fall and winter. They especially target people whose immune systems are depressed, whether from overwork, preexisting disorders, or a lack of good nutrition and exercise.

The best treatment for a cold is to stimulate your body's natural defenses as soon as the familiar symptoms first appear. Once the virus firmly establishes itself in your system, you can use natural therapies that have direct antiviral activity, as well as stimulate your immune system to eradicate the virus. Most colds last three to ten days. Do not take over-the-counter medications. These cold symptoms are your immune system's attempts to flush out the virus, so medications that suppress them can actually prolong your cold or cause a recurrence.

Colds can be difficult to distinguish from the flu. For adults, the presence of body aches and a fever usually indicates the flu, although a low-grade fever can sometimes exist alongside a cold. Children, on the other hand, may experience fevers as a normal part of a cold. For more information about the flu, see Flu. If your cold symptoms persist, or if they are accompanied by yellow or green mucus, call your doctor. You may have allergies or a different infection, such as sinusitis.

For adults, more than two colds a year may be an indication of underlying toxicity in the body. Some researchers feel that the body uses the cold virus as a way of detoxifying itself through mucus elimination and reduced appetite. In many cases, this could certainly be true. Also, a weakened immune system due to poor lifestyle habits and nutritional deficiencies could be at the root of reoccurring colds.

SYMPTOMS

- Runny nose
- Sneezing
- Congestion
- Cough
- Sore throat

- Swollen lymph glands
- Fatigue
- Loss of appetite
- Mild fever (occasionally, fevers can be higher in children)

ROOT CAUSES

- Toxicity in the body
- A deficient immune system due to

lifestyle factors, nutritional deficiencies, and high stress levels.

TREATMENT

Diet

Recommended Food

Eat lightly. Steamed vegetables, soups and broths, and herbal teas will let your body focus on healing, instead of on digestion. If you lose your appetite, don't force yourself to eat.

Stay hydrated. Drink plenty of clean water and other fluids (but see the note in the next section about sugar and juice) to cleanse away toxins and to keep the respiratory tract from drying out.

Increase your consumption of ginger, onions, and garlic. Try adding one or both to chicken soup or miso.

Hot water with lemon, honey, and cinnamon is a traditional cold remedy. Drink a cup every two hours to soothe your throat and chest, prevent mucus buildup, and encourage a cleansing sweat.

Food to Avoid

Sugar decreases the number of white blood cells that your body produces and depresses your immune system, so eliminate refined sugars from your diet for the duration of your illness. Also be wary of fruit juices. Although they are a traditional treatment for colds, fruit juices—especially orange juice—usually contain far more sugar than they do vitamin C. If you want to drink juice, dilute it first.

Avoid milk and other dairy products while you're sick. They encourage the production of mucus and will only make you feel worse.

℞ Super Seven Prescriptions—Common Cold

Super Prescription #1   Homeopathic Combination Cold Remedy
At the first signs of a cold, take a dose of the Combination Cold Remedy four times daily for three days. Then if you notice improvement, stop taking the remedy, unless symptoms return. If your symptoms do not improve within twenty-four hours, pick the remedy that best matches your symptoms under Homeopathy in this section.

Super Prescription #2   Echinacea (*Echinacea purpurea*) and **goldenseal** (*Hydrastis canadensis*)
Echinacea and goldenseal combinations are herbs that enhance immune function,

and echinacea has antiviral properties. *Note:* If you do not have any mucus production, use only echinacea. Take 500 mg or 2 to 4 ml of tincture four times daily.

Super Prescription #3   Lomatium dissectum

Take 500 mg or 2 to 4 ml of the tincture four times daily. Lomatium has strong antiviral effects.

Super Prescription #4   Vitamin C

Take 1,000 mg three to four times daily. Reduce the dosage if diarrhea occurs. Vitamin C supports immune system function through increased white blood cell activity.

Super Prescription #5   Zinc

Take 15 to 25 mg in zinc lozenge form (zinc gluconate or acetate) every two waking hours for four days. Zinc supports immune function and may have antiviral effects. Zinc nasal sprays may be even more effective. Take as directed on the container.

Super Prescription #6   Ginger (*Zingiber officinale*)

Take 500 mg of the capsule or drink the fresh tea four times daily. Ginger helps with a sore throat and chills.

Super Prescription #7   Astragalus (*Astragalus membranaceus*)

Take 500 to 1,000 mg or 3.0 ml of a tincture two to three times daily. Astragalus is an excellent treatment for preventing the common cold. Do not take astragalus if you have a fever.

Studies on the effectiveness of echinacea for the common cold have been mixed. It appears that the type of standardization and the potency of the product are important for achieving therapeutic effects. One randomized double-blind clinical study looked at the effectiveness of *Echinacea purpurea* for 120 patients with initial symptoms of acute, uncomplicated upper airway infection (in other words, the common cold). Echinacea (20 drops every two hours for the first day and thereafter three times daily) or a placebo was administered for up to ten days, after which patients were questioned about the intensity of their illness, time to improvement, and time until cessation of treatment. The time taken to improve was significantly shorter in the echinacea group, at four days, while people in the placebo group took an average of eight days to recover. No specific adverse events were reported.

General Recommendations

Oregano (*Origanum vulgare*) oil has powerful antiviral effects. Take 500 mg of the capsule form four times daily or as directed on the container.

Elderberry (*Sambucus nigra*) is useful for the common cold and the flu. Adults can take 10 ml and children 5 ml three times daily.

Garlic (*Allium sativum*) combats infection and supports the immune system. Take 300 to 500 mg or the liquid form three times daily. It can also be used on a long-term basis for preventing colds.

Thymus extract (*Thymus vulgaris*) optimizes immune activity. Take 1 to 2 capsules twice daily or as directed on the container.

Homeopathy

At the first signs of a cold, take 2 pellets of a 30C potency four times daily for three days of the remedy that best matches your symptoms in this section. Then if you notice improvement, stop taking the remedy, unless symptoms return. If your symptoms do not improve within twenty-four hours, pick another remedy.

Aconitum Napellus is for colds that come on suddenly after exposure to dry, cold weather. There is a scratchy throat and a thin discharge from the nose. You probably feel anxious, restless, and chilly, with a great thirst. This remedy is best taken within four hours of developing cold symptoms.

A review of twenty-one placebo-controlled studies found that "in each of the twenty-one studies, vitamin C reduced the duration of episodes and the severity of the symptoms of the common cold by an average of 23 percent." A dosage of 1,000 to 8,000 mg was used in these studies.

Allium Cepa is helpful when a person has a clear, burning nasal discharge that irritates the nostrils and the upper lip. The eyes water and have a stinging pain. The nose runs more when indoors and stops when outdoors.

Arsenicum Album is for a cold with a profuse, clear, watery discharge from the nose that makes the upper lip red. The nose may be stuffed but still runs. The person feels chilly, is thirsty for sips of water, and feels anxious and restless.

Ferrum Phosphoricum helps when a person feels feverish but does not act sick. The throat may be sore, and the face is flushed. It's best used at the onset of a cold.

Gelsemium (*Gelsemium sempervirens*) is for a cold accompanied by chills and muscle ache. The person feels drowsy and fatigued and has droopy eyelids. There may be a headache at the back of the neck.

Mercurius Solubilis or Vivus is helpful when the person is sensitive to both hot and cold temperatures. The tongue has a thick coating, and the person has bad breath, has excessive saliva production, and drools on pillow. The throat is often raw and sore.

Natrum Muriaticum is for colds that begin with sneezing and produce a thin clear or white discharge. The person may have a headache that is worse in the sun or the light. The cold may be accompanied by cold sores around the mouth and chapped lips.

Nux Vomica (*Strychnos nux vomica*) is for a person who is very chilly and irritable. Sneezing and coughing, along with a congested nose and sore throat, are common.

Pulsatilla (*Pulsatilla pratensis*) is helpful when there is thick yellow or green nasal mucus. The person has a low thirst and feels warm. The person also feels congested and is better outdoors or with fresh air. There is a desire to be comforted.

Acupressure

See pages 668–675 for information about acupressure points and administering treatment.

- Large Intestine 4 is a general tonic for colds and a specific remedy for headaches and congestion.
- If you have a sore throat, a cough, or chest congestion, use Kidney 27.
- Bladder 2 and Large Intestine 20 work on sinus congestion and pain.
- For head pain and congestion, use Gallbladder 20 and Governing Vessel 16 and 24.5.

Bodywork

Massage

If you are very congested, try a percussive massage to break up mucus. Percussive motions are best used on people who are relatively strong and healthy. Otherwise, a simple back rub may ease some of the congestion.

Reflexology

See pages 686–687 for information about reflexology areas and how to work them.

Work all the toes, as well as the areas corresponding to the lungs, the adrenal glands, the lower spine, the pituitary glands, and the lymph system.

If you have a sore throat, also massage the neck area.

Hydrotherapy

Hot baths, showers, and steams all help drain phlegm and detoxify the body. For extra benefits, add any of the essential oils listed in this entry under Aromatherapy.

If you're chilled, take frequent hot foot baths; otherwise, alternating hot and cold foot baths are excellent.

Aromatherapy

Any of the following oils can be added to baths or steam inhalations.

Lavender has immune-boosting properties and will also help you get to sleep. It's especially soothing if you have a cough.

Eucalyptus and peppermint relieve congestion and stimulate circulation.

Tea tree and melissa oils fight viruses and also work against any secondary bacterial infections that may develop.

Stress Reduction

Stress lowers your resistance and makes you much more susceptible to colds. If you get colds frequently, read the chapter on stress reduction in Part Two of this book and incorporate at least one of the techniques discussed there into your daily routine.

Bach Flower Remedies

For chronic stress problems that lead to colds, see the chart on pages 648–650 to find the remedy that best suits your personality and tendencies. Once you've chosen a remedy, place 10 drops of the liquid under your tongue. Hold the drops in place for thirty seconds and swallow. Use as often as needed.

Rescue Remedy is for physical crises, as well as emotional ones. It will bolster your defenses when you feel a cold coming on or when you're under a great deal of stress and surrounded by sick people in the office or at home.

Some people make little effort to get better when they have a cold; they even seem to welcome the illness. If you fall into this category, take Clematis to increase your resolve.

Other Recommendations

- Get plenty of sleep and rest.
- Unless you have a fever, take a brisk walk to keep mucus from settling into your body and to chase away the blues. Don't engage in any vigorous exercise, however.
- Keep a humidifier in your room. The moist air will thin secretions.
- If you have a sore throat, gargle with salt water.
- Colds can circulate through an entire family—and even come back to you. Break the cycle by keeping your hands clean and flushing tissues after you use them. Encourage your family members to eat well, to get rest, and to wash their hands often during your illness.

REFERENCES

Heisel, O., et al. 1997. Echiniguard treatment shortens the course of the common cold: A double-blind, placebo-controlled clinical trial. *European Journal of Clinical Research* 9:261–68.

Hemilä, H. 1994. Does vitamin C alleviate the symptoms of the common cold?—a review of current evidence. Scandinavian Journal of Infectious Diseases 26:1–6.

Constipation

In a healthy body, waste travels through the digestive tract in a predictable, regular cycle, usually taking between six and twenty-four hours to pass. Sometimes, however, waste matter passes through the large intestine too slowly, and the result is called constipation. When the bowels are constipated, it may be difficult or impossible to pass stools; in fact, the urge to pass may be absent altogether. Sometimes constipation has no signs other than the lack of bowel movement, but, usually, it is accompanied by a host of uncomfortable symptoms, ranging from a general feeling of malaise to a distended abdomen and painfully hard stools.

A healthy person generally has one to three complete bowel movements daily.

Although constipation is the number-one gastrointestinal disorder in the United States, its unwelcome effects are actually rather easy to avoid. Our Western diet—high in fat and low in fiber and fluids—is the cause of most constipation. When fiber and fluids are lacking, the contracting motions of the large intestine are not stimulated in a regular fashion, and waste is therefore not propelled through the tract. Treatment, then, relies largely on dietary changes. Other factors, such as stress, inactivity, and certain medications, can cause or contribute to constipation as well. Dietary changes are still encouraged in these cases, along with the removal, when possible, of the offending factor. No matter how much or how little discomfort you have, it is always important to address the causes of constipation. When waste matter remains in the colon for a long period of time, recent studies show that bacteria and other harmful matter can be reabsorbed back into the bloodstream.

Stress or suppressed emotions are often overlooked factors with constipation. There is a direct connection between perceived stress levels and gut motility. In addition, people with hectic lifestyles often do not take the time for regular bowel movements. And sometimes children hold back on stool movements for fear of pain or inconvenience.

A poorly functioning digestive system can also be a major contributor to constipation. This is particularly true with deficient bile flow from the liver and the gallbladder. Herbal therapies in this chapter work to improve bile production and flow.

The use of over-the-counter laxatives is a significant problem for many people with constipation. Although these medications relieve constipation, many of them make the bowels lazier over time.

Occasionally, constipation signals a more serious condition. If you have bloody stools, intense abdominal pain, or a cut near your rectum, see your doctor. And since chronic constipation can cause other illnesses, make an appointment if you have constipation that recurs or a single episode that lasts longer than a week.

Many people think of constipation as an uncomfortable but essentially harmless condition. In reality, recurring long-term bouts can lead to other problems, some merely distressing and others very serious. Constipation has been linked to the following disorders:

Arthritis

Skin disorders

Bad breath

Mood disorders, including depression

Headaches

Irritable bowel syndrome

Fatigue

Hemorrhoids

Hernias

Insomnia

Malabsorption syndrome

Weight gain

Varicose veins

SYMPTOMS

- Difficulty passing stools
- Decreased frequency passing stools
- Bloated, tender abdomen
- Loss of appetite
- Flatulence
- Malaise

ROOT CAUSES

- Poor diet (low fiber, low water intake)
- Stress
- Inactivity
- Medications
- Intestinal parasites
- Lack of beneficial intestinal flora
- Laxative or enema abuse
- Magnesium deficiency
- Colitis
- Underactive thyroid
- Liver problems

TREATMENT

Diet

Recommended Food

If you're unaccustomed to a high-fiber diet, move into these recommendations slowly. A sudden increase of dietary fiber can be quite a shock to the system and can even cause further digestive problems.

The basic, wholesome diet recommended at the beginning of this book is an excellent source of fiber. Eat lots of whole grains, especially brown rice; raw or lightly cooked fruits and vegetables; and beans, nuts, and seeds. Chew thoroughly, and don't eat too much at one sitting, even of healthful foods.

People with constipation often have a magnesium deficiency. Green leafy vegetables are high in this mineral, as well as in fiber, so now you have another reason to eat kale, broccoli, spinach, brussels sprouts, and the like.

Prunes and figs are time-honored sources of dietary fiber. You may want to plan on making one of these items a regular part of your breakfast.

Flaxseeds are a lesser-known but highly concentrated source of fiber. Don't cook with flaxseeds or subject them to heat; instead, sprinkle them on cereals or salads. Adults should take 1 to 2 tablespoons of ground flaxseeds daily, along with 10 ounces of water. Children can take 1 to 2 teaspoons.

Hot cereals or warm liquids at breakfast can stimulate contractions of the lower intestine. Enjoy some hot oatmeal or herbal tea, or do as our grandmothers did and add lemon juice to a glass of warm water.

Consume fermented products on a regular basis to keep your intestinal flora in balance. Kefir and sauerkraut are good choices, as is live unsweetened yogurt once the acute constipation is relieved.

Drink plenty of water to keep stools soft. A glass of clean water every two waking hours is usually an adequate amount.

Food to Avoid

Do not eat foods that are fried or otherwise high in saturated fat. Fat slows travel time through the intestines.

Avoid mucus-forming foods, which also slow the transit time of waste matter. Foods that encourage mucus production include all dairy products, fried and processed foods, refined flours, and chocolate.

A *New England Journal of Medicine* study of children with chronic constipation reported that cow's milk was the cause of it for two-thirds of the children involved in the study.

Caffeine and alcohol are hard on the digestive system and are dehydrating as well. During an episode of constipation, avoid them entirely. When you're regular again, consume them only in small quantities.

Detoxification

In severe or recurring cases of constipation, you may wish to undertake a three-day vegetable juice fast. See page 548 for details on the vegetable juice fast. Juices that are especially supportive of a cleanse for constipation include aloe, cabbage, apple, and green drinks. You still need fiber during a constipation cleanse, so add psyllium husks or flaxseeds to your juices.

Testing Techniques

The following tests help assess possible metabolic reasons for constipation:

Stool analysis for good bacteria levels, parasites, and infection

Thyroid hormones—blood, saliva, or urine

℞ Super Seven Prescriptions—Constipation

Super Prescription #1   Flaxseed oil
Take 1 to 2 tablespoons daily for adults and 1 to 2 teaspoons for children. Flaxseed oil lubricates the colon for an easier passage.

Super Prescription #2   Probiotic
Take a product containing at least 4 billion active organisms daily. Friendly bacteria (*Lactobacillus acidophilus, bifidus)* help with digestion and elimination.

Super Prescription #3   Cascara sagrada
Take 250 mg or 2.5 ml of tincture two to three times daily for the relief of acute constipation. This herb should not be used as a long-term solution for constipation.

Super Prescription #4   Dandelion root (*Taraxacum officinale*)
Take 250 to 500 mg or 2 ml with each meal. Dandelion stimulates bile flow and improves constipation.

Super Prescription #5   Psyllium
Take 1 teaspoon or 5 grams of psyllium husks twice daily or as directed on the container. Take it with 10 ounces of water. Psyllium acts as a bulk-forming laxative.

Super Prescription #6   Homeopathic Nux Vomica (*Strychnos nux vomica*)
Take a 30C potency twice daily for relief of acute constipation. See the homeopathic description further on of Nux Vomica, as well as of other indicated remedies.

Super Prescription #7   Magnesium
Take 250 mg two to four times daily for the relief of acute constipation. Magnesium improves gut motility and retains water in the colon. Do not use on a long-term basis, as it can lead to malabsorption and electrolyte imbalance.

General Recommendations

Milk thistle (*Silybum marianum*) improves liver function and bile flow. Take 200 to 250 mg of a product standardized to 80 percent silymarin with each meal.

Fenugreek (*Trigonella foenum-graecum*) is an herb that improves bowel contractions. Take 250 mg or 2 ml twice daily with meals.

Aloe vera juice improves bowel movements. Take a quarter cup twice daily or as directed on container.

Gentian root (*Gentiana lutea*) improves overall digestive function. Take 300 mg or 10 to 20 drops five to fifteen minutes before meals.

Enzymes improve digestive function. Take 1 to 2 capsules with each meal.

Homeopathy

Pick the remedy that best matches your symptoms in this section. Take a 6x, 12x, 6C, or 30C potency twice daily for two weeks to see if there are any positive results. After you notice improvement, stop taking the remedy, unless symptoms return. Consultation with a homeopathic practitioner is advised.

Alumina is for someone who goes many days without a stool. Stools are hard and dry. The person must strain to pass even a soft stool, and the person may have memory problems.

Bryonia (*Bryonia alba*) is helpful when there is no desire to pass stool. The stool is dry and hard. The person has a great thirst, is irritable, and may have a headache.

Calcarea Carbonica is for the chronically constipated person who feels chilly, with clammy hands and feet. The person feels overwhelmed.

Lycopodium (*Lycopodium clavatum*) is helpful when a person has constipation and problems with gas and bloating. There is a craving for sweets, and symptoms are worse in the late afternoon. The digestive system feels better with warm drinks.

Natrum Muriaticum is for people with constipation who have a strong craving for salt and water. The person may suffer from depression and is often sensitive to the sun or the light.

Nux Vomica (*Strychnos nux vomica*) is helpful when one has an urgent feeling but can't pass stools or stools are never completed. The person feels irritable and overstressed. Nux Vomica works well for people who work too hard, exercise too little, and eat and drink too much. It also helps those who have become addicted to laxatives.

Sepia is for constipation accompanied by hormonal issues, such as PMS and menopause. The person feels irritable and chilly and has stools that are hard to pass. A heavy sensation in the rectum and the lower abdomen may be present.

Silica (*Silicea*) helps when a person strains for a long time to have a bowel movement. Stool may come a little way out and then recede back in. The person is generally chilly and thin.

Sulphur is helpful if you have constipation alternating with diarrhea. The stool is often dry and hard, and the rectum is inflamed and burning. The person has a strong thirst for ice-cold drinks.

Acupressure

Use these points twice a day until you get relief. For chronic, recurring cases, you may have to work these points for several weeks before the fundamental problem is addressed. For more information about acupressure points and administering treatment, see pages 668–675.

- In acupressure, the most effective point for constipation and abdominal cramps is Conception Vessel 6.
- Another point that stimulates intestinal contractions is Large Intestine 4.

- Large Intestine 11 will strengthen the colon.
- Stomach 36 is a good general toner that strengthens the digestive system.

Bodywork

Massage

A self-massage of the abdomen feels quite relieving if you're constipated. Better yet, it can induce intestinal contractions. Lie down with your knees bent, and massage your abdomen with the flat of your hand, using pressure that's firm but gentle. Add the stimulating oils listed under Aromatherapy in this section for a more potent effect.

If you prefer, you can also get a professional massage of your lower back and pelvis.

Reflexology

See pages 686–687 for information about reflexology areas and how to work them.

Work the areas corresponding to the colon, the liver, the gallbladder, and the adrenal glands.

If stress is a cause or a result of constipation, also work the area that corresponds to the solar plexus.

In cases of chronic constipation, massage the entire foot and hand to address the systemic damage.

Hydrotherapy

Constitutional hydrotherapy is excellent to help with long-term and acute problems with constipation. See pages 676–677 for directions.

Aromatherapy

Black pepper and marjoram stimulate and warm the digestive system. Add them to a carrier oil, and use it in an abdominal massage or a bath.

If you need to relieve stress, you can experiment with many different oils and rotate your favorites so that you don't build up a tolerance to them. See page 658 for details on oils; you may want to start off with bergamot, jasmine, lavender, rose, sandalwood, or ylang ylang. Use them in any preparation you like.

Stress Reduction

General Stress-Management Therapies

Yoga and Pilates can be a wise choice for people suffering from constipation.

Laugh often. Laughter produces endorphins, the feel-good hormones, and takes you away from your worries, even if just for a few moments. It also stimulates and strengthens your digestive organs.

Bach Flower Remedies

Select the appropriate remedy, and place 10 drops of the liquid under your tongue. Hold the drops in place for thirty seconds and swallow. Use as often as needed.

If you feel tense but try to hide it, and if you often give in to others in hopes of avoiding conflict, use Agrimony.

Mimulus is the remedy for people whose fear, shyness, and sensitivity leave them too upset to act.

If you are stubborn, with a strong sense of duty that often leads you to ignore your own needs, take Oak.

Other Recommendations

- Exercise helps to stimulate intestinal contractions. You don't need to run a marathon: mild to moderate aerobic exercise should be enough. A brisk walk, taken thirty minutes every morning, is a goal most of us can easily achieve. Crunches done properly are also helpful to strengthen the abdominal muscles.
- Beware of over-the-counter laxatives. They are extremely harsh and can create an unhealthful dependency.
- Never repress the urge to defecate. When you hold back, you are actually training your bowels to misbehave. The result is often chronic—even lifelong—constipation.
- It is possible to retrain your bowels, if necessary. Sit on the toilet at the same time every day, even if you don't have an urge. Early morning or directly after exercise are usually good times. Do not strain—you'll only create hemorrhoids or varicose veins. Instead, breathe deeply, using your abdominal muscles, and try to relax.

REFERENCES

Iacono, G., F. Cavataio, G. Montalto, A. Florena, M. Tumminello, M. Soresi, A. Notarbartolo, and A. Carroccio. 1998. Intolerance of cow's milk and chronic constipation in children. *New England Journal of Medicine* 339(16):1100–4.

Cough

Coughing is a normal part of the body's immune system and respiratory defense system. Quick, sudden bursts of air and fluids from the respiratory tract help expel microbes, dust, chemicals, and other irritants, as well as foreign objects, from the airway.

Coughing can be a symptom of an underlying infection of the bronchial tubes or lungs, such as bronchitis, pneumonia, or croup. In some cases, it can suggest more serious diseases, such as asthma, lung cancer, or heart problems.

The goal in treating a cough is to address the underlying cause. For example, with infections, the immune system must be stimulated, and for allergy-produced coughs, the allergen must be removed or you must become desensitized to it. In any case, remember not to suppress a cough too much. In cases of infection, this is particularly true. The goal is to allow the body to expel foreign matter and to detoxify, while simultaneously soothing the cough to make a person more comfortable. This will prevent suppression of the disease, so that it doesn't turn into something more serious (such as bronchitis becoming pneumonia).

Be aware that certain drugs, such as some blood pressure medications, are known to cause coughing as a potential side effect.

If a cough lasts more than two weeks or if you have difficulty breathing or blood in the sputum, consult a doctor immediately.

SYMPTOMS

- Dry or wet cough

ROOT CAUSES

- Infection
- Allergens (environmental or food)
- Obstruction in the airway
- Anxiety

Testing Techniques

The following tests help assess possible metabolic reasons for coughing:

Food and environmental allergy testing—blood or electrodermal

Infection—blood work

Obstruction of airway—x-ray

TREATMENT

Diet

Recommended Food

To thin mucus secretions, drink a glass of clean water every two waking hours.

Homemade chicken soup also thins mucus. Add garlic or ginger for flavor and immune support.

To reduce phlegm, have some hot barley soup.

Onions are an old folk remedy and have anti-inflammatory properties, so eat them often.

If you have bacterial bronchitis and are taking antibiotics, consume nondairy sour products, such as kefir or sauerkraut, daily to replenish disease-fighting bacteria.

Food to Avoid

Eliminate foods that encourage mucus production: dairy products, chocolate, and bananas, as well as processed, refined, fried, and junk foods. Avoid simple sugars, as they suppress immune function.

Detoxification

Fast on water, soup, juice, and herbal tea for a few days to let your body turn its full attention to fighting the infection. Fasting will also speed the elimination of mucus, especially when expectorant herbal teas are part of the regimen. (See the following herbal recommendations.)

℞ **Super Seven Prescriptions—Cough**

Super Prescription #1   Homeopathy

Use a combination cough remedy, as directed on the container, or pick the remedy that best matches your symptoms under Homeopathy in this section. For acute coughs, take a 30C potency four times daily. For chronic coughs, take twice daily for two weeks to see if there are any positive results. After you notice improvement, stop taking the remedy, unless symptoms return. Consultation with a homeopathic practitioner is advised.

Super Prescription #2   Licorice (*Glycyrrhiza glabra*)

Licorice reduces coughing, enhances immune function, and soothes the respiratory tract. Use caution when supplementing licorice root if you have high blood pressure. It is best used short term under the guidance of a holistic doctor. Take 500 mg of the capsule or 1 ml of the tincture four times daily.

Super Prescription #3   Cherry bark

This reduces coughing, especially for wet coughs. Take 500 mg of the capsule or 1 ml of the tincture four times daily.

Super Prescription #4   N-acetylcysteine (NAC)

NAC reduces the viscosity of sputum so that it is easier to expectorate. It's useful for acute and chronic wet coughs (especially for smokers or people with asthma or emphysema). Take 300 to 500 mg twice daily.

Super Prescription #5   Mullein (*Verbascum thapsus*)

Take 500 mg of the capsule or 2 ml of the tincture four times daily. This herb promotes the discharge of mucus and has soothing and anti-inflammatory effects for the respiratory tract.

Super Prescription #6   Echinacea (*Echinacea purpurea*) and **goldenseal** (*Hydrastis canadensis*)

For acute bronchitis with a wet cough, take 500 mg or 2 ml of this combination four times daily. Both herbs enhance immune function, and goldenseal works to dry up mucus.

Super Prescription #7   Astragalus (*Astragalus membranaceus*)

Astragalus is an excellent treatment for chronic, as well as acute, bronchitis. It strengthens weak lungs and increases the body's general resistance to infection. Take 500 to 1,000 mg or 3.5 ml of a tincture two or three times daily. Do not take astragalus if you have a fever.

General Recommendations

Vitamin C enhances immune function for acute bronchitis and has anti-allergy benefits for chronic bronchitis. Vitamin C is particularly important for smokers. Take 500 to 1,000 mg three times daily.

Garlic (*Allium sativum*) has antimicrobial effects. Take 300 to 600 mg of garlic extract twice daily.

Bromelain has a natural anti-inflammatory effect and enhances the effectiveness of some antibiotics. Look for products standardized to 2,000 M.C.U. (milk-clotting units) per 1,000 mg or 1,200 G.D.U. (gelatin-dissolving units) per 1,000 mg. Take 500 mg three times daily between meals or along with antibiotic therapy.

Colloidal silver has an antimicrobial effect, especially for bacteria. Take ½ to 1 teaspoon, or as directed on the container, three times daily for five days.

Vitamin A enhances immune function. Take 25,000 to 50,000 IU daily for five days.

Ivy leaf (*Hedera helix*) may be helpful for chronic bronchitis for both children and adults. Take as directed on the container.

Other herbs that are useful and can be found in respiratory formulas include horehound, pleurisy root, plantain, marshmallow, ginger, peppermint, and cherry bark.

Homeopathy

Antimonium Tartaricum is for a congested, wet cough that produces a rattling noise in the chest. The person has trouble expectorating and may find it hard to breathe at times. The person feels better in a cool room and with the windows open.

Arsenicum Album is for a cough with a burning pain that feels better with sips of warm drinks. The person feels anxious and restless and may be very fatigued. Symptoms are worse from 12 A.M. to 2 A.M.

Bryonia (*Bryonia alba*) will treat a dry cough that causes stitching pain in the throat or the chest and that is worse at night. Movement of any type feels worse. The person has a great thirst and prefers to be left alone.

Coccus Cacti is for a cough that produces stringy mucus. The person feels a need to constantly clear the throat. Coughing often leads to vomiting.

Drosera is for a dry, barking cough that may end in gagging. The cough is worse lying down and worse after midnight.

Hepar Sulphuris (*Hepar sulphuris calcareum*) is for a rattling, barking cough that comes on after exposure to dry, cold air. The person coughs when uncovered and feels chilly and irritable. There is often yellowish mucus.

Kali Bichromium is for a hoarse cough that produces thick, stringy, yellow mucus. The cough is worse from eating and drinking.

Phosphorous is for a dry, tickling cough that is worse in the cold air, with talking or laughing, and when lying on the left side. The person may have a burning sensation in the chest and feels better with cold drinks.

Pulsatilla (*Pulsatilla pratensis*) will clear up a cough with yellow or green phlegm that is looser in the morning and drier at night. The person has a low thirst and feels better near an open window. The cough is worse when the person lies down.

Rumex Crispus is for a dry cough that begins as soon as a person lies down. The person feels a tickling sensation in the throat that leads to a cough. The cough is worse in cold air.

Silica (*Silicea*) is for a person who seems to have bronchitis all winter long. The person has weak immunity and low stamina and feels chilly. Coughing up mucus takes a lot of effort.

Spongia Tosta is helpful when someone has a dry, barking cough that is better with warm foods or liquids.

Sulphur is for bronchitis with burning pains that feel better with cold drinks. The person feels warm and desires a cool room. Sulphur is often used after a long bout of bronchitis, for complete recovery.

Acupressure

See pages 668–675 for information about pressure points and administering treatment.

- To relieve chest congestion, massage Kidney 27, Conception Vessel 22, and Lung 1 and 7.
- If you have difficulty breathing and need to calm your emotions, use Bladder 38.

Bodywork

Massage

A back massage will break up excess phlegm. If you have chronic coughing, you might want to schedule regular sessions with a professional massage therapist. If you're generally a strong and healthy person, ask your therapist to use percussive motions, which are highly effective at releasing phlegm. People who suffer from an occasional bout of acute bronchitis might prefer to rely on a loved one to perform this task each evening.

Hydrotherapy

Sit in a hot, steamy bath or a sauna to thin mucus secretions and sweat out toxins. If you have hypertension, do not use saunas.

Constitutional hydrotherapy works well for acute and chronic coughs. Follow the directions for treatment on pages 676–677.

Aromatherapy

Add eucalyptus, peppermint, lemon balm, or tree tea oil to a hot bath or a steam inhalation to drain congestion. You can also add any of these oils to a base oil and rub it directly onto your chest.

Stress Reduction

General Stress-Reduction Therapies

Stress can weaken your immune system and leave your lungs open to infection. If you're vulnerable to frequent bouts of bronchitis or suffer from chronic bronchitis, experiment with the techniques in the Exercise and Stress Reduction chapter until you find one or two that you like. Then practice them on a daily basis, or more often as needed.

Bach Flower Remedies

Select the remedy that meets your needs, place 10 drops of the liquid under your tongue. Hold the drops in place for thirty seconds and swallow. Use as often as needed.

Take Clematis if you tend to give in when feeling a respiratory infection coming on.

Red Chestnut is for people who worry a greating deal about their loved ones, even to the extent of neglecting themselves.

Other Recommendations

- Rest, preferably in bed, while the illness is at its worst. When you feel better, move around to keep the infection from settling into your lungs, but continue to rest after periods of activity.
- Don't take a cough suppressant. The lungs must expel phlegm to get healthy; suppressants keep them from doing so. Consistent suppressant use can lead to worse cases of acute bronchitis or even to chronic bronchitis or pneumonia.
- Encourage expectoration by applying warm compresses to your chest.
- Don't smoke or expose yourself to secondhand smoke.
- If you have chronic coughing and live in a damp, cold climate, you may have to move to another location that's dry and warm. You should have your doctor consider mold allergies as a cause of chronic coughing.
- People with chronic bronchitis need to keep their lungs as elastic and strong as possible. Exercise, breath deeply, and, if you enjoy music, take up a wind instrument.

Crohn's Disease

Crohn's disease is an inflammatory disorder that leads to severe ulceration of the digestive tract. This disease generally occurs in the last portion of the small intestine (ileum) and the beginning of the large intestine, but it can occur in any part of the digestive tract, from the mouth to the anus. Crohn's disease can affect the small intestine alone (35 percent), the large intestine alone (20 percent), or both—the last portion of the small intestine and the large intestine (45 percent). There may be just one ulceration or several, and they may skip areas of the digestive tract. When these ulcerations heal, they can leave behind scar tissue that narrows a portion of the gastrointestinal passageway.

As its sufferers know, symptoms of Crohn's disease can be exceedingly unpleasant. The most common symptoms include intense abdominal pain and chronic diarrhea, fever, loss of appetite, and weight loss. Other common symptoms include nausea, mouth and anal sores, fatigue, and a general sense of malaise. Crohn's can also lead to other disorders. The chronic diarrhea prevents the absorption of vital nutrients, with malnutrition as a frequent result. Persistent bleeding within the intestines can cause anemia, which only compounds the existing fatigue and the nutritional deficiencies. People with Crohn's may also develop fistulas, abnormal tunnels that connect one part of the intestine to the other, or even to other organs. Sometimes the scar tissue is so thick, it partially or completely obstructs the bowels, a dangerous condition that is always a medical emergency.

The onset of Crohn's disease usually takes place during adolescence or young adulthood, with most cases occurring before age thirty-five, although it can affect the elderly, too. In some cases, the disease strikes once and never returns. For most people, however, Crohn's is a chronic condition that may flare up every few months or every few years. The condition must always be taken very seriously—indeed, the symptoms make it hard to ignore—and sufferers must be under the care of a good doctor, preferably a gastroenterologist with experience in treating the disease. If Crohn's is left untreated, the bowels may eventually stop functioning altogether. Yet natural medicine has a lot to offer for people with this disease, and many find that they can keep the disease under control with a comprehensive natural approach, as described in this chapter.

As with many other intestinal disorders, no one is entirely sure what causes Crohn's disease. Crohn's disease is rare in "primitive" societies that follow diets based on whole, unprocessed food. In fact, the disorder was practically unheard of in the United States until the middle of this century, when consumption of refined and chemically treated products skyrocketed. Food allergies—which tend to afflict societies that rely on unnatural foods—are also thought to play a significant factor in this disorder, as are free radicals, which, again, are best counteracted with good nutrition. Dietary therapy is a crucial component of any treatment plan for Crohn's disease. Good eating habits will prevent many of the secondary disorders, like malnutrition and anemia, which Crohn's can cause; better yet, it will address the underlying problem. Although no one can officially claim a cure for this disease, many sufferers will testify that dietary changes have successfully eliminated their symptoms. Unfortunately, many doctors are unaware of the role that diet plays in this disorder.

Warning Signs of Bowel Obstruction

An obstructed bowel is a medical emergency. Crohn's sufferers are especially vulnerable to this disorder, because the scar tissue from ulcerated areas can partially or completely block the intestine. The classic indicators of bowel obstruction are vomiting and abdominal pain and distention. If you experience these symptoms, get medical help at once.

It is critical that digestive function also be improved with this condition. Increased intestinal permeability is an issue that needs to be addressed. As well, flora imbalance (dysbiosis) and undiagnosed intestinal infection from parasites, harmful bacteria, or yeast need to be tested and treated. Lifestyle is very important as well. Smokers are more likely to have Crohn's disease, and stress can be a powerful factor in the development of, as well as the recovery from, this disease.

For severe, acute flare-ups, your doctor may prescribe corticosteroids or other medications. The goal, though, is address the underlying causes with natural therapy so that you can heal the digestive tract and decrease the susceptibility to future attacks. Even if more aggressive measures are needed, the treatments described here can still reduce your suffering significantly.

SYMPTOMS

- Abdominal pain
- Chronic diarrhea
- Gas
- Loss of appetite
- Weight loss
- Nausea
- Fatigue
- Malaise
- Mouth and anal sores
- Headaches
- Low-grade fever
- Anemia

ROOT CAUSES

- Diet high in fatty and refined foods and low in fiber
- Food allergies
- Free radicals
- Nutritional deficiencies
- Stress
- Increased intestinal permeability
- Intestinal infection
- Poor lifestyle choices, such as smoking and drinking alcohol

---

Testing Techniques

The following tests help assess possible reasons for Crohn's disease:

Stool analysis—flora balance, possible infection, degree of inflammation

Food allergy test—blood or electrodermal

Vitamin and mineral analysis—blood or urine for nutritional deficiencies

Stress hormones—DHEA, cortisol

TREATMENT

Diet

Recommended Food

Good nutrition is important for everyone, but people with Crohn's must be especially diligent about eating wholesome meals. It's best to buy fresh ingredients (organic, if possible) and prepare them yourself.

Protein deficiency is common in people with Crohn's. Incorporate quality protein sources into your diet, such as organic chicken, legumes, turkey, and fish, for two meals a day. Soy is also an option unless you are sensitive to it.

Homemade soups and broths are excellent. These meals are liquefied and easy to digest. Use a variety of fresh vegetables and quality protein sources, as described previously. This is particularly helpful during the time of a flare-up.

Juices are ideal for Crohn's sufferers, because they require little work from the digestive system and their nutrients are easily absorbed. Drink vegetable juices every day. Cabbage juice is particularly effective in healing ulcerated areas.

Eat a cultured product like kefir or, if you're not allergic to dairy, live unsweetened yogurt every day. A deficiency of friendly intestinal bacteria is common in Crohn's patients.

Make proper hydration a priority. Drink at least one glass of clean water every two waking hours. You'll replenish the water lost to diarrhea, and you'll also help your bowels regulate themselves.

Food to Avoid

A study that reviewed the diets of people with Crohn's disease and ulcerative colitis found that the risk of Crohn's disease was highest in people who had a high sugar intake. The same study also reported that the consumption of fast foods twice a week tripled the risk of this disease.

Consumption of refined carbohydrates is strongly associated with Crohn's disease. Eliminate white flour, white rice, and both white and brown sugars from your diet. Almost all packaged products are made with at least one of these ingredients, so read labels carefully.

Foods that are high in saturated, hydrogenated, or partially hydrogenated fat will irritate your gastrointestinal tract and make diarrhea even worse. Avoid red meat, as well as any fried or greasy foods.

Many people with Crohn's disease have undetected food allergies; when they remove the allergens from their diets, the disease often completely disappears. To determine if a food or foods is causing your problem, read the Food Allergies section and follow the elimination diet that accompanies it. Dairy and wheat are common triggers for people with this disorder.

Be careful with high-fiber foods such as wheat bran, as it is too harsh for some people with this disease. Slowly increase fiber-rich foods in the diet.

Avoid alcohol, caffeine, carbonated drinks, and spicy foods. Although these products don't cause Crohn's disease, they irritate the gastrointestinal system and can make your symptoms worse.

Limit the use of fruit juices, which commonly irritate the digestive tract of people with this condition.

Detoxification

If you have Crohn's, chances are that your body has been exposed to toxic quantities of refined carbohydrates, fats, and possibly food allergens. Give your system a rest by going on a three-day juice fast. Drink a wide variety of juices, broths, and herbal teas, and try to include cabbage juice as well.

℞ Super Seven Prescriptions—Crohn's Disease

Super Prescription #1   Aloe vera
Take ¼ to ½ cup three times daily or as directed on the container. Aloe soothes and heals the lining of the digestive tract.

Super Prescription #2   DGL licorice (*Glycyrrhiza glabra*)
Chew 1 to 2 capsules or take 300 mg of a powdered form twenty minutes before each meal.

Super Prescription #3   Fish oil
Take a total daily dosage of an enteric-coated fish oil product containing at least 480 mg of EPA and 360 mg of DHA, spread out over three times a day. Fish oil reduces inflammation.

Super Prescription #4   Homeopathy
Use a combination digestive upset or cramping formula for the acute relief of symptoms, as directed on the container. Otherwise, see the description in the Homeopathy section for the most indicated remedy.

Super Prescription #5   Enzymes
Take 1 to 2 capsules with each meal. They aid in the digestion of food and are essential for all the metabolic activity in the body.

Super Prescription #6   Glutamine
Take 1,000 to 3,000 mg three times daily on an empty stomach. This amino acid is involved in the healthy turnover of cells that line the digestive tract.

Super Prescription #7   Probiotic
Take a product containing at least 4 billion active organisms daily. It supplies friendly bacteria such as *Lactobacillus acidophilus* and *bifidus*. A product containing *Saccharomyces boulardii* probiotic has proved to be helpful for diarrhea associated with this condition.

In a double-blind trial of people with Crohn's disease, researchers found that people who took an enteric-coated fish oil supplement had a recurrence rate of 26 percent after one year, while those taking a placebo had a 59 percent recurrence rate.

General Recommendations

Peppermint tea is an excellent tonic for Crohn's sufferers. It reduces nausea, relieves abdominal pain, and has a calming effect. Use with caution if you have reflux problems.

Chamomile (*Matricaria recutita*) will help reduce intestinal inflammation. This herb can be taken as a tincture at 4 to 6 cc three times a day.

Slippery elm (*Ulmus fulva*) is a traditional remedy for bowel disorders. It's high in mucilage, a substance that helps calm the intestines and reduce inflammation. Take 400 to 500 mg three or four times daily, or use 3 to 5 cc three times daily.

Cat's claw (*Una de bato*) has anti-inflammatory and antimicrobial effects. Take 500 mg three times daily.

Oregano (*Origanum vulgare*) oil can be taken for an infection that accompanies Crohn's disease. Take 500 mg of the capsule form three times daily or as directed on the container.

A high-potency multivitamin will supply a base of nutrients to guard against deficiencies that are common with this condition.

An antioxidant formula will reduce free radicals, which are often higher in people with Crohn's disease. Take as directed on the container.

Take a sublingual form of vitamin B12 and folic acid, to improve energy levels.

Chlorella, spirulina, or a greens formula will provide chlorophyll and other nutrients that promote digestive health. Use with caution, and slowly increase the dose to make sure they are not irritating.

Boswellia (*Boswellia serrata*) has a powerful anti-inflammatory benefit. Take 1,200 to 1,500 mg of standardized extract containing 60 to 65 percent boswellic acids two to three times daily.

Homeopathy

Pick the remedy that best matches your symptoms in this section. Take a 6x, 12x, 6C, or 30C potency twice daily for two weeks to see if there are any positive results. After you notice improvement, stop taking the remedy, unless symptoms return. Consultation with a homeopathic practitioner is advised.

Arsenicum Album is for burning pains in the abdomen that are made better in a warm environment or with warm drinks. The person feels anxious and restless.

Belladonna (*Atropa belladonna*) is the remedy for sudden abdominal pains and a fever that has a throbbing or burning pain. The symptoms are worse with motion.

Colocynthis is for sharp, colicky pains in the abdomen that feel better with pressure.

Ignatia (*Ignatia amara*) is for spasms of the digestive tract that come on after emotional stresses.

Magnesia Phosphorica is for cramping abdominal pain that is better with warm applications and worse from pressure.

Nux Vomica (*Strychnos nux vomica*) is for cramping pain. The person is irritable and chilly.

Pulsatilla (*Pulsatilla pratensis*) can be taken if rich, fatty foods give you diarrhea and if your symptoms are worse at night.

Sulphur can be taken if you are awakened by diarrhea that's urgent and explosive. Burning pain is often present, which feels better with cold drinks. The person may crave spicy foods and alcohol.

Acupressure

See pages 668–675 for information about acupressure points and administering treatment.

- Work Stomach 36 to increase your body's ability to absorb nutrients into the bloodstream.
- Improve the strength of your colon by working Large Intestine 11.
- If you suffer from painful abdominal cramps, use Spleen 16.
- Conception Vessel 6 will ease diarrhea and gas.

Bodywork

Massage

To ease pain in the stomach and the intestines, try an abdominal self-massage. Lie down in a comfortable place, bend your knees, and use the flat of your hand to press against the skin of the abdomen gently but firmly. This technique also encourages good digestion. If you like, you can use the antispasmodic oils suggested in the Aromatherapy section.

For stress relief, it's hard to beat a full-body massage. You or your partner can also practice some effective home-care techniques for stress reduction, like a neck or a foot rub.

Reflexology

See pages 686–687 for information about reflexology areas and how to work them.

To regulate peristalsis, work the colon.

Work the liver area to encourage detoxification.

For stress relief, stimulate the solar plexus.

Hydrotherapy

Constitutional hydrotherapy is excellent for improving circulation and enhancing the healing of the digestive tract. It can be used for acute bouts of Crohn's disease and for long-term prevention.

Aromatherapy

Chamomile and lavender are antispasmodic oils that relax abdominal cramps. Dilute some in a carrier oil and use in a massage, or add a few drops to a warm bath. Each oil is also a pleasant stress reducer.

Ginger will soothe an upset stomach. You can use it in a bath, a massage, or a warm compress. If you like, you can combine ginger with chamomile or lavender for a highly potent effect.

Stress Reduction

General Stress-Reduction Therapies

Anxiety and tension play a significant role in every bowel disorder, and Crohn's is no exception. Since the disease itself usually causes further stress, it's important to make time every day to relax. Note that any stress-reduction technique is likely to help.

Bach Flower Remedies

If none of the following suggestions apply to you, consult the chart on pages 648–650 to find the remedy best suited to your individual needs. Once you have chosen a remedy, place 10 drops of the liquid under your tongue. Hold the drops in place for thirty seconds and swallow. Use as often as needed.

If you are prone to panic attacks or high levels of anxiety, keep a bottle of Rescue Remedy on hand. It will help calm you down in an emergency and keep the emotional problem from affecting your intestines. Rescue Remedy is also useful when you have an acute attack of the disease itself, as it can stave off the tension that's often produced by extreme physical distress.

Vine is for people whose strong drives and ambition lead to intolerance of others.

If you have suffered much and are bitter and resentful as a result, Willow will help you regain an appreciation for life.

White Chestnut helps to quiet minds that are plagued by constant, repetitive worries.

Mimulus will help people who are plagued by very specific fears.

For a more generalized anxiety, caused by fears you can't name, take Aspen.

Other Recommendations

- If you smoke, it is important that you break the habit. And everyone with Crohn's disease must avoid smoky rooms.
- Since intestinal bleeding is a real danger in Crohn's disease, always check your stools for signs of blood, especially if it looks like tar. If you see any, call your doctor at once.
- Exercise promotes bowel health and also helps bring stress under control. Take a thirty-minute walk every day, or find some other aerobic activity you enjoy enough to perform regularly.

REFERENCES

Belluzzi, A., C. Brignola, M. Campieri, et al. 1996. Effect of an enteric-coated fish-oil preparation on relapses in Crohn's disease. *New England Journal of Medicine* 334:1557–60.

Persson, P. G., A. Ahlbom, and G. Hellers. 1992. Diet and inflammatory bowel disease: A case-control study. *Epidemiology* 3(1):47–52.

Cystitis. *See* Bladder Infection

Depression

Like many other chronic illnesses, depression can be caused by a wide variety of factors and is characterized by several out of a long list of symptoms. It affects people of all ages, races, and nationalities and, according to the World Health Organization (WHO), is the most costly of all diseases, largely because it disables people who would otherwise be productive. It is estimated that 10 percent of the U.S. population experiences depression severe enough to require medical attention, with women twice as likely as men to develop depression.

A major depressive episode is diagnosed when a patient suffers from a combination of psychological and physical symptoms that are a significant change from the person's prior level of functioning. It requires more than just a sad mood for the diagnosis to be made. A major depressive episode can be devastating and often affects every aspect of a person's life. Beyond a sad mood, there is often great fatigue and apathy, an inability to enjoy once-pleasurable activities, disturbed sleep, increased or decreased appetite, and a low sex drive. Depression generally leaves its sufferers feeling worthless, hopeless, guilty, irritable, or angry. Even a touch of the blues can impair the immune system, and serious cases often go hand-in-hand with other chronic illnesses. People with severe cases have constant thoughts of death and suicide. Depression can be deadly. Approximately one out of eight people will kill themselves during a major depressive episode.

Although it is often normal and healthy to experience sad moods in response to a trauma, such as the loss of a loved one, a major depressive episode is characterized by inappropriate sadness that persists or is out of proportion with its apparent cause. Clinical depression can further be categorized into unipolar depression, marked by recurring episodes of sadness, and bipolar depression, in which the sadness alternates with periods of elation and mania. Unipolar depression is by far the more common of the two. Both kinds of clinical depression can be caused by a number of factors, including constant tension and unresolved stress, genetics, chemical or hormonal imbalances, chronic illness, poor diet, food allergies, nutritional deficiencies, and even inadequate sunlight.

If your depression is clearly reactive to stresses or events in your life, many of the following therapies may ease some of your discomfort and help you work your way through the source of your sadness. Professional counseling is also a good idea. If you suspect that you are clinically depressed, first consult a doctor to rule out any underlying illness (such as a thyroid problem), then see a psychologist or a psychiatrist for a diagnosis and appropriate treatment. Obviously, it is best to work with a doctor who embraces natural therapies and will work with you to find the cause of your depression. The suggestions here will support your therapy and will also point you toward possible causes or aggravating factors of your disorder.

SYMPTOMS

A depressed person will usually have several of the following symptoms:

- Inability to enjoy things
- Fatigue

- Mood swings, at times characterized by unexplained weeping

- Feelings of apathy, worthlessness, helplessness, hopelessness, irritability, or guilt
- Sleep problems (either insomnia or sleeping too much)
- Appetite disturbances (eating too little or too much)
- Headaches, backaches, and digestive problems
- Difficulty concentrating or making decisions
- Increased anxiety
- Decreased sex drive
- Avoiding social situations
- Recurrent thoughts of death or suicide

ROOT CAUSES

Any of the following can cause depression by itself, but most depressed people are affected by more than one factor.

- Tension and stress
- Unresolved emotional issues
- Chronic illness or pain
- Neurotransmitter imbalance
- Hormonal imbalance, especially after childbirth or as a result of oral contraceptives and other synthetic hormone medications; commonly occurs with PMS and menopause
- Preexisting conditions—most commonly, hypoglycemia, anemia, sleep apnea, low adrenal function, and thyroid gland malfunction
- Alcohol and recreational drug use
- Poor diet
- Food allergies
- Nutritional deficiencies (particularly of B12, folic acid, B6, B1 tyrosine, and tryptophan)
- Lack of sunlight
- Medications, including corticosteroids, antihistamines, blood pressure medications, anti-inflammatory drugs, narcotics, and some pharmaceutical antidepressants
- Heavy metal toxicity
- Candidiasis
- Sleep disturbances

Testing Techniques

The following tests help assess possible reasons for depression:

Yeast overgrowth—stool analysis, blood, or urine

Food allergy test—blood or electrodermal

Hormone testing (thyroid, DHEA, cortisol, testosterone, IGF-1, estrogen, progesterone)—saliva, blood, or urine

Detoxification profile—urine

Vitamin and mineral analysis (especially magnesium, B12, folic acid B6, B1)—blood

Anemia—blood test (CBC, iron, ferritin, % saturation)

Food and environmental allergies/sensitivities—blood, electrodermal

Blood-sugar balance—blood

Toxic metals—urine or hair analysis

Amino acid analysis—blood or urine

TREATMENT

Diet

Recommended Food

Depression is often caused by inadequate nutrition. Even if that's not the case with you, a sound diet will help create healthier brain chemistry. Eat a good diet balanced with complex carbohydrates from sources like whole grains, vegetables, and legumes. Complex carbohydrates are high in serotonin, a deficiency of which can cause depression and insomnia.

Soy, beans, lean poultry, eggs, nuts (walnuts are excellent), and seeds are excellent sources of protein, which will boost your energy levels. Have some several times a day.

Consume cold-water fish, such as salmon, mackerel, and cod, three times a week.

You need to keep your sugar levels regulated, so instead of eating three large meals a day, try five to six smaller ones.

Consume 1 tablespoon of ground-up flaxseeds daily. This is a good source of fiber and essential fatty acids. Sprinkle on a salad or mix in a shake.

Add 1 tablespoon of flaxseed oil or an oil blend to your salad daily for healthful essential fatty acids.

Food to Avoid

Many depressed people have hidden food allergies. See the Food Allergies section and use the elimination diet on page 253 to determine which foods, if any, may be causing or aggravating your disorder. Any food is a potential allergen, but wheat is the product most often linked to depression.

Dramatically reduce your intake of hydrogenated and saturated fats, which only increases fatigue and sluggishness.

Caffeine and refined sugar may make you feel temporarily better, but your body soon "crashes" from the high, leaving you even more exhausted or irritable. They also deplete vital nutrients from your system. Eliminate these substances from your diet.

Alcohol is a depressant, so avoid wine, beer, and liquor. If you are so unhappy that you feel you need alcohol, talk to a doctor or a therapist. You may have a drinking problem—or you might be headed for one.

Detoxification

If you've been following a diet that's high in saturated fats and refined sugars, or if you've unknowingly been eating foods that have caused allergic reactions, some or even all of your symptoms may be caused by toxic buildup. A detoxification program will help cleanse your body.

If you feel sluggish and dull, and if your doctor has ruled out an underlying disease as the cause, a three-day juice and liquid fast may refresh you. See page 548 for further information.

℞ Super Seven Prescriptions—Depression

Super Prescription #1   S-adenosylmethionine (SAMe)
Take 200 mg of an enteric-coated form two times daily on an empty stomach for two weeks. If you notice improvement, stay on this dosage. If there is little improvement, then increase to 400 mg two to three times daily. SAMe increases

the concentration of brain neurotransmitters that are responsible for your mood. Take a 50 mg B-complex, as B6, folic acid, and B12 are involved with proper SAMe metabolism. *Note:* People with bipolar disorder should use this supplement only with medical supervision.

Super Prescription #2   5-hydroxytryptophan (5-HTP)

Start with 50 mg taken three times daily on an empty stomach. Dosage can be increased to 100 mg three times daily if necessary. Note that 5-HTP is a precursor to the neurotransmitter serotonin. Take a 50 mg B-complex, as B6 is required for the proper metabolism of 5-HTP. *Note:* Do not take in conjunction with pharmaceutical antidepressants or antianxiety medications.

Super Prescription #3   Saint-John's-wort (*Hypericum perforatum*)

Take 300 mg of a product standardized to 0.3 percent hypericin three times daily (total of 900 mg). Saint-John's-wort has been shown in numerous studies to be effective for mild to moderate depression.

Super Prescription #4   B-complex

Take a 50 mg B-complex one to two times daily. B vitamins such as B12, folic acid, and B6 are intricately involved in neurotransmitter metabolism. Sublingual B12 and folic acid supplements are useful for seniors or those with absorption difficulties.

Super Prescription #5   Fish oil

Take a product containing a daily dosage of 500 to 1,000 mg of EPA/DHA. Essential fatty acids such as DHA improve neurotransmitter function.

Super Prescription #6   Ginkgo biloba

Take 60 to 120 mg twice daily of a standardized product containing 24 percent flavone glycosides and 6 percent terpene lactones. Ginkgo improves blood flow to the brain and enhances neurotransmitter activity.

Super Prescription #7   High-potency multivitamin

This provides a base of the nutrients involved with brain function.

Well-designed studies have shown that SAMe is equal to or, in some cases, more effective than pharmaceutical antidepressants. It has also been studied in combination with pharmaceutical antidepressants and was found to quicken the therapeutic effects. A double-blind study at the University of California Irvine Medical Center found that 62 percent of people taking SAMe and 52 percent of those taking a pharmaceutical antidepressant improved significantly.

A review of twenty-three randomized clinical studies involving 1,700 people found that Saint-John's-wort (*Hypericum perforatum*) was equally as effective as pharmaceutical therapy for mild to moderate depression. One well-publicized study found that Saint-John's-wort was ineffective for major depression. The same study also found the pharmaceutical medication Zoloft ineffective, yet the press focused on the negative aspect of Saint-John's-wort and ignored the fact that health professionals recommend Saint-John's-wort for mild to moderate depression.

General Recommendations

DL-phenylalanine (DLPA) is an amino acid used by the brain to manufacture neurotransmitters. Take 500 to 1,000 mg on an empty stomach each morning. It should be avoided by people with anxiety, high blood pressure, or insomnia. Do not take in combination with pharmaceutical antidepressants or antianxiety medications.

L-tyrosine is an amino acid that also helps depression. Take 100 to 500 twice daily on an empty stomach. Do not take in combination with pharmaceutical antidepressants or antianxiety medications.

L-tryptophan has been a historic favorite of nutrition-oriented doctors for the treatment of depression. It acts as a precursor for the neurotransmitter serotonin. Take 500 to 1,000 mg three times daily on an empty stomach. This amino acid requires a prescription from your doctor and is available from compounding pharmacies.

Ashwagandha (*Withania somniferum*) improves stress hormone balance and relaxes the nervous system. Take 1,000 mg two to three times daily. This nutrient requires a prescription from a doctor.

DHEA is a hormone that, if you are low in, you should work with a doctor to normalize your levels; 5 to 15 mg is a good starting dosage.

Phosphatidylserine improves memory, and studies show that it's helpful for depression. Take up to 300 mg daily.

Vitamin D has been found in studies to help improve mood. It is particularly important for people who do not get regular sunlight, especially seniors. Take 400 to 800 IU daily.

Acetyl-L-carnitine has been shown to be helpful for seniors with depression. Take 500 mg three times daily.

If you feel tense and on edge, several herbal teas can help you calm down. Peppermint and chamomile have mild relaxing properties, but if you need something a little stronger, try hops (*Humulus lupulus*) or passionflower (*Passiflora incarnata*).

Oatstraw (*Avena sativa*) tea is a good tonic for the nerves. Drink a cup as needed.

For insomnia that accompanies or causes depression, valerian (*Valeriana officinalis*) or kava (*Piper methysticum*) tea, taken before bedtime, can be quite helpful.

Homeopathy

Pick the remedy that best matches your symptoms in this section. Take a 6x, 12x, 6C, or 30C potency twice daily for two weeks to see if there are any positive results. After you notice improvement, stop taking the remedy, unless symptoms return. Consultation with a homeopathic practitioner is advised.

Arsenicum Album is for people susceptible to depression who also suffer from anxiety and insecurity. They are often perfectionists who may have severe phobias. Restlessness and insomnia between 12 and 2 A.M. are common.

Aurum Metallicum is for deep depression, where there are thoughts of suicide. The person feels no joy and is in despair. There is relief from being in the sun.
Note: Suicidal tendencies should always be discussed with a doctor.

Ignatia (*Ignatia amara*) eases depression brought on by grief or emotional trauma and characterized by rapid mood swings. Frequent sighing and a sensation of a lump in the throat are characteristics of people who benefit from this remedy.

Kali Phosphoricum is for depression as a result of overwork. Mental fatigue is a common symptom that this remedy helps.

Natrum Muriaticum is for depressed people who do not reveal their emotions and who hold their feelings inside. They feel emotionally reserved and withdrawn. Deep inside, they want people to be with them, but then they feel aggravated when others console them. There is often a strong craving for salt and an aversion to sunlight.

Pulsatilla (*Pulsatilla pratensis*) is for people who burst into tears at little or no provocation. They may also be driven to seek constant comfort and reassurance. They are very sensitive and feel better from crying, attention, sweets, and being in the open air. Symptoms are worse in a warm environment. Depression is often worse for women around the menstrual cycle or with menopause.

Sepia is for women who feel indifferent to their families. There are feelings of depression, fatigue, and irritability and a low sex drive. They feel worse when consoled and better from exercise. They are usually chilly and have a strong craving for sweets (chocolate) and salty/sour foods. Depression associated with hormone imbalance, as seen with PMS and menopause, is a strong indication for this remedy.

Staphysagria is for people who have suppressed emotions (such as anger) that contribute to depression. They are usually quiet and do not stand up for themselves, which leads to shame and resentment. Headaches and insomnia are also common.

Acupressure

- Lung 1 is the point of choice to ease anxiety and depression. You can work the point as you would any other, but see the sidebar for a special technique that is especially effective for immediate relief.
- Stomach 36 is a good point for everyone with depression. It restores energy and well-being and soothes digestive troubles.
- For depression accompanied by fear or fatigue, use Bladder 23.
- Conception Vessel 17 will help relieve depression caused by grief or made worse by anxiety.

Bodywork

If you are depressed, you may find that for many reasons—strained relationships, an inhibited sex drive, a decreased desire for stimulation in general—you are touched less than usual. Because touch is necessary for well-being, this situation can lead to further depression. Try one or more of the following techniques and practice them on a regular basis.

Massage

Any massage can help you feel better, but a full-body treatment can be a highly effective way to release stress that has built up in your muscles. You can add any of the oils listed in the Aromatherapy section for added benefit.

People need to touch as much as they need to be touched, so learn some basic techniques and give massages to your loved ones. Hand, neck, shoulder, and foot rubs are easy to give.

Reflexology

See pages 686–687 for information about reflexology areas and how to work them.

For depression in general, work the areas of the foot that correspond to the head, the endocrine glands, the solar plexus, and the pancreas.

If you feel fatigued, working the adrenals, the diaphragm, the glands, and the spine will energize you.

For quick relief of stress or tension, massage the entire foot with rhythmic strokes that are firm but not deep.

Acupuncture

Treatments from a qualified practitioner can help relax the nervous system.

Hydrotherapy

A hot bath or a sauna can relax edgy nerves; the steam will also help detoxify your body. Essential oils can be added to your hot bath as you like. If you have high blood pressure, do not take saunas.

The following technique produces an immediate sense of calm. Practiced regularly over a long period of time, it can have a more permanent effect.

1. Sit comfortably in a chair with your back straight. Cross your arms in front of your chest so that your wrists overlap at your heart.
2. Place your middle finger in the soft area below the collarbone and near the top of the armpit. Apply light pressure.
3. Bend your head slightly toward your chest and inhale through your nose for three short breaths. Take a fourth breath; this time, fill your lungs with air and hold for a moment. Exhale slowly through your mouth.

Practice this entire sequence for three minutes every day or more often if you like.

Aromatherapy

Depression can manifest itself in a variety of moods, so you may want to refer to page 658 to find the oils best suited for your particular needs. Following are some suggestions; you can prepare them according to any of the methods as described in the Aromatherapy chapter.

To combat fatigue, use geranium, jasmine, neroli, bergamot, or rose.

If you need to calm down, lavender and melissa will have a soothing, quietly uplifting effect.

Ylang ylang and patchouli are also calming, and they have the additional benefit of stimulating your sex drive.

Stress Reduction

General Stress-Reduction Therapies

If you're depressed, you're experiencing powerful and probably continuous levels of stress. It is vital for your emotional and physical health that you find at least one way to control anxiety, fear, or tension. Prayer, counseling, and positive mental imagery are all helpful.

If you sense that your depression is more than you can handle, don't hesitate to seek help from a psychotherapist, a religious adviser, or a support group. It helps a great deal to talk to people who have worked with others in great emotional pain.

Make an effort to stay in contact with beauty. If you have a garden or live near a nice park, spend as much time there as possible. And try to bring some of that beauty indoors: buy yourself a bouquet of flowers, listen to a favorite CD, or hang a watercolor of a nature scene on the wall in your office.

Regular exercise has been shown to be effective in improving depression. Try to get some physical activity every day for thirty minutes.

It may sound facile, but one quick way to feel better, at least temporarily, is to go dancing. Dancing releases endorphins, powerful hormones that will raise your spirits, and you'll benefit from the touch of other people, not to mention the pleasure of losing yourself in the music.

Helping others with their problems is a great way to relieve depression.

Bach Flower Remedies

The chart on pages 648–650 will help you determine the remedy most suited to your needs. A few suggestions are listed here. Once you've chosen a remedy, place 10 drops of the liquid under your tongue. Hold the drops in place for thirty seconds and swallow. Use as often as needed.

Rescue Remedy is good in any crisis, whether emotional or physical. Use it when you feel an overwhelming mood coming on.

For rapidly changing moods or paralyzing indecision, take Scleranthus.

If you have given up hope of your depression ever lifting, Gorse will revive your spirits.

If you are burned out and exhausted at the thought of any activity, whether mental or physical, take Hornbeam.

Olive is for extreme apathy; if you cannot summon up interest in anything, it can help.

REFERENCES

1994. *Acta Scandinavica Neurologica* 89(154):19–26.

Davidson, J. R. T., et al. 2002. Effect of *Hypericum perforatum* (St. John's Wort) in major depressive disorder: A randomized controlled trial. *Journal of the American Medical Association* 287:1807–14.

Linde, K., et al. 1996. St. John's Wort for depression—An overview and meta-analysis of randomized clinical trials. *British Medical Journal* 313:253–58.

Diabetes

Diabetes is a chronic health problem that involves elevated blood sugar levels. The metabolism of carbohydrates, proteins, and fats directly or indirectly leads to the production of the substance glucose, also known as blood sugar. Glucose is needed to supply energy to every cell in the body. If glucose levels become too elevated, then they become toxic to the brain and other body organs. With diabetes, two main problems can occur. One is a deficiency of insulin, a hormone produced by the pancreas that transports glucose into cells. The second is the resistance of the cells to insulin so that blood sugar cannot enter the cells. According to the American Diabetes Association, 6.2 percent of the population has diabetes, with one third of the people (5.9 million) unaware that they have the disease.

Diabetes is categorized into three main types. In type 1 diabetes, also known as juvenile or insulin-dependent diabetes, the production and the secretion of insulin by the pancreas are severely deficient. Type 1 diabetes usually develops during childhood or adolescence. Because insulin levels are absent or dramatically low, people with type 1 need to inject themselves with insulin and monitor their blood sugar daily. This condition is thought to involve an autoimmune reaction, where the immune system attacks and damages its own pancreatic cells that produce insulin. Type 1 diabetes accounts for 5 to 10 percent of U.S. cases of diabetes.

Type 2 diabetes, often called adult-onset or non–insulin dependent diabetes, is by far the more common of the two: about 90 to 95 percent of the diabetes in the United States is type 2, affecting over 16 million people. It strikes during adulthood, most often in the elderly or in obese people over forty. It is becoming increasingly common with children, due to lack of exercise, obesity, and poor dietary habits. People with type 2 can produce sufficient insulin, but the insulin and the glucose it transports cannot effectively enter into the cells. This category of diabetes is most often linked to a diet that is high in refined carbohydrates and low in fiber, and it can usually be treated with an effective diet, exercise, and specific nutritional supplements.

The third category is known as gestational diabetes, diabetes that occurs during a woman's pregnancy.

All three types of diabetes are very serious medical conditions. When left unmonitored and untreated, blood-sugar levels can swing from dramatically low (hypoglycemia) to dangerously high (hyperglycemia). Hypoglycemia comes on quickly and leaves you feeling dizzy, pale, sweaty, and confused. You may feel uncoordinated or have palpitations. If your glucose levels are not raised, your symptoms could grow worse, and you could lapse into a coma. Hyperglycemia isn't much better. It may take hours or days to develop and can result in diabetic ketoacidosis, a life-threatening condition. Over the long term, both type 1 and type 2 diabetes can lead to heart disease, kidney and nerve disorders, loss of vision, and other problems. The high levels of blood sugar can also leave the body vulnerable to infection.

If you have type 1 diabetes, you must work very closely with a good doctor and follow a lifelong treatment plan that includes medication, diet, and exercise. Complementary therapies, while they may not substitute for conventional medical treatment, can provide helpful support to your taxed endocrine and other systems and help decrease the need for medications and reduce the long-term complications of the disease. In very rare cases some people are able to get off insulin therapy when a comprehensive natural approach is followed. This, of course, should never be tried without a doctor's supervision.

People with type 2 diabetes must also take their disease very seriously and consult a doctor on a regular basis; however, they will usually find that a comprehensive dietary, exercise, and supplemental program will reduce or eliminate the need for medication. No matter which kind of diabetes you have, you must always talk to your doctor about any therapies you plan to incorporate into your protocol. And never go off your medication without a doctor's consent.

SYMPTOMS

Because these symptoms may not seem serious, many people with diabetes remain undiagnosed. If they apply to you or to your child, see a doctor as soon as possible.

- Frequent urination (children may be constant bedwetters)
- Strong thirst
- Excessive appetite
- Weight loss
- Fatigue
- Irritability
- Blurred vision

ROOT CAUSES

- Heredity
- A poor diet (particularly in type 2)
- An autoimmune reaction (due to a viral infection, environmental toxin, food allergy) is one proposed theory as to the origin of some cases of type 1 diabetes.
- Chronic stress and the resulting stress hormone imbalance
- Nutritional deficiencies, especially of chromium, B vitamins, zinc, vanadium, and vitamin D
- Obesity

TREATMENT

Diet

The most important therapy for diabetes is a healthful diet. These dietary suggestions will help regulate your levels of sugar and also reduce your risk of complications, such as cardiovascular disease.

Recommended Food

Follow a diet that's high in fiber (vegetables, nuts, seeds, whole grains). Water-soluble fiber, as found in oat bran, beans, nuts, seeds, and apples, helps to balance blood sugar. Ground flaxseeds should be consumed daily. Consume 1 tablespoon with each

---

Testing Techniques

The following tests help assess possible reasons for diabetes:

- Hormone testing (thyroid, DHEA, cortisol, testosterone, IGF-1, estrogen, progesterone)—saliva, blood, or urine
- Intestinal permeability—urine
- Vitamin and mineral analysis (especially magnesium, chromium, vanadium, zinc, B vitamins)—blood
- Digestive function and microbe/parasite/candida testing—stool analysis
- Food and environmental allergies/sensitivities—blood, electrodermal

Your doctor makes a diagnosis of diabetes according to the symptoms you exhibit, in addition to the results of blood and urine tests. Testing will also help your doctor determine whether you have type 1 or type 2 diabetes.

meal or ¼ cup daily. Make sure to drink plenty of water when you start taking flaxseeds (10 ounces per tablespoon). A daily total of 50 mg of fiber daily is a great goal.

Consume vegetable protein (legumes, nuts, seeds, peas) or lean animal protein (turkey, chicken, fish) with each meal. Protein drinks that have low sugar levels can be consumed. Protein helps smooth out blood-sugar levels. Many people with diabetes benefit from increasing the relative amount of protein in the diet.

Focus on quality fats. Fish such as salmon is excellent, as are nuts and seeds. Use olive and flaxseed oil with your salads.

Instead of eating three large meals, have several smaller meals throughout the day to keep your insulin and blood-sugar levels steady. Or have three main meals with healthy snacks in-between. *Do not go longer than three hours without eating.*

Chromium deficiency has been linked to diabetes, so eat lots of brewer's yeast, wheat germ, whole grains, cheese, soy products, onions, and garlic. Onions and garlic will also help lower blood-sugar levels and protect against heart disease.

Enjoy plenty of berries, plums, and grapes, which contain phytochemicals that protect your vision.

Focus on foods with a low glycemic load value.

Sixty people with type 2 diabetes (30 men and 30 women) were divided randomly into six groups. Groups 1, 2, and 3 consumed 1, 3, or 6 grams of cinnamon daily, respectively, and groups 4, 5, and 6 were given placebo capsules corresponding to the number of capsules consumed for the three levels of cinnamon. The cinnamon was consumed for 40 days, followed by a 20-day washout period. Researchers found that after 40 days, all three levels of cinnamon reduced the mean fasting serum glucose (18–29%), triglyceride (23–30%), LDL cholesterol (7–27%), and total cholesterol (12–26%) levels. There were no significant changes found in the placebo groups.

Food to Avoid

Stay away from simple sugars. Obvious no-no's are candy, cookies, sodas, and other sweets.

White, refined bread also spikes blood-sugar levels. Whole grain breads, cereals, and pastas are better choices. Brown rice, barley, oats, spelt, and kamut are complex carbohydrates that are good choices.

Avoid cow's milk. Some studies have found a link between cow's milk ingestion and type 1 diabetes in children. It appears that some children, due to genetic reasons, react to the cow's milk protein (caseins), which causes an autoimmune reaction with the pancreas.

Eliminate alcohol and caffeine from your diet.

Cut back on your consumption of saturated fat. Found in red meat and dairy products, it has been shown to increase the risk of diabetes and heart disease.

Avoid artificial sweeteners. Instead, use diabetic-safe and more healthful natural sweeteners, such as stevia or xylitol.

Avoid high glycemic load foods.

Glycemic Index

Glycemic index (GI) has become a popular term, as it is more meaningful than the label "simple carbohydrate." GI refers to the rise of blood sugar after ingesting a specific food. This numerical value is compared to the GI of glucose at a value of 100. Lower glycemic values are recommended for people with obesity, diabetes, and insulin resistance. For example, a Coca-Cola soft drink has a glycemic index of 63, whereas a serving of kidney beans has a value of 23.

Glycemic Index Guidelines

GI of 70 or more is considered high.

GI of 56 to 69 is considered medium.

GI of less than 55 is considered low.

Glycemic Load

Recently, doctors and researchers have placed more value on the glycemic load (GL) value of foods. The glycemic load takes into account the amount of carbohydrates in a serving of a particular food. The glycemic index tells you how quickly a carbohydrate turns into blood sugar, but it neglects to take into account the amount of carbohydrates in a serving, which is important. The higher the glycemic load value, the greater the blood-sugar level and the resulting stress on insulin levels. This value is attained by multiplying the amount of carbohydrates contained in a specified serving size of the food by the glycemic index value of that food, and then dividing by 100. For example, an apple has a GI of 40, compared to glucose, which is the baseline at 100, but the amount of carbohydrates available in a typical apple is 16 grams. The GL is calculated by multiplying the 16 grams of available carbohydrate times 40 and then dividing by 100 to give a decimal number of approximately 6. Compare this to a serving of Rice Krispies that has a glycemic index of 82 and available 26 carbohydrates, making a glycemic load of 21. Another example would be macaroni and cheese, which has a glycemic load of 32.

Glycemic Load Guidelines

GL of 20 or more is considered high.

GL of 11 to 19 is considered medium.

GL of 10 or less is considered low.

Note: Glycemic index and glycemic load values for hundreds of different foods are available on numerous internet Web sites. These can be found at the *American Journal of Clinical Nutrition* Web site, http://www.ajcn.org (type in key word *glycemic load values*) or http://www.mendosa.com

Detoxification

Diabetics are particularly vulnerable to toxins. Although fasting is not an option if you have diabetes, other therapies will help flush out toxic build-up and reduce your risk of developing diseases.

Consume detoxifying super green foods, such as chlorella, spirulina, wheatgrass, barley grass, or a mixture of these super green foods.

The skin is the largest organ of elimination. Encourage it to expel toxins by giving yourself a dry brush from head to toe every morning or night.

Drink a glass of clean water every two waking hours to rid your body of toxins.

℞ Super Seven Prescriptions—Diabetes

Super Prescription #1   Chromium
Take a daily total of up to 1,000 mcg. Chromium improves glucose tolerance and balances blood-sugar levels.

Super Prescription #2   Gymnema sylvestre
Take 400 mg of a 25 percent gymneic acid extract daily. Gymnema improves insulin production in the pancreas, as well as insulin's ability to lower blood-sugar levels.

Super Prescription #3   Alpha lipoic acid
Take 300 to 1,200 mg daily. Alpha lipoic acid improves insulin sensitivity and reduces the symptoms of diabetic neuropathy.

Super Prescription #4   Vanadyl sulfate
Take 100 to 300 mg daily. It improves glucose tolerance in people with type 2 diabetes. Higher dosages should be used under the supervision of a doctor.

Super Prescription #5   Cinnamon extract
Take 500 mg twice daily. Cinnamon improves insulin sensitivity and utilization.

Super Prescription #6   High-potency multivitamin
This supplies many of the nutrients involved with blood sugar metabolism. Take as directed on the container.

Super Prescription #7   Essential fatty acids
Take a fish oil supplement with a combined total of 1,000 mg of DHA and EPA. Also take 1,500 mg of evening primrose oil daily. Essential fatty acids are needed for proper insulin function, and they support nerve health.

General Recommendations

Biotin is involved with glucose metabolism and is helpful for type 1 and type 2 diabetes. Take 9 to 16 mg daily.

An antioxidant formula supplies additional antioxidants, which are generally required in higher amounts in people with diabetes. Take as directed on the container.

B-complex vitamins are involved in blood sugar metabolism and help treat diabetic symptoms such as neuropathy. Take a 50 mg B-complex daily.

Vitamin B12 is helpful for the symptoms of diabetic neuropathy. Take 1,000 mcg sublingually or by injection from your doctor (1 cc twice weekly).

Vitamin C helps prevent the complications of diabetes. Take 1,000 mg two to three times daily.

Magnesium is involved with insulin production and utilization. Take a daily total of 500 to 750 mg. Reduce dosage if loose stools occur.

Studies have found chromium supplementation to be helpful for people with type 1 and type 2 diabetes, as well as for women with diabetes that occurs during pregnancy (gestational diabetes).

In one study, 22 people with type 2 diabetes were given 400 mg of gymnema extract daily for 18 to 20 months while they continued their diabetic medications. Researchers found a significant improvement in blood-sugar levels. Most people were able to reduce the amount of their medications, and 5 were able to discontinue their medications. Another controlled study of people with type 1 diabetes who supplemented gymnema extract found a decreased need for insulin and improved blood sugar control. Those taking a placebo showed no significant decrease in blood sugar or in insulin requirements.

CoQ10 tends to be low in people with diabetes. One study found that it has a blood sugar–lowering effect. CoQ10 prevents LDL cholesterol oxidation, which is more prevalent in people with diabetes.

Vitamin E improves glucose regulation and prevents cholesterol oxidation. Take 800 to 1,200 IU daily of a formula containing tocotrienols and tocopherols.

Banaba leaf has been shown in animal and human studies to lower blood-sugar levels. Take 16 mg three times daily.

Thymus (*Thymus vulgaris*) extract balances the immune system, which is important for type 1 diabetes. Take 500 mg twice daily on an empty stomach or as directed on the container.

Pancreas extract supports pancreatic function. Take 500 mg twice daily on an empty stomach or as directed on the container.

Adrenal extract supports adrenal gland function, which is also important for blood-sugar regulation. Take 500 mg twice daily on an empty stomach or as directed on the container.

DHEA is often low in people with diabetes. If tests show that you have low levels, take 5 to 25 mg daily under a doctor's supervision.

Psyllium has been shown to reduce blood-sugar levels. It is a good source of fiber. Take up to 5 grams daily.

Asian ginseng (panax ginseng) has been shown in a study to help improve blood-sugar levels in people with type 2 diabetes. Take 200 mg daily.

Bitter melon (*Momordica charantia*) can help balance blood-sugar levels. Take 5 ml twice daily of the tincture form or 200 mg in capsule form, three times daily of a standardized extract.

Garlic (*Allium sativum*) is an important herb for the diabetic. It stabilizes blood sugar and helps reduce your risk of heart disease and other circulatory disorders by improving blood flow, lowering elevated blood pressure, and reducing levels of "bad" cholesterol. Take 300 to 450 mg twice daily.

Bilberry (*Vaccinium myrtillus*) may help to prevent diabetic retinopathy and cataracts. Take 160 mg twice a day of a product standardized to 25 percent anthocyanosides.

Fenugreek (*Trigonella foenum-graecum*) is another herb that stabilizes blood sugar. Take a product with an equivalent dosage of 15 to 50 grams daily.

Gingko biloba stimulates blood flow. Find a brand that's standardized to 24 percent flavone glycosides, and take 60 to 120 mg twice daily.

Evening primrose (*Oenothera biennis*) oil may help prevent and treat diabetic neuropathy. Take a product containing 480 mg daily of GLA (the active essential fatty acid in evening primrose).

Teas made with peppermint, chamomile, and passionflower all have soothing properties and encourage relaxation.

Homeopathy

Consult with a homeopathic practitioner to individualize your homeopathic treatment.

Acupressure

See pages 668–675 for information about acupressure points and administering treatment.

- Governing Vessel 24.5 supports the endocrine system.
- To improve circulation, massage Gallbladder 21.

Bodywork

Massage

Diabetics often suffer from poor circulation, and a massage is a relaxing way to improve blood flow. Regular massages of the feet may be especially beneficial to help ward off foot ulcers.

Reflexology

See pages 686–687 for information about reflexology areas and how to work them.

Work the points that correspond to the pancreas, the liver, and the thyroid, pituitary, and adrenal glands. You will probably have to massage these points every day for several months to see an effect.

Hydrotherapy

Alternating hot and cold baths will stimulate circulation.

Aromatherapy

Have fun trying the many different relaxing oils. See page 658 for more information, but you may want to start with bergamot, jasmine, lavender, rose, sandalwood, or ylang ylang. Use them in a massage, a bath, lotions, or any of the other methods listed in the Aromatherapy chapter.

Stress Reduction

General Stress-Reduction Therapies

Diabetes puts additional stress on almost every part of your body and every area of your life. Keep your emotional health in balance by experimenting with the stress-reduction techniques discussed in the Exercise and Stress Reduction chapter. When you find one or two you like, practice them on a regular basis.

Other Recommendations

- Don't smoke or expose yourself to secondhand smoke. If you are diabetic, you are vulnerable to heart and kidney damage, both of which are linked to smoking. You may also have circulation problems, and smoking impairs blood flow.
- Poor circulation and nerve damage can lead to foot ulcers in diabetics. Keep the blood flowing through your feet by wearing comfortable shoes that fit well.
- If you're obese and have type 2 diabetes, you need to lose weight. The previous diet recommendations should help you take off the weight safely, as will the Obesity section in this book, but talk to your doctor about the best weight-loss plan for you.
- Alternating hot and cold compresses, applied to the abdomen, just over the pancreas and the kidneys, will encourage proper insulin production, along with regular elimination of fluids from the kidneys.
- Exercise regularly to maintain optimal blood-sugar levels. Walking after meals is effective for some people.
- If you're a woman and want to conceive, your blood-sugar levels must be under control before you get pregnant; otherwise, your baby will be at risk for developing birth defects. It often takes months of treatment before glucose levels become stable.

REFERENCES

Anderson, R. A. 2000. Chromium in the prevention and control of diabetes. *Diabetes Metabolism* 26:22–27 [review].

Baskaran, K., B. K. Ahamath, K. R. Shanmugasundaram, and E. R. Shanmugasundaram. 1990. Antidiabetic effect of a leaf extract from *Gymnema sylvestre* in non-insulin-dependent diabetes mellitus patients. *Journal of Ethnopharmacology* 30:295–305.

Foster-Powell, K., S. H. A. Holt, and J. C. Brand-Miller. 2002. International table of glycemic index and glycemic load values. *American Journal of Clinical Nutrition* 76:5–56.

Khan, Alam, M. S., Ph.D.; Mahpara Safdar, M. S.; Mohammad Muzaffar Ali Khan, M. S., Ph.D.; Khan Nawaz Khattak, M.S.; and Richard A. Anderson, Ph.D. 2003. Cinnamon improves glucose and lipids of people with type 2 diabetes. *Diabetes Care* 26:3215–18.

Shanmugasundaram, E. R., G. Rajeswari, K. Baskaran, et al. 1990. Use of *Gymnema sylvestre* leaf in the control of blood glucose in insulin-dependent diabetes mellitus. *Journal of Ethnopharmacology* 30:281–94.

Diarrhea

Acute diarrhea is a classic example of a poisoned, infected, or irritated digestive system. When the body is exposed to a toxic substance, its first priority is to expel that substance, and the digestive system has two basic strategies for performing the task. First, it secretes extra fluid to the intestines; second, it produces an unusual number of very strong intestinal contractions. As a result, loose watery stools of increased volume and frequency help propel the toxins out of your body.

Most often, the toxin that needs to be expelled is a bacteria or a virus, although parasites can definitely be the cause as well. These invaders can enter your body through contaminated food or water or through contact with an infected person. Diarrhea may also be your body's response to certain foods. An inability to digest milk and dairy products, called lactose intolerance, is a frequent cause of diarrhea, but many other foods can cause problems as well. You may also have diarrhea as a result of dietary overindulgence in general, even when the foods eaten do not usually give you trouble. In addition, anxiety and stress often play a role in all kinds of diarrhea.

While diarrhea is a useful and necessary response to poisoning—you certainly wouldn't want the toxins to remain in your body—it is often very uncomfortable and disruptive. However, for most cases of acute diarrhea (unless directed otherwise by your doctor), you should resist the temptation to take over-the-counter antidiarrhea medications, as they will only suppress the poisons and force your body to find some other way to get rid of them.

When it comes to most episodes of acute diarrhea, the best thing to do is allow your body to do its work. While no one enjoys the discomfort and the inconvenience, the symptoms usually run their course in a day or two. The main concern is that your intestines may be passing too much fluid, as well as vital nutrients like sodium and potassium, so you'll want to stay hydrated with plenty of fluids and electrolytes. Natural therapies can make you more comfortable and can reduce the intensity and the length of the illness.

Sometimes diarrhea can be a warning sign of a far more serious illness, such as bacterial enteritis, irritable bowel syndrome, colitis, Crohn's disease, celiac disease, hyperthyroidism, parasites, or even cancer. Call a doctor right away if your stools are bloody; if abdominal pain and cramping are not relieved by passing stools; or if the urge is so forceful that you fear incontinence. You should also seek medical help if the episode lasts longer than three days or if it recurs over a period longer than one week. Diarrhea in children under six always requires a doctor's attention.

SYMPTOMS

- Watery, loose stools of increased volume and frequency
- Abdominal pain and cramping
- Gas

ROOT CAUSES

- Viral infection
- Contaminated food or water
- Food allergy or intolerance
- Drug toxicity
- Bacterial or parasite infection
- Anxiety and stress
- Medications (such as antibiotics)
- Electrolyte imbalance and dehydration

TREATMENT

Diet

Although there are several important dietary strategies for diarrhea, the most critical are those to help you stay hydrated.

Recommended Food

While the attack is at its most acute, do not try to take in solid foods. Instead, focus on staying hydrated by drinking two cups of liquid every waking hour. Try water, diluted fruit and vegetable juices, electrolyte drinks, and broths. If you have a dry mouth or suddenly wrinkled skin that does not snap back when gently pulled, you may be on your way to severe dehydration. Drink a large glass of water or fresh vegetable juice immediately.

Food to Avoid

During the most intense stages of diarrhea, you will probably not feel much like eating. Do not force yourself to take in solid food during this time (although you should drink plenty of fluids).

Testing Techniques

The following tests help assess possible reasons for diarrhea:

Comprehensive stool analysis—bacterial and parasitic infection, flora balance

Food allergy/sensitivity testing—blood or electrodermal

Celiac disease testing for chronic cases—blood testing

As you feel better and regain your appetite, you should stay away from dairy products, fats, and oils, which will only upset your stomach again. If you do not have an intolerance to any of these foods, reintroduce them to your diet slowly.

Avoid sugar, especially if you have a bacterial infection. Bacteria feed on it. Even if a bacterium isn't the cause of your problem, keep sugar out of your diet; it promotes inflammation, which discourages healing.

Avoid caffeine and alcohol, which are too stimulating to the digestive tract.

If the cause of the problem is not clear, determine whether your diarrhea is caused by a food allergy or an intolerance. Once you feel better, use the elimination diet on page 253 to identify troublesome foods. Many cases of diarrhea can be traced to gluten intolerance, so make a special effort to examine the effects of wheat and seeds on your digestive system.

As you feel better, eat basic, simple foods that are easily absorbed. Soups, cooked fruits and vegetables, and brown rice are all good choices. Apples, bananas, carrots, and potatoes tend to taste especially good at this time, and for an excellent reason. They all contain an ingredient, pectin, that has a gentle binding quality.

One study has shown that roasted carob powder reduces the duration of diarrhea. Try a few tablespoons in some water.

Detoxification

Diarrhea is your body's method of self-detoxification. It's generally a good idea to fast on liquids for the first day; most likely, you will not want to eat solid foods anyway. See the dietary recommendations for details.

Tips for Travel

More than 50 percent of travelers to developing nations develop diarrhea from the microorganisms that are present in food and water. You can decrease your risk by taking the following steps:

- Prepare your body before you leave home. Six weeks before you leave, begin to eat lots of fresh garlic for its antibacterial and antiviral properties. You should also consume cultured products—live unsweetened yogurt, kefir, sauerkraut, and so on—to encourage the presence of friendly bacteria in your gut.

- When you arrive, continue eating garlic from your own supply, or take garlic capsules. We also recommend a probiotic supplement.

- This book generally recommends a diet that emphasizes raw plant foods. However, it may be wise to temporarily change your eating habits while traveling. Fried or chargrilled meats are often your best guarantee of thorough cooking. Avoid salads and raw foods, including fruits and vegetables, except those that have a thick outer skin, such as bananas and papayas.

- Use only bottled water, not just for drinking but also for brushing your teeth. Do not add ice to your drinks, unless you've made the ice yourself with bottled water.

- Don't eat at any restaurant or other establishment that is obviously unclean. Street food vendors are best avoided.

- When eating a food that is new food to you, try just a little at a time. Even if it is clean and free of microorganisms, your digestive system may not be able to handle large quantities of unusual foods right away.

Rx Super Seven Prescriptions

Super Prescription #1   Homeopathic Combination Diarrhea Remedy

For acute diarrhea, take a dose of a combination diarrhea remedy four times daily for twenty-four hours. If you notice improvement, stop taking the remedy unless symptoms return. If your symptoms do not improve within twenty-four hours, then pick the remedy that best matches your symptoms under Homeopathy in this section.

Super Prescription #2   Ginger (*Zingiber officinale*)

Drink a fresh cup of ginger tea, or take 500 mg in capsule form or 2 ml of tincture every two hours. Ginger reduces intestinal inflammation and lessens the effects of food poisoning.

Super Prescription #3   Probiotic

Take a product containing at least 4 billion active organisms two to three times daily. It contains friendly bacteria, such as *Lactobacillus acidophilus* and *bifidus,* which aid digestion and fight infection. Studies also show the probiotic *Saccharomyces boulardi* to be effective for diarrhea, especially for diarrhea associated with antibiotic use.

Super Prescription #4   Goldenseal (*Hydrastis canadensis*)

Take 1 ml of the tincture form or 300 mg in capsules four times daily. It helps improve diarrhea that is related to an intestinal infection.

Super Prescription #5   Enzymes

Take 1 to 2 capsules of a full-spectrum enzyme with each meal. Enzymes aid in the breakdown and the absorption of food.

Super Prescription #6   Oregano (*Origanum vulgare*) oil

Take 500 mg of the capsule form four times daily or as directed on the container. Oregano oil has powerful antimicrobial effects.

Super Prescription #7   Astragalus (*Astragalus membranaceus*)

This is an excellent treatment for chronic diarrhea. It has an astringent effect and improves digestion. Take 500 to 1,000 mg or 3.5 ml of a tincture two or three times daily. Do not take astragalus if you have a fever.

General Recommendations

Activated charcoal binds toxins in the digestive tract. Take 2 tablets three times in one day or as directed on the container for acute diarrhea.

Colostrum has been shown in studies to be effective for diarrhea. It also helps to heal the digestive tract. Take 500 mg three times daily.

Marshmallow (*Althea officinalis*) is soothing to the digestive tract. Take 500 mg in capsule form or 3 ml of the tincture three times daily.

Slippery elm (*Ulmus fulva*) is high in mucilage, which has a soothing effect on the intestines. Drink 3 to 4 cups each day. You can also use 5 ml of the tincture or 500 mg in capsules three times daily.

Cranesbill (*Germanium maculatum*) has an astringent effect on the colon for acute diarrhea. Take 3 to 5 ml of the tincture or 500 mg in capsule form three times daily.

L-glutamine is an amino acid that repairs the digestive tract. It is most useful for conditions associated with chronic diarrhea. Take 1,000 to 2,000 mg three times daily.

Lactase is an enzyme that digests milk sugar (lactose). If you are lactose intolerant and want to eat lactose-containing foods, take 1 to 2 lactase enzymes with each meal.

A study in the *Journal of Gut* reported that live probiotics interact with intestinal cells to protect them from the harmful effect of the bacteria *Escherichia coli* (EIEC 029:NM). Researchers found that these good bacteria prevented the *E. coli* from adhering to the cells and invading the body.

A randomized, placebo-controlled trial looked at the effect of probiotics on acute diarrhea in children from a daycare center. Probiotic supplementation was effective in reducing the duration of the diarrhea. The earlier the probiotics were begun, the more effective the results. In addition, a review of three double-blind clinical trials of diarrhea, which included 242 children, ages 6 months to 5 years, found "that individualized homeopathic treatment decreases the duration of acute childhood diarrhea."

Vitamin A and zinc have been shown to be helpful for children in Third World countries who suffer from infectious diarrhea. Take as directed by a doctor.

Red raspberry (*Rubus idaeus*) tea has historically been used for diarrhea. Drink 4 cups daily to reduce intestinal inflammation. If you prefer to take capsules, spread a dosage of 5 to 10 grams evenly throughout your day. Chamomile and peppermint teas are also good options.

Homeopathy

Aloe Socotrina is helpful when the diarrhea is characterized by rumbling and gurgling in the abdomen, followed by gushing stools. There are often yellow, mucus-filled stools.

Argentum Nitricum is for diarrhea that comes from anticipation anxiety before a stressful situation or event. It is also used for diarrhea that results from sugar ingestion.

Arsenicum Album helps when diarrhea and vomiting occur together. The person is anxious, restless, and chilly. It is good for diarrhea caused by food poisoning. There may be blood in the stool, and the person may feel better from sipping warm drinks.

Chamomilla (*Matricaria chamomilla*) is for green/yellow diarrhea that accompanies teething in infants.

China Officinalis helps when there is extreme exhaustion and weakness from diarrhea.

Ipecacuanha (*Cephaelis ipecacuanha*) is for diarrhea that is accompanied by nausea.

Mercurius Solubilis or Vivus is for burning and bloody diarrhea. The person often has extreme sweating and spasms of the intestines.

Phosphorous is for a watery stool. The person feels anxious and craves cold drinks.

Podophyllum is helpful when there is rumbling, gurgling, and cramping in the abdomen, followed by diarrhea. The diarrhea is painless, yet explosive, and is often worse in the morning.

Pulsatilla (*Pulsatilla pratensis*) is for diarrhea that results from eating greasy foods or fruits. The person feels better in the open air and worse in a warm room.

Sulphur is for burning, explosive diarrhea that wakes a person up in the morning. The stool has a very foul smell, like rotten eggs. The anus is red and excoriated. The person has a great thirst for cold drinks.

Veratrum Album is for painful, profuse diarrhea that resembles rice water. The person is very cold and desires drinks with ice.

Acupressure

See pages 668–675 for information about pressure points and administering treatment.

- Spleen 16 will relieve abdominal cramps associated with diarrhea.
- For diarrhea accompanied by gas, use Conception Vessel 6.
- Large Intestine 11 strengthens the colon.
- Stomach 36 is an excellent general toner that also strengthens the digestive system and improves the body's ability to absorb nutrients.

Bodywork

Massage

You may want to try a gentle self-massage of your abdomen. Lie down with your knees bent, and stroke the skin gently but firmly. For extra antispasmodic and soothing effects, use the essential oils recommended later in this entry.

Reflexology

See pages 686–687 for information about reflexology areas and how to work them.

Work the areas corresponding to the colon.

If your diarrhea is brought on or made worse by tension, also massage the area connected to the solar plexus.

Aromatherapy

Several oils have antispasmodic properties that will help relieve abdominal cramps. Chamomile, lavender, peppermint, and lemon balm are some good choices; in addition to soothing cramps, all these herbs will ease stress. Use any of these oils by themselves or in any combination in an abdominal self-massage.

Stress Reduction

General Stress-Reduction Therapies

Jon Kabat-Zinn, founder of the Stress Reduction Clinic at the University of Massachusetts, has discovered that patients with chronic nervous diarrhea improve greatly after learning meditation techniques. Meditation and other stress-reduction techniques, including biofeedback, can be helpful for people who are prone to diarrhea.

Bach Flower Remedies

Select the appropriate remedy, and place 10 drops of the liquid under your tongue. Hold the drops in place for thirty seconds and swallow. Use as often as needed.

For diarrhea brought on by an acute case of nervous tension, use Rescue Remedy.

If you are often fearful and anxious, Mimulus can have a calming effect.

Vervain is the remedy of choice for people who take on projects, especially charitable ones, with great zeal but who also have trouble keeping events in perspective. This difficulty often leads to great stress and tension.

Other Recommendations

- Constitutional hydrotherapy can be helpful for acute and chronic diarrhea. See pages 676–677 for directions.

REFERENCES

Jacobs, J., W. B. Jonas, M. Jimenez-Perez, and D. Crothers. 2003. Homeopathy for childhood diarrhea: Combined results and meta-analysis from three randomized, controlled clinical trials. *Pediatric Infectious Disease Journal* 22(3):229–34.

Resta-Lenert, S., and K. E. Barrett. 2003. Live probiotics protect intestinal epithelial cells from the effects of infection with enteroinvasive *Escherichia coli* (EIEC). *Gut* 52(7):988–97.

Rosenfeldt, V., et al. 2002. Effect of probiotic lactobacillus strains on acute diarrhea in a cohort of nonhospitalized children attending day-care centers. *Pediatric Infectious Disease Journal* 21(5):417–19.

Dizziness

Dizziness is the sensation that you are spinning or that your surroundings are spinning around you. Sometimes the sensation is mild and passes quickly, but it can also be so intense or prolonged that you may lose your balance and fall. Understandably, dizziness frequently produces nausea and vomiting.

Dizziness is not a disease in itself. Like pain, it's a symptom of an underlying problem, and any course of treatment for dizziness must begin with an investigation into the possible causes. Because the body keeps its balance through a complicated interplay of several organs, including the ears, the eyes, the nerves, and the muscles, finding the source of dizziness is not always easy.

Fortunately, dizziness often has its roots in a relatively minor cause. We've all experienced a spinning sensation when standing up too quickly after sitting or lying down for a long period of time; it may happen in airplanes, where there's less oxygen than most of us are used to. Occasional episodes of this kind are nothing to worry about. (If you experience it frequently, however, see a doctor.) Dizziness may also be the result of a fever, motion sickness, hyperventilation, a buildup of a wax in the ear canal, or a reaction to alcohol or drugs—factors that are either easily treated or temporary.

Sometimes, however, the underlying cause takes more effort to address. High blood pressure, anxiety, arteriosclerosis, food allergies, anemia, low blood sugar, hypothyroidism, and diabetes can all lead to dizziness. If nausea, vomiting, and a loss of hearing accompany the dizziness, you may have Ménière's disease, a disorder of the inner ear. In rare cases, dizziness is a warning sign of neurological disease or brain cancer.

If you experience dizziness, first rule out the obvious causes: motion sickness, fever and infection, and drug or alcohol use. In the case of motion sickness or fever, the dizziness will pass when travel or the illness ends. If your problem is related to alcohol or street drugs, stop using them; if you find that you can't, see the Substance Abuse section. For dizziness related to prescription medications, contact your doctor about alternatives.

If you can't immediately determine the cause on your own, see your doctor. He or she will take a thorough medical history to determine the most likely causes and will probably run a battery of tests. As you and your doctor search for the proper diagnosis, you can use the complementary therapies described further on to relieve your symptoms and reduce your chances of triggering an episode. In some cases, these therapies may resolve the problem altogether.

> Ménière's disease is an inner ear disorder characterized by vertigo (feeling as if the room around you is spinning around), tinnitus, and hearing loss.

SYMPTOMS

- Spinning sensation
- Nausea and vomiting
- Loss of hearing

ROOT CAUSES

Dozens of disorders and conditions can cause dizziness. Following are some of the most important.

- Returning to a standing position after a long period of sitting or lying down (orthostatic hypotension)
- Motion sickness
- Anxiety
- Fever
- Medications, street drugs, or alcohol
- Hyperventilation

- Wax build-up in the ear canal
- A disorder of the inner ear (such as Ménière's disease)
- Low blood sugar
- Circulatory disorders, such as high blood pressure or arteriosclerosis

- Anemia
- Hypothyroidism
- Diabetes
- Neurological disorders
- Brain tumors
- Allergies (environmental and food)

Testing Techniques

The following tests help assess possible reasons for dizziness:

Anemia—blood

Electrolyte imbalance—blood

Low or high blood sugar—blood, urine

Blood pressure—have your doctor check for orthostatic hypotension

Thyroid disorder—blood or saliva

Inner ear testing—by an ENT doctor

Food allergies/sensitivities—blood or electrodermal

TREATMENT

Diet

Recommended Food

Nutritional deficiencies can cause dizziness, and they can also cause some conditions that lead to dizziness. Eat meals that are based on a wide variety of basic, whole foods that you have prepared yourself. Keep your blood-sugar levels even by planning several small meals throughout the day, rather than three large ones. If you're nauseated, you may find that this strategy helps relieve your discomfort.

Some cases of dizziness have been linked to a deficiency of B vitamins, so add brewer's yeast to your meals. Other good sources of B vitamins are brown rice and leafy green vegetables. These vitamins will also help relieve anxiety.

Dizziness is sometimes caused by impaired circulation to the brain. Improve your blood flow by adding garlic, onions, and cayenne to your meals.

Food to Avoid

A response to a food allergen can cause dizziness. Read the entry on Food Allergies, and follow the elimination diet discussed there, to determine whether a food is the reason for your problem.

Even if your symptoms are not directly related to alcohol, avoid it. Alcohol can upset the inner ear and can aggravate other conditions that cause dizziness.

Excess sodium seems to affect the inner ear. Restrict your intake by avoiding processed, canned, or packaged foods, and don't use table salt to season your meals.

Avoid candy, cakes, cookies, and other sweets. These products will cause your blood-sugar levels to spike and then plummet, with dizziness as a possible result.

It's possible that chemicals added to food affect the intricate system that produces our sense of equilibrium. Avoid processed and junk food, along with any food made with additives.

℞ Super Seven Prescriptions—Dizziness

Super Prescription #1   Ginkgo biloba
Take 120 mg two to three times daily. Ginkgo improves circulation through the inner ear.

Super Prescription #2   Ginger (*Zingiber officinale*)
Take 300 to 500 mg or 2 to 3 ml three times daily. This ancient remedy is used for nausea and dizziness.

Super Prescription #3   Homeopathic Combination Dizziness and Nausea Formula
Take a 30C potency twice daily to see if there is improvement. If there are no changes within three days, pick another remedy that best matches your symptoms from the Homeopathy section.

Super Prescription #4   Ashwagandha (*Withania somniferum*)
Take 1,000 mg twice daily. If dizzy spells are related to nervous exhaustion or overwork, this tonic herb soothes and strengthens the frazzled mind.

Super Prescription #5   Panax ginseng
Take 100 mg two to three times daily of a product standardized to between 4 and 7 percent ginsenosides. This herb strengthens the adrenal glands. Low adrenal function may be the root problem, resulting in low blood pressure and the accompanying dizziness.

Super Prescription #6   B complex
Take a 50 mg complex twice daily. It combats the effects of stress that may be associated with dizziness.

Super Prescription #7   High-potency multivitamin
Take as directed on the container. If you are anemic, choose a formula that contains iron. It provides a base of nutritional support.

Homeopathy

Pick the remedy that best matches your symptoms in this section. Take a 6x, 12x, 6C, or 30C potency twice daily for two weeks to see if there are any positive results. After you notice improvement, stop taking the remedy, unless symptoms return. Consultation with a homeopathic practitioner is advised.

Aconitum Napellus is for sudden dizziness associated with anxiety, panic, or shock. Your pulse may be rapid, and you may even fear that you're going to die.

Bryonia (*Bryonia alba*) is for dizziness that occurs when you get up from a sitting position, turn your head, or bend over. You are irritable and have a great thirst for cold drinks.

Cocculus is for motion sickness and the dizziness that occurs from looking out the window. Nauseousness and/or vomiting may accompany the dizziness.

Conium is helpful when dizziness is worse from lying down or turning over in bed. Dizziness occurs from moving the head or the eyes.

Gelsemium (*Gelsemium sempervirens*) is for dizziness caused by a viral infection, making a person feel drowsy and droopy. It is also used for dizziness that follows stage fright.

Nux Vomica (*Strychnos nux vomica*) will ease dizziness that's brought on by a hangover or the ill effects of spoiled/contaminated food.

Pulsatilla (*Pulsatilla pratensis*) is for dizziness that comes on when you're in a warm or stuffy room. You feel worse when lying down. There is relief from walking or sitting in the open air.

Acupressure

See pages 686–675 for information about acupressure points and administering treatment.

When you feel dizziness coming on, sit down in a comfortable place, focus on a nonmoving object, and work the following points, all located at the top of your head: Governing Vessel 19, 20, and 21. Know these points so that you can use them whenever you need to, without having to look them up.

Bodywork

Massage

A general massage is an excellent way to stimulate circulation throughout the body. You can also practice a simple head and neck rub at home or see a massage therapist.

Reflexology

See pages 686–687 for information about reflexology areas and how to work them.

Work the areas corresponding to the eye/ear and the neck.

Hydrotherapy

Try constitutional hydrotherapy to improve circulation to the brain.

Aromatherapy

Lavender combats the sensation of vertigo. For immediate relief, place a vial of the oil directly under your nose and inhale deeply.

Ginger oil will reduce nausea. You can inhale the oil directly from the vial or use it in an abdominal massage.

Black pepper, eucalyptus, and rosemary increase circulation. You can use these oils separately or in combination; add them to a bath or dilute them with a carrier oil and use in a massage.

Essential oils are perhaps most famous for their stress-relieving properties. If you'd benefit from oils with calming properties, try the following: lavender, bergamot, ylang ylang, geranium, or rose. You can use these oils in any preparation you like, but you should avoid using any one for an extended period of time, as you may grow immune to its effects.

Stress Reduction

Anxiety and stress can cause dizziness. Even if your symptoms are caused by an underlying disorder like diabetes or hypothyroidism, stress can aggravate the problem and trigger an attack. That said, you should be wary of any doctor who diagnoses you with stress-related dizziness without first checking for physiological causes. This misdiagnosis frequently happens to women, who are told their dizziness is "just stress," when, in fact, an underlying disorder is at work.

General Stress-Reduction Therapies

Meditation, stretching, and mild exercise can help improve the symptoms of dizziness.

Bach Flower Remedies

Select the appropriate remedy, and place 10 drops of the liquid under your tongue. Hold the drops in place for thirty seconds and swallow. Use as often as needed.

If you are prone to panic attacks, keep a bottle of Rescue Remedy on hand. At the first sign of overwhelming stress or anxiety, a few drops will produce a calmer state of mind.

Aspen will help if your dizziness is produced by fears that you can't name. You may feel a generalized sense of anxiety, rather than stress over a specific problem.

If you are shy and withdrawn and are able to name your fears but are unable to talk about them with others, take Mimulus.

Those whose anxiety is caused by worries for other people will benefit from Red Chestnut.

Other Recommendations

- When you feel dizzy, sit down and focus your gaze on a fixed object until the sensation passes. This technique will shorten the duration of the dizziness and reduce nausea. Obviously, it will also prevent you from losing your balance and falling.
- Smoking inhibits circulation and can lead to dizziness. If you smoke, quit. Even if you don't smoke, you must avoid exposure to smoky rooms or bars.
- If you are prone to dizziness, avoid sudden changes in your posture. If you've been lying down or sitting for a long time, don't jump to your feet. Get up slowly.

Drug Addiction. *See* Substance Abuse

Ear Infection

While ear infections can occur at any age, they are most common in early childhood and infancy. In fact, ear infections are the reason for more than half the visits to pediatricians in the United States. Statistics show that acute ear infections affect two-thirds of American children under age two, while chronic ear infections affect two-thirds of children under age six!

There are two main categories of ear infection. The first is an outer ear infection, also known as swimmer's ear or otitis externa. It affects the ear canal, which runs from the ear opening to the eardrum, and happens when a substance (usually, water—hence the nickname) enters the ear canal and is trapped there by a build-up of wax. In this stagnant condition, bacteria breed and flourish. The body responds to the infection with inflammation, redness, pain, and sometimes a fever.

The second category, called a middle-ear infection or otitis media, is much more common, especially in very young children and infants. Most ear infections are usually associated with an upper respiratory infection or an allergy. Forty percent of cases involve bacterial infection, with the most common being *Streptococcus pneumoniae*. Many ear infections involve a viral infection that is unresponsive to antibiotics. Chronic middle ear infections (also known as serous otitis media or glue ear) refer

A comprehensive review of studies published in the *British Medical Journal* found that there was no significant difference in children with acute ear infections when antibiotics were given, as compared to a placebo.

to chronic swelling of the eardrum as a result of fluid accumulation. One of the reasons infants are more susceptible to ear infections is due to the fact that the eustachian tube (which drains fluid from the middle ear) is more horizontal than it is in adults and does not drain as efficiently. This tube becomes more vertical and drains better as children get older. The key is to prevent the build-up of this fluid with a proper diet. Food allergens, such as cow's milk and sugar, trigger a cascade of inflammation responses that often result in mucus and fluid. These foods are often the root problem. In addition, avoiding environmental allergens is important—particularly secondhand smoke. Addressing food allergies and environmental allergens is crucial so that "germs" do not have an environment to grow in. Of course, a healthy functioning immune system is also key in preventing infection.

Some infections are the result of a malfunctioning or still-developing eustachian tube, the passage that connects the three bones of the middle ear to the nose and the throat. When the eustachian tube isn't working properly, mucus isn't able to drain from behind the eardrum into the upper respiratory tract; instead, it remains trapped and causes pain and pressure. This situation often leads to infection, especially if there has already been a mucus-producing disease of the upper respiratory system, such as a cold or the flu.

Middle-ear infections can be quite painful. There may be a fever, perhaps a very high one, with some hearing difficulty or nausea and vomiting. If your child pulls or slaps at his or her ear, an infection is a strong possibility. Take all ear infections and ear pain seriously. The following treatments can be used to relieve pain, but do call a doctor for professional advice in the presence of a sustained fever or if the ear continues to hurt. If you or your child experiences severe ear pain, followed by a sudden relief and/or a discharge of blood or pus, consult a doctor immediately, even if you or the child feels well.

The prescribing of antibiotics for otitis media with effusion is controversial. This refers to the presence of fluid in the middle ear, in the absence of signs or symptoms of acute infection. According to the U.S. Agency for Health Care Policy and Research, most cases of otitis media with effusion resolve spontaneously. It must also be recognized that fluid left in the middle ear after antibiotic treatment is normal. Approximately 70 percent of children have fluid in the middle ear at 2 weeks, 50 percent have fluid at 1 month, 20 percent have fluid at 2 months, and 10 percent have fluid at 3 months after appropriate antibiotic therapy. According to studies, the fluid that remains does not need to be treated with antibiotics, as is typically done.

Conventional Treatment for Ear Infections

Ear infections have reached nearly epidemic proportions in the United States. In response, frustrated doctors have come up with aggressive treatments, usually in the form of heavy antibiotics and ear tubes. Sometimes these strategies are necessary and effective, but all too often doctors employ them as a first line of a defense, rather than as a last resort. Tubes in the ears, which relieve pressure on the eardrum and allow pus to drain, may seem like a good idea, but the tubes themselves often cause a great deal of damage. Interestingly, a study published in the *Journal of the American Medical Association* found that only 42 percent of these surgeries were appropriate. If your doctor recommends ear tubes, question him or her closely. Make sure that any treatment is tailored to your needs or your child's. And as always, try conservative measures—dietary changes, immune enhancement, homeopathy, and gentle herbals—before turning to harsh drugs or invasive procedures.

The over-prescribing of antibiotics for childhood ear infections has been a contributing factor to antibiotic-resistant bacteria. In addition, they put your child at risk for candida overgrowth (see Candidiasis).

SYMPTOMS

Not all of the following symptoms need to be present for a diagnosis of ear infection.

- Pain, often throbbing
- Fever
- Pressure or a feeling of fullness in the ear
- Pus from the ear
- Hearing difficulty in the affected ear
- Nausea and vomiting

ROOT CAUSES

- Buildup of wax, often the result of cleaning the ears with cotton swabs
- Upper respiratory infections
- Food allergies/sensitivities (especially, overconsumption of dairy products)
- Environmental allergies (molds, dust, animal dander, and hay fever)
- Smoking or secondhand smoke, which irritates the eustachian tube and causes inflammation behind the ear drum.
- Not being breastfed: Breastfeeding allows for the transport of immune factors from the mother to the child and matures the digestive tract so that the child is less susceptible to food allergies.
- Season: The incidence of earaches is highest in the winter. In northern climates, ear infections increase in frequency beginning in September.
- Fetal alcohol syndrome: More than 90 percent of children with fetal alcohol syndrome (which occurs from the mother drinking alcohol during pregnancy) have problems with ear infections.
- Genetic: Nearly 60 percent of all children with Down's syndrome experience problems with otitis media.
- Nutritional deficiencies of vitamins A and C and essential fatty-acid imbalance.
- Injuries: Children who suffered a trauma at birth (e.g., forceps delivery, vacuum extraction) and children with neck and head injuries are more susceptible (an indication for chiropractic, osteopathic, or craniosacral therapy).

TREATMENT

Diet

These dietary suggestions will help alleviate pain. More important, many of them will also prevent recurring infections. Significant changes in your child's diet may be necessary for optimal results. Work with a nutrition-oriented doctor.

Recommended Food
A good diet based on whole grains, high-quality protein, and fresh fruits and vegetables will build up the immune system and discourage infection.

Drink plenty of water to thin mucus secretions.

Essential fatty acids, found in cold-water fish, flaxseeds, and flaxseed oil, are useful in reducing the inflammation or the allergies that are often present.

Switch bottle-fed babies to a nondairy formula, with your doctor's supervision.

Breastfeeding mothers should avoid common allergens (e.g., cow's milk), in order to not pass the allergenic portion through the breastmilk. Food testing can be done with the mother.

Food to Avoid

Investigate the possibility of food allergies, especially to dairy, wheat, sugar, citrus fruits, soy, eggs, or chocolate. See the Food Allergies section, especially the elimination diet on page 253, for further advice. If you discover a trigger food, remove it from your diet.

If ear infections recur or are chronic, suspend the consumption of dairy products indefinitely. For infants and young children who are bottle-fed, replace the regular cow's milk formula with a hypoallergenic/predigested formula.

Simple sugars suppress the immune system, so stay away from refined carbohydrates.

Detoxification

A three-day juice fast can help break up excess mucus in the body. Use this therapy for adults only; children should never fast.

℞ Super Seven Prescriptions—Ear Infection

Super Prescription #1   Homeopathic Combination Earache Formula
Take a dose of the formula every thirty to sixty minutes for an acute earache. Improvements should be seen within two to four hours. Otherwise, see the remedies listed under Homeopathy in this section for a specific remedy.

Super Prescription #2   Garlic (*Allium sativum*) or **garlic/mullein drops**
Place 2 warm drops in the affected ear three times daily. Do not use if the eardrum is perforated or if fluid is draining out of the ear. These herbs have antibacterial/antiviral effects and natural pain-relieving qualities.

Super Prescription #3   Echinacea (*Echinacea purpurea*) and **goldenseal** (*Hydrastis canadensis*)
Adults can take 4 ml and children 2 ml four times daily or as directed on the container. Echinacea and goldenseal enhance immune function.

Super Prescription #4   Vitamin C
Adults should take 1,000 mg three to four times daily and children 500 mg three times daily. Reduce the dosage if diarrhea occurs. Vitamin C enhances immune function and reduces inflammation.

Super Prescription #5   Larix

Dissolve 1 to 2 teaspoons in a formula bottle for bottle-feeding infants or mix in water for older children and give it four times daily. Larix enhances immune function.

Super Prescription #6   Vitamin A

Give 2,000 to 5,000 IU daily (up to five days) for children up to six years of age. It's available in liquid form. Vitamin A supports immune function.

Super Prescription #7   Essential fatty acids

Adults should take 1 to 2 tablespoons of flaxseed oil or 3 grams of fish oil daily, or a formulation that contains a mixture of omega-3, 6, and 9 fatty acids. For children give a children's essential fatty acid formula or $\frac{1}{2}$ to 1 tablespoon of flaxseed oil daily. It can be mixed into the formula for bottle-fed infants. Reduce the dosage if loose stools occur. Essential fatty acids are helpful for the prevention of ear infections, as they reduce inflammation and allergic tendencies.

K. H. Friese, M.D., and his colleagues divided 131 young children (average age 5) into two groups. One group of 28 children received conventional treatment, such as decongestants, antibiotics, and fever-reducing medicines (12 different drugs in all), for ear infections. Another group of 103 children was treated with 1 or more of 12 homeopathic remedies. Children receiving the homeopathic treatment, on average, experienced 2 days of ear pain and required 3 days of therapy. Nearly 71 percent never had another ear infection after 1 year, and nearly 30 percent had a maximum of 3 recurrences. By contrast, children treated with conventional medicine, on average, experienced 3 days of ear pain and required 10 days of therapy. Nearly 57 percent did not have a recurrence after 1 year, while 43 percent experienced a maximum of 6 recurrences.

General Recommendations

Thymus (*Thymus vulgaris*) extract supports immune function. Take 250 to 500 mg twice daily on an empty stomach or as directed on the container.

Zinc supports immune function. Give 5 mg for children under two and 10 mg for those older than two. Adults should take 30 mg daily.

Chamomile tea is another way to help a child relax and sleep.

Because of its high mucilage content, marshmallow (*Althea officinalis*) is soothing to irritated ear membranes. Adults should take 2 grams three times a day; children six years and under can take 1 ml of the tincture three times daily.

Saint-John's-wort oil (*Hypericum perforatum*) relieves ear pain and fights infection. Place 2 warm drops in the affected ear three times daily. Do not use if the eardrum is perforated or if fluid is draining out of the ear.

Xylitol nasal spray and chewing gums prevent the buildup of bacteria that may cause ear infections. Use preventatively.

Homeopathy

Pick the remedy that best matches your symptoms in this section. For acute earaches, take a 30C potency (or the potency available to you) hourly, up to six doses. After you notice improvement, stop taking the remedy, unless symptoms return. Consultation with a homeopathic practitioner is advised.

Aconitum Napellus is helpful for a painful earache that comes on very quickly. The child experiences violent pain, restlessness, and great thirst. The earache often occurs after being out in the cold, dry wind. The ears are bright red. Aconitum is helpful only if used during the initial six hours of the ear infection.

Belladonna (*Atropa belladonna*) is for a sudden onset of earache, with high fever and a red face and eardrum. The right ear is more affected than the left. The pupils can be dilated, and child looks and feels hot, but the feet are cold.

Chamomilla (*Matricaria chamomilla*) is for a child with an ear infection, who is very irritable, angry, and hard to console. The child appears to be in a lot of pain, screaming and crying. The child wants to be carried, but it helps only for a short period of time. One cheek is often red, the other one pale. This is a great remedy for earaches that occur at the same time as teething.

Ferrum Phosphoricum is recommended for a child who has a fever and feels warm. The face and the affected ear are red (such as in Belladonna), but the child does not act sick.

Hepar Sulphuris (*Hepar sulphuris calcareum*) is helpful when the ears are very sensitive to the touch and to cold during an infection. The child is irritable and hard to console. There is a sharp pain in the ear that feels better with warm applications. There can be pus or discharge from the ear.

Lachesis is useful when the left ear is affected or when the infection starts in the left ear and moves to the right. The earache is worse with warm applications and at nighttime.

Lycopodium (*Lycopodium clavatum*) is helpful for right-sided ear infections. Ear symptoms are often worse from 4 to 8 P.M. and feel better with warm applications to the ear. The child is irritable and may have more gas and digestive upset than normal.

Mercurius Solubilis or Vivus is a great choice for an earache that has an offensive-smelling pus discharge. The child sweats more than usual. There is a thick coating on the tongue, along with bad breath and increased salivation. The symptoms are worse at night.

Pulsatilla (*Pulsatilla pratensis*) is for a child who has a fever, is weepy, and wants to be held and comforted. Ear pain feels better with cold applications or in the open air, and worse with warmth. The child has a low thirst. The fever and the ear infection often develop at night. There can be a yellow-green discharge from the nose and the ears.

Silica (*Silicea*) is used for children who are thin and frail, with weak immunity, and who suffer from chronic ear infections. It is also used for acute ear infections and for a ruptured eardrum with pus. Cold and wind bother the child.

Acupressure

See pages 668–675 for information about acupressure points and administering treatment.

Triple Warmer 21, Small Intestine 19, and Gallbladder 2 will ease ear pain.

Bodywork

Massage

Massage of the ear, the neck, and the temples is a gentle way to relieve a child's pain (or an adult's).

Reflexology

See pages 686–687 for information about acupressure points and how to administer treatment.

To reduce pain, work the ear/eye area.

Stimulate the lymph area to combat infection.

Hydrotherapy

Alternating hot (two minutes) and cold (thirty seconds) towels over the affected ear helps to relieve pain and inflammation.

Aromatherapy

Chamomile oil makes a gentle wash for the infected ear. First dilute the chamomile in a carrier oil, and place a couple of drops into the ear. After ten minutes, lie down on your side, with the infected ear turned toward the floor. Let the oil drain out (you may want to have a towel handy).

Other Recommendations

- Make sure not to bottlefeed while children are lying on their backs. They should be at a 30-degree angle or more to prevent fluid accumulation in the eustachian tube.
- Don't smoke or expose yourself or your children to secondhand smoke.
- Follow the old adage that says not to put anything into your ear that's smaller than your elbow. Cotton swabs pack wax into the ear canal.
- During the course of an infection, don't allow moisture into your ears. Put cotton gently in the outside of the ear while taking baths or showers or while washing your face. Don't go swimming until the infection has cleared.
- To reduce pain, apply heat locally. Try a hot water bottle wrapped in a towel or blow a hairdryer onto the affected ear.
- Chiropractic, osteopathy, and craniosacral treatments can be very helpful for some children with structural and motion abnormalities of the upper neck vertebrae. These abnormalities can cause fluid to build up and not drain properly, providing a breeding ground for infections. Many parents have reported that these types of treatments helped to prevent further ear infections with their children. Specific treatments by a practitioner can correct these imbalances.

REFERENCES

Friese, K. H., M.D., et al. 1997. "Acute otitis media in children: A comparison of conventional and homeopathic treatment. *Biomedical Therapy* XV:4, 113–16, 122.

Froom, J., et al. 1997. Antimicrobials for acute otitis media? A review from the international primary care network. *British Medical Journal* 315:98–102.

Kleinman, L. C., et al. 1994. The medical appropriateness of tympanostomy tubes proposed for children younger than 16 years in the United States. *Journal of the American Medical Association* 271:1250–55.

Eating Disorders (Anorexia Nervosa and Bulimia)

Eating disorders are characterized by a distorted body image and an intense fear of being fat. This abnormal mental state leads to extreme and sometimes life-threatening behavior. A person with an eating disorder may binge on large quantities of food and then vomit or use laxatives so that the food exits the body undigested, or the person may refuse to eat all. Although eating disorders can manifest themselves in many ways, they always result in an unhealthful, obsessive relationship with food. The best-known and most frightening kinds of eating disorders are anorexia nervosa and bulimia.

Anorexia nervosa occurs most frequently in teenage girls and college-age women, and it's estimated that about 1 percent of all young women in this age group suffer from the disease. It is here that eating disorders take their most disturbing form: slow, deliberate starvation. Despite their obviously emaciated bodies, anorexics believe that they are overweight. They refuse food, or they eat just enough to keep their systems minimally functioning. Some may eat occasionally, just to please their families or friends, but they often purge themselves of the food afterward. It's not hard to see that anorexia can lead to grave health problems. Weight loss, weakness, and fatigue are obvious early signs, but as the disease progresses, it can also lead to weak vital signs, irregular menstruation, and cold or tingling extremities. If the dieting continues, the person may go into cardiac arrest.

Bulimia is a more common disorder that affects a slightly older population, usually women in their twenties. Bulimics also have a distorted body image, but instead of dieting down to skin and bones, they use a cycle of bingeing and purging to maintain a relatively normal weight. Bulimics may eat thousands of calories at one sitting and then induce vomiting to expel the food from the body so that they can't gain weight. They may also use laxatives to keep the body from digesting the food. Because many bulimics are quite successful at hiding their purging, the disease may go unnoticed for years. In fact, bulimia is often diagnosed only when a doctor or a loved one notices a pattern of medical conditions associated with bulimia. The stomach acid produced by frequent vomiting often causes tooth decay or a chronically sore throat. Self-induced vomiting produces another telltale sign: sores on the knuckles or the fingers. Not surprisingly, bulimics also tend to suffer from nutritional deficiencies, as well as digestive disorders like constipation or diarrhea. In severe or long-term cases, the complications can be fatal. The stomach or the esophagus may rupture, or a potassium deficiency can lead to kidney failure or heart attack.

We do know that eating disorders are a recent and mostly Western phenomenon, rare before the latter half of the twentieth century and nonexistent in developing nations. Our culture's emphasis on dieting and thinness is one undeniable cause of the disorder; far too many girls—and an increasing number of boys—believe that they are unlovable and even unclean if they can't diet down to the current rail-thin standard. Even if these children don't intend to become anorexic or bulimic, it is highly likely that what starts out as "normal" dieting will disrupt the body's metabolism and chemistry and eventually lead to a serious disorder. Family dynamics also play a role: many sufferers come from families that place great pressure on their children to succeed. Although doctors used to believe that anorexia and bulimia were purely psychological in nature, it's now understood that chemical imbalances and the accompanying nutritional deficiencies may lead to eating disorders just as easily as they may to lead to depression.

An eating disorder must always be taken seriously. Even if a person does not meet the exact standards for an eating disorder, an obsession with food and dieting can pave the way for more serious problems. If you suspect that you have an eating disorder, find a counselor or a friend you can trust. Talking about the disorder is one of the first and best steps you can take toward healing it. See a doctor for assessment and treatment of any secondary disorders you might have developed; if your eating disorder is severe, you may have to be hospitalized so that your body can regain its strength and balance. Bulimics will need to see a dentist as well. Once you've talked to a doctor, you'll need to follow an eating plan that replenishes the nutrients in your body and helps you reestablish healthful patterns. If you're not already seeing a professional therapist, make an appointment. He or she can help you relearn good habits and thinking patterns.

If you are worried that a friend or a family member has an eating disorder, you may find that confronting the ill person results in the individual's denial or resistance. Sometimes the only way to help a victim of an eating disorder is to ask for professional help. Call a doctor or a psychologist and ask for advice; if you're on a college campus, the school may have an eating-disorder specialist you can talk to. In extreme cases, the person may need to be hospitalized.

SYMPTOMS OF ANOREXIA

- Unexplained and unnecessary weight loss
- Fear of being fat
- Obsession with preparing and serving food
- Obsessive dining rituals
- Fatigue
- Weakness
- Dizziness
- Mood swings
- Menstrual irregularities or delayed onset of menstruation
- Hair loss
- Cold or tingling extremities
- Irregular heartbeat
- Weak vital signs

SYMPTOMS OF BULIMIA

- Sores or calluses on knuckles
- Chronic sore or burning throat
- Erosion of tooth enamel, especially on the back teeth
- "Chipmunk" appearance from swollen salivary glands
- Digestive problems
- Weight fluctuation
- Menstrual irregularities
- Erratic heartbeat

ROOT CAUSES

- Weight-obsessed culture
- Dieting
- Family problems
- Chemical imbalance
- Low levels of serotonin
- Nutritional deficiencies (e.g., zinc)

Testing Techniques

The following tests help assess possible reasons for an eating disorder or imbalances that may aid in recovery:

Vitamin and mineral (especially zinc, iron, and B vitamins)—blood test

Blood-sugar balance—blood test

Stress hormone balance—saliva, urine, or blood

TREATMENT

Diet

The following suggestions will help you get back on track, but it is highly recommended that you work with a nutritional therapist. A professional can help you address the particular deficiencies your disorder has created and can show you how to develop eating habits that work for you.

Recommended Food

Instead of sitting down to a large breakfast, lunch, and dinner, eat small, nourishing meals throughout the day. This strategy will stabilize your blood sugar, and if you're bulimic, it will help you stop bingeing.

A high-fiber diet will restore regularity to your digestive system. Eat plenty of whole grains, oats, and vegetables. Green leafy vegetables are also a good source of potassium, a mineral that bulimics must replenish.

People with eating disorders are often lacking protein. Plan to have fish several times a week, and include servings of soy products or beans at most meals.

Anorexia nervosa has been linked to a zinc deficiency. Pumpkin seeds are an excellent source of this mineral. Eat a quarter to a half cup daily.

Many people with anorexia or bulimia have low levels of the neurotransmitter serotonin. Regulate your serotonin by eating complex carbohydrates like whole grains.

Food to Avoid

Some foods fool your appetite or tastebuds into feeling satisfied, when, in fact, you have received very little nutrition. A goal of your dietary therapy should be to relearn how to listen to your body's needs, so stay away from the following "tricky" products: processed food, junk food, sodas, and diet or "lite" foods.

Keep your blood-sugar levels steady by avoiding refined sugar. Do not eat candy, cake, cookies, ice cream, sodas, or other sweets.

Eliminate caffeine and alcohol, substances that upset the digestive system and sometimes produce anxiety.

℞ Super Seven Prescriptions—Eating Disorders

Super Prescription #1   High-potency multivitamin
Take as directed on the container. If you have been diagnosed as being iron-deficient anemic, choose a formula that contains iron. It will supply a base of vitamins and minerals for nutritional support.

Super Prescription #2   Homeopathy
Choose the remedy from the list in the Homeopathy section that best matches your situation.

Super Prescription #3   Zinc
Take 45 to 90 mg daily, along with 3 mg of copper. Studies have found that zinc deficiency is common in people with anorexia or bulimia. It is also required for the senses of taste and smell and for appetite.

Super Prescription #4   B-Complex
Take a 50 mg complex one to two times daily. Many of the B vitamins are depleted because of stress and are required for the formation of brain neurotransmitters that balance mood.

Super Prescription #5   5-Hydroxytryptophan (5-HTP)
Take 100 mg two to three times daily. It supports serotonin levels, which reduce anxiety and depression. Do not use in combination with pharmaceutical antidepressant or antianxiety medications.

Super Prescription #6   Gentian root (*Gentiana lutea*)
Take 10 drops in water or 300 mg fifteen minutes before each meal. It improves appetite and digestion.

One clinical trial of 20 women with anorexia looked at the effects of their supplementing 45 to 90 mg of zinc per day. As a result, 17 out of 20 women experienced weight gain within 8 to 56 months. Also, a double-blind study of 35 women hospitalized with anorexia found that supplementation of 14 mg of zinc per day resulted in a 10 percent increase in weight. This was twice as fast as with the group that received a placebo.

> **Super Prescription #7   Saint-John's-wort** (*Hypericum perforatum*)
> Take 300 mg of a 0.3 hypercin extract two to three times daily. This herb helps with depression and anxiety. Do not use in combination with pharmaceutical antidepressant or antianxiety medications.

General Recommendations

Vitamin B6 is important for the synthesis of neurotransmitters that improve mood and sense of well-being. Take 50 mg daily.

Essential fatty acids are often deficient in people with eating disorders. Take an essential fatty-acid complex, 1 tablespoon of flaxseed oil, or 3 grams of fish oil daily.

Chromium helps to balance blood-sugar levels. Take up to 1,000 mcg daily.

Homeopathy

Pick the remedy that best matches your symptoms in this section. Take a 6x, 12x, 6C, or 30C potency twice daily for two weeks to see if there are any positive results. After you notice improvement, stop taking the remedy, unless symptoms return. Consultation with a homeopathic practitioner is advised.

Ferrum Phosphoricum is helpful if you are pale, weak, and anemic.

Ignatia Amara is for people with an eating disorder who have emotional swings. They feel like crying easily, have anxiety and depression, yet are averse to consolation. It is useful for acute emotional upsets, such as grief, which contribute to the eating disorder.

Lycopodium (*Lycopodium clavatum*) is good for an upset stomach and bloating. The person tends to get low blood sugar and suffers from irritability and low self-esteem.

Natrum Muriaticum will help if you are often depressed and have long-standing grief associated with your eating disorder. You often crave salty foods, have a great thirst, and are averse to the sun.

Pulsatilla (*Pulsatilla pratensis*) is helpful if you tend to be sensitive and weepy and feel better with company. You also crave sweets and feel better in cool air.

Acupressure

See pages 668–675 for information about pressure points and administering treatment.

- Bring your appetite back to normal by working Spleen 16.
- Use Stomach 36 as a general tonic for all body systems and to improve your ability to digest and absorb nutrients.

Bodywork

Massage

A professional massage will help you get back in touch with your body.

Reflexology

See pages 686–687 for information about reflexology areas and how to work them.

Eating disorders wreak havoc on every body system. Work the entire foot for the full benefit. This treatment will also give you a quick mood lift.

To reduce anxiety, work the areas corresponding to the diaphragm, all the glands, the heart, and the solar plexus.

For depression, work the head, the endocrine glands, the solar plexus, and the pancreas.

Aromatherapy

Bergamot and peppermint oils encourage the appetite. Place the vial of oil directly under your nose and inhale deeply.

Stress Reduction

People who are anxious or depressed or exposed to high levels of stress are more vulnerable to eating disorders than others are. Many experts believe that eating disorders are a way of focusing on weight and food, instead of on complicated and unpleasant emotions. If you're trying to recover from anorexia or bulimia, you'll find that learning alternative ways to handle stress will reduce your need to exercise control via food.

General Stress-Reduction Therapies

For people who've considered themselves little more than an extension of their appetite, prayer and meditation can work wonders to restore a sense of wholeness.

If you are extremely anxious and nervous, consider EEG biofeedback. It will teach you how to recognize your body's panic signals and show you how to subdue them before they get out of control.

Bach Flower Remedies

If none of the following suggestions fits your personality, consult the chart on pages 648–650 to find the remedy that does. Once you've chosen a remedy, place 10 drops of the liquid under your tongue. Hold the drops in place for thirty seconds and swallow. Use as often as needed.

Rescue Remedy has a steadying effect during a physical or emotional crisis. Take it if you feel a panic attack about to start or if you are overwhelmed by a desire to binge or purge.

If you're a perfectionist and tend to be highly critical of others, Beech will help you see beauty in the world as it exists.

On the other hand, some hard-working perfectionists blame themselves for every problem that arises. Pine will help these people develop a clearer perspective.

Centaury is for people who are easily exploited and taken advantage of. This remedy can help you learn how to say no when necessary.

If having an eating disorder makes you feel ashamed, take Crab Apple.

For obsessive thoughts about food or about your eating disorder that just won't stop, take White Chestnut.

Other Recommendations

- People with eating disorders often become obsessed with burning off calories through physical activity. A far better option is to take a thirty-minute walk at a moderate pace. The mild exercise will boost your spirits, and if you can get out in the fresh air and sunshine, you'll feel even better.
- Girls who are just beginning puberty are particularly vulnerable to losing their self-esteem; they may also fear the upcoming body changes and natural weight gain. Both of these factors can set the stage for an eating disorder. You can help girls make a healthy transition into adolescence by encouraging them to develop a talent or an ability that improves self-esteem.
- It is imperative that a specialist in eating disorders manage the case of a person with an eating disorder.

REFERENCES

McClain, C. J., M. A. Stuart, B. Vivian, et al. 1992. Zinc status before and after zinc supplementation of eating disorder patients. *Journal of the American College of Nutrition* 11:694–700.

Safai-Kutti, S. 1990. Oral zinc supplementation in anorexia nervosa. *ACTA Psychiatrica Scandinavica* 361:14–17.

Eczema

Eczema is a troublesome but common skin disorder that affects up to 15 percent of the population. In its acute form, eczema causes inflamed red, dry, and itchy skin. Some patches may blister and weep, and, eventually, these areas may crust over. If the eczema is a chronic problem, the skin will continue to itch but may thicken and take on a leathery consistency. Usually, dry scales develop, and the skin's color may change.

Most acute cases are brought on by an allergic response. Sufferers may be allergic to a certain food or to other substances; in either case, it's quite possible to have a reaction from ingesting the allergen or just from touching it. If you can identify the irritant and remove it, the eczema will usually disappear. But if the skin continues to be exposed to the irritating factor, the rash may spread and develop into a chronic condition. Stress may aggravate acute eczema and keep it from resolving.

Eczema can appear in infancy or early childhood and most often develops on the face and the head or in the folds of the elbows, the knees, or the groin. In some cases, it will disappear as childhood progresses and either stay away for good or recur in adolescence or adulthood. Chronic eczema is a complex condition that usually involves a family history of eczema, asthma, or hay fever; difficulty handling stress; or food sensitivity. It has also been linked to abnormalities of the immune system, as well as to candidiasis and low levels of essential fatty acids and deficiencies of other nutrients that help keep down inflammation. Poor digestion and detoxification can also be at the root of eczema. Like most complicated ailments that involve the whole body and lifestyle, holistic treatment is the best approach for both relief and resolution. Conventional therapy for chronic cases is usually quite frustrating for the patient, as it generally just suppresses the skin problem and causes further spreading or intensifies the symptoms. Treating the root cause(s) with natural therapies, as described in this section, is, in our opinion, a superior way to help resolve this aggravating condition.

SYMPTOMS OF ACUTE ECZEMA

- Red, dry, swollen, and burning skin
- A strong, almost overwhelming desire to scratch
- Skin that blisters, oozes, and crusts over

SYMPTOMS OF CHRONIC ECZEMA

- Recurring cases of acute eczema
- Thick, dry skin with scaly patches
- Continued itching
- Color changes

ROOT CAUSES OF ACUTE ECZEMA

- Food allergies
- Contact with irritants (these can include but are not limited to dyes, perfumes, topical medications, plants, metals, soaps, wool, pollutants, and even sunlight)

ROOT CAUSES OF CHRONIC ECZEMA

- Suppressive treatments of acute eczema (such as long-term topical steroid treatment)
- Heredity
- Stress
- Food allergies or sensitivities
- An imbalanced immune system
- Deficiency of or inability to process essential fatty acids
- Candidiasis
- Low levels of stomach acid and poor digestion
- Poor detoxification

TREATMENT

Diet

Recommended Food

Eat a diet of basic, whole foods to encourage a healthy internal balance and a balanced immune system.

You should consume essential fatty acids every day. Flaxseeds and flaxseed oil are great sources; use the oil in dressings or sprinkle the seeds on cereal or salads. Flaxseeds and their oil change with heat, so do not bake with them or expose them to high temperatures. Cold-water fish, especially salmon, mackerel, and herring, are also good sources of EFAs.

Eat pumpkin or sunflower seeds daily. They are excellent sources of zinc, a mineral that encourages the proper metabolism of essential fatty acids.

Drink a glass of clean water every two waking hours to flush out toxins and to encourage skin health.

If you're constipated, your body will have to find another way to get rid of wastes—and that usually means that toxins are expelled through the skin. Eat plenty of whole grains, fruits, and vegetables. They're full of fiber and will keep your digestive tract clean.

Vitamin A and beta-carotene are necessary for good skin health, so eat your green

---

Testing Techniques

The following tests help assess possible reasons for eczema:

Intestinal permeability—urine

Detoxification profile—urine

Vitamin and mineral analysis (especially magnesium, B6)—blood

Digestive function and microbe/parasite/candida testing—stool analysis

Food and environmental allergies/sensitivities—blood, electrodermal

Essential fatty acid profile—blood

leafy and orange-yellow vegetables. Their nutrients are best delivered to your body when the food sources are raw, juiced, or lightly cooked.

Candidiasis is a possible cause of eczema, so eat cultured or sour products every day to stimulate the growth of "good bacteria." For more information, see Candidiasis.

Food to Avoid

Eliminate all additives from your diet. Not only are additives likely to cause a direct reaction, they contribute to a toxic internal environment that can manifest in the skin.

Determine whether you have an allergy or a sensitivity to any foods. See the Food Allergies section for further details. Common food triggers of eczema are dairy, citrus fruits, tomatoes, soy, shellfish, eggs, wheat, and gluten.

Do not eat saturated fat or solid fats, such as shortening or margarine. They interfere with the metabolism of essential fatty acids.

Stay away from inflammatory foods, especially sugar, spicy foods, dairy, caffeine, and alcohol. Sugar and caffeine also contribute to anxiety and stress, so you have an extra reason to avoid these substances.

Detoxification

Skin problems are usually a sign that the body is poisoned, perhaps from allergenic substances, toxic foods, or emotional stress. The following suggestions will help you release those poisons.

In cases of chronic eczema for adults, undertake a three-day juice fast once a month to sweep away toxic build-up. Green drinks with barley, spirulina, or blue-green algae detoxify the blood and are especially supportive of an eczema fast. Children over the age of five may use these green drinks under the guidance of a nutrition-oriented doctor.

℞ Super Seven Prescriptions—Eczema

Super Prescription #1   Homeopathic Combination Eczema/Rash Formula
Use a combination of the most common remedies indicated for eczema. Take as directed on the container three to four times daily for acute outbreaks and twice daily for chronic cases. If there is no improvement for acute eczema within forty-eight hours, switch to the indicated remedy listed under Homeopathy in this section.

Super Prescription #2   Essential fatty acids
Take a formulation that contains a mixture of omega-3, 6, and 9 fatty acids, as directed on the container. Or adults can take fish oil at a dosage of 1.8 grams of EPA daily or 2 tablespoons of flaxseed oil daily. Children can take fish oil at a daily dosage of 480 mg of EPA or ½ to 1 tablespoon of flaxseed oil. Essential fatty acids reduce inflammation and dryness, and studies show that they heal eczema.

Super Prescription #3   Vitamin C with bioflavonoids
Adults take 1,000 mg two to three times daily and children 500 mg two to three times daily. It reduces inflammation and promotes skin healing.

Super Prescription #4   Burdock root (*Arctium lappa*)
Adults should take 1 ml of the tincture form or 300 mg in capsules, while children can take 0.5 ml and 150 mg with each meal. Burdock root has a cleansing effect on the skin.

Super Prescription #5   Evening primrose oil (*Oenothera biennis*)
Adults can take 3,000 mg daily and children 1,000 mg daily. It contains GLA (gamma linoleic acid), which has anti-inflammatory effects on the skin. Some people with eczema need increased amounts of GLA. It's especially important if other essential fatty acids, such as fish or flaxseed oil, have not been helpful.

Super Prescription #6   Vitamin E
Adults should take 400 IU and children 200 IU daily. It promotes skin healing and prevents the oxidation of essential fatty acids.

Super Prescription #7   Probiotic
Adults should take a formula that contains at least 4 billion organisms per daily dosage and children at least 2 billion. Friendly flora such as *Lactobacillus* and *bifidobacterium* are involved with proper digestion, detoxification, and immune function.

A study in the *Journal of Clinical Allergy and Immunology* reported that breastfeeding mothers who supplemented with a probiotic were of great benefit to their infants with eczema after one month's period of time. It appears that this good bacteria reduces the effect of the infant's food allergy response.

General Recommendations

Zinc is needed for skin healing. Adults should take 30 mg twice daily, along with 3 mg of copper, and children can take 5 to 10 mg twice daily, along with 2 mg of copper.

Vitamin A promotes skin healing. It is particularly helpful for small bumps on the back of the arms. Adults should take 5,000 IU and children 2,000 IU daily.

Quercitin has anti-inflammatory effects. Adults should take 1,000 mg and children 500 mg three times daily.

Dandelion root (*Taraxacum officinale*) assists the liver in its detoxifying functions. Take 500 mg or 3 ml three times a day.

Many other herbs will reduce itching and swelling when applied topically. You can make a cream, a lotion, a cool compress, or a poultice with any of the following: comfrey, chamomile, calendula, chickweed, and witch hazel.

Red clover (*Trifolium pratense*) is beneficial for many skin disorders, although no one knows exactly how it works. Take 2 to 4 grams or 2 to 4 ml three times daily. If you have oozing skin or weeping blisters, you can also apply a cool infusion of red clover to the affected area.

Calendula (*Calendula officinalis*) heals broken or oozing skin and has an antiseptic quality. It's best used as a succus or cream.

Apply neem oil directly to the skin to heal and soothe patches of inflamed, red, and itchy skin.

If you are under stress, drink a cup of peppermint, chamomile, or passionflower tea to help you relax.

Homeopathy

Pick the remedy that best matches your symptoms in this section. Take a 6x, 12x, 6C, or 30C potency twice daily for two weeks to see if there are any positive results. After you notice improvement, stop taking the remedy, unless symptoms return. Consultation with a homeopathic practitioner is advised.

Arsenicum (Arsenicum Album) is for a chilly person who has very dry, itchy skin and swollen, tender skin eruptions. The eczema is worse in the winter, and the itching intensifies at night between midnight and 2 A.M. The person feels very restless, and the skin feels worse with warm applications.

Calcarea Carbonica is for people who are flabby and have clammy hands and feet.

Their eczema tends to be worse in the winter. They crave eggs and sweets. This is also a good remedy for infants who suffer from cradle cap.

Graphites is for people whose dry skin becomes thick and has a honeylike discharge. The itching is worse in a warm bed.

Medorrhinum is for eczema that has been a problem since birth or a very early age. The person craves oranges and ice, tends to be very warm, and sweats easily.

Mezereum is for eczema that blisters and oozes and then forms a thick crustlike layer. Cold applications and the open air make the skin feel better.

Petroleum is for eczema that is characterized by very dry, cracked skin, especially on the palms of the hands. The itching is worse at night and in the warmth of the bed.

Psorinum is for chronic eczema that causes people to scratch until they bleed. The symptoms are similar to those of people who should take Sulphur, except that in this case, the people are very chilly.

Rhus Toxicodendron is for blistery-looking eczema that is very itchy and feels better from warm applications and movement. The person may crave cold milk.

Sulfur is for dry, red, itchy skin that's made worse with bathing and warmth. The person who will benefit from this remedy feels hot, is restless, and generally has a thirst for cold drinks.

Acupressure

See pages 668–675 for information about pressure points and administering treatment.

- Spleen 10 clears heat from the blood.
- Bladder 23 and 47 will relieve eczema.
- Stomach 36 and Governing Vessel 24.5 both improve skin all over the body.
- If your eczema causes you stress, use Bladder 10 to soothe your nerves.
- Large Intestine 4 relieves constipation and depression.

Bodywork

Reflexology

See pages 686–687 for information about reflexology areas and how to work them.

Work the areas that correspond to the liver, the kidneys, the intestines, the endocrine glands, the lymph, and the solar plexus.

Hydrotherapy

Constitutional hydrotherapy is helpful for long-standing eczema. See pages 676–677 for directions.

Other Bodywork Recommendations

An oatmeal bath can be very soothing. Tie some oats in a cheesecloth or a leg from nylons, and let water run on the oats under the tap before you soak. This can be purchased as a powder, too. You can also use the wet ball of oats as compress directly on the affected area.

Aromatherapy

To soothe inflammation and itching and to relieve tension, add chamomile, geranium, or lavender to your bath or to a cream. These oils can be used separately or together.

If you want to relax, there are many oils you can try. See page 658 for information on oils; the following are all excellent: bergamot, jasmine, lavender, rose, sandalwood, or ylang ylang. Use them in a massage, a bath, lotions, or creams—but make sure you dilute them before applying them directly to the skin.

Stress Reduction

General Stress-Reduction Therapies

Any of the techniques in the Exercise and Stress Reduction chapter will help you control stress-related eczema. To help children, talk with them about how they are feeling and coping with their eczema, and what you are going to do naturally to help them heal.

Bach Flower Remedies

If none of the following suggestions seems to fit, see the chart on pages 648–650 to find the remedy that's best for you. Once you've chosen a remedy, place 10 drops of the liquid under your tongue. Hold the drops in place for thirty seconds and swallow. Use as often as needed.

If eczema is causing feelings of shame about your appearance, use Crab Apple.
If you've given up hope of finding a cure for your eczema, Gorse will help.
Larch is the remedy for people who lack self-confidence.

Other Recommendations

- If you have an acute case of eczema, you must avoid the offending irritant. If the source of the irritation is not obvious, review the possible triggers previously listed under "Causes of Acute Eczema," and try to avoid or treat each one. Exercise will help relieve stress and encourage detoxification.
- A little morning sunlight on your skin promotes healing, so take walks early in the day. If you live in a warm climate, be careful. Don't let your skin burn.

REFERENCES

Majamaa, H., and E. Isolauri. 1997. Probiotics: A novel approach in the management of food allergy. *Journal of Allergy and Clinical Immunology* 99:179–85.

Endometriosis

Endometriosis is a painful condition in which uterine tissue from the uterus attaches itself to other organs. The uterine tissue may appear in the fallopian tubes or the ovaries, or it may implant itself on the outer walls of the uterus itself. In rare cases, the tissue travels outside the pelvic region and appears in organs like the bladder, the lungs, and other areas.

These masses of tissue can be painful, in and of themselves, but to make matters worse, they continue to behave as if they're inside the uterus. They continue to fill up with blood over the course of the menstrual cycle, and every month, they shed blood just as the uterus does. Unlike normal menstrual blood, which leaves the body through the vagina, the blood from the abnormal growth has nowhere to go. Instead, it accumulates inside the pelvic cavity, where it often forms cysts. As menstrual cycles repeat themselves and the tissue continues to bleed each month, the cysts may grow so large that they bind organs together. Sometimes a cyst ruptures and leads to agonizing pain. Two out of three women have endometrial growth on the ovaries.

Pain in the pelvis and the lower back is the defining characteristic of endometriosis. The pain usually varies with the menstrual cycle and is at its worst during ovulation, menstruation, or sexual intercourse; sometimes it is so intense as to be incapacitating. A woman with endometriosis may experience heavy or prolonged menstrual bleeding, and this loss of blood can lead to anemia. Digestive problems are common in cases of endometriosis, as is nausea and vomiting. There is a strong connection between endometriosis and infertility, although it is unknown whether the excess tissue actually prevents conception, or if infertility somehow creates conditions hospitable to endometriosis.

No one knows for sure what causes endometrial tissue to leave the uterus and travel to other parts of the body. One prevailing theory is that the disorder is caused by retrograde menstruation, in which menstrual fluid fails to exit the body properly. Instead, some of the endometrial lining that is normally shed during menstruation backs up in the fallopian tubes and enters the pelvic cavity, where the tissue deposits itself and begins to grow. It is also possible that endometrial cells travel to the pelvic cavity via the bloodstream or the lymphatic system. Others believe that endometriosis is caused when the body is still an embryo. In a normal fetus, the cells that are meant to form the uterus differentiate themselves from others and begin to travel to the appropriate site. But according to this theory, the endometrial cells of some fetuses don't make the trip and end up in the wrong places. It is also thought that environmental estrogens may be a causative factor. These xenoestrogens are endocrine disrupters that have estrogenic effects in the body. This category of environmental estrogens includes plastics, detergents, household cleaners, pesticides, herbicides, and hormones found in meat products. In addition, studies have shown immune system imbalance to be a factor. Specifically, women with endometriosis have higher levels of antibodies that target their own ovaries and endometrial tissue. They also tend to have lower activity of the natural killer cells that usually keep abnormal cells in check. No matter what the cause, it does appear that all cases of endometriosis are linked to hormonal balance and that elevated estrogen levels are a problem.

It is important that liver function be optimized in women with endometriosis. The liver is responsible for breaking down estrogen (and other hormones) and secreting the metabolites into the large intestine for elimination. If the liver does not metabolize estrogen and its metabolites properly, they are recycled throughout the body.

While the liver is the dominant player in estrogen metabolism, the flora or "friendly bacteria" in the large intestine are also important in estrogen metabolism. They prevent the reactivation and the recycling of these unwanted estrogens. Conversely, "unfriendly bacteria" secrete an enzyme called beta-glucuronidase that causes estrogen to be recycled back through the body via the large intestine. A low-fiber and high-fat intake increases the activity of this enzyme.

While endometriosis is not a simple condition to treat, natural therapies often lead to significant improvement. The complementary treatments described here focus on regulating hormones and balancing the immune system and also suggest ways to provide gentle relief of pain and other symptoms.

SYMPTOMS

- Pain in the abdomen and the lower back, associated with menses
- Pain with sexual intercourse
- Prolonged or excessive menstrual bleeding
- Digestive problems
- Nausea and vomiting
- Anemia
- Infertility
- Pain with urination and bowel movements

ROOT CAUSES

- Retrograde menstruation
- Endometrial cells that travel through the bloodstream or the lymphatic system
- A genetic defect
- Hormonal imbalance (relatively high estrogen and low progesterone), due to poor liver function, diet, xenoestrogens, or ovulatory dysfunction
- Imbalanced immune system
- Flora imbalance (dysbiosis)

Testing Techniques

The following tests help assess possible reasons for endometriosis:

Immune system imbalance—blood

Hormone testing (especially for estrogen and progesterone)—saliva, blood, or urine

Detoxification profile—urine

Digestive function (particularly, flora balance and beta-glucuronidase activity)—stool analysis

Food and environmental allergies/sensitivities—blood, electrodermal

---

TREATMENT

Diet

It is important to eat certified organic foods as much as possible, due to the estrogenic effects of pesticides, herbicides, and hormone-laden meats.

Recommended Food

Whole grains, beans, and vegetables should form the basis of your diet. All these foods are high in fiber and will help to balance the friendly bacteria involved with estrogen metabolism.

Eat plenty of cold-water fish like salmon, tuna, and mackerel. These fish are good sources of essential fatty acids (EFAs), substances that reduce inflammation and pain. For additional EFAs, add 2 tablespoons of flaxseeds to your daily protocol, along with 10 ounces of water. Flaxseeds have been shown to help balance estrogen levels.

Eat fruits and vegetables, such as apples, cherries, broccoli, cauliflower, and brussels sprouts. They contain the phytochemical indole-3-carbinol, which supports the liver's detoxification of estrogen.

Regularly consume beets, carrots, artichokes, dandelion greens, onions, and garlic, as these foods stimulate liver detoxification.

Eat organic cultured yogurt to increase the levels of friendly flora in the large intestine.

Once a day, have a green drink to support detoxification.

Drink a glass of clean water every two to three waking hours to support detoxification.

Food to Avoid

Avoid red meat and dairy products, all of which contain high levels of dioxins that act as environmental estrogens.

affeine consumption appears to be a risk factor for endometriosis. According to researchers at the Harvard School of Public Health, women who consume 5 to 7 grams of caffeine a month had a significantly greater incidence of endometriosis. This is equivalent to about 2 cups of coffee a day.

To keep pain under control, stay away from inflammatory substances like sugar, caffeine, and alcohol.

Don't eat anything that depresses your immune system. Processed foods, fried food, refined sugar, and alcohol all limit your body's ability to fight your disorder.

℞ Super Seven Prescriptions—Endometriosis

Super Prescription #1   Natural progesterone
This balances out estrogen, regulates the menses, and relieves pain. Apply ¼ teaspoon (20 mg) to your skin twice daily from days 6 to 26 of your cycle (stopping during the week of your menstrual flow. It is best used under the care of a healthcare professional.

Super Prescription #2   Vitex (chasteberry)
Vitex balances the estrogen/progesterone ratio. Take 160 to 240 mg of a 0.6 percent aucubin standardized extract or 80 drops daily. Do not use Vitex if you are currently taking the birth control pill.

Super Prescription #3   Indole-3 carbinol
Take 300 mg daily. It assists the liver in estrogen detoxification.

Super Prescription #4   Dandelion root (*Taraxacum officinale*)
Take 300 to 500 mg in capsule form or 1 ml of tincture with each meal (three times daily). It improves liver detoxification.

Super Prescription #5   Vitamin E
Take 400 IU twice daily. It helps with estrogen metabolism and inflammation.

Super Prescription #6   Essential fatty acids
Take a daily combination of flaxseed (1 to 2 tablespoons) or fish oil (3,000 to 5,000 mg), along with gamma linoleic acid (GLA) from evening primrose oil or borage oil at a dose of 300 mg. These essential fatty acids decrease inflammation.

Super Prescription #7   D-glucarate
Take 500 mg daily. This phytochemical assists the liver in estrogen breakdown.

General Recommendations

B-complex vitamins are involved in estrogen metabolism. Take a 50 mg complex twice daily.

A high-potency multivitamin supplies many of the nutrients required for hormone metabolism. Take as directed on the container.

Vitamin C improves autoimmunity. Work up to 6 grams daily. Reduce the dosage if diarrhea occurs.

Motherwort (*Leonurus cardiaca*) is a good herb to use for acute uterine pain. Take 5 ml three times daily.

Red raspberry (*Rubus idaeus*) is an astringent herb that may help uterine inflammation and pain. Drink it as a tea, three cups daily.

If you have heavy menstrual bleeding, take nettle (*Urtica dioica*), a blood-building herb, to prevent anemia. Begin using the herb after the last day of your menstrual cycle, and take 500 mg two or three times daily for two weeks. Women with severe endometriosis often find that the pain keeps them up at night. If you need to get to sleep, try tea made with skullcap (*Scutellaria lateriflora*), passionflower (*Passiflora incarnata*), or valerian (*Valeriana officinalis*).

Homeopathy

Many sufferers report long-lasting results from constitutional homeopathic remedies, so it is highly recommended that you see a licensed professional for an individual assessment and remedy. For immediate relief of pain or other symptoms, use one of the following remedies, as appropriate. Take a 6x, 12x, 6C, or 30C potency twice daily for two weeks to see if there are any positive results. After you notice improvement, stop taking the remedy, unless symptoms return.

Arnica (*Arnica montana*) is for a deep, bruising pain.

Colocynthis will reduce cramping pain in the lower abdominal. The person feels better with pressure on the abdomen and when lying with the knees drawn up.

Dioscorea Villosa is for uterine pain that radiates out from the uterus. The woman arches her back with the pain and feels better standing up and worse lying down.

Cimicifuga Racemosa is for severe menstrual pain that gets worse as the flow increases. There are shooting and cramping pains that radiate across the pelvis or into the thighs.

Lachesis is helpful for menstrual pain and large, purplish clots. The woman feels warm and jealous.

Magnesia Phosphorica is for pelvic pain, cramping, and bloating that feel better when heat is applied. The woman feels worse in the cold air or when the painful area is touched.

Pulsatilla (*Pulsatilla pratensis*) is for menstrual pain when the pain is changeable. The woman feels weepy and better when comforted and has a strong craving for sweets.

Sepia is for hormone imbalance, where the woman feels irritable, has pain with intercourse, and craves sweets, as well as salty and/or sour foods.

Acupressure

See pages 668–675 for information about pressure points and administering treatment.

- Large Intestine 4 is a powerful point for relief of pain anywhere in the body.

Bodywork

Massage

Although it can't cure endometriosis, a massage of the belly and the lower back is an effective means of easing an acute attack of pain. Find a massage therapist whom you like and trust; if flare-ups occur at a predictable point in your cycle, you may want to make a standing appointment for treatment.

Reflexology

See pages 686–687 for information about reflexology areas and how to work them.

Work the areas corresponding to the uterus, the fallopian tubes, and the ovaries.

Hydrotherapy

A hot bath can help relieve digestive problems, as well as pain. Depending on your particular needs, you can add any of the essential oils listed under Aromatherapy in this section for additional potency.

Other Bodywork Recommendations

When you feel an acute episode of pain coming on, lie down and rest, with a hot compress on the affected area.

One study found that auricular (ear) acupuncture was as effective as hormone therapy in treating infertility due to endometriosis.

Acupuncture is highly recommended to help reduce the pain associated with endometriosis. In addition, Chinese herbal therapy from a qualified practitioner can be very helpful.

Aromatherapy

To relieve general endometrial pain not caused by a digestive problem, use rosemary or marjoram. Both of these herbs have a pleasant warming effect on the body. Add either of the oils to a bath, or dilute them in a carrier oil and use in an abdominal massage.

If you're constipated, black pepper can revive your digestive system.

For stomach cramps caused by diarrhea or other gastrointestinal problems, use neroli or chamomile to relax your muscles.

Many women with endometriosis come to dread sexual intercourse, as it often provokes severe pain. A few drops of ylang ylang or patchouli in a bath or a massage oil can help you relax, both emotionally and physically. (You may want to try different sexual positions until you find one that's most comfortable for you. But if sex continues to hurt, stop. Never force yourself—you'll only cause greater problems for you and your partner in the long run.)

Lavender encourages a good night's sleep. You can use this oil in any preparation you like; many people place a sachet filled with the dried flowers under their pillows.

Stress Reduction

People who suffer from chronic pain live with constant stress—more than their friends and family realize. Stress, too, can contribute to painful flare-ups. If you have endometriosis, it's important that you devote time every day to managing the tension that accompanies a chronic illness.

General Stress-Reduction Therapies

Yoga is an excellent stress reliever, and the gentle motions will also contribute to pain relief.

Pilates offers a gentle way to stretch and reduce stress.

One of the best ways to handle pain is to so thoroughly engage your mind that you're distracted from the bodily agony. Find a hobby or an activity you like, such as cooking or singing in a choir, and participate in it regularly. Some people find that writing in a journal can distract them for hours.

Bach Flower Remedies

Select the appropriate remedy, and place 10 drops of the liquid under your tongue. Hold the drops in place for thirty seconds and swallow. Use as often as needed.

If you are overwhelmed by fatigue, take Hornbeam.

Holly will reduce anxiety and anger.

Other Recommendations

- Moderate exercise is a natural pain reliever. Try to take a walk every morning, or find some other activity you like well enough to perform regularly.
- Use sanitary napkins instead of tampons. Tampons may encourage retrograde menstruation.

REFERENCES

Gerhard, I., and F. Postneek. 1992. Auricular acupuncture in the treatment of female infertility. *Gynecological Endocrinology* 6:171–81.

Grodstein, F., M. B. Goldman, L. Ryan, and D. W. Cramer. 1993. *American Journal of Epidemiology* 137(12):1353–60.

Fever

A fever is usually regarded as a symptom of an acute infection or an underlying illness. It is the body's way of stimulating the immune system or accelerating detoxification. Anyone with an elevated body temperature at least 1 degree above 98.6 degrees F is said to have a fever. However, in babies, the healthy body temperature can vary from 97 to 100 degrees F because their body temperatures are not yet developed. In healthy children, body temperatures can fluctuate by 2 degrees above or below 98.6 degrees F. The amount of clothing one is wearing, as well as the amount of activity, can influence one's body temperature. Often, a fever is accompanied by a flush to the face and sweat beads on the forehead.

Fevers are often a cause for worry, especially for parents, but they should be regarded as both friend and foe. When a child has a mild fever, it could be a signal that the child's natural defense system is waging a war against an invading microbe. As the army of white blood cells battles, the cells release chemicals called pyrogens. These pyrogens activate the hypothalamus, a part of the brain that serves as the body's thermostat regulator, to turn on the internal heat and raise the body temperature to fight off invaders (many microbes start to die at around 102 degrees F). When this occurs, heat is lost through the skin, and the blood vessels dilate.

The onset of a high fever may lead to a febrile seizure in some children and adults. Their muscles become rigid, and they experience convulsions or even loss of consciousness for up to fifteen minutes. This is an emergency situation that requires immediate medical attention. Upon recovering, a child may sleep for a long time. As horrific as these are to witness, febrile seizures rarely develop into epilepsy or cause permanent harm to the child.

People with temperatures above 102 degrees F may require medical intervention. If your child is younger than three months of age, notify your doctor about the fever. Be sure to get checked by a doctor if you or someone you are caring for experiences any of these symptoms:

- Acts confused, lethargic, or delirious
- Experiences a seizure
- Vomits or has diarrhea
- Complains of a stiff neck or has dilated pupils
- Has had the fever for more than seventy-two hours

And for infants and children, also be aware of these additional signs and symptoms:

- Cries continuously
- Is difficult to awaken
- Has a significant decrease in urine output or appears dehydrated
- Has trouble breathing

Conventional treatment focuses on fever-reducing medications, such as acetaminophen. From a holistic perspective, we look at fever as a generally positive thing, since it activates the immune system. We try to work with a fever and not necessarily suppress it, unless it is too high or the patient is very uncomfortable.

Note: Never give aspirin to a child who has a fever. This can cause an immune reaction, leading to the development of Reye's syndrome, a potentially fatal illness where vomiting and liver damage can occur.

SYMPTOMS

- Flushed face, elevated temperature

ROOT CAUSES

- Infection
- Detoxification reaction
- Systemic illness (cancer, etc.)

TREATMENT

Diet

Recommended Food

Eat lightly. Steamed vegetables, soups, broths, and herbal teas will let your body focus on healing, instead of on digestion. If you lose your appetite, don't force yourself to eat.

Stay hydrated. Drink plenty of clean water and other fluids (but see the note about sugar and juice further on) to cleanse away toxins and to keep the respiratory tract from drying out.

Increase your consumption of ginger, onions, and garlic. Try adding one or both to chicken soup or miso.

Regular water intake is important to prevent dehydration. Herbal teas and highly diluted fruit juices can also be given. Fruit juice popsicles are popular with kids.

Breastfeeding should be maintained for nursing infants.

Food to Avoid

Sugar decreases the number of white blood cells your body produces, and it depresses your immune system, so eliminate refined sugars from your diet for the duration of your illness. Also be wary of fruit juices. Although they are a traditional treatment for colds, fruit juices—especially orange juice—usually contain far more sugar than they do vitamin C. If you want to drink juice, dilute it first.

Avoid milk and other dairy products while you're sick, as they tend to suppress immunity.

℞ Super Seven Prescriptions—Fever

Super Prescription #1   Homeopathic Combination Fever Remedy
To reduce the effects of a fever, take a combination fever remedy four times daily for two days. Then if you notice improvement, stop taking the remedy, unless symptoms return. If your symptoms do not improve within twenty-four hours, pick the remedy that best matches your symptoms under Homeopathy in this section.

Super Prescription #2   Yarrow (*Achillea millefolium*)
Take 300 mg in capsule form, 2 ml of the tincture, or 1 cup of fresh tea four times daily or until the fever breaks. Yarrow induces a sweat to help break high fevers.

> **Super Prescription #3 Homeopathic Ferrum Phosphoricum**
> Take a 30C potency four times daily for two days. Then if you notice improvement, stop taking the remedy, unless symptoms return. If your symptoms do not improve within twenty-four hours, pick the remedy that best matches your symptoms under Homeopathy in this section.
>
> **Super Prescription #4 Echinacea** (*Echinacea purpurea*)
> Take 500 mg of the capsule form or 2 to 4 ml of the tincture four times daily. Echinacea stimulates immune function and reduces fever.
>
> **Super Prescription #5 Ginger** (*Zingiber officinale*)
> Take 500 mg of the capsule form or 2 ml of the tincture or drink the fresh tea four times daily. Ginger helps break a fever, especially for people who have a sore throat and chills.
>
> **Super Prescription #6 Elderberry** (*Sambucus nigra*)
> Adults should take 10 ml and children 5 ml three times daily. It's useful for fever related to the flu or other viral infections.
>
> **Super Prescription #7 Vitamin C**
> Take 500 to 1,000 mg three to four times daily. Vitamin C supports immune system function through increased white blood cell activity. Reduce the dosage if diarrhea occurs.

General Recommendations

Oregano (*Origanum vulgare*) oil has powerful antiviral effects. Take 500 mg of the capsule form four times daily or as directed on the container.

Garlic (*Allium sativum*) combats infection and supports the immune system. Take 300 to 500 mg in capsule or liquid form three times daily.

Thymus extract (*Thymus vulgaris*) optimizes immune activity. Take 1 to 2 capsules twice daily or as directed on the container.

Homeopathy

At the first signs of a fever, take 2 pellets of a 30C potency four times daily for two days of the remedy that best matches your symptoms in this section. Then if you notice improvement, stop taking the remedy, unless symptoms return. If your symptoms do not improve within twenty-four hours, pick another remedy.

Aconitum Napellus is useful at the very beginning of a fever, when there is a sudden onset. This often occurs after a person has been exposed to the cold or the wind. The person is restless and fearful, and children cry with the onset of the fever. This remedy is most useful in the first few hours of a sudden fever. One cheek may be red and the other pale during a fever.

Arsenicum Album is for a fever that occurs or increases between 12 and 2 A.M. The person is chilly, along with having a burning fever. Anxiety and restlessness are usually present. The symptoms are better with warm sips of water.

Belladonna (*Atropa belladonna*) is for a sudden, intense fever. The body feels very hot (especially the face), but the feet are cold. The pupils may be dilated, and the cheeks and the face are often bright red. The person is sensitive to light and has a throbbing headache. Some people may become delirious and hallucinate from the fever.

Bryonia (*Bryonia alba*) is for people who have a high fever with a tremendous thirst. They are very irritable and do not want to move.

Chamomilla (*Matricaria chamomilla*) is specific for a fever that accompanies teething. One cheek is red, while the other is pale. The child is very irritable.

Ferrum Phosphoricum is used as a general fever remedy. The person has a fever but does not act sick. The face is red and the body warm.

Gelsemium (*Gelsemium sempervirens*) is for a fever accompanied by chills and muscle aches. The person feels drowsy and fatigued and has droopy eyelids. There is often a headache at the back of the neck.

Mercurius Solubilis or Vivus is helpful when a person has a fever and is sensitive to both hot and cold temperatures. The tongue has a thick coating, and the person has bad breath, has excessive saliva production, and drools on the pillow. The throat is often raw and sore.

Pulsatilla (*Pulsatilla pratensis*) is for someone who has a fever with a low thirst. A feverish child wants to be held and is very clingy. Symptoms are better with the window open or when the person is out in the open air.

Pyrogenium is used when there is a high fever, and the person appears very sick. His or her body aches and feels bruised. The person has a high fever but a slow pulse.

Sulphur is for acute or long-lasting fevers when the whole body is warm. A body rash may accompany the fever. There is a tremendous thirst for cold drinks.

Acupressure

Large Intestine 4 is located between the webbing of the thumb and the index finger. Gently push on this spot on both hands to reduce fever.

Bodywork

Hydrotherapy

Constitutional or foot hydrotherapy works very well in helping to control fevers and fight infections. See the Hydrotherapy section for directions.

Fibroids, Uterine

Contrary to their name, fibroids are not fibrous at all. Rather, they are growths of smooth muscle and connective tissue that most often appear on the walls of the uterus. Although it can be frightening to hear that you have a growth of any kind, rest assured that fibroids are noncancerous and usually harmless. They are also quite common: Fibroids affect more than 50 percent of women overall and are the most common reason for major surgery. For reasons that we don't yet understand, they appear much more often in women of African or Caribbean descent than in any other group. Most women with the condition tend to have several fibroids at once.

Many women who have fibroids experience no symptoms at all; the growths are usually discovered in the course of a routine exam or an ultrasound. In some cases, however, fibroids inside the uterus wear away the organ's lining, resulting in heavy or prolonged menstrual periods, bleeding between periods, or pain and bleeding during sexual intercourse. Persistent blood loss can cause anemia. A fibroid may also grow so large that it distends the abdomen as it presses on the bladder or the intestines. A woman with a large fibroid may feel pain in her back or lower abdomen; if the growth distorts the bladder, she may feel a frequent urge to urinate. Sometimes the fibroid doesn't cause any pain but simply gives the abdomen a distended appearance. Women may also feel pressure, heaviness, and pain with sexual intercourse, as well as increased urinary frequency. Occasionally, a fibroid will block the fallopian tubes and lead to infertility or compress the ureters (the urinary tract from the kidneys to the bladder), causing impaired kidney function. In some instances the fibroids become calcified.

Fibroids are thought to be dependent upon estrogen; they tend to grow during the reproductive years and pregnancy, and they shrink with menopause, when estrogen levels recede. Fibroids often increase in size during perimenopause, when women do not ovulate regularly and thus have relatively higher estrogen levels (as ovulation increases progesterone). Thus hormone balance is the key factor with this condition.

Although estrogen is obviously an important factor in the development of fibroids, doctors do not know why the growths appear in some women and not in others. A tendency toward fibroids may run in families; the disorder is also more common in women who are obese or who have an underactive thyroid (which contributes to estrogen excess).

It is important that liver function be optimized in women with fibroids. The liver is responsible for breaking down estrogen (and other hormones) and secreting the metabolites into the large intestine for elimination. If the liver does not metabolize estrogen and its metabolites properly, then it is recycled throughout the body.

While the liver is the dominant player in estrogen metabolism, the flora or "friendly bacteria" in the large intestine are also important in estrogen metabolism. They prevent the reactivation and recycling of these unwanted estrogens. Conversely, "unfriendly bacteria" secrete an enzyme called beta-glucuronidase that causes estrogen to be recycled back through the body via the large intestine. A low-fiber and high-fat intake increases the activity of this enzyme.

Conventional medical treatment for fibroids has long been surgical removal of the uterus, a drastic option that should be considered only in those few cases in which fibroids cause severe pain or bleeding or pose a significant health threat. For mild to moderate cases, it is usually far wiser to follow a treatment program of conservative, noninvasive therapies until menopause is reached and the fibroids abate on their own.

SYMPTOMS

In most women with fibroids, the condition is asymptomatic, especially in the early stages when the fibroids are small. If symptoms do appear, they usually take the following forms:

- Heavy or prolonged menstrual bleeding
- Bleeding or unusual discharge between periods
- Pain and bleeding during intercourse
- Anemia
- Swelling in the lower abdomen
- A frequent urge to urinate
- Back or abdominal pain
- Constipation

ROOT CAUSES

- Relatively high levels of estrogen and low levels of progesterone, due to:
  —Environmental estrogens
  —Obesity
  —Underactive thyroid
  —Ovulatory dysfunction
  —Perimenopause
  —Low-fiber, high-fat diet

Caution: If you bleed so much that you need to change tampons or sanitary pads more than once every hour, see your doctor.

Testing Techniques

The following tests help assess possible reasons for fibroids:

Hormone testing (especially for estrogen and progesterone)—saliva, blood, or urine

Detoxification profile—urine

Digestive function (particularly, flora balance and beta-glucuronidase activity)—stool analysis

---

TREATMENT

Diet

It is important to eat certified organic foods as much as possible, due to the estrogenic effects of pesticides, herbicides, and hormone-laden meats.

Recommended Food

Since diet affects hormone balance, it's wise to give your body good general support with wholesome, freshly prepared meals. Base your diet around whole grains, vegetables, fruits, fish, beans, and soy products. To limit your exposure to pesticides, buy organic food wherever possible, and always wash your produce thoroughly.

Soy products and flaxseeds are good sources of phytoestrogens, substances that regulate the body's estrogen production.

Vitamin K will encourage proper blood clotting and may reduce an excessive flow of menstrual blood. Green vegetables are high in this nutrient.

Include sea vegetables like kelp (*Ascophyllum nodosum*) in your diet. These foods are high in iodine, a mineral that's necessary for a healthy thyroid.

If you have heavy or prolonged periods, you need extra iron to ward off anemia. Take a spoonful of unsulfured blackstrap molasses every day. For more suggestions, see Anemia.

For additional EFAs, add 2 tablespoons of flaxseeds to your daily protocol, along with 10 ounces of water. Flaxseeds have been shown to help balance estrogen levels.

Eat fruits and vegetables such as apples, cherries, broccoli, cauliflower, and brussels sprouts. They contain the phytochemical indole-3-carbinol, which supports the liver's detoxification of estrogen.

Regularly consume beets, carrots, artichokes, dandelion greens, onions, and garlic, as these foods stimulate liver detoxification.

Eat organic cultured yogurt to increase the levels of friendly flora in the large intestine.

Once a day, have a green drink to support detoxification.

Drink a glass of clean water every two waking hours. Water will help flush impurities from your body and reduce pain.

Food to Avoid

Avoid red meat and dairy products, all of which contain high levels of dioxins, which act as environmental estrogens.

To keep pain under control, stay away from inflammatory substances like sugar, caffeine, and alcohol.

Don't eat anything that depresses your immune system. Processed foods, fried food, refined sugar, and alcohol all limit your body's ability to fight your disorder.

Detoxification

Many fibroid sufferers have found that regular fasting results in significant relief of pain. Plan a three-day juice fast every three months; be sure to drink a wide variety of vegetable juices and green drinks during the three-day period.

℞ Super Seven Prescriptions—Fibroid

Super Prescription #1   Natural progesterone
This balances out estrogen, regulates the menses, and relieves pain. Apply ¼ teaspoon (20 mg) to your skin twice daily from days 6 to 26 of your cycle (stopping during the week of your menstrual flow. It is best used under the guidance of a health-care professional.

Super Prescription #2   Vitex (chasteberry)
This balances the estrogen/progesterone ratio. Take 160 to 240 mg of a 0.6 percent aucubin standardized extract or 80 drops daily. Do not use Vitex if you are currently taking the birth control pill.

Super Prescription #3   Indole-3-carbinol
Take 300 mg daily. It assists the liver in estrogen detoxification.

Super Prescription #4   Dandelion root (*Taraxacum officinale*)
Take 300 to 500 mg of the capsule form or 1 ml of the tincture with each meal (three times daily). It improves liver detoxification.

Super Prescription #5   Vitamin E
Take 400 IU twice daily. It helps with estrogen metabolism and inflammation.

Super Prescription #6   Essential fatty acids
Take a daily combination of flaxseed (1 to 2 tablespoons) or fish oil (3,000 to 5,000 mg), along with gamma linoleic acid (GLA) from evening primrose oil or borage oil at a dose of 300 mg. These essential fatty acids decrease inflammation.

Super Prescription #7   D-glucarate
Take 500 mg daily. This phytochemical assists the liver in estrogen breakdown.

General Recommendations

- B-complex vitamins are involved in estrogen metabolism. Take a 50 mg complex twice daily.
- A high-potency multivitamin supplies many of the nutrients required for hormone metabolism. Take as directed on the container.
- Red raspberry (*Rubus idaeus*) is an astringent herb that may help uterine inflammation and pain. Drink it as a tea, three cups daily.
- If you have heavy menstrual bleeding, take nettle, a blood-building herb, to prevent anemia. Begin using the herb after the last day of your menstrual cycle, and take 500 mg two or three times daily for two weeks.

Homeopathy

Pick the remedy that best matches your symptoms in this section. Take a 6x, 12x, 6C, 12C, or 30C potency twice daily for three weeks to see if there are any positive results.

After you notice improvement, stop taking the remedy, unless symptoms return. Consultation with a homeopathic practitioner is advised.

Calcarea Carbonica is for overweight women who get chilly and fatigued easily. They crave sweets and eggs. They have a tendency to get overwhelmed easily and struggle with anxiety. It is used for uterine fibroids that are sometimes characterized by uterine hemorrhage.

Fraxinus Americanus is a specific lesional remedy for uterine fibroids.

Lachesis is for women who experience surges of heat and aggravation from heat. They experience abdominal and uterine pain that improves once menstrual flow begins. They feel anger and suspiciousness.

Phosphorous is for women who have heavy bleeding from fibroids, characterized by bright red blood and clotting. They crave ice-cold drinks.

Pulsatilla is a good choice when there is fibroid pain and menstrual flow that changes. These women feel better having someone around, comforting them. There is a craving for sweets. Symptoms are worse in a warm room and better in the fresh air.

Sabina is for fibroids that cause pain in the lower back and sacrum that extends to the pubic bones. There is heavy uterine bleeding, with clots.

Sepia is for women with fibroids when their uterus feels like it is bearing down and will fall out. They feel irritable and want to be left alone. There is a strong craving for sweets and salty and sour foods.

Sulphur is for fibroids in women who get overheated easily. They desire a cool environment. There is a strong craving for ice-cold drinks.

Acupressure

See pages 668–675 for information about pressure points and administering treatment.

- To stop fibroid pain, work Large Intestine 4.

Bodywork

Acupuncture is highly recommended to help reduce the bleeding associated with fibroids. In addition, Chinese herbal therapy from a qualified practitioner can be very helpful.

Reflexology
See pages 686–687 for information about reflexology areas and how to work them.

- Work the areas that correspond to the uterus, the fallopian tubes, and the ovaries.

Hydrotherapy
Regular sitz baths in hot water will improve circulation to the pelvic region and will soothe pain in the abdomen and the lower back.

Constitutional hydrotherapy is helpful to reduce congestion in the area containing the fibroid. See pages 676–677 for directions.

Aromatherapy
Warming oils like rosemary, marjoram, and black pepper increase blood flow and relieve pain. If you're constipated, black pepper will also stimulate digestion. You can use these oils separately or in combination. Add a few drops to a sitz bath, or use them in a hot compress.

Stress Reduction

General Stress-Reduction Therapies

For overall hormone balance, utilize techniques such as exercise, yoga, and prayer.

Bach Flower Remedies

Select the appropriate remedy, and place 10 drops of the liquid under your tongue. Hold the drops in place for thirty seconds and swallow. Use as often as needed.

If you are panicked and very upset, take Rescue Remedy to induce a sense of calm. Aspen is for people who have intense, unexplained feelings of dread or fear.

Other Recommendations

- If you have fibroids, you should not take estrogen-replacement therapy.
- Moderate exercise like walking will stimulate blood flow to the pelvic region and will help relieve pain.

Fibromyalgia

Fibromyalgia is the name given to chronic, widespread muscular pain that has no obvious cause. The pain—usually described as aching, stiff, burning, or throbbing—may appear in any location of the body, but for a diagnosis of fibromyalgia to be made, you must have pain in at least eleven of eighteen specific "tender points." The pain from tender points and elsewhere in the body usually feels most severe upon waking and gradually lessens as the day goes on.

Although the pain of fibromyalgia alone can be so severe as to render its victims disabled, the disease can be complicated by any of several other problems. Fibromyalgia is closely linked to chronic fatigue syndrome, and many of its sufferers experience symptoms similar to those of CFS (see the symptom list further on). Irritable bowel syndrome, premenstrual syndrome, palpitations, and temporomandibular joint syndrome (TMJ) may also be present.

As with CFS, there is currently no one agreed-upon cause for this disease. In most cases, many factors combine to produce the varied components of fibromyalgia. Disordered sleep is a very common problem with this condition. The length and the quality of sleep must be improved for long-term success in most cases of fibromyalgia. Also, hormone imbalance is quite common. Particularly, low thyroid function and imbalances in estrogen/progesterone, as well as in the stress hormones DHEA and cortisol. Digestive function and detoxification usually need improvement to help people with fibromyalgia. Along with this digestive weakness come leaky gut syndrome and candida overgrowth, as well as general dysbiosis. Chronic infections that include viruses can be a factor. Food allergies are a significant contributor for

The tender points for fibromyalgia exist in pairs (one on the right side of your body and one on the left) at the following locations:

- Base of the skull
- Base of the neck
- Upper chest, a little more than an inch below the collarbone
- Along the top of the shoulder
- Upper back, close to the spine and about an inch below the preceding set of points
- Inside of the elbows
- Lower back, close to the dimples above the buttocks
- Upper outside edge of the thigh
- Inside of the knees

If you are testing yourself for a reaction to these points, you must touch them with enough pressure to whiten your fingernail. A doctor who is knowledgeable in the diagnosis of this condition can test these points for you.

some people, especially allergies to wheat, sugar, and cow's milk. As well, nutritional deficiencies, of magnesium, B vitamins, coenzyme Q10, L-carnitine, and several others, are very common. We have also found that many people with fibromyalgia have a brain chemistry imbalance. Using natural therapies to balance serotonin and other neurotransmitters results not only in a better mood but in less muscular pain. Toxic elements, such as lead, mercury, arsenic, and others, can also be one of the root contributors to fibromyalgia. These toxic elements interfere with the normal enzyme and cell function in the body. In addition, blood-sugar imbalances worsen pain and inflammation. Many people develop symptoms of fibromyalgia after a car accident, and thus structural abnormalities must be addressed through physical therapies. Chiropractic, osteopathic, and craniosacral therapy; physiotherapy; and sometimes massage are very helpful in reducing pain.

In essence, all of these potential imbalances lead to a defect in how the cells produce energy. Normally, the "energy-producing plant" of the cells, known as the mitochondria, produces efficient energy for the cells of the body. When a defect occurs in mitochondrial metabolism, it can lead to a shortage of energy for the muscle cells and other tissues of the body, resulting in fatigue and pain. Mitochondria require organic acids that are intermediaries in metabolic pathways in the body that create energy. Researchers have found that people with fibromyalgia often have imbalances in these organic acids. To correct this problem, one must address the root causes, as have been described. Fortunately, a comprehensive natural approach to fibromyalgia is very effective in eliminating the pain or greatly improving it.

SYMPTOMS

For a diagnosis of fibromyalgia to be made, two factors must be present:

- Unexplained, widespread pain that lasts at least three months
- Pain in at least eleven of the eighteen tender points when gentle pressure is applied

Many other symptoms may exist alongside the pain, including the following:

- Fatigue
- Sleep disturbances
- Irritable bowel syndrome
- Anxiety
- Depression
- Difficulty concentrating
- Memory problems
- Dizziness
- Tingling of the skin or other odd sensations
- Premenstrual syndrome (PMS)
- Temporomandibular joint syndrome (TMJ)
- Heart palpitations
- Heightened sensitivity to loud noises, bright lights, and changes in the weather
- Headaches

ROOT CAUSES

- Sleep disorder (including apnea)
- Allergies or sensitivities to certain chemicals, food, or the environment
- Chemical imbalance in the brain, especially of serotonin
- Virus (especially Epstein-Barr, HHV-6, cytomegalovirus)

- Hormone imbalance
- Damage to cells by free radicals (oxidative stress)
- Poor digestion and detoxification
- Toxic metals
- Blood-sugar imbalance
- Candidiasis and parasites
- Nutritional deficiencies, especially of minerals
- A build-up of phosphate or uric acid
- Structural abnormalities (spine and soft tissues)
- Emotional stress
- Overexertion

Testing Techniques

The following tests help assess possible reasons for fibromyalgia:

Chronic infection (human herpes virus type 6 [HHV-6], cytomegalovirus [CMV], Epstein-Barr virus [EBV]—blood

Blood pressure—blood pressure cuff

Hormone testing (thyroid, DHEA, cortisol, testosterone, IGF-1, estrogen, progesterone)—saliva, blood, or urine

Intestinal permeability—urine

Vitamin and mineral analysis (especially for magnesium, B1, B12, iron, and CoQ10)—blood

Digestive function and microbe/parasite/candida testing—stool analysis

Food and environmental allergies/sensitivities—blood, electrodermal

Blood-sugar balance—blood

Toxic elements (such as mercury, arsenic, etc.)—urine, hair

Cellular energy (organic acids)—blood or urine

Amino acids—blood or urine

Detoxification profile—blood or urine

TREATMENT

Diet

Recommended Food

Follow a sound diet that is based on whole, unprocessed foods. Emphasize raw or lightly cooked vegetables, especially greens, and other foods that are high in nutrients and fiber.

To keep up a steady supply of energy to your muscles, eat lots of lean protein—beans, raw nuts, soy products, fish, chicken, and turkey are all good sources—and plan on several meals throughout the day, instead of three large ones.

Eat some live unsweetened yogurt or other cultured food daily to combat candidiasis.

Omega-3 fatty acids help the body create prostaglandin, a hormone that reduces inflammation. Flaxseeds and flaxseed oil, as well as fatty fish, are excellent sources of omega-3 fatty acids.

Fibromyalgia has been linked to a magnesium deficiency, so make sure to consume foods that are high in this mineral, including green leafy vegetables, kelp, soybeans, cashews, and almonds.

Vitamins A, C, and E together help fight free radicals, whose presence may inhibit cells' ability to produce energy. For vitamin A, eat plenty of colored vegetables (especially the green, leafy ones) and skim milk. Good sources of vitamin E are soybeans, broccoli, brussels sprouts, whole grains, and, again, green leafy vegetables.

Drink a glass of clean water every two waking hours. You'll flush out toxins and reduce pain.

Food to Avoid

Determine whether a food allergy is causing or contributing to your pain. Read the Food Allergies section and follow the elimination diet there or have a nutrition-oriented doctor test your food sensitivities or allergies.

Mineral deficiencies have been linked to fibromyalgia, so avoid caffeine, which interferes with their proper absorption. Caffeine also contributes to sleep disturbances.

Reduce or cut out meat, fried and junk foods, high-fat dairy products, and other foods that are high in saturated fats. They contribute to inflammation and pain, as well as to insomnia; in addition, they slow your circulation and deplete your stores of energy.

Avoid sugar. It increases pain, weakens the immune system, disturbs sleep, saps your energy, and encourages the growth of *Candida albicans,* a fungus that some believe is a cause of fibromyalgia. The most common sources of sugar are sodas and processed food, but you also need to severely restrict your intake of natural sugars, like honey and even fruits.

Dramatically reduce your intake of processed food and carbonated drinks. These items are full of food additives that will only aggravate your condition.

Detoxification

A detoxification program can help improve cellular energy production. Follow the previous dietary suggestions, especially regarding fiber and water intake, and try these additional recommendations:

Follow a juice fast for three days for an initial cleanse, but limit your intake of sweet fruit juices. Instead, use vegetable and green drinks, along with unsweetened lemon or cranberry juice.

℞ Super Seven Prescriptions—Fibromyalgia

Super Prescription #1   Magnesium
Take 250 mg two to three times daily. Magnesium glycinate and magnesium aspartate are the preferred forms. Magnesium is important for cellular energy production and relaxes the nerves and the muscles.

Super Prescription #2   Malic acid
Take 1,000 to 1,200 mg twice daily. Malic acid is important for cellular energy production.

Super Prescription #3   5-Hydroxytryptophan (5-HTP)
Take 50 to 100 mg three times daily. This amino acid is a precursor used by the brain to manufacture the neurotransmitter serotonin, which reduces pain, improves sleep, and improves mood.

A double-blind, placebo-controlled study of fifty people with fibromyalgia looked at the effect of 100 mg of 5-HTP, taken three times daily for thirty days. In people supplementing with 5-HTP, significant improvement was found in their pain severity, morning stiffness, sleep patterns, anxiety, and fatigue.

Super Prescription #4   Methylsulfonylmethane (MSM)

Take up to 10,000 mg daily in divided doses. Start with 1,000 mg three times daily, and increase the dosage until pain relief is evident. Reduce the dosage if diarrhea occurs.

Super Prescription #5   S-Adenosylmethionine (SAMe)

Take 400 mg twice daily. SAMe is a naturally occurring nutrient that improves the balance of neurotransmitters such as serotonin; improves detoxification; and helps with cartilage formation.

Super Prescription #6   Vitamin B12

Have your doctor inject you with 1 cc twice weekly for four weeks and then once weekly or as needed. It can also be taken in the sublingual form, up to 1,000 mcg daily of the methylcobalamin form.

Super Prescription #7   Enzymes

Protease enzymes taken on an empty stomach have an anti-inflammatory and pain-relieving effect. Take as directed on the container.

A double-blind trial involving 800 mg of SAMe (S-adenosylmethionine) per day for six weeks found significant benefit for people with fibromyalgia in regard to pain, fatigue, stiffness, and mood. SAMe has been shown in numerous studies to also be effective for depression and osteoarthritis.

General Recommendations

A high-potency multivitamin provides a base of nutrients required for cellular energy production. Take as directed on the container.

Coenzyme Q10 supports cellular energy production. Take 200 to 300 mg daily.

Acetyl-L-carnitine supports cellular energy production. Take 500 to 1,000 mg daily.

Calcium relaxes the nerves and the muscles. Take 500 mg twice daily, along with 400 IU of vitamin D.

Milk thistle (*Silybum marianum*) supports liver detoxification. Take 250 mg of a 80 to 85 percent silymarin extract three times daily.

Vitamin E has anti-inflammatory benefits. Take 800 IU daily.

Vitamin C has anti-inflammatory and immune-enhancing benefits. Take 1,000 mg two to three times daily.

Grape seed extract or maritime pine bark improves circulation and has anti-inflammatory effects. Take 100 mg two to three times daily.

Alpha lipoic acid is an antioxidant that supports detoxification. Take 100 to 200 mg daily.

N-acetylcysteine supports detoxification and helps produce glutathione. Take 500 mg daily.

NADH supports cellular energy production. Take 10 to 20 mg on an empty stomach.

Passionflower (*Passiflora incarnata*) relaxes the nerves. Take 300 to 500 mg in capsule form or 1 ml of tincture three times daily. It can also be taken before bedtime to help with sleep.

Valerian (*Valeriana officinalis*) relaxes the nerves. Take 300 to 500 mg in capsule form or 1 ml of tincture three times daily. It can also be taken before bedtime to help with sleep.

Olive leaf extract (*Olea europa*) is good if you have a chronic viral infection. Take 500 mg three times daily.

A probiotic is important for digestive function and immunity. Take a product containing at least 4 billion active organisms daily.

Thyroid controls cellular energy and mood. If your levels are low, work with a knowledgeable doctor to use natural thyroid hormone (such as Armour or compounded T4/T3 or T3).

DHEA reduces stress and inflammation. If your levels are low, work with a doctor to normalize your levels. The normal starting dosage is 5 to 15 mg daily.

Natural progesterone can be helpful for women with fibromyalgia. Premenopausal women should apply ¼ teaspoon (20 mg equivalent) to the inside of their forearms one to two times daily on days 14 to 28 of their cycle. Menopausal women should apply ¼ teaspoon (20 mg equivalent) to the inside of their forearms twice daily for three to four weeks of the month. Postmenopausal women should apply ⅛ teaspoon (10 mg equivalent) to the inside of their forearms once daily for 3 weeks of the month.

Estrogen, cortisol, and testosterone need to be prescribed, based on your levels, by a doctor who is knowledgeable in natural hormone replacement.

Ginkgo biloba improves circulation and memory. Take 60 to 120 mg of a 24 percent flavone glycoside extract three times daily.

Fish oil supplies pain-relieving omega-3 fatty acids. Take a fish oil product containing at least 480 mg of EPA and 360 mg of DHA twice daily.

Flaxseed oil supplies pain-relieving omega-3 fatty acids. Take 1 to 2 tablespoons daily.

Evening primrose (*Oenothera biennis*) oil contains gamma linoleic acid (GLA), which decreases inflammation and pain. Take 2,000 mg daily.

A greens drink containing super green foods, such as chlorella, spirulina, barley grass, and others, supports detoxification and energy production. Take as directed on the container.

Melatonin promotes sleep. Take 0.3 to 0.5 mg a half hour before bedtime.

Black cohosh (*Cimicifuga racemosa*) is a good hormone balancer and relaxes spasms of the muscles. Take 40 mg of a 2.5 percent triterpene glycoside extract twice daily.

Cordyceps sinensis supports adrenal gland function. Take 800 mg twice daily of a standardized product.

Arnica (*Arnica montana*) oil relieves muscle pain and tenderness. Apply the oil to painful areas twice daily.

Homeopathy

Pick the remedy that best matches your symptoms in this section. Take a 6x, 12x, 6C, or 30C potency twice daily for two weeks to see if there are any positive results. After you notice improvement, stop taking the remedy, unless symptoms return. Consultation with a homeopathic practitioner is advised.

Arnica (*Arnica montana*) is the top choice for pain that feels deep and bruised and for all-over tenderness. Symptoms are worse after exertion.

Bryonia (*Bryonia alba*) is for pain that is aggravated by the slightest movement. Muscles feel better with cool applications and pressure and feel worse with warmth. The person is irritable and does not want to be touched.

Calcarea Carbonica is for people who get muscle soreness from exertion and cold, damp climates. They are usually chilly, with clammy hands and feet. There is a craving for sweets and eggs. There are often symptoms of anxiety and a feeling of being overwhelmed and easily fatigued.

Causticum is helpful when the muscles and the joints become stiff and sore from overuse and from the cold or dry weather. Symptoms are improved with warm applications. The muscles and the joints feel contracted.

Cimicifuga is for muscles that feel sore and bruised and worse in the cold. The back of the neck is sore and stiff. The person is prone to depression and hormone imbalance.

Ignatia (*Ignatia amara*) is for tight, spasmodic, or cramping muscles and fibromyalgia that comes on from stress or emotional upset.

Magnesia Phosphorica is for cramping or spasming muscles that feel better with warm applications.

Nux Vomica (*Strychnos nux vomica*) is for tight muscles that spasm. The person is chilly, and the symptoms are worse in cold weather and better with warm applications. Digestive problems, such as stomach ache or heartburn, are often present. The person is irritable and fatigued.

Pulsatilla (*Pulsatilla pratensis*) is helpful if your pain moves from joint to joint, and if you feel tearful and depressed. Fibromyalgia is often connected to the menstrual cycle or hormone imbalance.

Rhus Toxicodendron is for pain and stiffness that's worse in the early morning or after resting and during cold, rainy weather. Symptoms ease with continued movement and warm applications. The person feels restless.

Acupressure

See pages 668–675 for information about pressure points and administering treatment.

- Conception Vessel 17 supports the immune system and also eases depression and anxiety.
- Stomach 36 improves the body's ability to absorb nutrients. It will also lend general support to the digestive system, a helpful quality if you have irritable bowel syndrome.
- To relax cramped muscles and soothe your nerves, use Liver 3.
- Pericardium 6 relieves anxiety, indigestion, and heart palpitations.
- Bladder 38 quiets tension and promotes sleep.

Other Recommendations

Acupuncture has a good track record of relieving fibromyalgia pain. See the appendix for agencies that can provide you with lists of qualified acupuncturists in your area.

Bodywork

Many fibromyalgia sufferers have found that bodywork is quite helpful for easing pain and stress. Try several of the following techniques, as everyone responds differently.

Chiropractic or Osteopathic Manipulation
This improves structural alignment and nerve flow.

Massage
A gentle all-over massage eases pain and brings down stress levels.

Lymphatic drainage massage supports the immune system by detoxifying the tissues. This kind of massage is especially supportive during a fast.

Reflexology
See pages 686–687 for information about reflexology areas and how to work them.

Because fibromyalgia is a systemic, whole-body disease, it is best to work the entire foot, with special attention to the parts corresponding to the areas of your body that hurt.

Hydrotherapy

Hot or warm water can feel wonderful to fibromyalgia sufferers. Try taking a hot shower in the morning, when the pain is likely to be at its worst; at night, when you might have trouble sleeping, try a warm bath. Saunas and heated compresses are other pleasant ways to relax your muscles.

Constitutional hydrotherapy is a good long-term treatment. See pages 676–677 for directions.

Other Bodywork Recommendations

Postural therapies, such as the Feldenkrais method and the Alexander technique, help you move with greater ease and less strain. They are a good option for sufferers who can tolerate only the gentlest treatments. Contact a local specialist to learn more.

Aromatherapy

Add oils to a bath for additional pain-relieving qualities. Chamomile, lavender, and rosemary will reduce inflammation, and black pepper, ginger, and eucalyptus stimulate circulation and blood flow to the muscles.

If you don't have access to a bathtub, here's another way to use any of the previous oils: Add 25 drops of the oil to 2 quarts of boiling water. Soak several strips of cloth in the mixture, and let them cool to a comfortably warm temperature. Wrap the cloths around the painful area.

Juniper and melissa oils help break down toxins. Add them to a base oil, and use it as a detoxifying supplement to a lymphatic massage.

To reduce stress, experiment with a number of oils until you find the ones you like best, then alternate them so that you don't become inured to their effects. Some good choices to begin with are chamomile, jasmine, lavender, and rose. Almost any preparation method will work (except a straight application to the skin), but for all-day stress relief, you might like to diffuse the oil into the air of your office or room.

Stress Reduction

General Stress-Reduction Therapies

Consider positive mental imagery, meditation, and prayer a first line of defense against the symptoms of fibromyalgia. Regular meditation is both refreshing and calming. It improves your concentration and memory and, when used just before bedtime, can help you sleep. Biofeedback helps you learn to improve the way your body responds to stress.

It's not a bad idea to supplement your daily meditation with a yoga class once or twice a week. Yoga relaxes your body and mind, improves digestion, and can ease both joint and muscle pain.

Bach Flower Remedies

Consult the Bach Flower Remedy chart on pages 648–650 to find the best remedy for your personal situation. Once you've chosen a remedy, place 10 drops of the liquid under your tongue. Hold the drops in place for thirty seconds and swallow. Use as often as needed.

Rescue Remedy is available in cream form. When your pain is particularly acute, rub a little of the cream onto the affected area.

If you are overexerted and burned out, take Hornbeam.

Aspen is for people with vague, unnamable fears that result in insomnia or nightmares.

Olive is the remedy for people who are so exhausted that daily life is robbed of all pleasure.

If you have given up the belief that you'll ever feel better again, try Gorse.

Other Recommendations

- Magnet therapy can be helpful to reduce pain. Work with a practitioner who is knowledgeable in this area.
- Moderate, nonjarring exercise is one of the best treatments for fibromyalgia. Daily exercise for half an hour (a brisk walk or a swim are excellent choices) is far preferable to less frequent but more vigorous workouts. Studies show that people with fibromyalgia who exercise regularly have less symptoms than those who are inactive. Get adequate rest. Most of us need at least eight hours a day; if you need more, however, by all means take it. Overexertion will only aggravate your symptoms.

REFERENCES

Caruso, I., P. Sarzi Puttini, M. Cazzola, and V. Azzolini. 1990. Double-blind study of 5-hydroxytryptophan versus placebo in the treatment of primary fibromyalgia syndrome. *Journal of Internal Medicine Research* 18(3):201–9.

Jacobsen S., B. Danneskiold-Samsoe, and R. B. Andersen. 1991. Oral S-adenosylmethionine in primary fibromyalgia: Double-blind clinical evaluation. *Scandinavian Journal of Rheumatology* 20:294–302.

Flu

The flu, more properly called influenza, is an acute viral infection of the upper respiratory tract. Many people have difficulty distinguishing between the flu and the common cold, and, indeed, many of the symptoms are the same. Colds, however, tend to come on slowly and produce symptoms restricted to the chest, the neck, and the head; in contrast, the flu attacks swiftly and is accompanied by body-wide symptoms, including fever, aches, and general fatigue. While most people recover from colds within a few days, it may take weeks before the lingering fatigue and the cough of a flu completely disappear.

The three classifications of the influenza virus are A, B, and C. The most common virus is influenza A. It often occurs in epidemics during the late fall or the early winter. The highest incidence of the flu is in schoolchildren. It generally takes forty-eight hours after initial exposure for symptoms to begin occurring. Chills, a fever, a headache, and muscular aches and pains are the most common initial symptoms followed by a severe cough. Acute symptoms usually subside in two to three days. People who are most at risk for serious complications include those with chronic pulmonary or heart disease.

The influenza viruses mutate constantly, changing their structure just enough so that it is more difficult to build up immunity to them. These viruses are also highly contagious. They are communicated via coughs and sneezes, which propel infected droplets into the air and onto surfaces. Most communities see an outbreak of at least one flu virus every winter; every two to three years, the flu reaches epidemic proportions.

As with the common cold, there is no conventional cure for the flu. However, specific natural therapies described in this section have the potential to abort a flu in its early stages. The wisest course of action is to keep your immune system strong and healthy during the winter months, thereby reducing the virus's ability to take hold in your body. Eat well, exercise, rest, and follow the other general recommendations for health outlined in Part Two.

A note of caution: For most of us, a bout with the flu is highly unpleasant but temporary. However, it can sometimes develop into pneumonia, a serious disease that may be fatal: In people over sixty-five, this flu-related pneumonia is one of the leading causes of death. If you are in this age group, or if you have a compromised immune system or a chronic chest condition (such as asthma, emphysema, or cardiovascular disease), see a doctor immediately if you catch the flu. Very young children should also receive medical care right away. No matter what your age or physical condition, if a case of the flu leads to difficulty breathing or tightness in the chest, call your doctor.

SYMPTOMS

Most people with the flu experience the following symptoms:

- Fever
- Aches in the muscles and joints
- Fatigue and weakness
- Sore throat
- Dry cough

The following symptoms may also accompany the flu:

- Sneezing and runny nose
- Nausea and vomiting
- Swollen glands in the neck
- Insomnia
- Depression

Testing Techniques

The following tests help assess possible reasons for reoccurring influenza infections:

Immune system imbalance or disease—blood

Hormone testing (especially for thyroid, DHEA, cortisol)—saliva, blood, or urine

Intestinal permeability—urine

Detoxification profile—urine

Vitamin and mineral analysis (especially vitamins C and B12, iron, and CoQ10)—blood

Digestive function and microbe/parasite/candida testing—stool analysis

Anemia—blood test (CBC, iron, ferritin, % saturation)

Food and environmental allergies/sensitivities—blood, electrodermal

Blood-sugar balance—blood

ROOT CAUSES

- If overwork, stress, poor diet, or another illness has run down your immune system, you are much more likely to catch the flu during a community outbreak.

- Similar to the common cold, the flu acts as a means of detoxification for a toxic body.

TREATMENT

Diet

Recommended Food

Eat lightly to allow your body to focus on healing, rather than on digestion. During the first two to four days, when you are likely to feel the worst, your diet should consist mainly of liquids—clean water, hot broths, green drinks, herbal teas, and juices—to flush your body of toxins. If you feel like eating, you should have a variety of fruits, especially citrus and berries. These fruits are high in vitamin C and bioflavonoids, which stimulate the production of white blood cells.

After the most acute stage of the illness has passed, continue with the liquids and the fruits but also start eating salads, steamed or lightly cooked vegetables, and whole grains. If you have the stomach for them, nuts are an excellent source of zinc, a mineral that strengthens the immune system. However, if you still don't have an appetite, don't force yourself to eat. Remain on the liquid diet until you're hungry again.

Warmed applesauce or apple juice is soothing and provides high levels of vitamin C. Make sure the sauce or juice isn't overheated or boiled, however, or it will lose some of its potency.

Eat lightly. Steamed vegetables, soups, broths, and herbal teas will let your body focus on healing, instead of on digestion. If you lose your appetite, don't force yourself to eat.

Stay hydrated. Drink plenty of clean water and other fluids (but see the note about sugar and juice further on) to cleanse away toxins and to keep the respiratory tract from drying out.

Increase your consumption of ginger, onions, and garlic. Try adding one or both to chicken soup or miso.

Hot water with lemon, honey, and cinnamon is a traditional cold remedy. Drink a cup every two hours to soothe your throat and chest, prevent mucus buildup, and encourage a cleansing sweat.

Food to Avoid

Eliminate dairy and refined sugar products from your diet for the duration of your illness. These foods will only contribute to the formation of mucus and make the virus harder to expel. Sugar also has the extremely undesirable effect of depressing your immune system.

Caffeine depletes the body's stores of zinc, a mineral necessary for healing. Avoid coffee, black teas, and chocolate until the flu passes.

Detoxification

A bout of influenza generally forces its sufferer into a detoxification program by making it nearly impossible to tolerate food. A liquid and lighter diet, as described earlier, will flush out toxins, especially when combined with some of the detoxifying teas listed in the herbal sections.

Lomatium (*Lomatium dissectum*) was a life-saving remedy for Native American Indians living in the Nevada desert during the Spanish flu epidemic that killed over 500,000 people in the United States and 22 million worldwide. A local medical doctor noted that Native American Indians were recovering from the Spanish flu by ingesting boiled lomatium root. It is believed that phytochemicals found in lomatium root inhibit viruses from replicating and stimulate white blood cell activity.

℞ Super Seven Prescriptions—Flu

Super Prescription #1   Homeopathic Combination Flu Remedy
At the first signs of a flu, take a dose of the combination flu remedy four times daily for three days. This contains the most common remedies used for the flu. Another alternative is a flu remedy containing *Anas barbariae*. Then if you notice improvement, stop taking the remedy, unless symptoms return. If your symptoms do not improve within twenty-four hours, pick the remedy that best matches your symptoms under Homeopathy in this section.

Super Prescription #2   Lomatium dissectum
Take 500 mg in capsule form or 2 to 4 ml of the tincture four times daily. Lomatium has strong antiviral effects and has traditionally been used by herbalists to treat the flu.

Super Prescription #3   Elderberry (*Sambucus nigra*)
Adults should take 1 tablespoon four times daily and children 1 tablespoon twice daily. Elderberry inhibits influenza viral replication and reduces coughing.

Super Prescription #4   Echinacea (*Echinacea purpurea*) and goldenseal (*Hydrastis canadensis*)
Echinacea and goldenseal combination: Take 500 mg in capsule form or 2 to 4 ml of tincture four times daily. Both herbs enhance immune function, and echinacea has antiviral properties. *Note:* If you do not have any mucus production, use only echinacea.

Super Prescription #5   Oregano (*Origanum vulgare*) oil
Take 500 mg of the capsule form four times daily or as directed on the container. Oregano oil has powerful antiviral effects.

Super Prescription #6   Vitamin C
Take 1,000 to 2,000 mg three to four times daily. Reduce the dosage if diarrhea occurs. Vitamin C supports immune system function through increased white blood cell activity.

Super Prescription #7   Ginger (*Zingiber officinale*)
Take 500 mg of the capsule form or drink the fresh tea four times daily. Ginger helps with a sore throat and chills.

A double-blind, placebo-controlled study in the *Journal of Alternative and Complementary Medicine* reported that people who received elderberry extract (4 tablespoons a day for adults and 2 tablespoons for children) for three days significantly improved their flu symptoms. Ninety percent of people taking this herbal extract were completely well in two to three days, as compared to six days for those taking a placebo.

General Recommendations

Garlic (*Allium sativum*) has powerful antiviral and detoxification properties. Add it raw to broths, juices, soups, or vegetable dishes. You can also take 300 to 450 mg of garlic in capsules twice a day.

Astragalus (*Astragalus membranaceus*) is an excellent treatment for preventing the flu. Do not take astragalus if you have a fever. Take 500 to 1,000 mg in capsule form or 3.0 ml of a tincture two to three times daily.

Thymus (*Thymus vulgaris*) extract optimizes immune activity. Take 1 to 2 capsules twice daily or as directed on the container.

Homeopathy

At the first signs of a flu, take 2 pellets of a 30C potency four times daily for three days, of the remedy that best matches your symptoms in this section. If you notice improvement, stop taking the remedy, unless symptoms return. If your symptoms do not improve within twenty-four hours, pick another remedy.

Aconitum Napellus is for a flu that comes on suddenly after exposure to dry, cold weather. There is a scratchy throat and a thin discharge from the nose. You probably feel anxious, restless, and chilly, with a great thirst. This remedy is best taken within four hours of developing flu symptoms.

Arsenicum Album is for a cold with a flu in which a person feels exhausted, anxious, restless, and chilly and is thirsty for sips of warm water. Diarrhea and vomiting occur with the flu.

Belladonna (*Atropa belladonna*) is for the beginning phase of a flu characterized by a high fever that comes on suddenly. The face is flushed and the skin is hot, but the feet are cold. The pupils are dilated. A throbbing headache is common.

Bryonia (*Bryonia alba*) is for a flu with severe aching of the joints. The person feels worse from the slightest movement and may have a hard, dry cough. There is a great thirst for cold drinks. The person feels very irritable and does not want to move. The joints ache.

Eupatorium Perfolatum is helpful when there is a high fever and tremendous, deep aching of the bones and the muscles. The person has a great thirst for cold drinks.

Ferrum Phosphoricum helps when a person feels feverish but does not act sick. The throat may be sore, and the face is flushed. It's best used at the onset of a flu.

Gelsemium (*Gelsemium sempervirens*) is for a cold accompanied by chills and muscle aches. The person feels drowsy and fatigued and has droopy eyelids. There may be a headache at the base of the head.

Mercurius Solubilis or Vivus is helpful when the person is sensitive to both hot and cold temperatures. The tongue has a thick coating, and the person has bad breath, has excessive saliva production, and drools on the pillow. The throat is often raw and sore. Profuse sweating occurs.

Nux Vomica (*Strychnos nux vomica*) is for a person who has a digestive upset, such as stomach cramping and nausea, with the flu. There is great chilliness and irritability.

Rhus Toxicodendron is for extreme stiffness in the muscles and the joints that feels better with warm applications and when moving around. It is hard to find a comfortable position, so there is a lot of restlessness.

Sulphur is for the end stages of a long flu. Burning in the lungs may occur, as well as fever and sweating. The person has a great thirst for ice-cold drinks.

Acupressure

See pages 668–675 for information about pressure points and administering treatment.

- Large Intestine 4, Governing Vessel 24.5, and Gallbladder 16 and 20 all ease headache and head congestion.
- To reduce fever and strengthen the immune system, massage Large Intestine 11.
- Kidney 27 relieves a sore throat and chest congestion.

Bodywork

Massage

When most of your symptoms have passed and you're ready to resume a more normal schedule, an all-over massage will help you make the transition more smoothly.

Massage will break up the remaining toxins, relax muscles that may have tightened, and help you reconnect with your body.

If you have a lingering cough following an episode of the flu, a percussive massage will help break up the mucus. Percussive motions are best used on people who are relatively strong and healthy.

Reflexology

See pages 686–687 for information about reflexology areas and how to work them.

Work the areas corresponding to the chest and the lungs, the intestines, the diaphragm, the lymph system, and all the glands.

Massage the cervicals if your flu is accompanied by a sore throat.

For clogged sinuses, work all the toes.

Hydrotherapy

Constitutional hydrotherapy done each day relieves congestion and stimulates the immune system. See pages 676–677 for directions.

Aromatherapy

Add any of the following oils to baths or steam inhalations.

Tea tree oil has strong infection-fighting properties. Add to a bath, or mix a few drops of the oil with warm water and gargle with it. (Tea tree oil is quite concentrated, so add no more than 2 or 3 drops to a cup of water for gargling.) To prevent the infection from spreading to the rest of your household, use some in diffusers in the common rooms.

Use lavender in any kind of preparation to strengthen your immune system and help you sleep.

Add eucalyptus and peppermint—either alone or in combination—to a bath, in steam, or in an inhalation to relieve congestion.

Stress Reduction

If chronic stress leaves you constantly vulnerable to the flu and other upper respiratory infections, take some time out every day to detach yourself from any tension you might be experiencing.

Regular stress-management practice can also help you handle future difficult situations with a calm disposition.

General Stress-Reduction Therapies

Regular exercise and a positive attitude and mental imagery improve immune function and may help prevent a flu.

Bach Flower Remedies

See the chart on pages 648–650 to find the remedy that best suits your personality and tendencies.

Once you've chosen a remedy, place 10 drops of the liquid under your tongue. Hold the drops in place for thirty seconds and swallow. Use as often as needed.

When you first feel the flu coming on, immediately take a combination of Clematis, Crab Apple, Olive, and Walnut to increase your reserves of strength.

If you feel an overwhelming need for comfort, take Chicory, in addition to the four previously mentioned flowers.

Other Recommendations

- Rest is absolutely critical to the healing process. As soon as you feel the symptoms strike, get into bed and stay there for several days or even a week, if necessary. If you try to exert yourself during a bout of the flu, you may wind up with a secondary infection, such as pneumonia.
- Gargle with warm salt water to reduce sore throat pain.

REFERENCES

Alstat, E. K. 1987. Lomatium dissectum—An herbal virucide! *Complementary Medicine* 2(5).

Zakay-Rones, Z., N. Varsano, M. Zlotnik, O. Manor, L. Regev, M. Schlesinger, and M. Mumcuoglu. 1995. Inhibition of several strains of influenza virus in vitro and reduction of symptoms by an elderberry extract (*Sambucus nigra L.*) during an outbreak of influenza B Panama. *Journal of Alternative and Complementary Medicine* 1(4):361–69.

Food Allergies/Sensitivities

Food allergies and food sensitivities (also referred to as intolerances) are terms often used interchangeably. Technically, a food allergy is a measurable immune response to a normally harmless food. Symptoms include itchy hives, lip swelling, nausea, vomiting, diarrhea, wheezing, and difficulty breathing. Common food allergies are to peanuts, wheat, milk, eggs, MSG, and shellfish. Scientists are not sure what exactly causes food allergies. Since many allergies tend to run in families, there apparently is a genetic component. There is also evidence that some allergies are the result of exposure to a certain food or foods too early in life, before the immune system is fully developed. Many infants who are given cow's milk instead of breast milk in the first months develop an allergic reaction; the same goes for children who are fed wheat, eggs, peanut butter, or other products before they are ready. At any age, the overconsumption of a food is thought to lead to allergies. Wheat, for example, is a common allergen in the United States, because most people eat it at every meal and snack.

Food sensitivities are reactions to food where there is not necessarily an immune response, as measured by standard lab tests. These symptoms are not life threatening but are bothersome. These include, but are not limited to, abdominal cramps, bloating, headache, mood swings, reoccurring infections, joint pain, runny nose, skin rashes, dark circles under the eyes, and fatigue. Symptoms may occur up to thirty-six hours after ingesting the offending food. Common food sensitivities that we see with patients are to cow's milk, wheat, corn, soy, chocolate, citrus fruit, and artificial sweeteners and preservatives. Most food sensitivities are acquired throughout life. A lack of variety in the diet, poor digestion and detoxification, and genetics are often the underlying causes. Most people who have multiple food sensitivities have an underlying condition known as leaky gut syndrome. This means that foods are not being broken down effectively (especially proteins), and once absorbed, they cause a heightened immune reaction. The key to these cases is to heal the gut lining and improve food breakdown, something that natural medicine is very effective for. Many cases of food sensitivities can be eliminated or improved with natural therapies.

Do be aware that hundreds of conditions can be at least in part caused or worsened by food allergies or sensitivities. Common examples include

Arthritis

Asthma

Attention-deficit hyperactivity disorder

Bedwetting

Canker sores

Colic

Constipation

Depression

Diarrhea

Ear infections

Eczema

Gallbladder disease

Headaches

High blood pressure

Hives

Hypoglycemia

Irritable bowel syndrome

Inflammatory bowel diseases (Crohn's, ulcerative colitis)

Multiple chemical sensitivity

Overweight

Psoriasis

Reflux and ulcers

Sinusitis

Weakened immunity

Food allergies and sensitivities can sometimes be difficult to identify. Immune responses to food may take hours or days to develop, and they may be mistaken for seasonal allergies or for other diseases associated with their symptoms: colds, flu, skin problems, chronic fatigue, and many others. And allergies aren't just triggered by the consumption of large quantities of a problem food: you can have a reaction from a minute quantity or even from simply touching or inhaling an allergen. Use the elimination diet given here to determine which food or foods, if any, you are allergic to.

Also, specific testing with blood, electrodermal, skin scratch, or applied kinesiology by a holistic practitioner or a doctor can help you quickly identify your problem foods. They can then be avoided or you can desensitize yourself to them.

SYMPTOMS

Food allergies can produce a number of symptoms. The most common are listed as follows:

- Nasal congestion
- Sneezing
- Coughing
- Red, itchy, or watery eyes
- Dark circles or puffiness under the eyes
- Wheezing
- Sore throat
- Difficulty swallowing

- Hives, rashes, eczema, or other skin eruptions
- Nausea or vomiting
- Headache
- Fatigue
- Fluid retention
- Swelling of the throat and the tongue

Common symptoms of food sensitivities:

- Abdominal cramps and bloating
- Headache
- Mood swings
- Reoccurring infections
- Joint pain

- Runny nose
- Skin rashes
- Dark circles under the eyes
- Fatigue

ROOT CAUSES

- Overconsumption of a certain food
- Introduction of a food too early in infancy or childhood
- Stress, which depresses the immune system

- Poor digestion and detoxification
- Heredity

TREATMENT

If you experience difficulty breathing or develop hives that spread rapidly, *get emergency help at once.* Allergic reactions like these can be quickly fatal. If you know you have severe reactions to certain substances, talk to your doctor about emergency adrenaline kits you can keep on hand.

Diet

Obviously, the most important step in treating allergies is identifying them. Once you've identified the offending substances, adhere to the following suggestions to keep

Elimination Diet to Detect Food Allergies

Although it takes some time and dedication, an elimination diet is the best way to uncover any hidden food allergies. The first step is to come up with a list of possible trigger foods. Do this by keeping a food diary, writing down everything you eat each day for a week (or longer, if you sense that one week can't adequately represent your eating habits). At the end of the week, note the foods you've consumed most often during the week. This is your list of possible triggers.

Next, you should eliminate all the suspect foods on your list from your diet for a total of two weeks. For most people, this stage is difficult, as you're asked to give up the foods you love and rely upon the most; try to keep in mind that you'll be able to return to your usual diet, perhaps with a few modifications, soon.

If, after two weeks, your symptoms have disappeared, you know that you are allergic to at least one of the foods on your list. To identify which food or foods is the culprit, reintroduce the suspect foods to your diet one at a time. When reintroducing foods that have been eliminated, be sure to use the purest form of the food. For example, if milk is on your list of suspects, add whole milk back to your diet, not skim. If you've eliminated wheat, reintroduce it by eating cream of wheat or shredded wheat. Allow two full days to pass between reintroducing foods, as it may take a while for symptoms to manifest themselves. Should your symptoms reappear, you can assume that the food most recently reintroduced is an allergen, and you should banish it from your diet or work to have your immune system desensitized to it. Continue to make your way through the list, however, as you may be allergic to more than one food. Wait at least forty-eight hours after the onset of symptoms before reintroducing the next eliminated food.

At the end of the elimination diet, you will know which, if any, foods produce an allergic response in your body. Depending on your reaction, you can avoid or reduce your intake of this food.

them out of your diet and to reduce your chances of having a bad reaction, should you be accidentally exposed. Food sensitivities can generally be improved or cured by rotating foods in the diet, improving digestion and detoxification, and using the desensitization techniques described in this chapter.

Recommended Food

Fortify your immune system with a healthful, wholesome diet. Eat foods that are high in immune-building nutrients: seafood, beans, and nuts for magnesium; green leafy vegetables and brewer's yeast for B vitamins; and plenty of fresh fruits and vegetables for vitamin C.

A varied diet will discourage the development of allergies, so try to eat different foods every day.

Breast milk is best for infants. If, for some reason, you are unable to provide your baby with mother's milk, use a cow's milk alternative or a predigested, hypoallergenic formula.

Drink a glass of clean water every two waking hours to flush allergens out of your body and to encourage overall health.

Food to Avoid

Of course, you must avoid the foods that trigger a severe allergy response. In general, it is best to buy whole foods and prepare them yourself, so that you are aware of their content, but if you must buy packaged food, learn how to read labels and scrutinize

> ## Testing Techniques
>
> The following tests help assess possible reasons for food allergies/sensitivities, as well as determine the offending foods:
>
> Intestinal permeability—urine
>
> Detoxification profile—urine
>
> Digestive function and microbe/parasite/candida testing—stool analysis
>
> Food allergies/sensitivities—blood (IgE and IgG4), electrodermal, skin scratch
>
> Hormone testing (DHEA, cortisol)—saliva, blood, or urine

them carefully. Food preservatives and artificial colorings or flavorings can be at the root of food reactions.

Food sensitivities can generally be rotated in the diet, until you become desensitized to the offending food.

Detoxification

If you have recently suffered an allergy attack, go on a short, twenty-four-hour juice fast to cleanse the body of allergens. For chronic allergies, undertake a one- to three-day cleanse every three months.

℞ **Super Seven Prescriptions—Food Sensitivity**

Super Prescription #1   Digestive enzyme complex
Take a full-spectrum digestive complex with each meal.

Super Prescription #2   Protease enzymes
Take 1 to 2 protease enzyme capsules between meals two to three times daily. When taken on an empty stomach, protease enzymes are believed to metabolize food antibody complexes that cause symptoms. Do not use if you have an ulcer or gastritis.

Super Prescription #3   Homeopathic Desensitization Drops
Take a homeopathic dilution of the food(s) you are sensitive to, up to three times daily or as directed on the container. This approach of like cures like helps desensitize the immune response to sensitivity reactions.

Super Prescription #4   Probiotics
Take a product that contains at least 4 billion active organisms daily, thirty minutes after a meal. These good bacteria favorably alter the way the immune system perceives foods and also helps with their metabolism and digestion.

Super Prescription #5   Gentian root (*Gentiana lutea*)
This improves stomach-acid levels and overall digestive function. Take 300 mg in capsule form or 10 to 20 drops five to fifteen minutes before meals. It can also be used as part of a digestive bitters formula.

Super Prescription #6   Thymus (*Thymus vulgaris*) **extract**
Take 1 to 2 capsules or as directed on the container three times daily on an empty stomach. Thymus extract balances an overactive immune system.

Studies done with infants and nursing mothers have found that probiotics help improve food allergies. It appears that probiotics directly reduce the immune response to food allergens and indirectly improve symptoms, due to improved food digestion.

> **Super Prescription #7   Methylsulfonylmethane (MSM)**
> Take 1,000 mg twice daily. MSM has a natural antiallergy benefit that includes food sensitivities.

General Recommendations

L-glutamine repairs the lining of the small intestine for improved absorption. Take 500 mg three times daily.

An adrenal glandular supplement supports adrenal gland function and allergy control. Take 1 capsule three times daily between meals.

Pantothenic acid (vitamin B5) supports adrenal gland function and allergy control. Take 500 mg three times daily.

Milk thistle (*Silybum marianum*) supports liver function and detoxification. Take 250 mg of a 85 percent silymarin extract with each meal.

Betaine hydrochloric acid improves stomach-acid levels. Take 1 to 2 capsules with each meal.

Quercitin has antiallergy benefits. Take 500 mg three times daily.

Vitamin C with bioflavonoids reduces allergy reactions. Take 1,000 mg two to three times daily.

Homeopathy

Pick the remedy that best matches your symptoms in this section. For acute food reactions, take a 30C potency four times daily. For chronic food sensitivities, take 6x, 12x, 6C, 12C, or 30C potency twice daily for two weeks to see if there are any positive results. After you notice improvement, stop taking the remedy, unless symptoms return. Consultation with a homeopathic practitioner is advised.
Note: Homeopathy is not a replacement for medical treatment for serious acute food allergy reactions.

Lycopodium (*Lycopodium clavatum*) is for people who have problems with food reactions and also suffer tremendous bloating and gas. They crave sweets. Symptoms are usually worse in the early evening.

Nux Vomica (*Strychnos nux vomica*) is for people with multiple food sensitivities and digestive problems, such as heartburn, reflux, constipation, or stomach cramps. They tend to be chilly and irritable.

Urtica Urens is helpful if you have welts or hives with itchy, burning skin, especially after eating shellfish. If your hives or welts are rapidly spreading, get emergency help at once.

Acupressure

See pages 668–675 for information about pressure points and administering treatment.

- Large Intestine 4 relieves headaches and sneezing.
- If you have fatigue, swollen eyes, or head pain, use Bladder 10.
- Triple Warmer 5 fortifies the immune system.
- Stomach 36 strengthens the entire body and promotes a healthful balance.

Bodywork

Massage

If food allergies have left you chronically or severely congested, consider a percussive massage to help break up mucus.

Percussive motions are best used on people who are relatively strong and healthy. If you are frail, thin, or elderly, check with your massage therapist about the suitability of this treatment for you.

To reduce stress, get a relaxing massage that incorporates any of the soothing essential oils listed in the Aromatherapy recommendations.

Reflexology

See pages 686–687 for information about reflexology areas and how to work them.

To ease allergic reactions in the upper respiratory tract, work the big toes and the inside of the heels.

If you have been exposed to an allergenic food, work the liver and the colon to speed the processing and the release of toxins.

Aromatherapy

Use melissa in a bath, an inhalation, or a massage oil to reduce the intensity of an allergic attack.

Lavender and chamomile will relax and soothe the body after the stress of an allergic reaction. Use either oil according to your particular symptoms. If you have acne, mix into a lotion and apply directly to the skin. For other reactions, you can use a compress to apply the oil to a specific body part, add to a bath, or use in a massage for all-over relief.

If you're congested, try any of the following oils in a steam inhalation, a bath, a diffuser, or a massage: eucalyptus, peppermint, melissa, and tea tree.

Stress Reduction

General Stress-Reduction Techniques

Stress can impact your immune and digestive systems and can contribute to food sensitivities. Read the exercise and stress reduction section in Part Two and choose a couple of stress-reduction techniques you'd like to try. Once you've found one or two that you like, incorporate them into your daily routine. Regular practice will help you handle daily tension with detachment and equanimity.

Bach Flower Remedies

According to Bach Flower Remedy philosophy, intolerance of other people is a cause of most allergic conditions. If you have little patience for others, use Beech or Impatiens to expand your sense of goodwill. To take Beech or any other Bach remedy, place 10 drops of the liquid under your tongue. Hold the drops in place for thirty seconds and swallow. Use as often as needed.

REFERENCES

Laiho, K., A. Ouwehand, S. Salminen, and E. Isolauri. 2002. Inventing probiotic functional foods for patients with allergic disease. *Annals of Allergy, Asthma, & Immunology* 89(6 Suppl 1):75–82.

Majamaa, H., and E. Isolauri. 1997. Probiotics: A novel approach in the management of food allergy. *Journal of Allergy and Clinical Immunology* 99:179–85.

Food Poisoning

One of the most unpleasant and certainly potentially dangerous conditions is food poisoning. A person's body reacts to toxins produced by bacteria that contaminate food. The most common types of food poisoning result from the bacteria of salmonella, campylobacter, and staphylococcus.

Symptoms range from nausea, overall body weakness, fever, and abdominal cramps to violent episodes of vomiting and diarrhea as the body tries to rid itself of the contaminated food.

Most cases of food poisoning can be avoided. Food poisoning occurs as a result of improper handling, storing, or cooking of food. That is why it is important for people to always wash their hands thoroughly with soap before eating and especially before preparing a meal.

It is important to refrigerate foods like mayonnaise, egg salad, potato salads, rice puddings, and fried rice. These foods can be easily contaminated. Another common mistake is not to cook foods thoroughly and at high-enough temperatures. This is especially true with meats.

Follow the old adage in deciding whether or not to eat leftovers: "When in doubt, throw it out."

Food poisoning can also occur from eating plants that contain toxic chemicals (certain types of mushrooms) or foods contaminated with chemicals (e.g., heavy metals like lead). If you suspect that your child has eaten a poisonous plant, seek medical attention immediately.

Fortunately, most cases of food poisoning are short-lived, and your appetite will return within one to two days. However, head to the emergency room if you or your child has a medical condition that impairs the immune system (e.g., HIV, hepatitis) or displays any of these severe symptoms:

- Violent vomiting
- A fever exceeding 102 degrees F
- Vision problems
- Severe diarrhea that lasts more than one day or contains blood
- Trouble breathing or talking
- Headache and dizziness
- Dehydration

EXAMPLES OF FOOD POISONING

Staphylococcus

Foods that have been handled by people with skin infections can be contaminated when left at room temperature. The classic example is a potato salad left out for a long time at a picnic. Symptoms usually come on very quickly, within 2 to 8 hours, and usually begin to resolve within 12 hours. Symptoms may include

- Severe nausea and vomiting
- Abdominal cramps
- Diarrhea
- Headache and fever

Campylobacter

This infection usually results from poultry that has been infected and not cooked properly. It can also occur from unpasteurized milk and contaminated drinking water. Symptoms usually begin 2 to 5 days after exposure. Symptoms may include

- Diarrhea
- Nausea and vomiting
- Fever
- Abdominal pain and cramping

Salmonella

Infection is by one of the many types of salmonella bacteria. The most common contaminated foods include unpasteurized milk and undercooked poultry and eggs. This infection causes acute intestinal distress, with a sudden onset of headache, fever, abdominal pain, diarrhea, nausea, and sometimes vomiting. Dehydration in infants can be severe. Symptoms start 16 to 48 hours after eating and can last up to 7 days.

Botulism

Home-canned foods are the most common source of the spores that cause toxicity to the nervous system. Commercially prepared foods can also be at fault. The botulinum spores are very resistant to heat. It is recommended that canned foods be exposed to moist heat at 212 degrees F (120 degrees C) for 30 minutes to kill the spores. The toxins that are produced by the spores can be killed through heat by cooking the food at 176 degrees F (80 degrees C) for 30 minutes. Symptoms usually come on 18 to 36 hours after ingestion of the botulinum toxin. This can be a very severe and potentially fatal poisoning. Symptoms can include

- Nausea, vomiting, and abdominal cramps, followed by neurological symptoms such as
  - Vision changes
  - Muscle weakness
  - Difficulty breathing
  - Constipation

Note: Infant botulism occurs most often in children who are less than six months old. Botulinum spores may be present in honey, so it is recommended that children under one year of age not be given honey (as their immune systems may not be able to handle it).

E. Coli

This infection usually occurs as a result of undercooked beef or unpasteurized milk or through fecal-oral contamination. This bacterium infects the digestive tract and typically leads to bloody diarrhea and possibly kidney failure. Young children (younger than five years old) and the elderly are most susceptible to the damaging effects of this infection. Symptoms usually include

- Severe abdominal cramps
- Watery diarrhea, followed by bloody diarrhea (usually lasts 1 to 8 days)
- Fever is usually absent or low grade

Clostridium Perfingens

This bacterium is found in feces, water, soil, air, and water. Contaminated meat left at room temperature is the main source of infection. Symptoms usually begin 6 to 24 hours after ingestion and resolve within 24 hours. Common symptoms include

- Watery diarrhea
- Abdominal cramps

Traveler's Diarrhea

Bacteria endemic to the local water cause this infection. Viruses or bacteria can also cause it. It occurs in areas that lack adequate water purification. Common symptoms include

- Nausea and vomiting
- Loud gurgling noises in the abdomen
- Abdominal cramps
- Diarrhea beginning 12 to 72 hours after ingesting the contaminated water or food

Parasitic Infections

Giardia is the most common example. This parasite is transmitted through the fecal-oral route, mainly through water contamination. In most cases there are no symptoms, and symptoms usually take one to three weeks after exposure to appear. In cases where symptoms occur, the most common are

- Watery, malodorous diarrhea
- Abdominal cramps and distention
- Flatulence and burping
- Nausea
- Low-grade fever
- Fatigue

Chemical Food Poisoning

Plants or animals that contain a naturally occurring poison fall under the heading of chemical food poisoning. Common examples include

- Wild mushrooms (e.g., Amanita phalloides)
- Wild and domestic plants (yew, nightshade, castor bean, morning glory, and many others)
- Fish
- Shellfish

In addition, fruits and vegetables sprayed with insecticides or other chemicals can cause chemical poisoning if the foods are not washed.

Obviously severe cases require conventional treatment that focuses on identifying the type of infectious organism and then prescribing an antimicrobial medicine (e.g., antibiotics for bacterial infections). However, natural therapies are often effective for mild cases and can be used adjunctively for more severe cases.

TREATMENT

Diet

Recommended Food

The most important thing is to keep hydrated by drinking two cups of liquid every waking hour. Try water, diluted fruit and vegetable juices, electrolyte drinks, and broths. If you have a dry mouth or suddenly wrinkled skin that does not snap back when gently pulled, you may be on your way to severe dehydration. Foods that are easy to digest, such as soup, broths, and steamed vegetables, are recommended.

Food to Avoid

During the most intense stages of diarrhea, you will probably not feel much like eating. Do not force yourself to take in solid food during this time (although you should drink plenty of fluids).

As you feel better and regain your appetite, you should stay away from dairy products, fats, and oils, which will only upset your stomach again. If you do not have intolerance to any of these foods, reintroduce them to your diet slowly.

Avoid sugar, especially if you have a bacterial infection. Bacteria feed on it. Even if bacteria aren't the cause of your problem, keep sugar out of your diet; it promotes inflammation, which discourages healing.

Avoid caffeine and alcohol, which are too stimulating to the digestive tract.

If the cause of the problem is not clear, determine whether a food allergy or intolerance caused your diarrhea. Once you feel better, use the elimination diet on page 253 to identify troublesome foods. Many cases of diarrhea can be traced to gluten intolerance, so make a special effort to examine the effects of wheat and seeds on your digestive system.

As you feel better, eat basic, simple foods that are easily absorbed. Soups, cooked fruits and vegetables, and brown rice are all good choices. Apples, bananas, carrots, and potatoes tend to taste especially good at this time, and for an excellent reason. They all contain an ingredient, pectin, that has a gentle binding quality.

One study has shown that roasted carob powder reduces the duration of diarrhea. Try a few tablespoons in some water.

Detoxification

Diarrhea is your body's method of self-detoxification. It's generally a good idea to fast on liquids for the first day; most likely, you will not want to eat solid foods anyway. See the dietary recommendations for details.

℞ Super Seven Prescriptions—Food Poisoning

Super Prescription #1   Homeopathic Combination Diarrhea Remedy and Homeopathic Combination Nausea/Vomiting Remedy
For acute diarrhea and nausea/vomiting, alternate doses of a combination diarrhea and combination nausea/vomiting remedy four times daily for twenty-four hours. Then if you notice improvement, stop taking the remedy, unless symptoms return. If your symptoms do not improve within twenty-four hours, pick the remedy that best matches your symptoms under Homeopathy in this section.

Super Prescription #2   Ginger (*Zingiber officinale*)
Drink a fresh cup of ginger tea, or take 500 mg in capsules or 2 ml of a tincture

every two hours. Ginger reduces intestinal inflammation and lessens the effect of food poisoning.

Super Prescription #3   Probiotic
Take a product containing at least 4 billion active organisms two to three times daily. It contains friendly bacteria, such as *Lactobacillus acidophilus* and *bifidus,* which fight intestinal infection.

Super Prescription #4   Goldenseal (*Hydrastis canadensis*)
Take 1 ml of the tincture or 300 mg in capsule form four times daily. It helps improve diarrhea that is related to an intestinal infection.

Super Prescription #5   Oregano (*Origanum vulgare*) **oil**
Take 500 mg of the capsule form four times daily or as directed on the container. Oregano oil has powerful antimicrobial effects.

Super Prescription #6   Peppermint (*Mentha piperita*)
Take 1 ml of a tincture or 250 mg in capsule form or drink 1 cup of fresh tea every two hours. Peppermint reduces nausea and cramping.

Super Prescription #7   Activated charcoal
Take 3 capsules every two hours for three doses. Activated charcoal capsules taken internally can help to absorb toxins from food poisoning. Charcoal works best when taken in the first stages of food poisoning (when you first realize you have food poisoning).

A study in the *Journal of Gut* reported that live probiotics interact with intestinal cells to protect them from the harmful effect of the bacteria *Escherichia coli* (EIEC 029:NM). Researchers found that these good bacteria prevented the *E. coli* from adhering to the cells and prevented invasion.

GENERAL RECOMMENDATIONS

Parasite Blend

If your doctor suspects that you have a parasite infection, take a herbal parasite blend with herbs such as garlic, black walnut (*Juglans nigra*), wormwood (*Artemisia absinthium*), and grapefruit extract. Take as directed on the container.

Homeopathy

Pick the remedy that best matches your symptoms in this section. For acute symptoms, take a 30C potency four times daily. After you notice improvement, stop taking the remedy, unless symptoms return. Consultation with a homeopathic practitioner is advised.

Arsenicum Album is the most common remedy for food poisoning. Symptoms include diarrhea (especially burning diarrhea), vomiting, chilliness, anxiety, and restlessness. Symptoms tend to be worse between midnight and 2 A.M. The person experiences burning pains in the abdomen. Symptoms are better from warm drinks.

China (*Chinchona*) is a good remedy for diarrhea and bloating that has led to exhaustion and weakness. It is useful to take after an acute bout of food poisoning, to regain strength.

Testing Techniques

The following test helps assess possible reasons for food poisoning:
   Comprehensive stool analysis—bacterial and parasitic infection, flora balance

Ipecacuanha (*Cephaelis ipecacuanha*) is for extreme nauseousness and vomiting. The person experiences a sinking sensation in the stomach. Vomiting does not relieve the symptoms.

Mercurius Corrosivus is for food poisoning that causes bloody, burning diarrhea. The person may alternate between feeling chilly and sweaty.

Nux Vomica (*Strychnos nux vomica*) is for food poisoning that causes heartburn, cramping, and painful diarrhea that feels better temporarily from passing stool or from warm applications. The person is chilly and irritable. This is also a good general remedy to use for the ill effects from food, such as spicy or rich foods.

Phosphorous is a remedy for burning diarrhea, abdominal pain, and vomiting that feel better with cold drinks or cold food.

Podophyllum is for profuse, watery, explosive diarrhea with gas. Stool may contain yellow mucus.

Veratrum Album is indicated when there are profuse, rice-water stools that occur simultaneously with forceful vomiting. The person experiences violent cramping and feels very cold.

Acupressure

Work Stomach 36—four finger widths below the kneecap and one finger width toward the outside of the leg (outside of the shin bone on the muscle).

Bodywork

Hydrotherapy

Constitutional hydrotherapy helps relieve abdominal pain and bring good immune cells into the digestive tract to fight the infection.

Aromatherapy

Add 2 drops of German chamomile and 1 drop of black pepper into a carrier oil, and rub over the person's abdomen.

REFERENCES

Resta-Lenert, S., and K. E. Barrett. 2003. Live probiotics protect intestinal epithelial cells from the effects of infection with enteroinvasive *Escherichia coli* (EIEC). *Gut* 52(7):988–97.

Gallbladder Problems

The gallbladder is a digestive organ located in the upper right portion of the abdomen, directly underneath the liver. It is responsible for storing and concentrating bile that is produced by the liver. Bile is a greenish-yellow color and is composed of bile acids, water, electrolytes, bilirubin, cholesterol, and phospholipids. As food enters the small intestine, hormonal and nervous system activity causes the gallbladder to contract and sends bile through the common bile duct into the beginning portion of the small intestine, known as the duodenum. Bile has several different functions, which include the digestion and the absorption of fats, and the absorption of fat-soluble nutrients, the retention of water in the colon to promote bowel movements, the excretion of bilirubin (degraded red blood cells), the elimination of drugs and other compounds in the body, and the secretion of various proteins involved in gastrointestinal function. As you can see, dysfunction in bile production and secretion can result in many different health problems.

The most common problem associated with the gallbladder is gallstones. It is estimated that 20 percent of people over the age of sixty-five have gallstones. Every year, more than 500,000 people have surgery to remove their gallbladders. The symptoms of gallstones can greatly vary, from person to person. Most people with gallstones often have no symptoms throughout their lives, as the stones pass without problems. Symptoms may include right-sided abdominal pain (or pain anywhere in the abdomen) and radiating pain that goes to the right shoulder blade. Abdominal bloating, gas, belching, and recurrent pain are common, too. Most often, gallstones have been found with a routine exam, and if they are causing no symptoms, they are left alone. Gallstones that cause pain and other symptoms are treated conventionally, with surgery (often using laparoscopy), bile acids taken orally (for stones that are noncalcified), or, more commonly, lithotripsy, the use of shock waves to fragment the stones so that they will pass.

Gallstones are formed as a result of the bile becoming saturated with cholesterol. This can be due to an increase in cholesterol secretion or decreased bile and lecithin secretion. This then causes other particulate matter to attract cholesterol and sets the stage for stone formation. As you will read in this chapter's treatment section, there are natural ways to decrease the saturation of cholesterol in the bile via diet and nutritional supplementation.

Risk factors for gallstones include

Sex: Women are two to four times more likely than men to have gallstones. This, in part, may be due to the use of oral contraceptives and synthetic hormone replacement.

Race: Gallstones are more common in women of North American Indian ethnicity.

Obesity causes an increased secretion of cholesterol into bile. Also, it should be noted that rapid weight loss (during the initial phases) can contribute to gallstone formation.

Age: The frequency increases with age.

A Western diet is a contributing factor.

A positive family history predisposes one to this problem.

Digestive tract diseases, such as Crohn's disease, increase one's risk.

A persistent obstruction of the bile duct can also result in fever, nausea, and vomiting. At this point, the condition is termed acute cholecystitis. This is an acute inflammation of the gallbladder wall as a response to the gallstone obstruction. In rare cases, infection and pus may fill the gallbladder or cause perforation of the gallbladder wall. These situations are dangerous and require immediate surgery. While most cases of acute cholecystitis are surgically treated, people who improve greatly within one to two days may not require surgery if the gallstones are small enough to pass through into the intestinal tract. Ultrasound and X-rays are used to diagnose gallstones and acute cholecystitis.

The natural approaches in this chapter are highly successful in preventing further gallstone formation and gallbladder inflammation/attacks, as long as the present stones are not too large. People with asymptomatic or "silent" gallstones should not require surgery, if the proper diet and supplemental measures are followed.

SYMPTOMS (GALLSTONES AND ACUTE CHOLECYSTITIS)

- Right-sided abdomen pain (or pain anywhere in the abdomen) and radiating pain that goes to the right shoulder blade
- Fever
- Nausea
- Vomiting

ROOT CAUSES

- Drugs, such as oral contraceptives and synthetic hormone replacement and some cholesterol-lowering drugs
- Race (more common in women of North American Indian ethnicity)
- Obesity
- Rapid weight loss
- Constipation
- Western diet (high in saturated fat, low in fiber, alcohol)
- Food allergies/sensitivities (root cause for gallbladder attacks)
- Positive family history
- Increased risk from digestive tract diseases, such as Crohn's

TREATMENT

Diet

Recommended Food

Fiber-rich foods are important in reducing the likelihood of gallstones. A variety of fruits, vegetables, whole grains, and oat bran is recommended. Include five to seven servings of fruits and vegetables a day.

Regularly eat beets, globe artichokes, and organic dandelion greens, as they improve bile flow.

Olive oil has historically been used by nutritionists and naturopathic doctors to improve bile flow. Use it on salads regularly.

Flaxseeds are a highly concentrated source of essential fatty acids, the "good" fats that reduce inflammation. Add flaxseeds to juices, salads, or fruit plates, or use the oil as a salad dressing.

Studies have shown that vegetarians are at a lower risk for gallstones. This does not mean you need to be a strict vegetarian if you have gallstones, but you should greatly increase the amount of plant foods in your diet.

Food to Avoid

Avoid the use of fried foods and foods with a high percentage of saturated fat (dairy products and red meat).

It is important to limit your intake of simple carbohydrates and sugars. Researchers have found that gallstones are rare in countries like Africa, where the diet is low in refined sugars and high in fiber. In one study, 13 people with gallstones ate a diet containing refined carbohydrates for 6 weeks, then consumed a diet of only unrefined carbohydrates for an additional 6 weeks. The cholesterol-saturation index of bile (indicating a tendency to form gallstones) was higher in 12 of the 13 people during the period of time they ate refined carbohydrates.

Food allergies or sensitivities can be a root cause of gallbladder attacks. Since the 1940s, James Breneman, M.D., the former chairman of the Food Allergy Committee of the American College of Allergists, reported that food allergies can initiate gallbladder attacks and gallbladder disease. One study found that 100 percent of a group of patients were symptom free after following an elimination diet that included beef, rye, soy, rice, cherries, peaches, apricots, beets, and spinach for one week. Foods that were most likely to cause gallbladder symptoms in this study included eggs, pork, and onions. Other common triggers included fowl, citrus fruits, milk, coffee, corn, beans, and nuts. Dr. Breneman believes that food allergies cause inflammation and swelling of the bile duct, which restricts bile flow from the gallbladder.

One study found that men who drank coffee had a lower risk of gallstones than men who did not drink coffee. However, coffee initiates gallbladder contractions, so people with known gallstones should avoid its use.

Testing Techniques

The following tests help assess possible reasons for gallstone attacks:

Food allergy/sensitivities—blood or electrodermal

Stool analysis—analyze fat digestion

Essential fatty-acid balance—blood test

℞ Super Seven Prescriptions—Gallbladder Problems

Super Prescription #1   Wild yam root (*Dioscorea villosa*)
Take 2 to 3 ml or 500 mg of the capsule form every hour for the relief of gallbladder spasms and pain. Wild yam root has an antispasmodic effect on the bile duct.

Super Prescription #2   Milk thistle
Take a milk thistle extract standardized to contain a daily total of 420 mg a day. Milk thistle increases bile flow and decreases bile cholesterol saturation.

Super Prescription #3   Lipase enzymes
Take 1 to 2 capsules of lipase enzymes with each meal to improve fat digestion.

Super Prescription #4   Homeopathic China
Take a 30C potency twice daily for two weeks and then stop using it, unless symptoms return. This remedy is helpful for people with gallstones and gallbladder disease that causes bloating, nausea, flatulence, and diarrhea, as well as gallbladder pain.

Super Prescription #5   Dandelion root (*Taraxacum officinale*)
Take 2 ml of tincture or 500 mg of the capsule form with every meal. Dandelion root improves bile flow.

Super Prescription #6   Turmeric (*Curcuma longa*)
Take a product standardized to contain 150 mg of curcumin with each meal. Turmeric has anti-inflammatory properties, improves bile flow, and relaxes the bile duct.

Super Prescription #7   Globe artichoke (*Cynara scolymus*)
Take 1 to 2 ml of the tincture or 500 mg of the capsule form with each meal. Globe artichoke improves bile flow.

General Recommendations

Bile salts are particularly helpful for someone who has had his or her gallbladder removed. Take 1 to 2 tablets of bovine bile salts with each meal to improve digestion and the absorption of fats.

Vitamin C is required to convert cholesterol into bile. Take 500 to 1,000 mg three times per day with meals.

Phosphatidylcholine is a component of lecithin that helps increase the solubility of cholesterol. Take 1,000 mg twice daily.

Fish oil reduces inflammation, and animal studies show that a deficiency of essential fatty acids predisposes you to gallstones. Take a daily dosage of an enteric-coated fish oil product containing at least 480 mg of EPA and 360 mg of DHA twice daily.

Full-spectrum digestive enzymes aid in the digestion of food and make food sensitivities less likely. Take 1 to 2 capsules with each meal.

A probiotic supplies friendly bacteria, such as *Lactobacillus acidophilus* and *bifidus*. These good bacteria are involved with cholesterol and bile acid metabolism. Take a product containing at least 4 billion active organisms daily.

Homeopathy

Pick the remedy that best matches your symptoms in this section. For acute gallstone pain, take a 30C potency four times daily. For chronic gallstone pain, take a 6x, 12x, 6C, 12C, or 30C twice daily for two weeks to see if there are any positive results. After you notice improvement, stop taking the remedy, unless symptoms return. Consultation with a homeopathic practitioner is advised.

Berberis Vulgaris is for sharp, stitching, or colicky pains that radiate from the gallbladder to the stomach or the shoulder. Abdominal pain makes you double over in pain.

Calcarea Carbonica is a good remedy for people with a predisposition to gallbladder problems. The abdomen feels swollen on the right and is sensitive to pressure. The person feels worse from standing, worse from exertion, and better from lying on the painful side. People requiring this remedy are usually overweight and chilly and tire easily. They also tend to feel anxious and overwhelmed. There is a craving for sweets, eggs, and dairy products.

Chelidonium Majus is used when there is pain in the right upper abdomen that radiates to the right shoulder blade. Symptoms are worse from eating fatty foods and better from warm drinks.

China Officinalis is a remedy that is helpful for people with gallstones and gallbladder disease who experience bloating, nausea, flatulence, and diarrhea, as well as gallbladder pain.

Colocynthis is for cramping pains that make a person double over or lie down and apply pressure on the abdomen. Symptoms may come on after anger or suppressed emotions.

Dioscorea is a specific remedy for when people bend backward to relieve the gallbladder pain. Their symptoms are worse from lying down or bending forward. This remedy is indicated when abdominal pain from gallstones is relieved by bending backward and is worse when the person bends forward or lies flat.

Lycopodium is a remedy for gallbladder pain accompanied by bloating and a distended abdomen that feel better from warm drinks or warm applications and from rubbing the abdomen. Gas often occurs in evening (4 to 8 P.M.). People requiring this remedy are often chilly and crave sweets.

Magnesia Phosphorica is helpful for right-sided abdomen pain and gas pains that feel better with warm drinks or warm applications. It is also used for gallbladder spasms.

Nux Vomica is for stitching pains and cramps, accompanied by nausea or heartburn. Symptoms may come on after the consumption of spicy foods, coffee, alcohol, or other stimulants. The person feels chilly, impatient, and irritable.

Pulsatilla is specific for gallbladder pains that come on after eating rich or fatty foods like ice cream. The person feels better in the fresh air and desires consolation when not feeling well.

Acupressure

See pages 668–675 for information about acupressure points and administering treatment.

- Work Stomach 36 to improve digestion.
- Liver 21 and 34 improve gallbladder function.

Bodywork

Reflexology

See pages 686–687 for information about reflexology areas and how to work them.
Work the gallbladder and the liver area to reduce pain and spasm.

Hydrotherapy

Constitutional hydrotherapy is excellent for improving and reducing gallbladder pain and spasms. It can be used for acute bouts and for long-term prevention.

Aromatherapy

Chamomile and lavender are antispasmodic oils that relax abdominal cramps. Dilute some in a carrier oil and use in a massage, or add a few drops to a warm bath. Each oil is also a pleasant stress-reducer.

Stress Reduction

General Stress-Reduction Therapies

For some people, anger and anxiety worsen existing gallbladder problems. Take time to meditate and relax.

Bach Flower Remedies

If none of the following suggestions apply to you, consult the chart on pages 648–650 to find the remedy best suited to your individual needs. Once you have chosen a remedy, place 10 drops of the liquid under your tongue. Hold the drops in place for thirty seconds and swallow. Use as often as needed.

If you are prone to panic attacks or high levels of anxiety, keep a bottle of Rescue Remedy on hand. It will help calm you down in an emergency and keep the emotional problem from affecting your intestines. Rescue Remedy is also useful when you have an acute attack of the disease itself, as it can stave off the tension often produced by extreme physical distress.

Vine is for people whose strong drives and ambition lead to an intolerance of others.

If you have suffered much and are bitter and resentful as a result, Willow will help you regain an appreciation for life.

White Chestnut helps to quiet minds that are plagued by constant, repetitive worries.

Mimulus will help people who are plagued by very specific fears.

For a more generalized anxiety, caused by fears you can't name, take Aspen.

Other Recommendations

Exercise should be part of a program to prevent gallstones.

In a study of over 60,000 women, an average of two to three hours per week of exercise reduced the risk of gallbladder surgery by approximately 20 percent. Choose an exercise system you like and be consistent with it.

REFERENCES

Breneman, J. C. 1968. Allergy elimination diet as the most effective gallbladder diet. *Annals of Allergy* 26:83–87.

Leitzmann, M. F., E. B. Rimm, W. C. Willett, et al. 1999. Recreational physical activity and the risk of cholecystectomy in women. *New England Journal of Medicine* 341:777–84.

Leitzmann, M. F., W. C. Willett, E. B. Rimm, et al. 1999. A prospective study of coffee consumption and the risk of symptomatic gallstone disease in men. *Journal of the American Medical Association* 281:2106–12.

Thornton, J. R., et al. 1983. Diet and gallstones: Effects of refined carbohydrate diets on bile cholesterol saturation and bile acid metabolism. *Gut* 24:2–6.

Gastritis. *See* Ulcers

Glaucoma

Glaucoma affects more than two million Americans and is the second leading cause of blindness in this country. This can be a very serious disease that must be given medical care as soon as possible, if permanent vision loss is to be avoided. In the healthy eye, fluid is produced and drained at equal rates. If the fluid cannot drain properly, it builds up and puts pressure on the optic nerve, the retina, and the lens. This pressure can partially damage or even completely destroy the retina and the optic nerve.

If the outflow channels are open and become blocked with debris, the disorder is called open-angle glaucoma. Chronic open-angle glaucoma is the most common form and usually occurs over the years. Fluid drains too slowly from the anterior chamber of the eye and pressure builds up. At first, increased pressure in the eyes produces no symptoms. As the disease progresses, symptoms may include narrowing peripheral vision, mild headaches, and vague visual disturbances, such as seeing halos around electric lights or having difficulty adapting to darkness. At some point, tunnel vision—where the visual field narrows and makes it hard to see anything on either side when looking forward—may develop.

If the channels are blocked by the iris, the disorder is called closed-angle glaucoma. Fluid pressure increases quickly and causes intense pain in one eye, along with headaches and vision problems, including blurring or a "halo effect" around lights. The eyeball feels hard to the touch, and the pain may be so severe that it causes nausea and even vomiting. The eyelid swells, and the eye becomes red and watery. These symptoms are warning signs that you must receive medical care immediately.

Permanent vision loss and even total blindness can settle in after just a few days. Fortunately, acute glaucoma is rather rare and accounts for only 10 percent of all glaucoma cases. Certain medications, long periods spent in darkness, and stress are all potential triggers for an attack.

Since the disease targets older people most frequently, anyone over sixty-five should make glaucoma tests part of their annual eye exam. African Americans, who have a much higher incidence of glaucoma than the rest of the population does, should start getting annual tests after the age of forty, as should anyone with diabetes. If at any age you experience a loss of peripheral vision, constant low-level headaches, eye pain, or blurred vision that is not corrected with one new lens prescription, see a doctor at once. If you test positive for glaucoma, you may not be able to recover the damage that's already been done, but there's a good chance that you can significantly slow the progress of the disease.

There does not seem to be one single cause of glaucoma. Most likely, a variety of factors come into play. A good strategy for prevention, as well as treatment in conjunction with a doctor's care, incorporates reducing the general number of toxins in the body, eating foods that support the eye, correcting nutritional deficiencies associated with glaucoma, enhancing digestion, avoiding medications that predispose one to glaucoma, and reducing stress.

SYMPTOMS OF OPEN-ANGLE GLAUCOMA

- Narrowing peripheral vision
- Mild headaches
- Vague visual disturbances
- Tunnel vision

SYMPTOMS OF CLOSED-ANGLE GLAUCOMA

Chronic glaucoma is usually asymptomatic until irreversible damage has already been done. Signs that chronic glaucoma has already progressed include the following:

- Intense pain in one eye, with vision problems
- Nausea and vomiting
- Swollen eyelid
- Red, watery eye
- Vision loss

ROOT CAUSES

- Accumulation of wastes and metabolic slowdown related to aging
- High blood pressure
- Some prescription drugs, including corticosteroids, antidepressants, and blood pressure medication
- Certain illness, such as other eye disorders (especially macular degeneration) and diabetes
- Nutritional deficiency
- Heredity

TREATMENT

If you have glaucoma of either kind, you must be under a doctor's care. The therapies listed here will complement and support your conventional treatment. Natural therapies work very well for chronic and open-angle glaucoma.

Testing Techniques

The following tests help assess possible reasons for glaucoma:

Blood pressure

Hormone testing (thyroid)—saliva, blood, or urine

Intestinal permeability—urine

Detoxification profile—urine

Vitamin and mineral analysis (especially magnesium, vitamin C)—blood

Food and environmental allergies/sensitivities—blood, electrodermal

Blood-sugar balance—blood

Diet

Recommended Food

Eat a basic, wholesome diet based on whole grains and fresh fruits and vegetables.

Carotenoids are essential for optimum eye health. Consume plenty of orange, yellow, and green leafy vegetables. It is also highly recommended that you drink live juice made from these and other fruits and vegetables several times a day.

The bioflavonoid anthocyanidin fights free radicals and helps keep the collagen around the eye healthy and flexible. Blueberries and cherries are excellent sources.

Drink a glass of clean water every two waking hours to flush out toxins and to keep the eye tissues supple. Spread your consumption of water and other liquids out across the day, so that you do not build up pressure in your eye.

Some studies have shown fish oils to lower eye pressure. Incorporate fatty fish such as salmon, mackerel, and cod into your meals two or three times a week.

Chromium and magnesium both have beneficial effects on glaucoma. Brewer's yeast is the best source of chromium; kelp, leafy greens, apples, and safflower and sesame oils will provide you with magnesium.

Food to Avoid

If you have glaucoma, do not take the herb ephedra (*Ma huang*), which dilates the pupils and may increase eye pressure.

Fluid retention in the eye may be a response to food allergies. See the Food Allergies section to determine whether a food is contributing to your problem. If you find that consumption of a certain food makes your eyes red, irritated, painful, or tender, you must avoid that product from now on.

Caffeine has been shown to reduce blood flow to the eye, so avoid coffee, chocolate, and caffeinated teas and sodas.

A toxic liver may be related to eye problems. Avoid alcohol, which puts a terrible burden on this essential organ.

℞ Super Seven Prescriptions—Glaucoma

Super Prescription #1   Magnesium
Take 250 mg twice daily. Magnesium relaxes the blood vessel walls and improves blood flow to the eye.

Super Prescription #2   Vitamin C
Take 1,000 mg two to four times daily. Studies show that vitamin C supplementation reduces eye pressure.

Super Prescription #3   Fish oil

Take a formula containing a daily dose of 600 mg of EPA and 400 mg of DHA. Animal studies using this supplement show a significant drop in intraocular pressure.

Super Prescription #4   Alpha lipoic acid

Take 100 mg twice daily. This antioxidant has been shown to improve vision for some people with this disease.

Super Prescription #5   Bilberry (*Vaccinium myrtillus*)

Take 160 mg twice daily of a 25 percent anthocyanosides extract. Bilberry improves blood flow and contains flavonoids that support eye structure and function.

Super Prescription #6   Ginkgo biloba

Take 60 mg three times daily of a 24 percent flavone glycoside extract. Ginkgo has been shown to be helpful for glaucoma. It improves blood flow and contains flavonoids that support eye structure and function.

Super Prescription #7   Chromium

Take 250 to 500 mcg twice daily. It is particularly important for people with diabetes to supplement for blood-sugar balance and the prevention of glaucoma.

Studies using 2,000 mg or more a day of vitamin C demonstrate that this nutrient lowers intraocular pressure in people with glaucoma. One study found that vitamin C reduced intraocular pressure by a whopping 16 mm Hg. An even more aggressive approach is to consult with a physician who uses intravenous vitamin C. The benefits of vitamin C are only present as long as one is supplementing this nutrient.

General Recommendations

Grape seed extract or maritime pine bark improves circulation. Take 100 to 200 mg daily.

Rutin is a bioflavonoid that has been shown in older studies to help glaucoma. Take 20 mg three times daily.

Homeopathy

Chronic glaucoma is a constitutional disorder, so see a homeopathic practitioner for a specific remedy that suits your individual tendencies and needs.

Acupressure

These points are especially helpful for people who use their eyes a great deal and suffer from eyestrain. For information about pressure points and administering treatment, see pages 668–675.

- Stomach 3 relieves pressure on the eyes.
- Bladder 10 soothes eyes that are tired and red from eyestrain.
- Improve blood flow to your head and eyes by working Large Intestine 3 and 4.

Bodywork

Massage can't relieve glaucoma directly, but neck and head massage will ease stress and improve circulation to the eye area.

Chiropractic, craniosacral, or osteopathic treatments may also be helpful.

Reflexology

See pages 686–687 for information about reflexology areas and how to work them.

Work the areas corresponding to the eyes, the neck, and the kidneys.

Aromatherapy

Stress is a trigger for acute glaucoma and may be a contributing factor in the chronic version. Many oils can help you handle tension and anxiety, but here are some good ones to start: bergamot, jasmine, lavender, rose, sandalwood, or ylang ylang. You can use them in any preparation you like, but do be sure not to rely on just one oil, as it might lose some of its effects from overuse.

Stress Reduction

General Stress-Reduction Therapies

Stress may contribute to glaucoma, and it's definitely caused by glaucoma: For many people, vision problems mark a significant change of life. Consider learning to meditate. You'll reduce daily tension, and you can practice the technique for the rest of your life, no matter what the condition of your eyes.

Bach Flower Remedies

Select the appropriate remedy and place 10 drops of the liquid under your tongue. Hold the drops in place for thirty seconds and swallow. Use as often as needed.

For an attack of acute glaucoma, Rescue Remedy can help you handle the pain calmly as you seek professional help. Do not use Rescue Remedy in place of medical care.

Within the Bach remedy philosophy, eye problems are thought to be connected to clouded internal vision and a refusal to see the world as it is.

If you tend to be dreamy and live in a fantasy world, try Clematis.

Honeysuckle is for people who want to avoid present concerns and spend a great deal of time in nostalgia for the past.

If you have vague, general fears that you can't name, let alone confront, take Aspen.

Other Recommendations

Avoid eyestrain from reading or working at computer terminals for long periods. Take frequent breaks and look away from the screen or your reading material often.

Don't watch television in the dark. Prolonged periods in the darkness with the pupils dilated can bring on acute glaucoma.

Tobacco smoke reduces blood flow to the retina, so don't smoke. You must also avoid smoky rooms, bars, and restaurants.

Mild to moderate aerobic exercise can reduce eye pressure, so find an activity you enjoy and make it a daily habit.

Wear sunglasses that block UVA and UVB rays; both kinds of light create free radicals that have been linked to glaucoma.

REFERENCES

Filina, A. A., N. G. Davydova, S. N. Endrikhovskii, et al. 1995. Lipoic acid as a means of metabolic therapy of open-angle glaucoma. *Vestnik Oftalmolgii* 111:6–8.

Ringsdorf, W. M., Jr., and E. Cheraskin. 1981. Ascorbic acid and glaucoma: A review. *Journal of Holistic Medicine* 3:167–72.

Virno, M., et al. 1967. "Oral treatment of glaucoma with vitamin C." *Eye Ear Nose Throat Monthly* 46:1502–8.

Gout

Gout is an intensely painful disorder caused by the buildup of uric acid. Although it affects both sexes, men are much more likely—by a factor of ten—to suffer from gout. The condition was once known as the "rich man's disease," and, in fact, it often strikes people who eat heavy, fatty foods and who overindulge in alcohol. Although this kind of diet was once solely the province of the wealthy, one no longer has to be rich to eat poorly. Today, the disease affects people across the entire spectrum of economic classes.

Uric acid is a metabolic by-product of protein breakdown. Purines raise uric acid levels in the body. Most purines are created by the body, but a few are taken in through food and drink. Since purines can't be absorbed, they are normally broken down by a digestive enzyme that allows them to be dissolved and passed out of the body in urine. If there is more uric acid than the enzymes can break down, the acid accumulates in the tissues and the bloodstream. Eventually, it crystallizes into needle-shaped deposits. These sharp crystals of uric acid poke their way into the tissue that surrounds a joint and ultimately penetrate the joint itself. The resulting pain is extreme and is usually followed by redness and swelling of the joint, which may be highly sensitive to the touch. The pain may go on for days or even weeks, and unless the cause of gout is addressed, the attack is likely to recur. A person with gout is also more likely to suffer from uric acid kidney stones. Gout most often occurs in the joint at the base of the big toe, but it may also appear in other locations like the ankle, the thumb, the wrist, the elbow, and even the earlobe.

Newer research is demonstrating that people with insulin resistance are more susceptible to gout. It is estimated that 76 percent of people with gout have insulin resistance. With this condition, the cells become resistant to the hormone insulin, and blood glucose levels remain high. This in turn leads to increased insulin levels and a resulting uric acid increase. If you follow a syndrome X–type diet (one rich in plant foods, moderate protein consumption—especially fish—and low in saturated fat and refined carbohydrates), uric acid decreases and the resultant gout flare-ups can be prevented. This, along with a calorie-restricted diet and exercise, should be the primary plan for people with gout.

Conventional medicines that lower the levels of uric acid are available, but you should consider them a last resort. For hundreds of years, the best way to treat gout has been with diet and detoxification therapies. Sometimes doctors automatically prescribe medication for gout because they don't believe their patients will commit to changing their diets. If your doctor suggests medication for you, explain to him or her that you're willing to try a new eating plan. You may find that you can forgo harsh medicines entirely.

SYMPTOMS

- Sharp pain, usually in a single joint and most often in the big toe
- Inflamed, red joints that feel hot and are tender to the touch
- Fever

ROOT CAUSES

- A diet high in saturated fats, refined carbohydrates, and alcohol
- Insulin resistance

- Dehydration (in people susceptible to gout)
- Obesity
- Kidney disease
- Surgery
- Joint injury
- Stress

- Pharmaceutical medications that increase uric acid (e.g., aspirin, diuretics, and high-dose niacin therapy)
- Lead toxicity
- High blood pressure
- Acidic system

South African researchers placed men with a history of gout on a nonconventional diet more suited for people with insulin resistance. The diet was higher in protein, complex carbohydrates (instead of refined carbs), and polyunsaturated and monounsaturated fats (instead of saturated fats). High purine foods, such as poultry and fish, were not restricted. After four months on this diet, the average number of gout attacks fell by two thirds. The average decrease in uric acid was 18 percent. In addition, there was an average loss of seventeen pounds and improvements in lipid markers such as lowered LDL cholesterol and triglycerides, and improved good HDL cholesterol.

TREATMENT

Diet

Recommended Food

For the first stages of an attack, see the detoxification suggestions further on.

After the pain has subsided, introduce whole grains, nuts, seeds, and soy products into your meals. These foods are high in fiber, which encourages the elimination of uric acid, and soy products are excellent vegetarian sources of protein. Continue to eat several helpings of raw fruits and vegetables daily.

Berries, especially cherries, strawberries, and blueberries, neutralize uric acid. Eat fresh berries as snacks or for dessert, and drink a glass of cherry juice every day.

Flaxseeds are a highly concentrated source of essential fatty acids, the "good" fats that reduce inflammation. Add flaxseeds to juices, salads, or fruit plates, or use the oil as a salad dressing.

One of the most important foods you can eat to prevent gout is fish. Eat fish such as salmon, cod, halibut, and sardines, as they reduce inflammation.

Drink as much clean water as you can. One glass every two waking hours should be your minimum consumption.

Food to Avoid

The traditional approach for treating gout has been to eliminate from your diet foods that are high in purines: red meat, meat broths and gravies, bouillon, consommé, sweetbreads, shellfish, anchovies, sardines, herring, mushrooms, asparagus, brewer's yeast, fish, poultry, eggs, dried beans, peas, lentils, cooked spinach and rhubarb. However, this is not only not necessary but for people with insulin resistance (the majority of gout sufferers), this can make your gout problem worse. Instead, focus on eating the foods in the recommended food list.

Rich foods aggravate gout pain. Stay away from saturated, hydrogenated and partially hydrogenated fats and oils, and do not eat products made with refined flour or sugar.

Alcohol increases uric acid levels. If you suffer from gout, you must not drink alcohol in any form.

Detoxification

During an acute episode of gout, you may not feel much like eating. This response is useful, as it helps your body focus on eliminating the uric acid and discourages you from eating foods that may make the condition worse. When the pain begins, start a three-day juice fast; drink large quantities of cherry juice and green drinks (wheatgrass, chlorella, spirulina, etc.) and include plenty of clean water and herbal teas. This fast will help speed the elimination of uric acid and reduce inflammation. Do not fast for more than three days, however, as prolonged periods without food can have a reverse effect and actually raise the levels of uric acid in your body.

After the fast, limit yourself to raw fruits and vegetables (along with juices, herbal teas, and water) for several days or until the pain subsides. These foods will encourage further elimination of uric acid and will realkalinize your body's internal environment.

A study of twelve people with gout found that eating one-half pound of fresh or canned cherries or drinking a full quart of cherry juice prevented gout attacks. In all twelve people, uric acid levels returned to normal, and the gout attacks ceased. Black, sweet yellow, and red sour cherries were all effective.

Testing Techniques

The following tests help assess possible reasons for gout:

   Urinary pH—urine

   Blood pressure

   Detoxification profile—urine

   Vitamin and mineral analysis (especially magnesium, folic acid, B6, B12)—blood

   Food and environmental allergies/sensitivities—blood, electrodermal

   Blood-sugar balance—blood

℞ Super Seven Prescription—Gout

Super Prescription #1   Homeopathic Colchicum
Take a 30C potency every waking two hours for two days. This homeopathic remedy is specific for gout pains that are worse with any motion.

Super Prescription #2   Celery seed extract
Take 450 mg two to three times daily to treat and prevent gout. Celery seed extract has anti-inflammatory effects and may reduce uric acid levels.

Super Prescription #3   Nettle root (*Urtica dioica*)
Nettle root encourages the elimination of uric acid from the kidneys. Select a product made with the concentrated root extract, and take 250 mg three times a day.

Super Prescription #4   Fish oil
Take a daily dosage of a fish oil product containing at least 480 mg of EPA and 360 mg of DHA. Fish oil reduces inflammation in the joints.

Super Prescription #5   Chlorella
Take 500 mg four times daily. Chlorella is rich in chlorophyll and works to alkalinize the body.

Super Prescription #6   Bromelain
Take 500 mg three times daily between meals. Look for products standardized to 2,000 M.C.U. (milk-clotting units) per 1,000 mg or 1,200 G.D.U. (gelatin-dissolving units) per 1,000 mg. Bromelain has a natural anti-inflammatory effect. Protease enzyme products also have this benefit.

Super Prescription #7   Folic acid
Take 10 to 40 mg daily, under the supervision of a doctor. High doses of folic acid may help reduce uric acid levels.

People with gout should avoid high doses of niacin (more than 1,000 mg), as it can increase uric acid in some individuals.

General Recommendations

Quercitin has natural anti-inflammatory effects. Take 500 to 1,000 mg three times daily.

Devil's claw (*Harpagophytum procumbens*) should not be taken if you have a history of gallstones, heartburn, or ulcers. Take 1,500 to 2,500 mg of the standardized powdered herb in capsule or tablet form daily, or use 1 to 2 ml of a tincture three times a day.

Dandelion root (*Taraxacum officinalis*) cleanses the kidneys. Take 500 mg or 1 to 2 ml three times daily. Be sure the preparation you use is made from the dried root.

A cream made with capsicum (cayenne pepper) has a remarkable and documented ability to relieve pain. You can find capsicum cream at most health food stores. Apply the cream to the affected area two to four times daily for symptomatic relief. Choose a cream standardized to 0.025 to 0.075 percent capsaicin. Capsaicin depletes the nerves of substance P, a neurotransmitter that transmits pain messages.

Homeopathy

Pick the remedy that best matches your symptoms in this section. For acute gout pain, take a 30C potency four times daily. For low-grade gout pain, take a lower potency, such as 6x, 12x, or 12C, twice daily for two weeks to see if there are any positive results. After you notice improvement, stop taking the remedy, unless symptoms return. Consultation with a homeopathic practitioner is advised.

Arnica (*Arnica montana*) is for deep, bruising pain.

Belladonna (*Atropa belladonna*) is for intense, throbbing, and burning pain that comes on quickly. The joint looks red and is worse from jarring.

Bryonia (*Bryonia alba*) is for pain that intensifies with the slightest touch or movement. The person becomes very irritable.

Ledum (*Ledum palustre*) is the remedy for throbbing pain that is better from ice and cold-water applications. The knees and the feet are affected.

Pulsatilla (*Pulsatilla pratensis*) will ease pain that moves around within the joint and that improves with gentle motion and the application of a cold compress.

Rhododendron is for gout of the big toe that flares up before a storm. Warm applications feel better.

Sulphur is for gout where there is a burning sensation and itching of the skin. Symptoms are better with cold applications and worse from any heat.

Acupressure

No matter where gout surfaces in your body, you can use Large Intestine 4 to significantly reduce the pain.

Bodywork

Massage

Do not rub the painful joint, as a local massage will only aggravate the pain. (During an acute attack, you probably won't even want to touch the area.) However, a lymphatic massage for the rest of the body will help break down toxins, and it will help distract you, albeit temporarily, from the gout. Add juniper oil to the massage for added detoxification benefits.

Reflexology

See pages 686–687 for information about reflexology areas and how to work them.

Work the areas corresponding to the kidneys and to the body part affected by gout.

Hydrotherapy

Some people find that cold water is welcome relief for a "hot" joint; others find that warm or hot hydrotherapy is more soothing. You will probably know instinctively which is best for you, so choose between the following suggestions accordingly.

During an acute attack, hold the joint under cold running water. Follow up with a cool bath.

Constitutional hydrotherapy can be used to help with acute gout and prevent further problems, due to its detoxifying qualities.

Other Bodywork Recommendations

Apply a hot or cold compress to the affected joint. To speed up the expulsion of uric acid, you can add juniper oil to the compress.

Acupuncture can be very helpful for acute gout.

Aromatherapy

Juniper oil helps break down toxic deposits and carries them away from the body. Add it to a hot sitz bath or a compress, or dilute it in a carrier oil and use in a massage (but don't rub the affected joint directly).

Stress Reduction

Meditation is an excellent therapy for people suffering from gout. With practice, you can learn how to focus so intensely that you can switch your attention away from pain. And since stress and tension often trigger attacks of gout, regular stress-reduction techniques such as positive imagery may help reduce your chances of a recurring episode.

Bach Flower Remedies

See the chart on pages 648–650 to find the remedy that best suits your personality and tendencies. Once you've chosen a remedy, place 10 drops of the liquid under your tongue. Hold the drops in place for thirty seconds and swallow. Use as often as needed.

Rescue Remedy is for any emotional or physical crisis. Take it when gout pain starts up, or when you experience some emotionally stressful event that might trigger the pain.

If you tend to be frustrated by people who don't share your way of doing things, take Beech. It will help develop your tolerance.

Gorse is for people who are overwhelmed by their illness and who feel that nothing can be done to improve their condition.

Holly will help people who project a confident, even aggressive, image, but who are eaten up inside by feelings of insecurity or jealousy.

If you are a busy, quick-thinking sort who cannot tolerate slow-moving people, Impatiens will help.

If you feel apathetic and resigned to having gout, Wild Rose would be a good selection.

Other Recommendations

- Exercise will stimulate blood flow and decrease pain. Try a nonimpact sport like swimming.
- Magnet therapy can be effective in alleviating the pain of gout. Use as directed by a knowledgeable practitioner.
- People who are overweight are more vulnerable to gout than others are. If you need to lose weight, the dietary suggestions here can help. For further suggestions, see Obesity.

REFERENCES

Blau, L. W. 1950. Cherry diet control for gout and arthritis. *Texas Reports on Biology and Medicine* 8:309–11.

Dessein, P. H., E. A. Shipton, A. E. Stanwix, B. I. Joffe, and J. Ramokgadi. 2000. Beneficial effects of weight loss associated with moderate calorie/carbohydrate restriction, and increased proportional intake of protein and unsaturated fat on serum urate and lipoprotein levels in gout: A pilot study. *Annals of the Rheumatic Diseases* 59(7):539–43.

Hair Loss

As part of the body's renewal process, most of us lose 50 to 100 hairs every day. The average rate of growth is approximately ½ inch per month. Interestingly, hair grows fastest in the summer, as heat and friction speed up growth. Conversely, it grows slower in the cold and the winter months. More rapid hair loss begins in both sexes by age fifty and tends to accelerate once people reach their fifties. A human adult body has an average of 5 million hairs, with 100,000 to 150,000 of those located on the scalp.

Since most of us also grow new strands to replace the ones that have been shed, there's usually no reason to worry about a few stray hairs that come out with a good brushing or that swirl down the drain after a shower. Hair loss poses a potential problem only if it leads to noticeable thinning or balding, and even then, it is often a normal part of life.

Genetics and hormones determine the most common reasons for hair loss. Male pattern baldness is characterized by a receding hairline and loss of hair, especially on the crown of the head. By age forty, two-thirds of Caucasian men are noticeably bald. Female pattern baldness is characterized by a general thinning of the hair all over the head and a moderate loss of hair on the crown or the hairline. It also occurs between the ages of thirty and forty and often becomes more apparent during and after menopause. About 50 percent of children with a balding parent of either sex will inherit the dominant baldness gene.

Besides age and genetics, the main culprit in balding appears to be an overabundance or overactivity of the male hormone dihydrotestosterone (DHT) within the hair follicle. DHT is a derivative of testosterone and is driven by an enzyme called 5-alpha reductase, which is produced in the prostate, the adrenal glands, and the scalp. The activity of this enzyme tends to increase as people, especially men, age. It also causes the hair follicle to degrade, and it shortens the growth phase. Some follicles die, but most shrink and produce weaker hairs that become thinner, many to the point where they fall out from daily activities. Another important hormone is progesterone. Menopausal women commonly find improvement with the use of natural progesterone for excessive hair loss.

Other physiological factors might cause hair loss. Recently, a group of Japanese researchers reported a correlation between excessive sebum in the scalp and hair loss. Excessive sebum, often accompanying thinning hair, is attributed to an enlargement of the sebaceous gland. The researchers believe that excessive sebum causes a high level of 5-alpha reductase and pore clogging, thus malnutrition of the hair root. Animal fat in the diet is believed to increase sebum production. Medical researchers in Asia also believe that hair loss is caused mainly by an insufficient blood supply to the scalp.

The effects of stress can be a cause of hair loss and thinning in both men and women. Generally, this type of hair loss or thinning is reversible once the levels of stress have calmed down or the person has dealt with the stress sufficiently.

In addition, various autoimmune and other systemic diseases can lead to hair loss. The list includes many conditions, ranging from psoriasis and thyroid disease, to cancer.

Other reasons for hair loss and thinning may include strict dieting (the loss is due to malnutrition), heavy metal toxicity (e.g., arsenic), chemotherapy, and severe illness. Several different nutrient deficiencies can contribute to hair loss, brittleness, or thinning. When it comes to hair loss, the most common in women is iron deficiency. You will need a blood test by your doctor to see if this is occurring.

Genetic Baldness . . . or Medication?

If you experience thinning or receding hair, chances are that you're seeing the first signs of genetic pattern baldness. Before you come to a conclusion, however, you should run a check of any medications you might be taking. Many pharmaceutical medications cause hair loss, such as the following:

Cholesterol-lowering drugs:

clofibrate (Atromid-S) and gemfibrozil (Lopid)

Parkinson medications:

levodopa (Dopar, Larodopa)

Ulcer drugs:

cimetidine (Tagamet), ranitidine (Zantac), and famotidine (Pepcid)

Anticoagulents:

Coumarin and heparin

Agents for gout:

allopurinol (Loporin, Zyloprim)

Antiarthritics:

penicillamine, auranofin (Ridaura),

indomethacin (i\Indocin), naproxen (Naprosyn), sulindac (Clinoril), and methotrexate (Folex)

Drugs derived from vitamin A:

isotretinoin (Accutane) and etretinate (Tegison)

Anticonvulsants for epilepsy:

trimethadione (Tridione)

Antidepressants:

tricyclics, amphetamines

Beta-blocker drugs for high blood pressure:

atenolol (Tenormin), metoprolol (Lopressor), nadolol (Corgard), propranolol (Inderal), and timolol (Blocadren)

Antithyroid agents:

carbimazole, iodine, thiocyanate, thiouracil

Others:

Blood thinners, male hormones (anabolic steroids), and chemotherapeutic agents

It is common for women who are going through menopause to experience hair loss and thinning. This is due to the fluctuating changes in many of their hormones. Natural hormone-balancing protocols, administered by a knowledgeable doctor, can reverse this hair loss. Also, low levels of thyroid hormone can result in hair loss in women and men of all ages. This can include thinning of the eyebrows. Hypothyroidism often develops around menopause or during pregnancy. On the other hand, hyperthyroidism can be the cause of hair loss as well.

No matter whether you have a temporary or permanent condition, many complementary therapies exist that can help you improve your hair and scalp health. While they can't completely reverse permanent baldness, many treatments can encourage small but significant regrowth.

SYMPTOMS

- Receding hairline
- Thinning hair
- Hair that falls out in patches

ROOT CAUSES

- Heredity
- Hormone imbalance (particularly, thyroid)
- Serious illness, especially with a high fever
- Pregnancy
- Menopause
- Stress
- Chemotherapy
- Hypothyroidism
- Autoimmune disorders
- Crash or fad diets
- Syphilis
- Extremely high doses of vitamin A
- Nutritional deficiencies
- Heavy metal toxicity
- Poor scalp circulation
- Malabsorption, parasites

TREATMENT

Diet

Recommended Food

Hair loss can be caused or aggravated by poor diet. Make sure to eat varied, well-rounded meals made from basic foods. Include plenty of whole grains, vegetables, and quality protein (such as beans, nuts, fish, and lean poultry).

Biotin promotes hair and scalp health and, in some cases, can even prevent hair loss. The best sources of biotin are nuts, brown rice, brewer's yeast, and oats. Many of these foods are also high in B vitamins, which promote hair growth.

Iron is essential for hair growth. Take a spoonful of unsulfured blackstrap molasses every day, and include several of the following foods in your meals: green leafy vegetables (except spinach), leeks, cashews, berries, dried fruits, and figs.

Your body needs vitamin C to absorb iron; eat citrus fruit after an iron-rich meal.

Testing Techniques

The following tests help assess possible reasons for hair loss:

Hormone testing (thyroid)—saliva, blood, or urine

Intestinal permeability—urine

Vitamin and mineral analysis (especially iron)—blood

Heavy metal toxicity—hair or urine

Stool analysis—parasites

Eat nuts, seeds, and avocados for vitamin E, a nutrient that keeps the scalp in good condition. Olive oil is another excellent source.

Foods containing essential fatty acids, as found in nuts (walnuts), flaxseeds, and fish, are important.

Food to Avoid

Avoid foods that deplete your system of nutrients and impair circulation, such as saturated and hydrogenated fats, refined flour and sugar, and processed food.

℞ Super Seven Prescriptions—Hair Loss

Super Prescription #1   Saw palmetto (*Serenoa repens*)
Take 320 to 400 mg daily of an 85 percent liposterolic extract.
This herb has historically been used by herbalists for hair loss in men and women. Recent research shows it to be effective for men.

Super Prescription #2   Essential fatty acids
Take a combination formula containing a blend of omega-3 and omega-6 fatty acids. Take 4,000 mg of fish or flaxseed oil and evening primrose or borage oil containing 200 mg of GLA daily.

Super Prescription #3   Biotin
Take 2,000 to 3,000 mcg daily.

Super Prescription #4   Methylsulfonylmethane (MSM)
Take 3,000 mg daily. It contains the mineral sulfur, which helps promote hair development.

Super Prescription #5   Fo Ti (*Polygonum multiflorum* or He shou-wu)
Take 500 mg three times daily. This Chinese herb is used by practitioners of Oriental medicine to slow or stop hair loss, although it is mainly used in formulas with other herbs.

Super Prescription #6   Silica (*Silicea*)
Take 500 mg twice daily. This mineral fosters hair development.

Super Prescription #7   Rosemary essential oil
Apply 3 to 5 drops per 1 ounce of shampoo daily to improve scalp circulation.

General Recommendations

Zinc is a mineral required for hair development. Take 30 mg daily, along with 3 mg of copper.

Natural progesterone cream can be helpful for women with low levels, particularly women in menopause. See the Menopause section for proper use.

Enzymes improve the absorption of foods and nutrients. Take a full-spectrum complex with each meal.

Take a high-potency multivitamin daily to provide a base of the nutrients required for healthy hair.

A B-complex supplement combats the effects of stress and contains vitamins in the B family that contribute to healthy hair. Take a 50 mg complex twice daily.

A greens formula that includes super green foods, such as chlorella, spirulina, barley, and wheatgrass, provides a host of hair-healthy nutrients. Take as directed on the container.

A study in the *Journal of Alternative and Complementary Medicine* reported that a product containing saw palmetto (*Serenoa repens*) and a plant compound called beta-sitosterol (also found in saw palmetto and other plants) may increase hair growth in men. This study included 19 men between the ages of 23 and 64 years who had mild to moderate hair loss. They were given either a placebo or a supplement containing 400 mg of a standardized extract of saw palmetto and 100 mg of beta-sitosterol per day. After about five months, hair growth in 60 percent of the men taking the herbal combination had improved, compared with their initial evaluation. Only 11 percent of those receiving the placebo had any improvement.

A vitamin B12 deficiency may be at the root of hair loss. Take as part of a B-complex or take 200 to 400 mcg of the sublingual form daily.

Homeopathy

Pick the remedy that best matches your symptoms in this section. Take a 6x, 12x, 6C, 12C, or 30C potency twice daily for two weeks to see if there are any positive results. After you notice improvement, stop taking the remedy, unless symptoms return. Consultation with a homeopathic practitioner is advised.

Arsenicum Album is helpful when hair loss is the result of stress. The person is very fearful and restless.

Ignatia (*Ignatia amara*) is for hair loss that comes on with acute grief or an emotional trauma.

Lycopodium (*Lycopodium clavatum*) is for premature balding and graying of the hair. People who require this remedy often have digestive problems and crave sweets.

Natrum Muriaticum is for hair loss accompanied by depression, a strong salt craving, and an aversion to being in the sun.

Phosphoric Acidum is for hair loss that is accompanied by fatigue and mental debility. Hair loss may come after grief or sorrow. There is often a craving for carbonated beverages.

Sepia is helpful when there is a hormone imbalance–related hair loss, as seen during menopause or after using the birth control pill.

Silica (*Silicea*) is helpful when there has been a chronic illness, accompanied by hair loss. The hair is brittle, and the person tends to be thin, chilly, and easily fatigued.

Acupressure

See pages 668–675 for information about pressure points and administering treatment.

- If you have been eating poorly or have suffered from an illness, work Stomach 36 to encourage maximum absorption of nutrients into your bloodstream.

Bodywork

Massage
A scalp massage will increase circulation to the head and will help hair follicles receive nutrients from the blood.

Aromatherapy
Rosemary oil will stimulate hair growth. Take a few minutes before a shampoo to rub some into your hair and scalp.

If you need to reduce stress, essential oils can help. Lavender, chamomile, jasmine, rose, and geranium all have relaxing properties, as do many others. See page 658 for more suggestions. Find a few that you enjoy and use them in baths, massages, or diffusers, or just hold the bottle under your nose and inhale deeply.

Stress Reduction

If you experience so much stress that your hair is falling out, you may need a therapist to help you cope. Hair loss is often related to shock or grief; look for a professional who has experience with your particular problem.

Any of the strategies in the Exercise and Stress Reduction chapter can help you with long-term stress management. Find the therapy you like best and practice it regularly.

Bach Flower Remedies

See the chart on pages 648–650 to find the remedy that best suits your personality and tendencies. Once you've chosen a remedy, place 10 drops of the liquid under your tongue. Hold the drops in place for thirty seconds and swallow. Use as often as needed.

Rescue Remedy is the treatment of choice for cases of shock or panic.

If you have recently been in an accident, or if a natural disaster has brought grief to you or your family, take Rock Rose.

If you have been mourning for a long time and tend to retreat into the happier times of the past, Honeysuckle will help you come to terms with your present situation.

Other Recommendations

- Exercise increases circulation everywhere, including the scalp. Talk a walk daily.
- Be gentle to your hair. When it's wet, use a wide-toothed comb to separate the strands, or, if possible, let your hair dry completely before combing it into place. Do not use a blow dryer, and don't dye your hair or use bleach on it. If you want to pull your hair back, do so loosely, and use a special coated elastic that won't grip the individual strands and pull them out.
- Sleep is essential for hair renewal and growth. Try to get eight hours a night, or more, if that's what your body needs.

REFERENCES

2002. *Journal of Alternative and Complementary Medicine* 8:143–52.

Prendiville, J. S., and L. N. Manfredi. 1992. Skin signs of nutritional disorders. *Seminars in Dermatology* 11(1):88–97.

Halitosis. *See* Bad Breath

Headache

Headaches are one of the most frequently occurring disorders; they're more prevalent than even the common cold. Most of us have experienced headaches of varying intensity and kind, and most of us will continue to have them now and then.

The vast majority of headaches are caused by tension in the muscles of the head, the shoulders, and the neck. If you have a tension headache, you may feel tightness, pressure, or throbbing anywhere in your head or neck. Often the pain is worse as the day goes on but disappears upon waking the next day.

Migraine headaches are another matter. They account for only 6 percent of headaches, but what they lack in numbers, they make up for in severity. They are intensely painful and are often accompanied by vision disturbances, extreme sensitivity to light, nausea, and vomiting. A migraine episode, which is usually

*W*arning: Sometimes headaches signal a medical emergency. If you have a headache that is much more severe than any you've ever felt before, or if you experience a headache along with any of the following symptoms, seek medical help at once:

Double vision

Confusion or disorientation

A stiff neck

Projectile vomiting

Paralysis

Vertigo

Fever

Deafness in one ear

Extreme fatigue or weakness

incapacitating, may last a few hours, or it can go on for several days. Unlike tension headaches, migraines are not caused by muscular tension but by disturbances in blood flow to the head. In addition, it is rare to have just one migraine; most migraine sufferers get them at least once a month. The disorder can run in families and affects far more women and girls than it does men or boys.

Cluster headaches are a different type of headache, characterized by painful one-sided headaches that usually occur in clusters of several headaches in a short period of time. There may be no headaches for weeks or months.

Headaches can be triggered by a variety of factors, most often stress and anxiety but also allergies, hormone imbalance, poor digestion and detoxification, low blood sugar, fatigue, and drugs (including caffeine and alcohol). Most headaches are best addressed by identifying and removing the trigger or triggers, along with implementing strategies for natural pain relief.

If you have recurring or extremely severe headaches, however, you should consult a doctor to rule out any serious underlying causes, which can range from glaucoma to high blood pressure to brain tumors. Check with your doctor before combining herbs with prescription headache medications.

SYMPTOMS OF A CLUSTER HEADACHE

- One-sided headaches that are intense for a number of days or weeks and then disappear and reappear later

SYMPTOMS OF A TENSION HEADACHE

- Sensation of a tight band around the head
- Pressure or throbbing anywhere in the head or the neck
- Tension in the neck or the shoulder

SYMPTOMS OF A MIGRAINE HEADACHE

- Severe pain, usually on one side of the head
- Vision disturbances that precede or accompany head pain
- Sensitivity to light
- Nausea and vomiting
- May last for several days

ROOT CAUSES

- Emotional stress
- Fatigue
- Allergies (food or environmental)
- Sinusitis
- Eyestrain
- Poor posture and spinal misalignment, especially of the neck and the jaw (TMJ)

- Excessive intake or withdrawal from drugs, like alcohol, caffeine, nicotine, or illegal substances
- Low blood sugar
- Hormonal imbalance

- Constipation and poor digestion/detoxification
- Nutritional deficiencies (especially of magnesium, B6, essential fatty acids)

Testing Techniques

The following tests help assess possible reasons for headaches:

Blood pressure

Hormone testing (thyroid, cortisol, estrogen, progesterone)—saliva, blood, or urine

Intestinal permeability—urine

Detoxification profile—urine

Vitamin and mineral analysis (especially magnesium, B6, iron)—blood

Digestive function and microbe/parasite/candida testing—stool analysis

Food and environmental allergies/sensitivities—blood, electrodermal

Blood-sugar balance—blood

Toxic metals—hair, urine

TREATMENT

Diet

Recommended Food

To avoid headaches caused by food additives, eat meals that you've prepared from whole foods. To keep your blood sugar steady, try to have five small portions throughout the day, instead of three large meals.

Make sure you get enough fiber to reduce the chance of headaches induced by constipation or toxic buildup. One to two tablespoons of ground flaxseeds, along with 10 ounces of water, is a good way to start the day.

Drink a glass of clean water every two waking hours. The fluid will keep the muscles in your head and neck supple and will also flush out toxins.

If you want to prevent headaches, include sources of both calcium and magnesium in your diet. Soy products, green leafy vegetables, and beans are all rich in calcium. Green leafy vegetables and beans are good sources of magnesium as well, as are nuts, bananas, and wheat germ. If food allergies keep you from eating these foods, take a good calcium/magnesium supplement every day to ensure adequate intake.

Fish such as salmon and mackerel are rich in omega-3 fatty acids that may help prevent migraine headaches. Consume a serving three to five times weekly.

Food to Avoid

If you suffer from migraines or recurring headaches, see the Food Allergies section and the accompanying elimination diet to determine whether your problem may be caused by an allergic reaction or a sensitivity. Common triggers of both tension and migraine headaches include foods that contain either tyramine or phenylalanine. Tyramine can be found in cheese, chocolate, citrus fruits, coffee, cold cuts, herring, smoked fish, wine, alcohol, sausage, sour cream, and vinegar.

Sources of phenylalanine include monosodium glutamate (MSG), the artificial sweetener aspartame, and nitrates, which can be found in processed meats, especially hot dogs. If you do have an allergy or a sensitivity, eliminate the troublesome food or foods from your diet.

Avoid caffeine, alcohol, and sugar products (including artificial sweeteners).

Do not consume sugary foods. They cause your blood-sugar level to rise sharply and then crash; often, the result is a headache.

Very cold foods can also cause headaches. Ice cream and cold drinks are frequent culprits, so avoid them.

Detoxification

In one study, forty-nine people with reoccurring migraines were given 400 mg of riboflavin daily for at least three months. The average number of acute migraine attacks decreased by 67 percent, and migraine severity was reduced by 68 percent. In a separate double-blind trial, 59 percent of patients assigned to receive vitamin B2 had at least a 50 percent reduction in the number of headache days, whereas only 15 percent of those taking a placebo experienced that degree of improvement.

If you suffer from chronic headaches, a detoxification program can be effective. Try a two- to three-day vegetable juice fast, unless low blood-sugar levels bring on your headaches.

Constitutional hydrotherapy can aid detoxification. See pages 676–677 for directions.

℞ Super Seven Prescriptions—Headache

Super Prescription #1   Homeopathic combination headache formula
This contains the most common homeopathic remedies for headaches. Take as directed on the container for the treatment of all three types of acute headaches. For an individualized remedy, see the Homeopathy section further on.

Super Prescription #2   Magnesium
Take 200 mg two to three times daily. Reduce the dosage if diarrhea occurs. Magnesium has been shown in several studies to be effective in alleviating migraine headaches, and we also find it very helpful in preventing tension headaches. Intravenous magnesium can be very effective for acute headaches. Consult with a nutrition-oriented doctor for intravenous treatments.

Super Prescription #3   Riboflavin (vitamin B2)
Take 400 mg daily for at least three months. Studies have shown it to be effective in preventing migraine headaches.

Super Prescription #4   Feverfew (*Tanacetum parthenium*)
Take a product standardized to contain 250 to 500 mcg of parthenolides daily. Several studies have shown it to be effective in reducing the severity, the duration, and the frequency of migraines.

Super Prescription #5   5-hydroxytryptophan (5-HTP)
Take 50 to 100 mg three times daily. Several studies have shown 5-HTP to be effective in preventing migraine and tension headaches. It has a direct effect on serotonin levels, which affect circulation in the blood vessels of the brain, and increases the body's endorphin levels (natural painkillers). Do not use if you are currently on a pharmaceutical antidepressant or an antianxiety medication.

Super Prescription #6   Essential fatty acids

Take 5,000 mg of fish oil or 1 tablespoon of flaxseed oil daily. Essential fatty acids improve circulation and reduce inflammatory prostaglandins that may contribute to migraine headaches

Super Prescription #7   Vitamin B6

Take 50 mg daily. Vitamin B6 is involved in the synthesis of neurotransmitters, such as serotonin, which may be deficient in migraine sufferers.

General Recommendations

Calcium relaxes the nervous system, the muscles, and the blood vessels, making it helpful for all types but especially for tension headaches. Take 500 mg twice daily.

Ginkgo biloba improves circulation to the brain and has anti-platelet activity. Take 60 mg two to three times daily of a 24 percent flavone glycoside extract.

Melatonin has been shown in preliminary research to help migraine headaches. This is a hormone supplement to consider, especially if you have insomnia. Take 0.3 to 0.5 mg before bedtime.

Peppermint or menthol cream applied to the temple area has been shown in studies to be helpful for tension headaches.

White willow bark (*Salix alba*) contains salicin, the ingredient from which aspirin is derived. White willow bark is a highly effective pain reliever that's much easier on the stomach and the entire body than its pharmaceutical counterpart is. Take 60 to 120 mg daily.

Take a few quiet moments with a relaxing cup of tea to reduce tension/stress headaches. Peppermint, chamomile, and passionflower are all good choices.

Enzymes taken with meals improve digestion and absorption. Take a full-spectrum enzyme with each meal or as directed on the container.

Homeopathy

Pick the remedy that best matches your symptoms in this section. For acute headaches, take a 30C potency four times daily. For chronic headaches, take a 6x, 12x, 6C, 12C, or 30C twice daily for two weeks to see if there are any positive results. After you notice improvement, stop taking the remedy, unless symptoms return. Consultation with a homeopathic practitioner is advised.

Belladonna (*Atropa belladonna*) helps when it is a right-sided headache that starts on the back of the head (right side) and extends to the right eye or the forehead. There is throbbing pain, as if the head would burst. The face is flushed and the skin feels hot, but the feet are cold. The person feels better lying down in a dark, quiet room.

Bryonia (*Bryonia alba*) is for pain in the left eye or the forehead that extends to the whole head. Symptoms are worse with any movement and feel better with pressure and stillness. Constipation may be associated with the headache. There can be nausea and a great thirst. The person is irritable and wants to be alone.

Calcarea Phosphorica is for schoolchildren who get chronic headaches and stomach aches. The pain is intense at the back of the head. The child craves smoked meats, may be homesick, and is often irritable.

Cimicifuga is helpful when there is severe neck stiffness and pain with the headache, which often occurs with the menstrual cycle or with hormonal changes during menopause.

Gelsemium (*Gelsemium sempervirens*) is for a dull, heavy pain at the back of the

In a double-blind trial of 81 people, ages 18 to 65, with migraines, a dose of 600 mg of magnesium per day was significantly more effective than a placebo at reducing the frequency of migraines. In weeks 9 through 12, the attack frequency was reduced by 41.6 percent in the magnesium group and by 15.8 percent in the placebo group.

neck, which then spreads like a tight band around the head. The person feels tired and dizzy and may have blurred vision. The headache improves after urinating.

Glonoinum is for a congestive headache with intense pounding. Symptoms are worse from the sun and from heat and better from cold applications.

Ignatia (*Ignatia amara*) is for headaches associated with neck or back spasms. It feels as if a nail were driven into the head. It's also good for headaches that begin after emotional grief or a trauma.

Iris (*Iris versicolor*) is for right-sided migraine headaches that feel as if the head is constricted. Nausea and vomiting occur with the headache. There is often blurry vision. The person feels better with movement.

Lachesis is for left-sided headaches, with a burning, congestive, pulsating feeling. The face can be flushed. The person wakes up with a headache. Heat and touch worsen the headache, and the open air improves it.

Lycopodium (*Lycopodium clavatum*) is for a right-sided headache in the temple or the forehead area. Symptoms are worse from 4 to 8 P.M. and from being overheated or going too long without eating.

Magnesia Phosphorica is for tension headaches. This remedy helps to relax tight muscles.

Natrum Muriaticum is a great remedy for migraine headaches caused by being in the sun or headaches that come on from stress or grief. The person feels better lying down in a dark, cool room.

Natrum Sulphuricum is for headaches that come on after a head injury.

Nux Vomica is for headaches caused by stress, overwork, and bad reactions to food. The headache feels better with cold applications. There is often a stomach ache and nausea. This remedy is used for headaches caused by alcohol or food allergies. The person is irritable from the headache and feels worse from noise, light, and opening the eyes. Nux Vomica is also useful for headaches caused by constipation.

Pulsatilla (*Pulsatilla pratensis*) is helpful when headaches occur around the menstrual cycle. The location of the headache changes rapidly. Symptoms are worse from the heat or from stuffy rooms and better in the open air.

Sanguinaria is for a headache that begins in the right side of the neck or the shoulder and radiates to the right eye. There is relief from vomiting.

Spigelia is for a stitching, sharp headache around the left eye. Symptoms are worse with movement or any jarring and better with heat or hot bathing.

Acupressure

See pages 668–675 for information about pressure points and administeing treatment.

- Large Intestine 4 is good for all kinds of aches, but it is especially successful at treating pain in the front of the head.
- For headaches accompanied by tired, painful eyes or sinus congestion, use Bladder 2.
- Gates of Consciousness 20 will ease headaches of any sort, including migraines.

Bodywork

Massage

For almost immediate relief, have someone rub the back of your neck and your upper back with ice.

If your headache is caused by sinus pain, you can practice an effective self-massage. Lean forward over a sink or a towel to allow the sinuses to drain, and gently rub the areas over and below your eye sockets. You can also extend out from beneath your eye socket in a straight line across your cheeks.

An all-over massage can help relieve stress before it turns into a headache. If you're prone to anxiety and tension, you may want to schedule regular sessions with a massage therapist.

Reflexology
See pages 686–687 for information about reflexology areas and how to work them.

Work the areas corresponding to the head, the neck, the spine, and the solar plexus.

Other Bodywork Recommendations
Postural problems are at the root of many recurring headaches. See a chiropractor or an osteopath for a diagnosis and, if necessary, an adjustment of your vertebrae.

Acupuncture can be very helpful for all three types of headaches.

Aromatherapy
Lavender and peppermint will soothe both head pain and stress. Add a few drops of either to a carrier oil, and massage the temples. You can also add these oils to a cold compress.

If your headache is brought on by sinusitis, use eucalyptus in a steam inhalation. The oil will open up your sinus cavities quickly.

Stress Reduction

General Stress-Reduction Therapies
Many headache sufferers experience excellent results with biofeedback. People with tension headaches tend to clench their head and neck muscles unconsciously throughout the day, but they can use EMG muscle biofeedback to learn how to spot this clenching reflex and how to stop it, thus avoiding headaches. People with migraines can learn to increase blood flow to their head via thermal biofeedback. If biofeedback is too expensive or too complicated for you, find another stress-management technique and practice it daily. Read the Exercise and Stress Reduction chapter and experiment with the therapies there until you find one or two you enjoy.

Bach Flower Remedies

Flower remedies are often an ideal way to address the causes of headaches, whether tension or migraine. Select the appropriate remedy, and place 10 drops of the liquid under your tongue. Hold the drops in place for thirty seconds and swallow. Use as often as needed.

If you suffer from migraines, keep a bottle of Rescue Remedy handy. When you feel one about to start, take some to ease the physical and emotional crisis.

Agrimony is a frequent choice for headache relief; most of us can benefit from it at some point in our lives. Take it when you feel you must repress your emotions and hide your concerns from other people.

Elm is for people who are overwhelmed. They may be overworked and fear failure.

Take White Chestnut to calm down an overactive brain and to free yourself from obsessive thoughts.

If hard work is making you feel grim and humorless, a combination of Oak and Vine will help.

When feeling weepy and blaming others for your problems, Willow would be helpful.

Other Recommendations

- Breathe deeply. Some headaches are caused or made worse by an inadequate supply of oxygen.
- To reduce muscular spasms, lie down in a darkened room and apply a cold compress to the painful area. Some people may find that a warm compress is more effective.
- A heating pad, a warm compress, or a hot towel on the neck or the shoulders is a relaxing way to ease muscular tension.
- Place an ice pack (wrapped in a thin towel) on the back of the neck and put the feet in a bucket of warm water for ten minutes.
- Poor posture and the resulting misalignment of the vertebrae can lead to headaches. Wear flat or low-heeled shoes that fit well, and if you work long hours at a telephone, ask your company to invest in a headset for you. Ergonomic chairs are also recommended for people who sit a long time during the day.
- Women on the birth control pill should consider discontinuing it to see if their migraine headaches improve. Also, women using synthetic hormone replacement should switch to natural HRT or nutritional supplements to see if their headaches go away. See the Menopause section for more information.
- Get checked for temporomandibular joint problems, which can be a cause of tension or migraine headaches.

REFERENCES

Peikert, A., C. Wilimzig, and R. Kohne-Volland. 1996. Prophylaxis of migraine with oral magnesium: Results from a prospective, multi-center, placebo-controlled and double-blind randomized study. *Cephalalgia* 16:257–63.

Schoenen, J., J. Jacquy, and M. Lenaerts. 1998. Effectiveness of high-dose riboflavin in migraine prophylaxis. A randomized controlled trial. *Neurology* 50:466–70.

Schoenen, J., M. Lenaerts, and E. Bastings. 1994. High-dose riboflavin as a prophylactic treatment of migraine: Results of an open pilot study. *Cephalalgia* 14:328–29.

Hearing Loss

Hearing loss is always a disturbing problem, but it's one that too often goes untreated. Many people who experience diminished hearing simply accept it as an unfortunate but normal part of life. While it's true that for some people, age-related hearing loss is unavoidable, the progression of many cases can be halted, significantly slowed, or even reversed with proper diagnosis and treatment. And with good nutrition and ear care, it's often quite possible to prevent hearing loss in the first place.

Hearing is a complex combination of many processes in the ear, the nerves, and the brain, and any disruption of these functions can lead to partial or complete deafness. Nevertheless, hearing problems can generally be categorized according to one of two types: conductive and sensorineural. Conductive hearing loss, which is caused by mechanical problems in the ear's structures, is by far the more common of the two. Although its tendency to come on suddenly can be frightening, it can often be resolved.

The most frequent cause of conductive hearing impairment is a buildup of wax in the ear canal. Normally, wax (or cerumen, to use its medical name) lines the ear canal and serves as a lubricant. When too much wax accumulates, it can block the canal and can lead to hearing loss, as well as to pain and ringing in the ears. A middle-ear infection can also cause a blockage, especially if the infected fluid remains in the ear for a long time and coagulates around the small bones (ossicles) that are responsible for transmitting sound waves. Ear infections and excessive ear wax are both readily treatable, often with home care, and several highly effective nutritional strategies can prevent the problem from recurring.

In some instances, conductive hearing damage is more serious. If you suffer hearing loss after a fall or a blow to the ear or the head, or if you experience a sudden, intense pain in your ear, see your doctor at once. You may have a ruptured ear drum or damage to the hearing sensor, called the organ of Corti. Even innocuous-looking cotton swabs can cause grave damage, including ruptures, when inserted deep into the ear canal. Some drugs can also affect the organ of Corti, so talk to your doctor if you experience hearing loss after starting a new prescription drug. Finally, some conductive hearing damage may simply be a part of aging. As the body gets older, the eardrum can thicken and other ear structures may grow weak, leading to partial loss of hearing. More than 40 percent of people seventy-five and older experience some degree of hearing problems.

Sensorineural hearing damage affects the nerves that receive sound waves and transmit their impulses through the ear and to the brain, where the impulses are registered as the sensory perception of sound. Almost all sensorineural hearing damage is due to high levels of noise. Loud concerts and stereos turned up to full volume may be the most obvious source of excessive noise, but sirens, airplanes, trains, jackhammers, and construction sounds are common culprits as well. Every time you're exposed to a loud noise, your auditory nerves are damaged; a lifetime of noises can add up to permanent hearing loss. In some cases, sensorineural hearing problems are caused by other disorders, including diabetes, arteriosclerosis, lupus, and hypothyroidism. And again, sometimes nerves simply weaken with age and lose their ability to conduct sound effectively. However, recent research has shown that loud noises form free radicals that damage the inner ear. Antioxidants such as vitamin E, zinc, NAC, magnesium, and vitamin A appear to protect against this cause of damage, although they have not been shown to reverse hearing loss. In some cases, tumor growths on the nerves involved with hearing are responsible for the hearing loss. One must also consider other structural possibilities, such as vertebral and soft tissue misalignment in the neck and the jaw (TMJ), as well as in cranial bones.

No matter what you suspect the source of your hearing problems to be, it's important that you consult a doctor about any sudden hearing loss or any gradual hearing damage that does not resolve itself within a few weeks. For one, the problem may be treatable. Even if you're older and believe that the hearing problem is due to age-related deterioration of ear structures or nerves, you may be surprised to find that the cause is actually wax buildup (something to which people over sixty-five are prone) or a side effect of medication. If the cause is not obvious to your doctor, he or she should run tests to rule out an underlying disorder. Finally, even hearing problems that are not reversible by natural means can often be significantly improved with hearing aids, electronic implants, or even surgery.

SYMPTOMS

- Hearing loss may occur gradually, or it may happen suddenly.
- Partial or total inability to hear

ROOT CAUSES

- Accumulation of ear wax
- Middle-ear infection
- Poor diet and nutritional deficiencies
- Food allergies
- Trauma to the ear
- Medication
- Loud noise

- Age-related weakening of the ear structures and the nerves
- Structural abnormalities (especially cervical spine, TMJ, and cranial bones)
- High cholesterol
- Other disorders that cause hearing loss

TREATMENT

For further information about treating infections of the middle ear, see Ear Infection.

Diet

Recommended Food

Although no one has proven (yet) that antioxidants can reduce or prevent hearing loss, we do know that they slow many aspects of the aging process. Increasing your antioxidant intake by consuming more deeply colored fruits and vegetables certainly can't hurt you, and it may prevent or slow hearing damage (along with many other disorders we tend to associate with old age).

Eat plenty of fiber at every meal. Good sources include whole grains, especially oats and brown rice; beans; nuts and seeds; and raw or lightly cooked fruits and vegetables. Fiber will improve circulation to your entire body, including your ears. Fibrous foods also tend to require chewing, an activity that discourages wax from accumulating in your ear canals.

Since hypothyroidism can lead to hearing loss, include sea vegetables such as kelp, in your diet. These foods are high in iodine, a mineral that's necessary for good thyroid health. You can easily incorporate sea vegetables into soups, especially miso broth, or add them to a stir-fry with brown rice and tofu.

Food to Avoid

If you experience frequent ear infections or a buildup of earwax, you may have a food allergy. Read the Food Allergies section, and follow the elimination diet there; if a certain food provokes ear problems or excess mucus (which can lead to infection), avoid it.

Even if you are not allergic to milk or dairy products, stay away from them for the duration of an infection or a wax problem. Dairy encourages mucus to accumulate, which can encourage infection or excess wax.

If you have a chronic hearing problem, eliminate saturated fat, especially red meat and fried foods, from your diet. Saturated fat contributes to earwax and slows circulation to the ear structures. Removing saturated fat from your meals and snacks will also help reverse arteriosclerosis, a disorder that may cause hearing loss.

Bacteria feed on sugar, so people who are prone to ear infections should radically reduce their consumption of it. The best course of action is to cut out all refined sugars and have fruit or naturally sweetened products for dessert.

Detoxification

If you have recurring ear infections or wax problems, a short juice fast will help clear your body of excess mucus. Fasting is also helpful for people whose hearing loss is connected to food allergens, as a three-day respite from solid food will rid your system of the toxic substance.

Testing Techniques

The following tests help assess possible reasons for hearing loss:

Specialized hearing tests by an otologist

Blood pressure

Vitamin and mineral analysis (especially magnesium, B12, and iron)— blood

Food and environmental allergies/sensitivities—blood, electrodermal

---

R Super Seven Prescriptions—Hearing Loss

Super Prescription #1   Ginkgo biloba
Take 60 to 120 mg twice a day of a 24 percent flavone glycosides standardized extract. This herb increases blood flow, which helps ear tissues receive the oxygen and the nutrients they need for good health.

Super Prescription #2   Vitamin B12
Take 200 to 400 mcg of sublingual B12 daily. This B vitamin is important for nerve health.

Super Prescription #3   High-potency multivitamin
Take as directed on the container.

Super Prescription #4   Vitamin E
Take 400 to 800 IU daily. It acts as an antioxidant and improves circulation.

Super Prescription #5   Cayenne (*Capsicum annuum*)
Take 300 mg twice daily. Cayenne improves circulation.

Super Prescription #6   Garlic (*Allium sativum*)
Take 300 to 600 mg of aged garlic twice daily. Garlic decreases cholesterol levels and improves blood flow.

Super Prescription #7   Bromelain
Take 500 mg three times daily between meals. Look for products standardized to 2,000 M.C.U. (milk-clotting units) per 1,000 mg or 1,200 G.D.U. (gelatin-dissolving units) per 1,000 mg. Bromelain has a natural anti-inflammatory effect. Protease enzyme products also have this benefit.

General Recommendations

If you have an ear infection, an herbal solution made from 3 or 4 drops of warm olive oil combined with oil of Kyolic garlic, mullein, or lobelia can work wonders. Either lie down on your side until the oil works its way into the ear, or place a cotton ball loosely in the outer ear to the keep the oil from running out.

Marshmallow will help drain excess mucus. Take 2.5 to 3.0 grams twice a day, or take 5 to 15 cc of a tincture three times a day.

Homeopathy

For prolonged hearing loss, it's best to see a homeopathic practitioner for a constitutional remedy.

Acupressure

See pages 668-675 for information about pressure points and administering treatment.

- To stimulate better hearing, work these two ear points: Gallbladder 2 (also known as Reunion of Hearing) and Small Intestine 19 (Listening Place).

Bodywork

Massage

A head rub will improve circulation; a gentle head massage will also help ease the pain caused by an ear infection.

Reflexology

See pages 686–687 for information about reflexology areas and how to work them.

To release pain and stimulate circulation, work the eye/ear area and the neck.

Other Bodywork Recommendations

Spinal and cranial treatments from a chiropractor, an osteopath, a craniosacral practitioner, or a naturopath can be helpful in improving nerve flow and circulation.

Aromatherapy

Several oils benefit circulation, including marjoram, ginger, rosemary, and black pepper. You can combine any of these with a carrier oil to use in a head massage. If you prefer not to get oil in your hair, you can add the oils to a steam inhalation.

Other Recommendations

- Protect your ears from loud noises. If you are outdoors and hear a loud sound such a siren or a train whistle, cover your ears; if you're in a car, roll up the windows.
- Play music at a low to moderate level, and wear earplugs if you must attend a loud concert.
- For those of you who cannot avoid exposure to noises because of your job, invest in earphones that cover your ears, and rest in a quiet place as often as you can.
- Excessive ear wax can often be treated successfully at home. Buy an over-the-counter preparation containing carbamide peroxide and gently squeeze a few

drops in your ear canal. This solution will help soften the wax so that it comes out easily. (You can also use hydrogen peroxide, if you prefer.) Allow the liquid to remain in your ear for a few minutes; for very hard wax, you may want to wait a day or two. Then use a bulb syringe filled with warm water to gently flush out the ear. If the plug of wax does not come out immediately, keep trying. It may take some time, but most people find that the wax does come out eventually.

Hemorrhoids

It is estimated that 50 to 75 percent of Americans will suffer from hemorrhoids at least once, and nearly one-third of the population has an ongoing problem with this often-painful condition. Hemorrhoids are usually caused by increased pressure on the veins of the anus and the rectum. This pressure inflames and swells the veins, much in the same way that pressure on the veins of the legs creates varicose veins. Increased pressure on the anal veins can occur for many reasons but is most commonly the result of constipation, especially straining to pass stools, and pregnancy and childbirth. There may also be a genetic component to this disorder.

Hemorrhoids can be divided into three categories. Internal hemorrhoids develop inside the rectum, where they cannot be seen. Because they are usually painless, you may not even be aware of them unless they bleed. External hemorrhoids are located at the lower end of the anal canal, at the opening of the anus and under the skin. They are likely to become inflamed; when they do, they turn blue or purple and feel tender to the touch. Because of the high number of nerves in the anus, these hemorrhoids can be quite painful.

If an internal hemorrhoid becomes enlarged, it may collapse and descend so that it partially protrudes outside of the anus. These lumpy-looking masses of tissue are called prolapsed hemorrhoids. They usually appear after a bowel movement and produce both mucus and heavy bleeding. Prolapsed hemorrhoids can be excruciating painful.

Most cases of hemorrhoids are linked in some way to a lack of dietary fiber. They are best treated at home with increased fiber intake, detoxification, and soothing treatments for the pain and the itching. If your hemorrhoids don't improve with these conservative strategies, see a doctor about more aggressive treatments. In rare cases, surgery is required to remove large and very painful hemorrhoids. If you have any rectal bleeding at all, consult with a doctor so that he or she can rule out a more serious underlying condition.

SYMPTOMS

- Pain, itching, burning, or bleeding in the anal area
- Blue or purple patches of hard skin near the anus
- Lumpy tissue protruding from the anus

ROOT CAUSES

- Constipation and straining
- Pregnancy and childbirth
- Lifting heavy objects
- Obesity

- Inactivity, especially standing or sitting for extended periods
- Food allergies
- Portal hypertension and poor liver function

- Poor anal hygiene
- Hypothyroidism

TREATMENT

If sluggish digestion is a cause of your hemorrhoids, you will find additional suggestions for relief in the Constipation section.

Diet

Almost everyone who suffers from hemorrhoids—even people who aren't constipated—will benefit from dietary changes.

Recommended Food

If you're unaccustomed to a high-fiber diet, incorporate these suggestions incrementally. If you try to introduce too much fiber at once, you'll only place more pressure on your digestive tract.

The best way to relieve hemorrhoids is to consume more fiber. Eat lots of whole grains, raw or lightly cooked fruits and vegetables, and beans, nuts, and seeds. Rather than sitting down to three large meals every day, plan on several smaller meals.

To allow stools to pass more easily, drink a glass of clean water every two waking hours.

Add prunes or figs to your breakfast to speed up a sluggish intestine.

Have a tablespoon of flaxseed oil every day to encourage elimination, or sprinkle 1 to 2 tablespoons of ground flaxseeds onto cereal or salads.

Vitamin K will help stop or prevent bleeding. Green leafy vegetables, especially kale, are good source of this nutrient, as are kelp and alfalfa sprouts.

An overgrowth of candidiasis is an often-overlooked aggravator of hemorrhoids. Consume soured food like unsweetened live yogurt, kefir, and sauerkraut to increase the numbers of friendly bacteria that inhibit this fungal growth. These products will also help you absorb vitamin K.

Eat wheat germ for its high level of vitamin E. You'll promote circulation and prevent blood clots in your already-stressed circulatory system.

Bioflavonoids have been shown to significantly reduce inflammation and to strengthen capillaries, so enjoy some berries a few times daily.

If you're pregnant, you have another reason to eat your leafy greens. These vegetables are high in B6, a vitamin that many pregnant women lack; a deficiency may contribute to hemorrhoids. Brewer's yeast and wheat germ are also good sources.

Food to Avoid

Fats and oils slow down the digestive system. Stay away from foods that are fried or otherwise high in saturated fat.

Caffeine and alcohol are dehydrating and worsen hemorrhoids.

Avoid sugars and spicy foods, as they also tend to worsen this condition.

Some cases of hemorrhoids are caused by food allergies. Read the Food Allergies section, and try the elimination diet to determine whether you need to remove certain foods from your diet. The most common ones that lead to hemorrhoids are cow's milk, wheat, citrus fruit, tomatoes, and peanuts.

Testing Techniques

The following tests help assess possible reasons for hemorrhoids:

Hormone testing (hypothyroid can contribute to sluggish bowel and liver function)—saliva, blood, or urine

Digestive function and microbe/parasite/candida testing—stool analysis

Food and environmental allergies/sensitivities—blood, electrodermal

---

Detoxification

If hemorrhoids result from constipation or straining on the toilet, go on a three-day juice fast to cleanse accumulated waste matter from your digestive tract. If you are constipated when you begin taking the fast, add psyllium husks or flaxseeds to your juices for fiber.

℞ Super Seven Prescriptions—Hemorrhoid

Super Prescription #1   Butcher's broom (*Ruscus aculeatus*)
Take a standardized extract that gives you 200 to 300 mg of ruscogenins daily. Ruscogenins are constituents within this herb that are believed to constrict and reduce inflammation of hemorrhoidal tissue.

Super Prescription #2   Horse chestnut (*Aesculus hippocastanum*)
Take a standardized extract that contains 100 mg of aescin daily. This herb improves circulation and reduces swelling.

Super Prescription #3   Collinsonia (stone root)
Take 500 mg three times daily. Collinsonia reduces hemorrhoid swelling.

Super Prescription #4   Witch hazel (*Hamamelis virginiana*)
Apply as a gel or a cream to external hemorrhoids, or add 1 ounce to a sitz bath daily.

Super Prescription #5   Flaxseed oil
Take 1 to 2 tablespoons daily. Flaxseed oil improves regularity and reduces straining. It also contains essential fatty acids that promote tissue healing.

Super Prescription #6   Bioflavonoid complex
Take 1,000 mg two to three times daily. Various flavonoids, such as rutin and hesperidin, have been shown to be effective in treating hemorrhoids. They reduce swelling and prevent bleeding.

Super Prescription #7   Bilberry (*Vaccinium myrtillus*)
Take a standardized extract containing 25 percent anthocyanosides at 160 mg twice daily. Bilberry improves circulation and strengthens capillary walls.

A study of fifty-one pregnant women found that supplementation of bilberry significantly improved the pain, the burning, and the itching associated with their hemorrhoids.

General Recommendations

Grape seed extract or maritime pine bark extract have anti-inflammatory effects and improve circulation. Take 100 mg twice daily.

A greens drink that contains a blend of super green foods, such as chlorella, spirulina, and so on, provides fiber and improves liver function. Take as directed on the container.

Aloe vera juice is healing and soothing to the entire digestive tract. Drink 4 ounces daily or as directed on the container.

Vitamin C strengthens the rectal tissue. Take 500 mg two to three times daily.

A probiotic contains friendly bacteria, such as lactobacillus and bifidobacterium, which improve digestion and constipation. Take a product that contains at least 4 billion active organisms daily.

Dandelion root (*Taraxacum officinalis*) promotes bile flow and improved regularity. Take 300 mg in capsule form or 2 ml of tincture three times daily.

Psyllium is a good fiber supplement and has been shown to reduce the pain and the bleeding associated with hemorrhoids. Take 5 to 7 grams daily, along with 10 ounces of water.

Homeopathy

Pick the remedy that best matches your symptoms in this section. Take a 6x, 12x, 6C, 12C, or 30C potency twice daily for two weeks to see if there are any positive results. After you notice improvement, stop taking the remedy, unless symptoms return. Consultation with a homeopathic practitioner is advised.

Aesculus (*Aesculus hippocastanum*) is for pain that feels as if the rectum is being poked with sticks. The pain extends to the back.

Aloe vera is for large, painful hemorrhoids. The doctor states that the hemorrhoids look like a "bunch of grapes." They feel better with cold compresses. The person may be prone to having diarrhea.

Calcarea Fluorica is helpful when bleeding and itching occur with the hemorrhoids. Often, lower back pain is present. The person may have problems with flatulence and constipation.

Ignatia (*Ignatia amara*) is for hemorrhoids that cause a stabbing or sticking pain, along with rectal spasms. The symptoms feel worse from emotional upset.

Nux Vomica is for painful hemorrhoids that come on as a result of chronic constipation and straining with bowel movements. The person is irritable and has a tendency to overuse alcohol, drugs, or medications.

Ratanhia is helpful when a person experiences a lot of pain after a bowel movement. There is a cutting pain that feels like one is sitting on broken glass.

Sulphur is for large, itching, burning hemorrhoids that tend to be worse at night. The anal area is red and inflamed, and there is often flatulence with a foul odor.

Acupressure

See pages 668–675 for information about pressure points and administering treatment.

- To relieve constipation, work Conception Vessel 6 and Large Intestine 4.
- Keep the colon strong and healthy by working Large Intestine 11 on a regular basis.
- Use Stomach 36 to improve the assimilation of nutrients into the body.

Bodywork

Massage

If you're constipated, a self-massage of the abdominal area can induce intestinal movement. Lie down with your knees bent, and massage your abdomen with the flat of your hand, using firm but gentle pressure.

A professional massage of your lower back and pelvis may also relieve constipation.

Reflexology

See pages 686–687 for information about reflexology areas and how to work them.

Work the areas corresponding to the sigmoid colon, the rectum, and the lower back.

If you are constipated, also work the areas related to the liver, the gallbladder, and the adrenal glands.

Hydrotherapy

Constitutional hydrotherapy is a good long-term treatment for hemorrhoids. See pages 676–677 for directions.

An alternating warm (one minute) and cold (thirty seconds) sitz bath offers relief and improves circulation.

Aromatherapy

Geranium relaxes your system by easing anxiety and depression, which often lead to constipation. Add it to your bath water or use a few drops in a compress.

Tea tree oil reduces the chances of infection. You can also add this to a bath or a compress. This is a potent oil, so start off with just 2 or 3 drops. If you don't have a reaction, you can increase the amount by a few more drops the next time you make a preparation.

If you need to stimulate your digestive system, marjoram and black pepper will help. Add either or both to a bath, or combine with a carrier oil and use it in a massage.

Stress Reduction

General Stress-Reduction Therapies

Give yoga a try. Not only will it reduce tension and relax your body, many of the breathing techniques and the postures are meant to exercise your digestive organs.

Regular exercise is very important to reduce the effects of stress and improve circulation.

Bach Flower Remedies

Select the appropriate remedy, and place 10 drops of the liquid under your tongue. Hold the drops in place for thirty seconds and swallow. Use as often as needed.

If you are quick to anger and sometimes fear you might become violent, use Cherry Plum.

People who pride themselves on getting the job done quickly and efficiently but who are frustrated by those who work at a slower pace should take Impatiens, which helps develop tolerance.

Other Recommendations

- If you're constipated, do not strain when sitting on the toilet. Try to relax and breathe deeply.

- Do not use laxatives. They only address the surface of the problem and can cause your bowels to become dependent on them. If you need temporary relief, see the Constipation section.

- Get regular exercise. Any kind will do, but a daily walk is always a good idea.

- For temporary relief of pain and itching, use any of the following as a topical lotion: cocoa butter, zinc oxide, olive oil, or calendula gel.

- If you must stand or sit for long periods of time, take frequent breaks to stretch and move around.

- Special foam-rubber pillows known as a "doughnuts" are helpful when you need to sit. They have a hole in the middle so there is less pressure on the hemorrhoids.

- If you're obese, losing weight will reduce or even eliminate your hemorrhoids. The dietary suggestions in this section should help you take the weight off safely, but if you'd like additional recommendations, see Obesity.

REFERENCES

Teglio, L., et al. 1987. Vaccinium myrtillus anthocyanosides (Tegens) in the treatment of venous insufficiency of lower limbs and acute piles in pregnancy. *Quadeni di Clinica Osterica e Ginecologica* 42(3):221–31.

Heart Attack and Heart Disease. *See* Cardiovascular Disease

Hepatitis

Hepatitis is the general term for the inflammation of the liver, which is the body's largest internal organ and is located beneath the breastbone, extending under the bottom of the right side of the rib cage. Hepatitis can result from the use of alcohol, drugs, and chemicals but is most commonly caused by one of several specific hepatitis viruses.

One of the liver's functions is to produce and metabolize bile, which is necessary to break down fats and expel toxins out of the body. With hepatitis, bilirubin, a pigment normally excreted in bile, builds up in the bloodstream and accumulates in the skin. This causes the characteristic yellowish color of the skin and the eyes, as well as dark urine. Classic symptoms of hepatitis include nausea, fatigue, loss of appetite, weight loss, clay-colored stools, fever, and diarrhea. Blood tests show an elevation of one or more liver enzymes.

At least six different viruses cause acute viral hepatitis. The main three are hepatitis A, B, and C. Other hepatitis viruses include D, E, and G.

Hepatitis A, which has a 15- to 45-day incubation period, is highly contagious and is spread mainly by fecal-tainted food or water. Epidemics are common in underdeveloped countries. Contaminated raw shellfish can be a causative factor. It can also be transmitted through blood or saliva secretions. Hepatitis A is an acute infection, and people do not become chronic carriers of the virus. It does not play a role in the development of chronic hepatitis or cirrhosis. A vaccine for hepatitis A is available.

Hepatitis B has an incubation period of 30 to 180 days. It is contracted by contaminated blood or blood products, as happens with drug users who share needles. It can also occur from sexual contact and, less commonly, from transfusions tainted with infected blood. People can become chronic carriers of this virus. A wide spectrum of liver diseases is associated with hepatitis B, including cirrhosis and liver cancer. A vaccine for hepatitis B is available.

Hepatitis C has an incubation period of 15 to 150 days. This is the most common form of viral hepatitis. In the past, it was more commonly contracted through contaminated blood. The main causes of hepatitis C infection worldwide include unscreened blood transfusions and the reuse of needles and syringes that have not been adequately sterilized. In developed countries, it is estimated that 90 percent of people with chronic HCV infection are current and/or former injecting drug users or those with a history of transfusion of unscreened blood or blood products. Hepatitis C can also be transmitted by sexual activity and from mother to infant. It is estimated that 3 percent of the world's population (170 million people) are chronically infected with hepatitis C virus. Most people with hepatitis C have no symptoms. According to the World Health Organization, about 80 percent of newly infected patients progress to develop the chronic infection. Cirrhosis develops in about 10 to 20 percent of people with chronic infection, and liver cancer develops in 1 to 5 percent of those with chronic infection over a period of twenty to thirty years. Currently, there is no vaccine to prevent hepatitis C. Antiviral drugs are the standard conventional treatment. Effectiveness of these drugs varies, but side effects prevent many people from continuing treatment.

Hepatitis D virus occurs only in the presence of acute or chronic hepatitis B virus infection. Drug addicts who share needles are at high risk for this infection. It is characterized by an unusually severe acute hepatitis B infection.

Hepatitis E virus is most commonly transmitted via contaminated water in developing countries. The infection can be severe but is not chronic.

Hepatitis G virus can be transmitted by blood. Currently, not a lot is known about this virus, although it can become chronic.

The early symptoms of acute hepatitis may include a loss of appetite, fatigue, nausea, vomiting, and fever. Hivelike eruptions and joint pains occasionally occur. After a period of three to ten days, the urine darkens and is followed by jaundice (yellowing of the skin). The liver is usually enlarged and tender, and the spleen may enlarge as well. Blood tests will show elevated liver enzymes from the beginning stage of the illness.

Hepatitis usually resolves within four to eight weeks, especially hepatitis A. However, 5 to 10 percent of hepatitis B infections become chronic, and up to 80 percent of hepatitis C infections become chronic. Hepatitis lasting for six months or longer is generally termed chronic.

Natural therapies can be very helpful in preventing liver damage and decreasing the viral load or the infectiousness of the hepatitis viruses. Holistic therapies are becoming very popular for people with hepatitis C—an emerging world epidemic. The effectiveness of conventional antiviral drug therapy varies, and side effects of these drugs can be severe. Natural treatment is used to augment the immune system to fight the viral infection and to improve and protect liver function. Our experience is that most cases can be helped with natural treatment, and sometimes the improvements are dramatic. Many natural therapies in this chapter can be combined with conventional therapy.

SYMPTOMS

- Nausea
- Fatigue
- Loss of appetite
- Weight loss
- Clay-colored stools
- Fever
- Diarrhea
- Dark urine
- Jaundice

ROOT CAUSES

- Viral infection
- Adverse reaction to drugs and other toxins
- Alcohol
- Weakened immune system

Testing Techniques

The following tests go beyond regular conventional testing and identify reasons for weakened immunity:

Blood work (conventional testing)—immune function, liver enzymes, viral load

Stool analysis—digestive health

Hormone analysis by saliva, urine, or blood (testosterone, DHEA, cortisol, melatonin, IGF-1, thyroid panel)

Toxic metal—hair or urine

Oxidative stress analysis—urine or blood testing

TREATMENT

Diet

Recommended Food

During the acute phase, it is recommended that you consume soups, broths, diluted vegetable juices, herbal teas, steamed vegetables, brown rice, and nonred meat protein sources, such as free-range turkey or chicken, legumes, and fish.

To promote healing of the liver and to provide a diet that is supportive to the immune system, consume lots of vegetables and moderate amount of fruits, whole grains, and legumes. Reduce or eliminate foods that are taxing to the liver, such as fried foods; refined sugar products; foods containing trans-fatty acids, such as margarine and vegetable shortening; and saturated fats, found in meat and dairy products. Make fresh juices out of foods such as apples, beets, and carrots. Start with small amounts to see how you tolerate them. Steamed artichokes are healing to the liver. Eating smaller and more frequent meals is recommended. Soups and stews are good, as they are easy to digest. Purified water should be consumed, an 8-ounce glass every two to three waking hours.

Food to Avoid

Cut out junk food, sugar, and alcohol, all of which suppress your immune system and tax your entire body.

Avoid saturated fats and hydrogenated oils, which stress the immune system and the liver. Stay away from fried foods and solid fats, such as margarine, lard, and vegetable shortening.

Find out now if you have any food allergies or sensitivities, because they weaken the immune system. See the elimination diet on page 253 for further details.

Detoxification

Every month consider doing a juice fast. Juices made from carrots, cabbage, greens, and apples help cleanse the body. Green drinks are another excellent way to purify the blood.

Rx Super Seven Prescriptions—Hepatitis

Super Prescription #1   Milk thistle (*Silybum marianum*)
Take a daily dosage of a product standardized with regard to silymarin, so that you supplement a daily total of 600 to 1,000 mg of the active constituent silymarin daily. This herb protects the liver, promotes liver cell regeneration, and helps reduce liver enzyme count.

Super Prescription #2   Vitamin C
Take 1,000 mg three to four times daily of a buffered (nonacidic) vitamin C. A more therapeutic technique is to keep gradually increasing the dosage until loose stools occur, and then cut back on the dosage. Intravenous vitamin C treatments from a holistic doctor are even more effective. Vitamin C improves immune function and has antiviral properties.

Super Prescription #3   Catechin
Take 750 mg three times daily. Catechin is a type of flavonoid that was shown in studies to be helpful for acute and chronic hepatitis. It is best used under the supervision of a doctor.

Super Prescription #4   Thymus extract
Take as directed on the container. Look for a high-quality purified thymus extract. A typical dose is 200 to 300 mg three times daily. Thymus extract has been shown to improve immune function and be helpful for people with hepatitis C.

Super Prescription #5   Licorice root (*Glycyrrhiza glabra*)
Take 500 mg three times daily. One of the active phytonutrients in licorice root, known as glycyrrhizin, has been used as part of injectable formulas to treat chronic hepatitis B and C, with favorable outcomes. Licorice root has been shown to have immune-enhancing and antiviral properties. Holistic doctors also administer glycyrrhizin intravenously for a strong therapeutic effect. *Note:* High doses of licorice root may cause high blood pressure. High doses, as recommended in this section, are best used under the supervision of a physician.

Super Prescription #6   Reishi extract
Take 3,000 to 6,000 mg daily of a standardized extract. Preliminary studies have shown Reishi extract to be effective for hepatitis B and elevated liver enzymes. Reishi is commonly used by health practitioners for liver support.

Milk thistle (Silymarin) was studied in a group of 21 people who had active liver disease (cirrhosis). People who took 420 mg of silymarin had a 15 percent reduction in the liver enzyme AST and a 23 percent decrease in the enzyme ALT.

Super Prescription #7   Schisandra extract (*Schisandra chinensis*)

Take 500 mg three times daily. Studies have found that this Chinese herb is effective in treating chronic hepatitis.

General Recommendations

Turmeric (*Curcuma longa*) (90 to 95 percent curcumin) has anti-inflammatory benefits for liver infection. Take 500 mg three times daily.

Alpha lipoic acid supports immune function and has anti-inflammatory properties. Take 300 mg twice daily.

Phosphatidylcholine helps the liver to process fats and protects the liver cells. One study demonstrated benefits for people who had chronic hepatitis B. Take 3,000 mg daily.

Astragalus is an excellent herb for long-term immune support and is used for chronic viral hepatitis. Take 2 ml of the tincture or 1,000 mg of the capsule form three times daily.

A high-potency multivitamin and mineral formula should be supplemented, for general immune system support.

Selenium is important, because a deficiency can make it easier for viruses to replicate. Make sure you are getting a total of 400 mcg daily.

Zinc supports immune function. Take a daily total of 30 to 50 mg.

Vitamin E-complex is important for protection against liver damage and to support immune function. Take 800 mg of a blended formula containing tocopherols and tocotrienols.

Phyllanthus (*Phyllanthus amarus*) was shown in one study to be effective for people who were chronic carriers of hepatitis B. Take 200 mg three times daily.

Dandelion root improves liver function. Take 3 ml of the tincture or 500 mg in capsule form three times daily with meals.

Liver glandular extract supports liver function. Take as directed on the container.

A greens drink that contains super green foods, such as chlorella, spirulina, and others, supports liver detoxification and immunity. Take as directed on the container.

Homeopathy

Pick the remedy that best matches your symptoms in this section. Take a 6x, 12x, 6C, 12C, or 30C potency twice daily for two weeks to see if there are any positive results. After you notice improvement, stop taking the remedy, unless symptoms return. Consultation with a homeopathic practitioner is advised.

Cardus Marianus is a specific remedy for inflammation of the left lobe of the liver. The person's symptoms are worse when lying on the left side. There is abdominal or liver pain that is worse from breathing in or from movement.

Chelidonium is used when there is pain under the right rib cage, radiating to the right shoulder blade. Abdominal pain is ameliorated after eating or by lying on the left side with the legs drawn up. The person feels better from warm drinks. Jaundice is usually present.

China is used when the liver is very sensitive to the touch. There is tremendous bloating of the abdomen, which is not relieved from passing gas.

Lycopodium is used for hepatitis in which bloating, indigestion, and flatulence are prominent symptoms. There is discomfort in the upper right area of the abdomen. The symptoms feel better from warm drinks. The person feels irritable and craves sweets.

Natrum Sulphuricum is used to treat jaundice that is accompanied by diarrhea. The tongue has a greenish coating. It is used for hepatitis that causes headaches, accompanied by nausea and vomiting. The person feels better from firm pressure or rubbing of the abdomen.

Nux Vomica is helpful when constipation, cramping, or reflux accompanies hepatitis. Common symptoms also include fatigue and irritability. The person is chilly and feels better from heat.

Phosphorous is indicated for hepatitis that occurs from solvent and toxin exposure. The person feels a thirst for ice-cold drinks but tends to vomit after drinking them.

Sulphur is a remedy for chronic hepatitis with jaundice and diarrhea. The person feels very warm and desires a cool environment.

Acupressure

Pericardium 6 is used to relieve nausea.

Stomach 36 is used for fatigue.

Stomach 37 is for diarrhea and abdominal cramps.

Acupressure and acupuncture can be very effective in treating hepatitis. See a practitioner of Asian medicine for a specific treatment.

Bodywork

Massage

Lymphatic massage detoxifies the body, while improving circulation. Consult with an experienced practitioner.

Reflexology

See pages 686–687 for information about reflexology areas and how to work them.

Massage the liver points to relieve liver congestion.

To detoxify cells and tissues, work the area corresponding to the lymph system.

Other Bodywork Recommendations

Constitutional hydrotherapy helps to improve liver detoxification and stimulate the immune system for viral hepatitis. See pages 676–677 for directions.

Aromatherapy

Add juniper to a carrier oil, and use it in a lymphatic massage. Juniper helps break down toxins that have built up as a result of compromised liver function.

General Stress-Reduction Therapies

A diagnosis of chronic hepatitis can be very stressful. Although family and friends are always a welcome source of strength, you may also want to recruit the help of a professional who has experience working with people suffering from chronic illness. A religious adviser, a psychotherapist, or a support group leader can offer you invaluable advice and help.

In a world of expensive and invasive medical treatments, meditation and positive mental imagery can come as a relief.

Exercise is a healthful way to relieve stress and improve immune function.

Bach Flower Remedies

Consult the chart on pages 648–650 to find the appropriate flower remedy for your particular condition. Once you've found the right remedy, place 10 drops under your tongue. Hold the drops in place for thirty seconds and swallow. Use as often as needed.

For fear of the unknown, try Aspen.

For exhaustion and fatigue, Hornbeam or Olive can be useful.

Rescue Remedy is excellent in any stressful crisis.

Other Recommendations

Avoid the use of acetaminophen and over-the-counter painkillers and other pharmaceuticals, if possible, as they stress the liver.

Chinese herbal therapy from a practitioner of Asian medicine can be highly effective.

REFERENCES

Chang, H. M., and P. But, (eds.). 1986. *Pharmacology and Applications of Chinese Materia Medica,* Vol. 1. Singapore: World Scientific.

Lirussi, F., and L. Okolicsanyi. 1992. Cytoprotection in the nineties: Experience with ursodeoxycholic acid and silymarin in chronic liver disease. *Acta Physiologica Hungarica* 801(1–4):363–67.

Herpes

The herpes family of viruses includes more than seventy known members. The most common ones that humans encounter include herpes simplex 1 and 2, Epstein-Barr virus, varicella zoster, and cytomegalovirus. This section contains information on herpes simplex 1 (HSV-1) and herpes simplex 2 (HSV-2).

Both of the herpes simplex viruses cause small, irritating, fluid-filled blisters or eruptions on the skin and the mucous membranes. Herpes simplex virus 1 is often at the root of cold sores, also known as fever blisters, since sun exposure can bring on an outbreak.

The initial symptoms of a cold sore include burning and tingling sensations around the edges of the lips and the nose, where itchy, painful blisters and/or small, red pimples will form within a few hours and last a few days. They usually dry up and crust over in eight to twelve days after onset, although natural and conventional therapy can often greatly reduce the healing time. A person may complain of localized pain, as well as have a mild fever and swollen lymph nodes in the neck.

Herpes simplex virus 2 causes blisters on the genitals and is typically spread through sexual contact (although herpes simplex virus 1 can also cause genital herpes and vice versa). The burning and tingling sensations surrounding the genital areas are its initial symptoms. The moist linings surrounding the sex organs will soon become the sites of blisters that later turn into sores or lesions that can easily become infected and irritating. It should be noted that a pregnant woman carrying the herpes simplex virus 2 may pass it along to her baby during birth, allowing the baby to form lesions from contact, as well as problems with its nervous systems, such as seizures and mental retardation. Women are screened for this infection during their pregnancy, and cesarean section birthing can prevent the transfer of herpes simplex 2.

Herpes simplex virus 1 and 2 are extremely common. Once they enter the body, herpes viruses can remain dormant in the nervous system for several years or life. Their outbreak is more likely when the immune system is under stress, such as during infectious illness (common cold), when under physical or emotional stress, from excessive exposure to sunlight, and from nutritional deficiencies and allergies to food or drugs.

Conventional treatment for a cold sore is to let it run its course, apply antiviral topical solutions, or use pain-relieving medications. The antiviral drug acyclovir (Zovirax) is used to suppress outbreaks of oral and genital herpes. Antibiotics may be given for secondary skin infections.

Natural therapy focuses on enhancing the immune system so that one is not as susceptible to a herpes outbreak. In addition, this section discusses some natural remedies that have direct antiviral effects. It has been estimated that 90 percent of the population has one or both herpes viruses. The key is to have a resilient immune system that can fight off and contain the herpes virus. In the case of genital herpes, the best approach is prevention through avoidance of casual sexual contact. However, natural therapies can make a dramatic impact in reducing outbreak recurrence and severity for people with genital herpes.

SYMPTOMS

- A burning, tingling sensation on reddened skin, accompanied by one or more clusters of small, fluid-filled vesicles

ROOT CAUSES

- Sexual contact
- Immune system suppression
- Nutritional deficiencies

TREATMENT

Diet

Recommended Food

Consume foods that are rich in the amino acid L-lysine, as they may inhibit herpes virus replication. These includes legumes, fish, turkey, chicken, and most vegetables.

Bell peppers, brussels sprouts, broccoli, potatoes, and other brightly colored vegetables and fruits provide vitamin C and bioflavonoids that help heal the skin.

Fish such as salmon, nuts like walnuts, and seeds such as flaxseeds provide essential fatty acids that are necessary for tissue repair.

Food to Avoid

Avoid foods that are high in the amino acid L-arginine, as it may stimulate HSV replication. These foods include peanuts, almonds, and other nuts, as well as whole wheat and chocolate.

Reduce or eliminate sugars, as they interrupt the healing of tissue and suppress immune function.

Acidic foods, such as grapefruit, tomatoes, oranges, and other citrus fruits, may aggravate cold sores and should be avoided during an outbreak.

Testing Techniques

The following tests help assess possible reasons for repeated herpes outbreaks:

Immune system imbalance or disease—blood

Hormone testing (thyroid, DHEA, cortisol, testosterone, IGF-1, estrogen, progesterone)—saliva, blood, or urine

Intestinal permeability—urine

Detoxification profile—urine

Vitamin and mineral analysis (especially iron)—blood

Digestive function and microbe/parasite/candida testing—stool analysis

Food and environmental allergies/sensitivities—blood, electrodermal

Amino acid imbalance—blood or urine

℞ Super Seven Prescriptions—Herpes

Super Prescription #1   L-lysine
Take 1,000 mg three times daily between meals for an acute outbreak. For preventative purposes, take 500 mg two to three times daily between meals. This supplement has been shown in some studies to help treat acute outbreaks and may reduce recurrence.

Super Prescription #2   Lemon balm extract (*Melissa officinalis*)
Apply a lemon balm topical cream four times daily to the affected area. It has mainly been studied for healing cold sores.

Super Prescription #3   Homeopathic Herpes Nosode
Take a 30C potency three times daily for three days. This remedy stimulates an immune response to the herpes virus. It can be used for both oral and genital herpes and is also used to prevent recurrences.

Super Prescription #4   Lomatium root (*Lomatium dissectum*)
Take 1 ml or 500 mg four times daily for acute outbreaks. Lomatium root has immune-enhancing and antiviral properties.

Super Prescription #5   Propolis
Apply propolis tincture or ointment four times daily to the affected area. Propolis has been shown to heal genital herpes and most likely helps cold sores.

Super Prescription #6   Vitamin C
Take 1,000 mg, along with 500 mg of bioflavonoids, three times daily. Vitamin C improves immune function and reduces the duration of the infection.

Super Prescription #7   Zinc
Take 30 mg twice daily, along with 3 mg of copper. Zinc supports immune function and has been shown in studies to reduce the frequency, the severity, and the duration of a herpes outbreak. Topical application of zinc sulfate has been shown to reduce the recurrence of herpes outbreaks.

General Recommendations

Licorice root extract (glycyrrhetinic acid) cream has been shown to be effective for herpes outbreaks. Apply to lesions four times daily.

In one double-blind trial, topical application of an extract of lemon-balm cream, applied four times daily for five days, led to significantly fewer symptoms and fewer cold sore blisters than experienced by people using a placebo cream. Lemon balm has also been shown to help prevent recurrence of cold sores.

B-complex is important for people who are prone to cold sore outbreaks. Take a 50 mg complex one to two times daily.

Take a probiotic product containing at least 4 billion active organisms twice daily, thirty minutes after meals. It supplies friendly bacteria, such as *Lactobacillus acidophilus* and *bifidus,* that are important for immune function.

Echinacea (*Echinacea purpurea*) supports immune function and has antiviral properties. Take 500 mg or 2 to 4 ml of a tincture three times daily.

A high-potency multivitamin provides a base of nutrients required for a healthy immune system. Take as directed on the container.

A super green food supplement, such as chlorella or spirulina, or a mixture of super green foods, supports immune function. Take as directed on the container.

Thymus (*Thymus vulgaris*) extract supports the activity of the thymus gland, an important component of the immune system. The dosage is 1 to 2 tablets/capsules twice daily between meals or as directed on the container.

Homeopathy

Pick the remedy that best matches your symptoms in this section. For acute herpes outbreaks, take a 30C potency four times daily. For chronic herpes infections, take a 6x, 12x, 6C, 12C, or 30C twice daily for two weeks to see if there are any positive results. After you notice improvement, stop taking the remedy, unless symptoms return. Consultation with a homeopathic practitioner is advised.

Arsenicum Album is for people with cold sores who have symptoms of burning herpetic lesions that feel better with warm applications and warm drinks. They tend to feel anxious and restless.

Hepar Sulphuris is for very painful and sensitive mouth sores. The lesions feel very sensitive and are aggravated from cold drinks and cold air. The person feels chilly and irritable.

Mercurius Solubilis or Vivus is helpful when bleeding gums, a thickly coated tongue, heavy salivation and drooling, and offensive breath accompany the cold sores. The lesions burn and are worse at night.

Natrum Muriaticum is a specific remedy for cold sores that break out from sun exposure, fever, or emotional stress. The lesions are often near the lips. The corners of the mouth are often cracked as well. There is often a strong craving for salty foods. This remedy is also used for cases of chronic genital herpes. The person has a tendency toward depression and avoids the sun.

Rhus Toxicodendron is helpful for painful, swollen, itchy vesicles that burn and break out quickly. The person feels restless. Symptoms are worse from the cold or the damp.

Sulphur is a useful remedy for red, inflamed, itchy, and burning herpetic lesions. Symptoms are better from cold applications or ice-cold drinks. People requiring this remedy are very warm, with a great thirst for cold drinks.

Bodywork

Aromatherapy

Mix 1 drop of lemon and 1 drop of myrrh in a carrier oil, and with a Q-tip, dab the oil onto the herpes lesion.

Research on the herpes virus shows that in a culture dish, the amino acid arginine stimulated growth of the virus, while the addition of lysine inhibited growth. In a study, forty-five patients who experienced frequent herpes outbreaks received 312 to 500 mg of L-lysine for two months to three years. The dosage was increased to 800 to 1,000 mg for acute outbreaks, and foods that are high in the amino acid arginine were restricted (chocolate, seeds, nuts). This therapy reduced the frequency of outbreaks and greatly accelerated the recovery from acute outbreaks. Another double-blind study found that 1,200 mg of L-lysine significantly reduced the recurrence of herpes simplex outbreaks.

In one study involving ninety men and women with genital herpes, investigators compared propolis ointment to the pharmaceutical acyclovir. The participants were examined during their course of treatment. The authors of the study concluded that propolis ointment appeared to be more effective than acyclovir and a placebo in healing genital herpes lesions.

Other Recommendations

Acupuncture is helpful for some people with recurrent herpes. See a qualified practitioner for treatment.

Magnet therapy can be effective in reducing pain and stimulating skin healing. Use under the guidance of a knowledgeable practitioner.

Applying ice to a cold sore at the first signs of symptoms can help prevent a full-blown outbreak. Apply for ten minutes and then stop. Repeat every hour. An adult should apply it to the lesion of a young child to prevent damaging the skin.

REFERENCES

Griffith, R. S., et al. 1978. A multicentered study of lysine therapy in herpes simplex infection. *Dermatologica* 156:257–67.

Koytchev, R., R. G. Alken, and S. Dundarov. 1999. Balm mint extract (Lo-701) for topical treatment of recurring herpes labialis. *Phytomedicine* 6:225–30.

McCune, M. A., et al. 1984. Treatment of recurrent herpes simplex infections with L-lysine hydrochloride. *Cutis* 34:366–73.

Vynograd, N., I. Vynograd, and Z. Sosnowski. 2000. A comparative multi-centre study of the efficacy of propolis, Acyclovir and a placebo in the treatment of genital herpes. *Phytomedicine* 7(1):1–6.

Herpes Zoster. *See* Shingles

Hiatal Hernia and Acid Reflux Disease

A person is said to have a hiatal hernia when part of the stomach protrudes, or herniates, through the opening of the diaphragm and into the chest cavity. While almost half of all Americans over the age of forty have this disorder, many of these people experience few, if any, symptoms. Hiatal hernias are generally not considered dangerous unless they produce persistent or severe symptoms.

The food you eat starts its digestive journey in the mouth and then slides down the esophagus, a long tube that leads to the stomach. Because food is meant to travel through the digestive system in one direction only, the base of the esophagus is outfitted with a ring of muscles that acts as a sentry. At the stomach entrance, the muscles relax and allow the food to pass into the stomach, where acids start to break it down into a digestible stew. Once you're finished eating and the esophagus is empty, the muscular rings and valves tighten. This action keeps the food and the acids from backing up out of the stomach and refluxing into the esophageal tube.

Hiatal hernias can keep this system from working properly. When part of the stomach slides out of place (herniates), the ability of the muscular rings to keep food and acid in the stomach may be inhibited. In a phenomenon known as acid reflux, food and acid splash up into the esophagus, causing heartburn, chest pains, and belching. A person with severe symptoms may regurgitate stomach acid into the throat and the mouth. Sometimes the acid reflux leads to angina-like chest pains and spasms; the symptoms may be so intense that they are mistaken for a heart attack. Over long periods of time, the constant irritation of the esophagus can lead to inflammation, scarring, ulceration, hemorrhaging, and even esophageal cancer.

As with almost all digestive disorders, poor diet plays a large role in the unpleasant symptoms of hiatal hernias. Anything that contributes to an overly full stomach—eating too much, or eating foods that are not easily digested—encourages the stomach's contents to back up. In many cases, food allergies make the condition worse. Stress can trigger severe gastric upset as well. Anything that traumatizes the stomach muscles, such as injury, surgery, or pregnancy, can lead to hiatal hernias, as can the general weakening of muscles most people associate with aging. Finally, some people inherit a genetic tendency to this condition.

Bodywork therapies can be utilized to improve the structural problem that occurs with this condition. This involves manipulating the soft tissue, as well as the stomach itself, in a downward direction. This is described further in this chapter.

Acid reflux can also be caused by being overweight, from stomach infections, and from the effects of stress.

No matter what the cause, hiatal hernias respond well to dietary, herbal, and stress-reduction therapies. If you have this disorder, you'll also want to get regular check-ups to monitor the health of your esophagus.

SYMPTOMS

- Symptoms are usually worse after eating.
- Heartburn that's worse when bending over or lying down
- Belching
- Pains and muscle spasms in the chest
- Acid reflux

ROOT CAUSES

- Poor diet
- Food allergies
- Weakness of stomach muscles
- Pregnancy
- Trauma to the stomach area
- Stress
- Inherited tendency

TREATMENT

Diet

Recommended Food
Eat basic, unrefined foods that have not been stripped of their natural fiber. Whole grains, raw vegetables, and raw nuts and seeds are all good choices.

Avoid overeating by planning several light meals throughout the day.

Testing Techniques

The following tests help assess possible reasons for hiatal hernia and acid reflux:

Hormone testing (progesterone for women)—saliva, blood, or urine

Digestive function and microbe/parasite/candida testing—stool analysis

Food and environmental allergies/sensitivities—blood, electrodermal

---

Drink plenty of water. To maintain good digestive health, you need to drink a glass of clean water every two waking hours. In addition, have a large glass or two whenever you feel symptoms coming on. The water will dilute and neutralize the rising stomach acids.

The powers of cabbage juice to soothe the digestive tract are extraordinary. Drink a glass every day.

Add flaxseeds or flaxseed oil to your meals every day.

Food to Avoid

Avoid overeating. Don't eat on the run; take time to enjoy your meals and to savor each bite. Stop eating before you feel full.

Do not eat just before bedtime. Allow two to three hours for your stomach to empty.

Stay away from foods that are hard to digest. Saturated, hydrogenated, and partially hydrogenated fats linger in the stomach and often lead to acid reflux. The most frequent culprits are fried and greasy foods, red meat, and heavy sauces.

Food allergies are linked to hiatal hernias, so see the Food Allergies section and follow the elimination diet given there. If a food causes you trouble, eliminate it from your diet. You may find that your symptoms improve significantly or even disappear.

Avoid caffeine, alcohol, chocolate, and spicy or minty foods. They irritate the stomach and can aggravate your symptoms.

Detoxification

If you have a hiatal hernia, a three-day juice fast with green drinks and vegetable juices will help alkalinize your system; include healing herbal teas as well. Do not drink citrus fruit juices during this time, as they will only acidify and irritate your stomach lining.

D GL is a special type of licorice root (*Glycyrrhiza glabra*) extract used by holistic doctors to relieve acid reflux and ulcer pain. DGL stimulates cell growth of the mucous layer that lines the stomach and the intestines. It also improves blood flow and reduces muscle spasms. A study involving one hundred people compared the effects of DGL to those of the pharmaceutical antacid drug Tagamet and found that both were equally effective for healing ulcers.

℞ Super Seven Prescriptions—Hiatal Hernia and Acid Reflux

Super Prescription #1   Licorice root (DGL)
Chew one to two 400 mg tablets (or take in powder form) twenty minutes before each meal. DGL is a special type of licorice extract that soothes and heals the stomach and the esophagus. It does not cause high blood pressure.

Super Prescription #2   Aloe vera juice
Take 1 to 2 tablespoons three times daily or as directed on the container. Aloe vera promotes healing and soothes the digestive tract.

Super Prescription #3   Homeopathic Nux Vomica
Take a 30C potency two to three times daily. This homeopathic is specific for heartburn and reflux.

Super Prescription #4   Slippery elm (*Ulmus fulva*)
Take 1 teaspoon, 300 mg of the capsules, or 3 ml of the tincture three times daily. This herb is used to soothe and reduce inflammation of the lining of the esophagus and the stomach.

Super Prescription #5   Digestive enzymes
Take 1 to 2 capsules of a full-spectrum blend with each meal. Enzymes help you to digest foods more effectively so that they are less likely to cause irritation. *Note:* Some people may need to use a formula that contains no protease, as this protein digestive enzyme may irritate the stomach for some individuals.

Super Prescription #6   Marshmallow root (*Althea officinalis*)

Take 300 mg of the capsule or 3 ml of tincture three times daily. Marshmallow root soothes and reduces inflammation of the lining of the esophagus and the stomach.

Super Prescription #7   Probiotic

Take a product containing at least 4 billion active organisms daily. It contains friendly bacteria, such as *Lactobacillus acidophilus* and *bifidus,* which improve digestive function.

General Recommendations

Gentian Root (*Gentiana lutea*) improves overall digestive function. Take 300 mg or 10 to 20 drops five to fifteen minutes before meals.

A super green food supplement, such as chlorella. spirulina, or a mixture of super green foods in a drink, helps to neutralize acidity. Take as directed on the container.

Chamomile tea is soothing to the digestive tract. Drink one to two cups daily.

Liquid calcium is soothing to the stomach. Take a formula containing 500 mg of calcium and 250 mg of magnesium twice daily. Magnesium helps to relax tightened muscles of the esophagus and the stomach.

Homeopathy

Pick the remedy that best matches your symptoms in this section. For relief of acute acid reflux, take a 30C potency every fifteen minutes up to four doses. For chronic acid reflux, take a 6x, 12x, 6C, 12C, or 30C dose twice daily for two weeks to see if there are any positive results. After you notice improvement, stop taking the remedy, unless symptoms return. Consultation with a homeopathic practitioner is advised.

Arsenicum Album is for a burning sensation in the esophagus or the stomach that is alleviated by drinking milk or frequently sipping on warm water and sitting up. The person feels anxious and restless.

Carbo Vegetabilis will help people whose sluggish digestion leads to flatulence, belching, and bloating in the upper abdomen. People who benefit from this remedy are often pale and cold. Despite their chilliness, they feel better with cool air and drinks.

Lycopodium (*Lycopodium clavatum*) is also for gas and bloating, but in this case the symptoms are usually brought on by anxiety and lack of confidence. The person feels worse when wearing tight clothes and better when sipping warm drinks. There may be a sour taste in the mouth. Symptoms are often worse in the late afternoon and the evening.

Natrum Carbonicum is for people who have trouble digesting most foods, especially milk.

Nux Vomica is for people with heartburn and reflux that occurs from stress, spicy foods, and alcohol. They are generally chilly, irritable, and oversensitive to stimuli (noise, light). Constipation is often a problem as well.

Pulsatilla (*Pulsatilla pratensis*) is helpful if you feel worse after eating rich and fatty foods. Symptoms are worse in a warm room and better with fresh air. You also tend to feel tearful when ill, and you greatly desire comfort.

Phosphorous helps when you have a burning pain in the stomach that feels better from cold drinks. However, soon after drinking, you feel nauseous and may vomit.

Sulphur is for burning pain and belching, accompanied by diarrhea. The person tends to be very warm and gets relief from ice cold drinks.

Acupressure

See pages 668–675 for information about pressure points and administering treatment.

- Strengthen your upper digestive tract and reduce tension by working Pericardium 6.
- Stomach 36 gives general support to the entire body while improving your ability to absorb nutrients.
- Lung 1 reduces stress.
- Conception vessel 12 reduces heartburn.

Bodywork

Reflexology

See pages 686–687 for information about reflexology areas and how to work them.

Work the areas corresponding to the stomach, the diaphragm, and the adrenal glands. To reduce stress, also work the solar plexus.

Other Bodywork Recommendations

A chiropractor, an osteopath, or a naturopath can perform a gentle manipulation of your stomach with a downward pull. This helps reduce the stomach protrusion and soft tissues that have gone too far up through the diaphragm. Noticeable improvements can be noted within a few treatments.

Also, acupuncture can be quite effective in managing the symptoms. See a qualified practitioner.

Aromatherapy

Add any of the following oils to a warm bath, or dilute them in a carrier oil and use them in a gentle massage of your abdomen or lower back.

If your digestive system is slow to break down the food in your stomach, black pepper will stimulate the process.

Chamomile and ginger oils will help soothe stomach pain.

Stress Reduction

General Stress-Reduction Therapies

Any stress-reduction technique will help calm your stomach, so feel free to use any of the strategies listed in the Exercise and Stress Reduction chapter. You may find that yoga is especially helpful, as it not only reduces stress but also builds up the abdominal muscles. Regular exercise and Pilates are excellent as well.

Bach Flower Remedies

See the chart on pages 648–650 to find the remedy that best suits your personality and tendencies. Once you've chosen a remedy, place 10 drops of the liquid under your tongue. Hold the drops in place for thirty seconds and swallow. Use as often as needed.

If you are a quick, efficient person who is easily angered by those who move more slowly, take Impatiens.

Rock Water is for opinionated people who keep tight control over their needs and desires.

If you're an ambitious person and tend to judge others rather harshly, take Vine.

Perfectionists who don't like to compromise will be helped by Beech.

White Chestnut will quiet obsessive thoughts.

If you feel turmoil due to not forgiving others and have a tendency to feel sorry for yourself, then Willow would be appropriate for you.

Other Recommendations

- If you are obese, your symptoms will greatly improve if you lose weight. The dietary suggestions here may help, but see the Obesity entry if you need further advice.
- Do not wear clothes that fit tightly around your midsection. Constrictive clothing can push the stomach even farther out of place.
- Smoking aggravates heartburn, so if you smoke, quit. If you don't, you must still avoid exposure to secondhand smoke.
- Do not bend over, lie down, or put any great strain on your body within a few hours after eating. Organize your activities so that you can perform them when your stomach is empty.

REFERENCES

Morgan, A. G., et al. 1982. Comparison between Cimetidine and Caved-S in the treatment of gastric ulceration, and subsequent maintenance therapy. *Gut* 23:545–51.

High Blood Pressure. *See* Blood Pressure, High

High Cholesterol. *See* Cholesterol, High

HIV. *See* AIDS and HIV

Hives

Hives, medically known as urticaria, are raised white or yellow bumps surrounded by red, inflamed patches of skin. Hives usually cause a burning sensation at first, which soon gives way to intense itching. Aside from these symptoms, the course of hives is unpredictable. The rash may erupt suddenly and then disappear almost as quickly, or it may linger for weeks or even longer. It most often appears on the arms, the legs, or the trunk, but it can develop on any part of the body; sometimes it erupts in one place and then vanishes, only to appear somewhere else.

Although we don't tend to think of skin as an excretory organ, it actually plays a significant role in allowing toxins to pass out of the body. During the flu, for example, the body's temperature rises so that the virus can be expelled through a cleansing sweat. Just as poisons leave the body through sweat, they can also be excreted via skin eruptions like hives. Hives, like the symptoms of the flu, are an indicator that your body has detected a toxin and is trying to eliminate it.

An episode of hives is most frequently a response to an allergen or an irritant, which in either case is a normally harmless substance that produces a toxic response in your body. Possible allergens and irritants include insect bites, cosmetics, perfumes, detergents, and household cleaners. Certain foods may also trigger an allergic response. Shellfish are notorious for causing hives, but dairy, meat, and poultry are frequent instigators as well. Any food made with additives, preservatives, or pesticides may also produce a reaction. Some people with chronic or recurring cases of hives find that their triggers are frustratingly ubiquitous: heat, cold, sunlight, and stress have all been known to bring on a rash.

Drugs and viruses can also cause hives. Antibiotics, especially penicillin, cause hives in some unfortunate people; during a bacterial infection, they will need to work closely with their doctors to determine the best course of medical action. Lately, doctors have linked viruses like hepatitis B and Epstein-Barr to hives, and the fungus *Candida albicans* has also been known to trigger the disorder.

Some people suffer from reoccurring hives due to the effects of stress. In these cases, it is important for them to incorporate stress-reduction techniques into their lifestyle. Also, hives can be symptoms of more serious conditions, such as parasitic infections, hepatitis, cancer, hyperthyroidism, and rare blood disorders.

Anyone who sufferers from chronic or recurring hives should consider that his or her digestive system may not be functioning properly, thereby forcing the skin to throw off toxins that would normally be excreted by the intestines. A close review of dietary and lifestyle habits is in order.

The good news is that hives, although irritating and itchy, rarely pose a significant health threat. In almost all cases, they disappear from the skin without leaving a scar or other marks, and they do not damage any other organs. The best treatment is to identify the irritant or the toxin and then avoid it; you'll also want to employ methods that help you speed up the detoxification process. Sometimes, however, hives can cause the tongue and the throat to swell up; breathing becomes difficult, if not impossible. If you have hives and experience any trouble breathing or swallowing, you have a medical emergency. Call for medical help immediately. If you know that you are prone to severe hives, keep an emergency adrenaline kit on hand.

SYMPTOMS

- Burning or itchy white bumps appear, surrounded by areas of redness and inflammation.

- Hives may appear anywhere on the body and may come and go without warning.

Testing Techniques

The following tests help assess possible reasons for hives:

Immune system imbalance or disease—blood

Hormone testing (thyroid, DHEA, cortisol)—saliva, blood, or urine

Intestinal permeability—urine

Detoxification profile—urine

Digestive function and microbe/parasite/candida testing—stool analysis

Food and environmental allergies/sensitivities—blood, electrodermal

---

ROOT CAUSES

- Response to an allergen or an irritant
- Certain drugs, especially antibiotics and aspirin
- Infectious agent
- Poor digestion

TREATMENT

Diet

Recommended Food

If you have a chronic case of hives and cannot identify the cause, it is highly recommended that you buy food in its natural state whenever possible and prepare it yourself. This eating plan will drastically reduce your chances of encountering a food allergen.

Everyone with hives should make it a priority to follow a high-fiber diet that includes oats, brown rice, beans, and raw fruits and vegetables. You'll improve your digestion and reduce the necessity of expelling toxins through your skin.

If your hives are triggered by sunlight, eat lots of deeply colored vegetables. They're high in carotenoids and will improve your skin's resistance to the sun.

Essential fatty acids reduce inflammation. Eat cold-water fish several times a week; if you're following a vegan diet, add flaxseeds to your salads, or use flaxseed oil as a dressing.

Candidiasis may be a factor in persistent hives. Although live active yogurt is generally recommended for people with candidiasis, you should stay away from it if you are allergic to dairy. Instead, try kefir or sauerkraut. Many people with dairy allergies choose to drink sauerkraut juice daily—an acquired taste, to be sure, but one that goes a long way toward replacing the friendly bacteria that fight *Candida albicans*.

Drink a glass of clean water every two waking hours. You'll flush out impurities and encourage the health of nearly every body system, including the skin.

Food to Avoid

Hives are often caused by a response to a food allergen or an irritant. Read the Food Allergies section and follow the elimination diet to find out if a certain food triggers hives for you; if so, it goes without saying that you must banish that food from your diet. Some people can't even come into contact with allergenic foods, let alone ingest them, so stay as far away from these as you can. Any food can conceivably cause hives, but shellfish, dairy, eggs, cured meats, citrus fruit, and peanuts are the most common triggers.

Avoid foods that prevent your body from functioning optimally. Processed, junk, and refined foods all depress your immune and digestive systems, even if you're not allergic to them.

Alcohol and caffeine are diuretics that pull nutrients out of your body. Since your poisoned system needs all the support it can get, stay away from these substances.

Digestive problems are linked to all skin disorders. Do not eat meat, fried foods, or foods high in saturated fat; they take too long to travel through the intestines and lead to constipation. Avoid dairy products, as they slow food down on its way through the digestive system.

Detoxification

People with chronic or recurring cases of hives should follow a detoxification program to encourage a faster elimination of toxins.

Go on a three-day juice fast. Concentrate on green drinks, especially those with barley, spirulina, and blue-green algae, as well as carrot, apple, and beet juices. (Be sure to include the beet tops while you're processing the vegetables through the juicer.)

As you fast, you may find that toxins rise to the skin at an increasing rate. Don't be concerned; it is normal for hives to get worse shortly before they get any better. To remove debris and dead skin cells, dry-brush your skin every morning. Do not brush areas where hives are present.

℞ Super Seven Prescriptions—Hives

Super Prescription #1   Homeopathic Apis (*Apis mellifica*)
Take a 30C potency every fifteen minutes, up to four doses. This remedy is specific for hive outbreaks where there is itching and swelling.

Super Prescription #2   Vitamin C
This nutrient reduces the effects of histamine, a chemical that is released by the body during an allergic reaction. Take 1,000 to 2,000 mg three times daily. Reduce the dosage if diarrhea occurs. Use a nonacidic vitamin C product.

Super Prescription #3   Quercitin
This nutrient reduces the effects of histamine, a chemical that is released by the body during an allergic reaction. Take 1,000 mg three times daily.

Super Prescription #4   Vitamin B12
Taking 1,000 mcg of the injected form (given by your doctor) one to three times weekly can help reduce the severity of acute hives. The oral form is not as effective, but you can take 400 mcg of sublingual B12 daily.

Super Prescription #5   Greens drink
Take daily, as directed on the container, a blend containing super green foods such as chlorella or spirulina. You can also take these supplements individually. They support detoxification and neutralize acidity.

Super Prescription #6   Burdock root (*Articum lappa*)
Take 300 mg or 3 ml three times daily to support detoxification of the skin.

Super Prescription #7   Nettle leaf (*Urtica diocia*)
Take 300 mg three times daily of a freeze-dried nettle product. Nettle leaf has an antihistamine effect.

General Recommendations

Aloe vera reduces inflammation and is soothing to the skin. You may smooth a cream or a lotion directly onto the hives for temporary relief; to address the body's imbalances more directly, drink aloe vera juice.

Chamomile (*Matricaria recutita*) is a good all-around tonic for hives. Used in a cream, it relieves itching. Drunk as a tea, it eases stress.

If you need more potent relief from stress or anxiety, drink valerian (*Valeriana officinalis*) tea once during the day and again just before bedtime.

People with skin disorders often have stressed livers. Milk thistle (*Carduus marianus*) will help cleanse this crucial organ. Find a product standardized for 70 to 80 percent silymarin, and take 200 to 250 mg twice daily.

Homeopathy

Pick the remedy that best matches your symptoms in this section. For relief of acute hive outbreaks, take a 30C potency every fifteen minutes, up to four doses. For chronic hives, take a 6x, 12x, 6C, 12C, or 30C twice daily for two weeks to see if there are any positive results. After you notice improvement, stop taking the remedy, unless symptoms return. Consultation with a homeopathic practitioner is advised.

Apis (*Apis mellifica*) is for red, swollen, burning hives that feel better with cold applications and in the fresh air.

Histaminum is a remedy used for general allergy reactions. It calms down the release of the chemical called histamine that leads to allergy reactions.

Rhus Toxicodendron is for hives that are caused by getting chilled in the rain or in dampness and that itch violently. They feel better when heat is applied.

Urtica Urens is for hives that feel like prickly heat and are caused by insect bites or from eating shellfish.

Acupressure

See pages 668–675 for information about pressure points and administering treatment.

- To remove heat from the blood, work Spleen 10.
- Other points that ease heat-related skin conditions are Bladder 23 and 47 and Stomach 2 and 3.
- If stress is a trigger for you, work Bladder 10 whenever you feel tense and likely to break out.
- Spleen 10 clears heat from the blood.
- If you are constipated, work Conception Vessel 6 and Large Intestine 4 to stimulate intestinal contractions.

Bodywork

Reflexology

See pages 686–687 for information about reflexology areas and how to work them.
    Work the liver and the colon to encourage detoxification.
    If you need to reduce tension, stimulate the solar plexus.

Hydrotherapy

A cool bath will not cure hives, but it can temporarily relieve the itching.

Aromatherapy

Chamomile, lavender, and melissa will reduce inflammation, itching, and stress. Use any one of the oils or all of them together in a bath, a compress, or a lotion. As it's possible that you'll have a reaction to one of these oils, start off by using them in small quantities, and test them on a small area of skin before plunging into a bath.

Stress Reduction

General Stress-Reduction Therapies

Folk wisdom has always noted the link between anxiety and hives, and now at least one scientific study seems to confirm this traditional knowledge. If you get hives frequently—even if they're caused by an identifiable trigger—you should seek out a relaxation therapy and practice it regularly.

Bach Flower Remedies

Consult the chart on pages 648–650 to determine the best remedy for your particular needs. Following are some suggestions. Once you've chosen a remedy, place 10 drops of the liquid under your tongue. Hold the drops in place for thirty seconds and swallow. Use as often as needed.

Rescue Remedy is for both physical and emotional crises. Take it when hives first appear or when you are under a heavy burden of stress that may lead to a breakout.

The Bach Flower philosophy considers allergies a manifestation of emotional intolerance. Beech will help you increase your sympathy for people who try your patience.

If you despair of identifying the substance that triggers your hives, take Gorse to refresh your optimism.

If hives make you feel ashamed, take Crab Apple.

Other Recommendations

- An oatmeal bath can reduce itching. Add a cup of oatmeal powder, such as Aveno, to a warm bath. The other alternative is to put oatmeal into a cheese-cloth bag and tie it with a string, hang it under the faucet or float it in the tub. Soak in the warm bath for five to fifteen minutes. When you're done, pat your skin dry so that a film of oatmeal is left on your skin. This film contains the anti-itch properties of the oatmeal.

Hypothyroidism (Underactive Thyroid)

The thyroid gland, situated at the base of the neck below your Adam's apple, secretes hormones that control metabolic activity in every cell of the body. In a condition called hypothyroidism or underactive thyroid, the thyroid fails to produce sufficient quantities of that hormone. This can be the result of the thyroid itself malfunctioning or due to the fact that it is not receiving the proper message from the brain to produce more hormones. As a result, all body systems function at a slower rate. If you suffer from this condition, you probably feel tired and weak most of the time. You move slower than you used to, and even relatively simple and routine activities, like preparing dinner, seem overwhelming; worse, you may not even be able to summon up any interest in trying. Most likely, you've gained weight and have a hard time digesting food. Your joints and muscles may ache, and because your body temperature has plummeted, you feel cold even when others are complaining of the heat. And those symptoms are just some of the most common. Others include recurring infections, hair loss, brittle nails, dry skin, menstrual problems, and high cholesterol levels. As you might imagine, hypothyroidism is often mistaken for other ailments, especially depression or even laziness.

Iodine deficiency was once the most frequent cause of hypothyroidism. Although today most Americans get plenty (and sometimes too much) of this trace mineral from iodized table salt, there still exists a significant minority who don't get enough or whose absorption is impaired. Nowadays, the most frequent cause of hypothyroidism is Hashimoto's disease, an autoimmune disorder in which the body manufactures antibodies that attack thyroid tissue and suppress production of the thyroid hormone.

There are other thyroid conditions that may also lead to hormonal underproduction. Stress, nutritional deficiencies, inactivity, some medications, and hormonal fluctuations as a result of pregnancy and menopause also have a role to play.

Hypothyroidism is more common in women. The balance of estrogen and progesterone can have an indirect influence on the thyroid glands. Most common is estrogen dominance, where relatively higher estrogen levels suppress thyroid function. This predisposition can occur throughout a woman's life. Women on synthetic estrogen therapy are particularly susceptible to decreased thyroid function.

The effects of stress and the balance of stress hormones are also important in thyroid function. Chronic elevation of the stress hormone cortisol suppresses thyroid function, while low levels of DHEA appear to make one more susceptible to hypothyroidism.

Toxic metals, such as mercury, lead, arsenic, and others, can also interfere with thyroid activity.

Although hypothyroidism can wreak havoc upon your entire body, it is easy to treat, especially if caught in its early stages. If you suspect that you have an underactive thyroid, follow the instructions given here for taking your basal body temperature. If your body temperature is consistently low, you should see a doctor for an evaluation. For mild cases, nutritional supplements can set you back on track quickly. For people with more severe cases, the use of thyroid hormone replacement may be required. Even if you require a thyroid hormone supplement, you should complement this regime of supplementation with dietary changes, stress-reducing activities, exercise, and general hormone balancing.

A word of caution: Many doctors rely on a blood test to diagnose hypothyroidism. Unfortunately, this test is extremely unreliable and often fails to catch mild to moderate cases of the disorder. If your basal body temperature is consistently low and if you experience the symptoms described here, but your blood test does not reveal hypothyroidism, consider working with a more holistic doctor for preventative care. Besides the basal body temperature, it may be of more help to run a saliva or urine thyroid test.

SYMPTOMS

- Fatigue
- Apathy
- Depression and irritability
- Weight gain
- Aches and pains
- Sensitivity to cold and heat
- Constipation
- Menstrual problems (irregular periods)
- Recurring infections
- High cholesterol
- Hair loss
- Dry skin and hair
- Brittle, peeling nails
- Infertility
- Insomnia
- Anxiety and panic attacks
- Poor memory and concentration
- Low libido
- Headaches
- Premenstrual syndrome
- Lowered immunity
- Carpal tunnel syndrome
- Raynaud's phenomenon
- Water retention
- Dry eyes/blurred vision
- Eyebrow loss (outer one-third)
- Anemia and easy bruising
- Slow healing
- Hoarse voice
- Tingling hands and feet

ROOT CAUSES

- Hashimoto's disease and other inflammatory disorders of the thyroid
- Iodine deficiency
- Stress
- Poor diet
- Inactivity
- Pregnancy

- Hormone imbalance (especially estrogen/progesterone, cortisol/DHEA)
- Surgery on or radiation of the thyroid
- Certain medications, most notably lithium and synthetic estrogen
- Failure of the pituitary gland

TREATMENT

Diet

Recommended Food

It stands to reason that hypothyroidism is most frequently found in landlocked regions, where iodine-rich foods from the sea are less available. If you have an underactive thyroid, it may be helpful to consume plenty of sea vegetables, such as kelp, nori, dulse, kombu, and wakame. Fish and sea salt are also good sources of iodine.

Essential fatty acids found in flaxseeds, walnuts, and fish are important for thyroid function.

Food to Avoid

Certain vegetables known as goitrogens may suppress thyroid function. These include kale, broccoli, cauliflower, cabbage, soy, and brussels sprouts. Cooking the vegetables inactivates the goitrogens, so that they are safe to eat for someone with low thyroid.

It's never advisable to drink tap water, but people with hypothyroidism must be especially wary of it. Most tap water is full of fluorine and chlorine, two chemicals that inhibit your ability to absorb iodine.

How to Take Your Basal Body Temperature

Basal body temperature is one of the most effective tools for diagnosing hypothyroidism, and it's easy to take and record your temperature at home. The night before you begin the recordings, assemble the following:

- A thermometer; if not digital, shake it down to 96 degrees F or lower
- Pen or pencil
- Paper
- Clock, watch, or stopwatch

Place these items on your bedside table, within easy reach of your usual sleeping position. When you wake up in the morning, place the thermometer under your armpit and lower your arm over it. Hold the thermometer tightly in place for ten minutes. You need to lie still for the entire seven to ten minutes, as even a small movement can disrupt the reading. When the ten minutes are over, note your temperature and record it, with the date, on the paper.

Repeat this procedure for three days. If you are a menstruating woman, you should begin taking your temperature on the second day of your period.

After three days, take the average of the readings. If it is below 97.7 to 98.2 degrees F (the normal range for a basal temperature), you probably have an underactive thyroid.

Testing Techniques

The following tests help assess possible reasons for hypothyroidism:

Thyroid hormone testing (thyroid: TSH, Free T4, Free T3, Reverse T3, anti-thyroglobulin antibodies, anti-thyroid peroxidase)—blood, saliva, urine

General hormone testing (DHEA, cortisol, testosterone, IGF-1, estrogen, progesterone, insulin)—saliva, blood, or urine

Intestinal permeability—urine

Toxic metals (e.g., mercury, lead)—hair or urine

Vitamin and mineral analysis (especially vitamin A, selenium, zinc, copper, magnesium)—blood

Amino acid analysis (especially L-tyrosine)—blood or urine

Digestive function and microbe/parasite/candida testing—stool analysis

Food and environmental allergies/sensitivities—blood, electrodermal

Hypothyroidism can also be traced to a deficiency of several other minerals, including zinc, selenium, and copper. A deficiency of the amino acid tyrosine is often present in those with hypothyroidism. To make sure you're getting enough of these nutrients, incorporate pumpkin seeds, beans, almonds, soy products, and fish into your diet.

A slow metabolism often means a slow digestive process. Encourage faster elimination of food by eating more fiber in the form of whole grains, beans, fruits, and vegetables.

You must stay adequately hydrated. Drink a glass of clean water every two waking hours.

℞ Super Seven Prescriptions—Hypothyroidism

Super Prescription #1   Bladderwrack (*Fucus vesiculosus*)
Take 100 mg or 1 ml twice daily.

Super Prescription #2   Thyroid glandular
Take 1 tablet/capsule three times daily on an empty stomach or as directed on the container. It stimulates and supports thyroid function.

Super Prescription #3   Pituitary glandular
Take 1 tablet/capsule three times daily on an empty stomach or as directed on the container. It stimulates thyroid function.

Super Prescription #4   L-tyrosine
Take 500 mg twice daily on an empty stomach. This amino acid is used in the synthesis of the thyroid hormone.

Super Prescription #5   Natural progesterone
This is for women who have low thyroid hormones and low progesterone levels. See the PMS and Menopause sections for the proper dosage.

Super Prescription #6   Guggul (*Commiphora mukul*)
Take a product containing 25 mg of guggulsterones three times daily.

Super Prescription #7   Homeopathic Thyroidinum 3x or **6x**
Take 3 pellets three times daily. This homeopathic preparation of thyroid is used to stimulate thyroid activity.

If you have had a blood TSH (thyroid-stimulating hormone) test, this refers to the hormone released by your pituitary gland in your brain. Its job is to stimulate thyroid hormone secretion when the brain senses your thyroid levels are getting low. A normal lab range is referenced as 0.5 to 5.5 uU/ml. We feel that 0.2 to 2.0 is an optimal TSH range. Furthermore, it is important to have your free thyroxine (T4) and free tri-iodothyronine (T3) levels tested, as these are the two most metabolically active thyroid hormones, especially the free T3. Also, since Hashimoto's thyroiditis is the most common cause of low thyroid, you should have your thyroid antibody levels tested.

Nori Rolls

If you don't live near a sushi bar, you can easily make these nori rolls at home. With a little practice, you can turn them out quickly for a light lunch or a sophisticated hors d'oeuvre. If you want to boost your meal's iodine quotient, serve miso soup sprinkled with toasted wakame alongside the nori rolls.

Ingredients

Use quantities that suit your needs and tastes.

Toasted nori

Brown rice, uncooked

Clean water

Brown rice vinegar

Salt

Carrots, green and red peppers, cucumbers, and avocado, cut into long, thin strips

Wasabi (optional)

Tamari soy sauce for dipping

Pickled ginger (buy a brand that doesn't add coloring; many companies add an artificial pink color to their product)

Equipment

Bamboo rolling mat

Cook the brown rice, using 1 cup of clean water for each cup of rice. Once the rice is done, toss in 2 tablespoons of brown rice vinegar for every cup of cooked rice. Set the rice and vinegar mixture aside until it is no longer hot to the touch and you are able to handle it without burning your hands.

Center a sheet of nori on the rolling mat. When the rice is ready, moisten your hands with water and pat a small handful of rice evenly across the nori. Leave an inch-wide strip at the top side of the nori sheet.

Take a very small amount of wasabi—around half a teaspoon—and spread it in a thin, horizontal line about two or three inches from the base of the nori sheet. Wasabi is a kind of Japanese horseradish that is extremely hot, so use caution. If you dislike hot food, you can omit this step.

Above the line of wasabi, make two more horizontal lines, this time with the vegetables. With your hands, press the vegetables firmly into the rice.

Grasp the bottom edge of the bamboo mat and use it to help you roll up the sheet of nori. Some rice may squeeze out of the sides, but you can fix that later. Stop when you reach the inch-wide border at the top of the sheet.

Press the border into the roll to seal it up. Most nori sheets will seal up on their own; if yours won't stick, dampen your fingers with a little water, run them along the bare strip, and try again.

Trim the edges of the roll with a sharp knife to neaten the presentation and to clean up any rice spillage, and then cut the roll into half-inch slices. (Some people prefer a wider slice; how you cut the roll is up to you.)

Serve the rolls with the pickled ginger. Offer small bowls of tamari soy sauce and wasabi on the side for dipping.

General Recommendations

A high-potency multivitamin provides a base of nutrients required for thyroid hormone synthesis. Take as directed on the container.

Essential fatty acids are important for thyroid function. Take 3,000 mg of fish oil or 1 tablespoon of flaxseed oil and 150 mg of GLA from evening primrose or borage oil.

Ashwagandha (*Withania somniferum*) has been shown to improve thyroid and stress hormone levels. Take 500 mg three times daily.

Take DHEA if tests show that your levels are low. Take 5 to 15 mg each morning, under the supervision of a doctor.

Homeopathy

Although homeopathic remedies are not a substitute for thyroid supplementation, they are quite useful for easing the symptoms of an underactive thyroid. In mild cases, these remedies may stimulate the thyroid enough not to require supplement thyroid hormone.

Pick the remedy that best matches your symptoms in this section. Take a 6x, 12x, 6C, 12C, or 30C potency twice daily for two weeks to see if there are any positive results. After you notice improvement, stop taking the remedy, unless symptoms return. Consultation with a homeopathic practitioner is advised.

Calcarea Carbonica is helpful when there is low thyroid function, accompanied by chilliness, fatigue, and a sense of being overwhelmed. The person tends to be flabby and may have excessive sweat on the head at nighttime. There is a craving for eggs and milk products.

Lycopodium (*Lycopodium clavatum*) is helpful if you have a right-sided enlargement of the thyroid. You also experience a tremendous amount of gas and bloating. There is a strong craving for sweets. You tend to be chilly and irritable.

Pulsatilla (*Pulsatilla pratensis*) is for women who are warm and who desire cool, fresh air. There is a craving for sweets, a low thirst, and symptoms of hormone imbalance, possibly due to PMS or menopause, that are characterized by weeping and sadness.

Sepia is for women with low thyroid hormone, who are irritable and chilly. They crave salty, sweet, and sour foods.

Nux Vomica is helpful if you suffer from fatigue and also feel chilly, achy, irritable, and constipated. It is good for thyroid burnout from overworking.

Acupressure

See pages 668–675 for information about pressure points and administering treatment.

- Triple Warmer 17 has a balancing effect on the thyroid.
- For depression, work Lung 1. You'll find yourself taking air more deeply into your lungs and relieving stress with each breath.
- If you feel weak and fatigued, work Bladder 23 and 47. Do not press on these points if you have severe back pain.
- Work Conception Vessel 6 to ease constipation.

Bodywork

Massage

A full-body massage will reduce stress, improve circulation, and lift your energy level. If you like, you can add any of the essential oils listed in the Aromatherapy section to further enhance the treatment.

Reflexology

See pages 686–687 for information about reflexology areas and how to work them.
   Work the area corresponding to the thyroid.

Aromatherapy

Geranium oil will regulate the thyroid hormone. Use it in a bath, or better yet, add to a carrier oil and incorporate into a massage. Geranium can also help lift fatigue and depression. So can jasmine, neroli, bergamot, and rose.

If your skin is dry, add chamomile (*Matricaria chamomilla*) to a lotion, a cream, or a carrier oil and apply the mixture to the affected area.

Oil of black pepper or marjoram will stimulate a sluggish digestive system and improve overall circulation.

Stress Reduction

General Stress-Reduction Therapies

High levels of stress inhibit the thyroid's ability to properly manufacture its hormone. Exercise has been shown to improve thyroid function and should be done on a daily basis.

Bach Flower Remedies

See the chart on pages 648–650 to find the remedy that best suits your personality and tendencies. Once you've chosen a remedy, place 10 drops of the liquid under your tongue. Hold the drops in place for thirty seconds and swallow. Use as often as needed.

If your illness makes you despondent or discouraged, take Gentian.

Olive and Hornbeam are the remedies for prolonged apathy or exhaustion. You may wish to take them in combination for a more potent effect.

People who tend to devote themselves to serving others will find that Centaury gives them the courage and the focus to pursue their own dreams.

Other Recommendations

- When it comes to prescription thyroid medication, some supplements are better than others. The most commonly prescribed, Synthroid, is a pharmaceutical product that contains only one active hormone, thyroxine. Far more effective are natural desiccated thyroid supplements, which are made with two active hormones—thyroxine and tri-iodothyronine—and sometimes more. Ask your doctor if you can take Armour Thyroid Extract, widely considered the best natural desiccated thyroid product on the market. Also, the use of compounded thyroid that contains exact doses of T4 and T3, or just T3 alone is equally beneficial when prescribed by an experienced doctor.
- Enzyme supplements improve the faulty digestion that is common in hypothyroidism; when inflammation is present, enzymes will aid in healing. If you're taking enzymes as a digestive aid, take the supplements before your meals. If you need to reduce inflammation, take them one or two hours after eating. Use the dosage amounts recommended on the product label.
- Antihistamines and sulfa drugs keep your body from absorbing iodine. If you take either of these medications, talk to your doctor about possible alternatives.

Impotence

Impotence, also referred to as erectile dysfunction, is a man's inability to attain or sustain an erection sufficient for normal, satisfying sexual intercourse. It was once thought that almost all impotence was caused by psychological factors, but we now know that as many as 85 percent of cases are brought on by physiological disturbances. No matter what the cause, it helps most men to realize that they are not alone. Nearly every man experiences impotence at some point, and almost 20 million have chronic or recurring problems.

Many physiological factors may contribute to impotence, but the most frequent are hormonal changes, medications, diet, and chronic illness. Low levels of testosterone, the male sex hormone, are a critical link to male impotence. The most common cause of impotence is atherosclerosis, which is hardening of the arteries with plaque build up. This causes a problem with blood flow to the penis. See the Cardiovascular Disease section for a comprehensive program to reverse this vascular problem. Also, dilation of the arteries and blood flow to the genital area are dependent on a chemical produced in the body known as nitric oxide.

In addition, many prescription drugs can cause reduced blood flow to the genitals or can interfere with brain activity, hormones, or nerve transmission. If you suffer from impotence and are on a prescription medication, talk to your doctor. He or she may be able to find alternatives for you.

Diet is another common cause. Just as a high-fat, low-fiber routine can inhibit blood flow to the heart, it can also block the arteries that lead to the penis. Men with high blood pressure or arteriosclerosis may have difficulty maintaining erections. Other chronic illnesses, especially diabetes, can take a toll as well.

It is important to note here that aging is not a cause of impotence. While it's true that impotence affects older people more frequently than it does the rest of the population, this situation can be attributed to the increased incidence of disease and medication in the elderly. And disease itself is not an inevitable part of aging; see Aging, for information about staying healthy throughout the full span of your life. If you are healthy and content, you can be sexually vigorous well into your eighties and beyond.

If you are not chronically impotent—that is, if you are impotent only in certain situations or can achieve an erection on your own or in your sleep, then it's likely that psychological factors are causing or contributing to your problem. Overwork and fatigue have reached epidemic levels in our society, and many men—especially those who have children—simply feel too tired to enjoy sex. Depression, anxiety, stress, fear of failure, and fear of pregnancy are other frequent causes.

The following drugs may cause impotence; popular brand names for those drugs are also given, where applicable.

Drug	Popular Brand Names (where applicable)
Alcohol	
Antidepressants and tranquilizers	Ativan, Paxil, Prozac, Valium, Xanax
Antihistamines	Most cold, flu, and allergy medicines
Antihypertensives	Cardizem, Inderal, Procardia
Antacids	Pepcid, Tagamet, Zantac
Cocaine	
Diuretics	Dyazid, Lasix
Narcotics	
Nicotine	

Many cases of impotence can be successfully treated with an improvement in lifestyle and dietary habits, as well as with nutritional supplements, but anyone with a chronic problem should see a doctor first to rule out underlying disorders.

SYMPTOMS

- Inability to achieve or maintain an erection

ROOT CAUSES

- Low levels of DHEA and testosterone
- Prescription medications
- Street drugs
- A diet that's high in fat and low in fiber
- Underlying illness (most often, arteriosclerosis, high blood pressure, and diabetes)
- Hormonal imbalance
- Fatigue
- Stress or anxiety
- Depression
- Other psychological factors (fear of pregnancy, fear of failure, lack of desire)
- Heavy metal poisoning

Treatment

If an underlying condition or a medication is causing impotence, check with a doctor before undertaking any changes in your diet, medication, or habits. If you have cardiovascular disease or diabetes, see the appropriate section in this book for further recommendations.

Diet

Recommended Food

Eat a healthful diet that's high in fiber and nutrients. Good sources of fiber include fresh raw vegetables, apples, oats, and whole grains.

Vitamin E dilates blood vessels and improves blood flow. Foods that are high in this nutrient include wheat germ, soy products, leafy green vegetables, and whole grain cereals.

Enjoy soybeans, pumpkin seeds, and sunflower seeds as snacks or in salads. They're excellent sources of zinc, which aids the prostate and improves testosterone levels.

Watercress leaves, sesame seeds, and bee pollen are libido enhancers. Add some to your meals every day.

Food to Avoid

Avoid foods that are high in saturated, hydrogenated, or partially hydrogenated fats, including red meat, butter, margarine, shortening, and refined vegetable oils. A high-fat diet causes circulatory problems and blocks the flow of blood to the genitals.

Eliminate junk and processed foods from your diet. Not only are they generally fatty and lacking in nutrition, they contain chemicals that might affect sexual performance.

Don't eat large meals just before sex. Your body will be too focused on digestion to concentrate on desire.

Testing Techniques

The following tests help assess possible reasons for impotence:

Immune system imbalance or disease—blood

Blood pressure

Hormone testing (thyroid, DHEA, cortisol, testosterone, IGF-1, estrogen, progesterone)—saliva, blood, or urine

Intestinal permeability—urine

Detoxification profile—urine

Vitamin and mineral analysis (especially magnesium, B12, iron, and CoQ10)—blood

Digestive function and microbe/parasite/candida testing—stool analysis

Anemia—blood test (CBC, iron, ferritin, % saturation)

Food and environmental allergies/sensitivities—blood, electrodermal

Blood-sugar balance—blood

Moderate your intake of caffeine and alcohol. While a cup of coffee or a glass of wine should not pose a problem for most people, overindulgence can lead to temporary or chronic impotence.

Detoxification

A three-day juice fast will help clear your body of toxins and generally improve your circulation.

R_X Super Seven Prescriptions—Impotence

Super Prescription #1   L-arginine
Take 1,000 mg three times daily on an empty stomach. This amino acid leads to blood vessel dilation and improved blood flow, which are required for an erection.

Super Prescription #2   *Cordyceps sinensis*
Take 800 mg twice daily of Cs-4 mycelium extract. Cordyceps has historically been used to treat low libido and impotence in men, and Chinese studies verify this effect.

Super Prescription #3   *Panax ginseng*
Take 100 mg two to three times daily of a product standardized to between 4 and 7 percent ginsenosides. This herb is revered in China for its ability to improve libido and sexual function for men.

Super Prescription #4   Ginkgo biloba
Take 120 mg twice daily of a standardized product containing 24 percent flavone glycosides and 6 percent terpene lactones. Ginkgo improves blood flow, and studies show it to be effective for erectile dysfunction.

Super Prescription #5   DHEA
If lab testing shows that your levels are low, take 25 to 50 mg daily under the supervision of a doctor. Studies show that some men who are low in this hormone improve their erectile function with supplementation. DHEA is also a precursor hormone to testosterone.

A double-blind, randomized, placebo-controlled study involving forty men who were confirmed to have low DHEA levels were given either 50 mg of DHEA or a placebo for six months. Men taking DHEA had a significant improvement in libido and erectile function.

A double-blind trial involving *Panax ginseng* for three months found that it significantly improved libido, the ability to maintain an erection, and patient satisfaction with sex.

Several studies have shown that gingko biloba extract improves erectile dysfunction in men. A study of men with impotence as the result of pharmaceutical medications (such as antidepressants) found that 200 mg of ginkgo biloba extract improved sexual function in 76 percent of the men.

Super Prescription #6   Potency wood (*Muira puama*)

Take 500 mg three times daily. Studies have shown this herb from South America to improve sexual desire and impotency.

Super Prescription #7   Oatstraw (*Avena sativa*)

Take 300 mg three times daily. Oatstraw relaxes the nervous system and is thought to increase libido.

General Recommendations

Niacin (vitamin B3) is a vasodilator and improves blood flow. Take 250 mg three times daily.

Zinc is a mineral that's required in the synthesis of testosterone. Take 30 mg twice daily, along with 3 to 5 mg of copper.

Tribulus terresteris ("Puncture Vine") is a folk remedy for improving libido and erectile function. Take 500 mg three times daily.

Damiana (*Turnera diffusa*) is a traditional remedy for impotence that improves blood flow to the genitals. Take 400 to 800 mg or 2 to 3 cc of the tincture three times daily.

Ashwagandha (*Withania somniferum*) is an ancient Ayurvedic medicine used to treat stress and impotence. Take 1,000 mg three times daily.

Yohimbe (*Pausinystalia yohimbe*) increases blood flow to erectile tissue and increases libido. Take a product standardized to yohimbine hydrochloride at a dosage of 10 mg three times daily. It should be used under the supervision of a doctor and should be avoided by people with high blood pressure, any cardiovascular condition, or kidney disease; by pregnant women; or by individuals being treated for a psychological disorder.

Homeopathy

Agnus Castus is a remedy for men who were involved in frequent sexual activity for many years. There may be a cold sensation in the genitals. Men requiring this remedy are often anxious about their health and may have problems with memory and concentration.

Caladium is a remedy for men who have an interest in sexual relations, but the genitals are completely limp. There may be frequent wet dreams without an erection. Men who require this remedy often crave tobacco.

Lycopodium (*Lycopodium clavatum*) is for men who have erection problems as a result of worry and low self-confidence. Digestive problems, such as gas and bloating, are common, and symptoms are worse in the late afternoon.

Selenium Metallicum is a remedy for men who have decreased sexual ability, especially after a fever or an exhausting illness. They feel weak and exhausted, but interest is usually still present. There may be unusual hair loss.

Staphysagria is for mild-mannered, shy men with deep emotions, such as suppressed anger. Their problems with impotence often begin after an embarrassing event.

Acupressure

See pages 668–675 for information about pressure points and administering treatment.

- To relieve stress and encourage calm, deep breathing, work Lung 1.
- Bladder Points 23 and 47—together they are known as the Sea of Vitality—will improve sexual potency and reduce fatigue.

Bodywork

Reflexology

See pages 686–687 for information about reflexology areas and how to work them.

Work the areas that correspond to the testes, the prostate, the pituitary and adrenal glands, and the solar plexus.

Hydrotherapy

Constitutional hydrotherapy can be used to improve circulation. See pages 676–677 for directions.

Some men find that hot baths and saunas lower their sex drive. Try taking warm— not hot—showers and baths. Stay away from saunas to see if your condition improves.

Aromatherapy

Several oils ease stress while stimulating sexual desire. Among the best are patchouli, ylang ylang, sandalwood, and jasmine. Try a few drops in a bath or add them to a carrier oil, and use this in a sensual massage.

Stress Reduction

General Stress-Reduction Therapies

Regular meditation can fit nicely into the schedule of almost anyone, including people who are overworked. Try to set aside twenty minutes every night after work, to detach yourself from the worries of the day.

Bach Flower Remedies

Select the appropriate remedy, and place 10 drops of the liquid under your tongue. Hold the drops in place for thirty seconds and swallow. Use as often as needed.

If you lack sexual confidence and feel inadequate, Larch will help you feel more secure.

Crab Apple is for people who feel inhibited because they've been taught that sex is dirty. This remedy will encourage a healthy attitude toward sexuality.

Pine will help people who feel that sex is shameful, sinful, or morally wrong. People who also worry that it is physically dirty should combine Pine with Crab Apple.

If you are utterly exhausted and drained, Olive will have a strengthening effect.

Other Recommendations

- Regular exercise stimulates blood flow, reduces stress, and helps unclog arteries. Moderate daily exercise has been strongly linked to better sexual performance.
- Don't smoke or expose yourself to secondhand smoke. Nicotine is a well-known cause of impotence.

REFERENCES

Choi, H. K., D. H. Seong, and K. H. Rha. 1995. Clinical efficacy of Korean red ginseng for erectile dysfunction. *International Journal of Impotence Research* 7:181–86.

Cohen, A. J., and B. Bartlik. 1998. Ginkgo biloba for antidepressant-induced sexual dysfunction. *Journal of Sex and Marital Therapy* 24:139–43.

Reiter, W. J., A. Pycha, G. Schatzl, et al. 1999. Dehydroepiandrosterone in the treatment of erectile dysfunction: A prospective, double-blind randomized, placebo-controlled study. *Urology* 53:590–95.

Infertility

To many couples, pregnancy seems like a simple matter—so simple that not getting pregnant is their chief concern. But after years of protected sex, men and women who decide they want children may discover that conception is a far more complex process than they realized.

Here's an extremely simplified version of what must happen: First, a woman secretes several hormones—each at the correct time—that cause one of the eggs in her ovaries to mature and to be released into the fallopian tube. A man must then contribute enough sperm (tens of millions of them) that have the ability to travel up into the tube, where the egg is fertilized. The egg makes it way to the uterus and implants itself in the uterine wall. If anything goes wrong with any one of these events, the couple will not conceive. Because the process is so complicated, it often takes a number of months of trying before a woman can become pregnant. But if a couple has had regular, unprotected sex for at least a year and still cannot conceive, the partners are considered infertile.

For the last few decades, the rate of infertility in the United States has increased. No hard statistics are available, but experts estimate that between 16 and 25 percent of all couples have serious difficulty getting pregnant. As with most other conditions that have been on the rise, many of today's infertility cases can be attributed to lifestyle changes in the latter half of the twentieth century. Poor nutrition, stress, eating disorders, extremely intense exercise, and exposure to environmental toxins all take a grave toll on the body. When one or both members of a couple have weakened body systems, the chances increase that something will go awry in the conception process. People today also have more sex partners than they used to, and with increased sexual activity comes a greater risk of contracting diseases that damage the reproductive organs. Finally, many couples now choose to delay childbearing until their thirties or even forties, when a woman's fertility begins to decline.

If you're having trouble getting pregnant, it's wise for both of you to take a break and spend a few months restoring and nourishing your bodies. Good nutrition, herbal supplementation, hormone-balancing protocols, and effective stress management help a great many couples conceive; these strategies will also increase the chances that your baby will be healthy. (Not to mention that you'll need those stress-management techniques when you're a parent!)

Hormone balance is particularly important for both sexes. We find that women with infertility problems often have low ovulatory progesterone levels or low thyroid function. Both of these hormones can be a limiting factor in conception. With men, low thyroid, as well as low testosterone, can be problematic.

Many couples are confused about when, during the woman's menstrual cycle, conception can occur. It is important to understand that the best chance of conception is to have sexual relations one to two days before ovulation occurs, not on the day of ovulation. Over-the-counter LH (luteinizing hormone) test kits are readily available to help determine when ovulation is going to occur. This hormone rises approximately forty-eight hours before an egg is released (ovulation). Basal body temperature can also be used to determine ovulatory patterns. This method must be used over many months to determine when a woman ovulates. Many practitioners and books explain how to properly use this technique.

Although a lot of focus with fertility is on the female partner, keep in mind that studies show that approximately 40 percent of infertility cases are due to men's sperm abnormalities. These include low sperm count, decreased sperm motility, or abnormal sperm shape.

One or both of you may have an anatomical abnormality: for example, many women suffer from blocked fallopian tubes, often as a result of a chlamydia infection, and men may have a varicose vein of the testicle, called a varicocele. In many cases, these conditions can be treated with surgeries and procedures. Couples that can't get pregnant in any other way may eventually consider in vitro fertilization, and an increasing number of women with ovary problems are turning to egg donors. Unfortunately, however, all the medical techniques in the world—complementary, conventional, and cutting-edge—can't guarantee that every couple that wants a baby will conceive. Before you begin a series of invasive and expensive procedures, be sure to speak frankly with your doctor about the risks involved and the chances of success. And take heart: many people, exhausted from years of diagnostics and surgeries, give up trying—only to discover that they've finally become relaxed enough to conceive.

SYMPTOMS

- Failure to conceive after twelve months of regular, unprotected intercourse that is timed with ovulatory patterns.

ROOT CAUSES

Dozens of factors can cause infertility. Following are some of the most common.

- Poor nutrition and nutritional deficiencies
- Stress
- Sexually transmitted diseases
- Environmental toxins
- Congenital abnormalities
- Hormonal problems (especially low thyroid or low progesterone)
- Medical conditions such as endometriosis, polycystic ovary syndrome, varicocele
- Eating disorders, especially anorexia
- Overly intense exercise
- Obesity
- Toxic metals

TREATMENT

Diet

Recommended Food

In general, you should eat wholesome meals made with organic vegetables, grains, and soy products. Eat fish several times a week, but be sure it's from a clean water source.

Vitamin E nourishes the endocrine system, so use cold-pressed nut and seed oils for cooking or as a base for salad dressings. Wheat germ is another good source of vitamin E; add it to smoothies, cereals, or salads.

Essential fatty acids promote gland health and are often lacking in people who follow radical low-fat diets. Incorporate cold-water fish, flaxseeds, or flaxseed oil into your meals daily.

Men should snack regularly on pumpkin seeds. They're an excellent source of zinc, a nutrient that's an important part of male reproductive fluids.

Testing Techniques

The following tests help assess possible reasons for infertility:

Hormone testing (thyroid, DHEA, cortisol, testosterone, IGF-1, estrogen, progesterone)—saliva, blood, or urine

Ovulation pattern—ovulation kit

Vitamin and mineral analysis—blood

Anemia—blood test (CBC, iron, ferritin, % saturation)

Food and environmental allergies/sensitivities—blood, electrodermal

Toxic metals—hair analysis or urine

Eat vegetables, fruits, beans, whole grains, and other sources of fiber at every meal, and drink a glass of clean water every two waking hours. You'll promote your overall health and sweep away toxins that may be suppressing your reproductive system.

Food to Avoid

Don't eat anything that depresses body systems or causes nutrient depletion. Cut out refined sugar and white flour, along with fried or processed food.

Animal meats are loaded with chemicals that mimic the effects of estrogen, a hormone that in excess can decrease sperm count and fertility. If you must eat meat, make sure it's organic.

Avoid alcohol, which reduces the number of normal sperm in men and generally weakens the health of both sexes.

Caffeine consumption has been linked to fertility problems, including miscarriage. Avoid coffee, soft drinks, chocolate, black and green teas, and pharmaceutical medications containing caffeine.

Detoxification

Drink purified water to avoid chlorine and other chemicals that may affect fertility.

℞ Super Seven Prescriptions—Infertility

Super Prescription #1   Vitex agnus-castus (chasteberry)
Women should take 160 to 240 mg of a 0.6 percent aucubin extract each morning. Vitex stimulates the ovaries to ovulate and normalizes progesterone levels.

Super Prescription #2   Natural progesterone cream
Women should apply ¼ teaspoon (20 mg) to the skin once daily. Make sure to start using this hormone after you ovulate. If you become pregnant, continue utilizing the progesterone until the third trimester or as directed by your doctor. *Note:* This treatment is best used under the guidance of a doctor who is knowledgeable about natural hormones.

Super Prescription #3   Vitamin C
Take 500 mg twice daily. Vitamin C prevents sperm agglutination in men and has been shown to be helpful with female infertility as well.

In one study, 48 women from ages 23 to 39 who were diagnosed with infertility took Vitex supplement once daily for three months. During the trial, 7 women became pregnant and 25 women experienced normalized progesterone levels, which, in theory, may increase the chances for conception.

Super Prescription #4   Vitamin E

Take 400 IU daily. Animal and human studies have shown this vitamin to be important for fertility.

Super Prescription #5   L-arginine

Men should take 2,000 mg twice daily on an empty stomach. This amino acid has been shown to increase sperm quality and count.

Super Prescription #6   *Panax ginseng*

Men should take 300 mg of a product standardized to between 4 and 7 percent ginsenosides daily. This herb has been shown to increase sperm count and motility.

Super Prescription #7   Zinc

Men should take 30 mg twice daily, along with 3 to 5 mg of copper. Studies show that this mineral improves sperm quality, count, and motility.

General Recommendations

L-carnitine or acetylcarnitine improves sperm motility. Take 1,500 mg twice daily.

Coenzyme Q10 improves sperm motility. Take 100 mg daily.

Selenium improves sperm motility. Take a daily total of at least 100 mcg.

A high-potency multivitamin provides a base of the nutrients that are important for fertility. Take as directed on the container.

Iron is important for women, if testing shows iron-deficiency anemia. Take 15 mg twice daily or as directed by your doctor.

PABA has been shown in studies to help women with chronic infertility. It is thought to improve the effects of estrogen. Take 100 mg four times daily, for up to seven months.

Vitamin B12 has been shown to increase sperm count. Men should take 1,500 mcg of oral B12 or 400 mcg of the sublingual form daily.

Homeopathy

Consult a homeopathic practitioner for a constitutional remedy.

Acupressure

You may need to use these points on a daily basis for several months before you see results. For information about pressure points and administering treatment, see pages 668–675.

- Both men and women should work Bladder 23 and 47 to build up vitality and encourage conception.
- To stimulate general wellness and the effective absorption of nutrients, work Stomach 36.
- If you need to relieve tension, use Lung 1. It will help you to breathe deeply and focus on the here and now.

Acupuncture

See a qualified practitioner for regular treatments, as studies have shown this therapy to be helpful for improving female fertility.

In a study, 178 men with low sperm counts or abnormal sperm function were given 4,000 mg of L-arginine daily for at least 2 months. As a result, 62 percent of the men had a marked increase in sperm motility and count, and 28 pregnancies occurred. Researchers also noted that men with very low initial sperm counts, of less than 20 million per ml, did not have as beneficial a response as men with higher counts did.

Bodywork

Massage

Massage won't magically make you fertile, but it is relaxing, and it has the additional benefit of stimulating blood flow to your entire body, including to your reproductive organs and endocrine system.

Reflexology

See pages 686–687 for information about reflexology areas and how to work them.

Work all the gland points to regulate hormone production.

Women should work the areas corresponding to the reproductive system. These points will help stimulate blood supply to the pelvis and will help relieve blockages.

To clear blockages, men should work the areas corresponding to the testes and the prostate.

For relief of tension and stress, both sexes should work the diaphragm/solar plexus point.

Hydrotherapy

Sitz baths, either hot or cold, will increase blood supply to the pelvic region.

Aromatherapy

Rose oil is said to improve sperm's ability to travel through the female reproductive organs to a waiting egg. Although no one has verified this via scientific method, it certainly can't hurt to use a little rose in a massage oil or a bath, especially since the essence also has calming and sensuous qualities.

If months of trying to conceive have sapped you or your partner of sexual desire, try using ylang ylang, sandalwood, or patchouli in a bath or a massage. Each of these oils is a renowned aphrodisiac and promotes a sense of quiet relaxation.

Note: If you become pregnant, stop using essential oils.

Stress Reduction

Tension and stress, whether about fertility or any other issue, have long been linked to an inability to conceive. It doesn't matter which stress-reduction technique you use, as long you find one that works for you and employ it frequently.

Bach Flower Remedies

See the chart on pages 648–650 to find the remedy that best suits your personality and tendencies. Once you've chosen a remedy, place 10 drops of the liquid under your tongue. Hold the drops in place for thirty seconds and swallow. Use as often as needed.

Some people feel embarrassed or ashamed over an inability to conceive. Crab Apple will help abate these feelings.

If you've tried conceiving for a few months and are already discouraged, take Gentian to regain your optimism.

Gorse will help people who feel that nothing will ever help them conceive.

People who are completely exhausted from work, rounds of doctor's appointments, or anything else should take Olive.

If you blame yourself for not being able to conceive, take Pine for a more balanced view of the situation.

Other Recommendations

- Smoke can dramatically reduce your fertility and will also harm a growing fetus. If you're trying to get pregnant, you must avoid smoke of all kinds.
- Exercise to improve your circulation and general health, but don't overdo it. People who overtrain find it difficult to conceive.
- Women who are obese need to focus on losing weight for optimal fertility. See the Obesity section.
- Men should know that sperm must stay relatively cool. That's why the testicles are apart from the rest of the body, not inside it. If the testicles are heated, sperm may die or be damaged. Stay away from saunas and hot tubs, and don't wear tight-fitting underwear.
- After sex, a woman should lie in bed for fifteen to twenty minutes with her knees up. To keep conception from seeming like a science project, the man should stay with her and hold her gently.

REFERENCES

Propping, D., and T. Katzorke. 1987. Treatment of corpus luteum insufficiency. *Zeitschrift für Allgemeinmedizin* 63:932–33.

Schacter, A., et al. 1973. Treatment of oligospermia with the amino acid arginine. *Journal of Urology* 110:311–13.

Influenza. *See* Flu

Insomnia

Insomnia is our nation's silent health crisis. Almost half of all adults report having difficulty sleeping, but less than 10 percent discuss the issue with their doctor. Almost everyone has suffered from temporary insomnia due to stress, overeating, or consuming stimulants before bed and knows how draining and exhausting sleep loss can be. But people who have chronic insomnia—a consistent inability to go to sleep or to stay asleep through the night—are at risk for far more than fatigue. Sleep deficiency suppresses the immune system and the libido, decreases productivity, and can lead to other disorders like depression, chronic fatigue, heart disease, and headaches.

Before the use of electric lighting, the average American got nine hours of sleep a night. Now the average is less than seven hours and still going down, as the distractions of twenty-four hour-shopping and entertainment becomes more widespread. How much sleep is enough? It has become fashionable to proclaim a need for very little sleep. However, studies involving mental function show that most adults do best with eight hours; some may need as many as nine or even ten. Children and teens need more sleep than adults do, and older people often find that they simply sleep less than they used to. If you nod off to sleep very quickly—within five minutes of putting your head on the pillow—or if you feel an urge to nap during the day, you probably need more sleep than you're getting.

Stress and anxiety are the most common causes of insomnia, but physiological factors often play a significant role as well. Stimulants, heavy metals, chronic pain, and breathing problems can keep you from sleeping, as can many medications and disorders.

Sleep apnea affects 5 percent of adults, but most of them will never be diagnosed. During this condition, a person repeatedly stops breathing during the night and wakes up to catch his or her breath. The two consequences of this are a significant drop in the blood's oxygen and severe sleep deprivation. Be suspicious of this condition if you snore, have daytime sleepiness, have high blood pressure, or are overweight. This condition is best identified during a sleep study that your doctor can order. The recommendations in this section—especially the dietary ones—may help to treat sleep apnea. Weight loss can be an important component, as can avoiding sleeping on your back. One standard treatment is a C-pap machine, which involves a mask that is kept over your face while you sleep. It keeps constant pressure in the airway so that it does not collapse. Orthodontic devices that keep the lower jaw and the tongue forward are sometimes useful. In rare cases, extremely large tonsils or abnormalities in the throat structure may need to be surgically corrected.

Restless leg syndrome is a disorder characterized by unusual or painful sensations in the legs, accompanied by an irresistible urge to move the legs. It's often brought on by rest and occurs most often in the evening. It can produce difficulty falling asleep. Many studies have shown that restless leg sufferers have low or low-normal iron levels. Iron supplementation has helped many people, but three months of treatment is usually needed before improvement is noted.

Hormone imbalance can be a root cause of insomnia. This can involve several different hormones. It is common for many women experiencing menopause to develop insomnia. This is generally due to changes in estrogen and progesterone levels. The obvious solution is to follow a hormone-balancing program. See the Menopause section for more information. Likewise, younger women with premenstrual syndrome can experience the same. In addition, low or hyper functioning thyroid can interfere with sleep. We also find that elevated levels of the stress hormone cortisol interfere with deep REM sleep, which studies confirm. It is not uncommon to find seniors with deficiencies in DHEA, testosterone, and growth hormone, which can be underlying causes as well. The sleep hormone melatonin can work wonders in selected cases, when supplemented correctly.

If you suffer from insomnia, you may find that the gentle treatments in this section help you get a good night's sleep. If they don't, talk to your doctor. He or she should review your general health and may also refer you to a sleep disorder specialist. It is not recommended, under any circumstance, that you take over-the-counter sleeping aids. They do not promote deep, restful sleep, and they may also create any of several side effects, including depression, confusion, and dry mouth. Worse, they can be addictive.

SYMPTOMS

- Inability to sleep or to sleep through the night

ROOT CAUSES

- Stress and anxiety
- Aging
- Stimulants, including caffeine, decongestants, and thyroid medications
- Sugar
- Indigestion
- Pain
- Alcohol
- Lack of exercise

- Restless leg syndrome
- Hormonal changes (e.g., menopause)
- Vitamin deficiencies (e.g., B12, iron)

- Breathing disorders, including asthma and sleep apnea
- Other disorders, such as hypothyroidism and hypoglycemia

Testing Techniques

The following tests help assess possible reasons for insomnia:

Sleep study—lab setting

Hormone testing (thyroid, DHEA, cortisol, testosterone, IGF-1, estrogen, progesterone)—saliva, blood, or urine

Vitamin and mineral analysis (especially magnesium, calcium, B12, iron)—blood

Anemia—blood test (CBC, iron, ferritin, % saturation)

Food and environmental allergies/sensitivities—blood, electrodermal

Blood-sugar balance—blood

TREATMENT

Diet

Recommended Food

At dinner, eat foods that are high in tryptophan, a chemical that stimulates serotonin, which in turn helps you sleep. Turkey, chicken, tuna, soy products, live unsweetened yogurt, and whole-grain crackers are all good, low-sugar sources.

Complex carbohydrates are also relaxing, so incorporate whole grains, especially brown rice or pasta, into your dinners.

This book does not generally recommend dairy products, aside from yogurt, but a glass of milk before bedtime is a time-honored sleep aid. Try this only if you do not have a sensitivity or an allergy to dairy products.

Deficiencies of calcium and magnesium can lead to insomnia. Be sure your diet is high in leafy greens, sesame and sunflower seeds, oats, almonds, and walnuts.

The B-vitamins are also essential for good sleep. Brewer's yeast is the best source. Sprinkle it on your dinner salad or add a teaspoon to a bedtime glass of water or a green drink.

Drink a glass of clean water every two waking hours so you won't wake up at night with a dry mouth. Have your last glass two hours before bedtime, or you'll be up for other reasons.

Food to Avoid

The first rule for insomniacs is to monitor caffeine intake strenuously. Do not have any products containing caffeine—such as coffee, black tea, or chocolate—for eight hours before you go to sleep.

Drink alcohol only in moderation, and don't have any within two hours of going to bed. While a drink might make you feel drowsy, the alcohol only disrupts the deep, late-night sleep that is so crucial to rest. If you have a chronic problem with insomnia, avoid alcohol completely.

The adrenal glands release cortisol as a response to stress. Cortisol is released by the body in a natural rhythm with the sleep-wake cycle. Levels increase and peak in the early morning hours as part of the body's physiological response to awakening. An oversecretion of cortisol at nighttime can interfere with sleep. This is because rapid eye movement (REM) sleep (a process that occurs during deep sleep) occurs primarily when cortisol levels are decreasing. Conversely, the adrenal hormone DHEA has a balancing effect on high cortisol levels and has been shown to significantly increase REM time during sleep.

Food allergies or sensitivities disrupt sleep for some people. See the Food Allergy section to identify possible offending foods.

Sugar is another common culprit in insomnia. After lunchtime, avoid sugary foods, even sweet fruits. Chocolate, with its double whammy of sugar and caffeine, should be considered an enemy of the sleep-deprived.

℞ Super Seven Prescriptions—Insomnia

Super Prescription #1   5-Hydroxytryptophan (5-HTP)
Take 100 to 200 mg one hour before bedtime. This supplement promotes serotonin production in the brain for relaxation. Do not use if you are currently taking pharmaceutical antidepressants.

Super Prescription #2   Melatonin
Take 0.3 to 0.5 mg one hour before bedtime. This hormone promotes sleep. It is best used on a short-term basis or under a doctor's supervision.

Super Prescription #3   Passionflower (*Passiflora incarnata*)
Take 500 mg or 1 to 2 ml a half hour before bedtime. Passionflower is a great sleep aid that relaxes the nervous system and does not cause drowsiness in the morning.

Super Prescription #4   Valerian (*Valerian officinalis*)
Take 600 mg or 2 ml a half hour before bedtime. Several studies show valerian to be effective for insomnia. *Note:* A small percentage of users may notice a stimulating effect from valerian.

Super Prescription #5   Calcium/magnesium
Take 500 mg of calcium and 250 mg of magnesium each evening. Both minerals help relax the nervous system. Some people have better results taking one of the minerals alone in the evening and the other earlier in the day. Experiment to see what works better for you.

Super Prescription #6   Hops (*Humulus lupulus*)
Take 500 mg or 1 to 2 ml a half hour before bedtime. Hops is a nervine that relaxes the nervous system.

Super Prescription #7   Vitamin B12
Take 1,500 mcg in capsules or 400 mg of the sublingual tablet form daily. This vitamin is more commonly deficient in seniors, and a deficiency may contribute to insomnia.

A double-blind trial found that 600 mg of valerian extract taken thirty minutes before bedtime was comparable in efficacy to oxazepam (Serax), a commonly prescribed pharmaceutical for insomnia. Studies have also found that the combination of valerian and lemon balm (*Melissa officinalis*) works well to treat insomnia, with a comparable effect to the pharmaceutical sleep medication triazolam (Halcion). A hangover sensation was noted in people taking the triazolam but not in the lemon balm/valerian users.

General Recommendations

Vitamin B6 is involved in the production of serotonin and other neurotransmitters that promote sleep. Take 50 mg daily.

Chamomile (*Matricaria chamomilla*) relaxes the nervous system. Drink a fresh cup of tea in the evening or take 300 mg of the capsule form.

Saint-John's-wort (*Hypericum perforatum*) acts as a nerve tonic and can ease mild cases of depression and related insomnia. Take 900 mg daily of a 0.3 percent hypericin extract. Do not take Saint-John's-wort if you are on medication for depression.

Homeopathy

Pick the remedy that best matches your symptoms in this section. Take a 6x, 12x, 6C, 12C, or 30C potency twice daily for two weeks to see if there are any positive results.

After you notice improvement, stop taking the remedy, unless symptoms return. Consultation with a homeopathic practitioner is advised.

Aconitum Napellus is a remedy for people who have just experienced a terrifying situation and who develop insomnia. Restlessness, fear, and panic attacks may wake a person up.

Arsenicum Album is for people who have tremendous anxiety and restlessness. They often wake up between the hours of midnight and 2 A.M. They tend to be perfectionists and have many insecurities and fears.

Cocculus is a good remedy for people who can't sleep after staying up too long. As a result, they may feel weak and dizzy, have trouble thinking, and be irritable, as well as sleepy.

Coffea Cruda is very specific for people with insomnia that's caused by overstimulation. They are wide awake at 3 A.M., with a racing mind.

Ignatia (*Ignatia amara*) is a specific remedy for insomnia caused by emotional upset—usually grief or a loss. There can be uncontrollable crying, loss of appetite, and mood swings. The person often sighs a lot during the day and muscles may twitch during sleep.

Kali Phosphoricum is for insomnia as a result of nervous exhaustion caused by overwork or mental strain. The person is extremely sensitive, and depression and anxiety are common.

Lycopodium (*Lycopodium clavatum*) is for people with insomnia as a result of fear and stress. They usually have poor confidence, which further worsens stress levels. Digestive problems, such as gas and bloating, are usually present. There is a craving for sweets.

Nux Vomica is for insomnia after indulging in rich, spicy food or alcohol. The sleep problem may be the result of overwork. The person is irritable and impatient, wakes at 3 A.M., thinking about business, and is highly sensitive to light, noise, sound, and other stimuli.

Sulphur is a good remedy for insomnia that comes on from itching at night or from feeling too heated at night. The person throws the covers off at night or sticks the feet out. There is a strong craving for ice-cold drinks and spicy foods.

Zincum Metallicum is for people who are very restless from being overworked. Their legs and arms are restless, and it's hard for them to lie still in bed.

Acupressure

See pages 668–675 for information about pressure points and administering treatment.

- Pericardium 6 and Lung 1 will reduce anxiety and heart palpitations.
- Another point to reduce tension is Conception Vessel 17.
- If indigestion is a problem, you should make it a habit to avoid greasy and spicy foods. If you do indulge, Spleen 16 will help you digest the food properly.
- Large Intestine 4 is a good general point for pain relief. Try it if arthritis or other aches keep you up at night.

Bodywork

Massage

Any kind of massage will help you relax and unwind. Most people with insomnia would benefit from a professional massage as well as home and self-care techniques. Use some relaxing essential oils for an even more potent effect.

Reflexology

See pages 686–687 for information about reflexology areas and how to work them.

To relax your nerves, work the diaphragm and the solar plexus.

Hydrotherapy

Before sleeping, take a ten-minute hot footbath to draw blood out toward your limbs and away from your head.

If you need to relax, take a hot bath—but make sure to do it at least two hours before bed. Otherwise, your body temperature will be too high to allow sleep.

Other Bodywork Recommendations

Many people who have trouble sleeping rub their heads in frustration. Try to avoid this temptation. You'll only increase the blood flow to your brain, which can make sleeping even more difficult.

Acupuncture and Chinese herbal therapy can be very effective for insomnia. See a qualified practitioner.

Aromatherapy

Essential oils can have a dramatic relaxing effect. Many can help you get to sleep, but lavender, neroli, chamomile, and ylang ylang are some of the best. Add some to a bath or a massage, or sprinkle a few drops on your pillow. You might also like to add the oil to a diffuser in your bedroom.

Marjoram is another sleep-inducing oil that has the additional benefit of warming and relaxing the muscles. You can use it in any of the previous preparations, but it may be most effective in a bath or a massage.

Lavender sachets are a time-honored sleep aid. Tuck one under your pillow for all-night insomnia relief.

Stress Reduction

General Stress-Reduction Therapies

Make nightly meditation sessions a habit. Try to devote twenty or thirty minutes (some of you may need even more) before bedtime to cultivating a relaxed focus and a sense of detachment from the day's worries. You'll find that you're much more likely to sleep.

Most of us have lain awake in bed at some point, trying to nod off by counting sheep. But, as you've probably experienced, unlimited counting can lead to panic, especially as you reach the higher numbers. By the time you've reached one hundred, you may be frantic with the awareness of how much sleepless time has passed since you've begun the exercise, and a sense of futility sets in. Instead, try this meditative technique when you can't sleep. Breathe calmly and deeply from your abdomen, and count each breath. Give one count to each inhalation and one count to each exhalation. When you reach ten, start again at one. Don't keep track of how many series of ten you've done; simply use the numbers as a means of focus, rather than as a means of marking time. This technique will help you avoid frustration and will often send even seasoned insomniacs off to sleep within minutes. And even if you can't get to sleep, you'll feel much more relaxed and rested than if you spent the night sweating over sheep counts.

Bach Flower Remedies

See the chart on pages 648–650 to find the remedy that best suits your personality and tendencies. Once you've chosen a remedy, place 10 drops of the liquid under your tongue. Hold them in place for thirty seconds and swallow. Use as often as needed.

Stress often triggers insomnia, but sometimes insomnia itself can bring on a panic attack. If this happens to you, take some Rescue Remedy for an instant calming effect.

For insomnia caused by the "mind chatter" of an overactive brain, take White Chestnut. It will release you from the grip of persistent, circular thoughts or worries.

If your sleeplessness is brought on by worries for other people, Red Chestnut will help.

Take Mimulus for generalized fears or fears you can't name.

Mustard will help relieve insomnia due to depression or sadness.

If you overwork yourself but still fear failure, take Hornbeam. It will help you face your daily challenges calmly.

If sleep evades you due to shock from a serious illness or an accident, use Star of Bethlehem.

Other Recommendations

- Get into a sleep routine. Create a bedtime ritual to help yourself quiet down and to signal your body that it's time to rest. Have a cup of herbal tea, or practice one of the relaxation techniques listed in this section. Go to bed at the same time every night, and wake up at the same hour each morning. Do not change this routine on the weekend.
- Keep your bedroom quiet, dark, and comfortable. Invest in a good mattress and pillow, and have several covers available to suit various nighttime temperatures.
- Use the bed for sleep and sex only. Everything else, including reading, writing letters, and making phone calls, should take place off the bed, preferably in another room.
- If you can't sleep, get out of bed and move to another room, if possible. Try not to dwell on your insomnia; instead, read a magazine or a light novel, or engage in some other quiet activity.
- Don't smoke or expose yourself to secondhand smoke. Nicotine, like alcohol, has an initial calming effect but ultimately disrupts sleep.
- Many nonaspirin pain relievers contain caffeine. If you have chronic pain and need relief to sleep, check for brands that don't list caffeine as an ingredient.
- Get exercise during the day, even if long nights awake have left you tired. People who exercise regularly report better and deeper rest than those who don't. Do not exercise within two hours before bed, however, as your body may be too stimulated to sleep.

REFERENCES

Dorn, M. 2000. Valerian versus oxazepam: Efficacy and tolerability in non-organic and non-psychiatric insomniacs: A randomized, double-blind, clinical, comparative study. *Forsch KomplementärmedKlass Naturheilkd* 7:79–84 [in German].

Dressing, H., D. Riemann, H. Low, et al. 1992. Insomnia: Is valerian/balm combination of equal value to benzodiazepine? *Therapiewoche* 42:726–36 [in German].

Irritable Bowel Syndrome

Although irritable bowel syndrome is now the standard term, there are many other names for this group of symptoms, including:

- Spastic colon
- Mucous colitis
- Gastric colitis
- Nervous indigestion
- Intestinal neurosis

Common Illnesses That Mimic IBS

- Cancer of the colon or the rectum
- Duodenal ulcer
- Diverticular disease
- Biliary tract disease
- Parasitic diseases, such as amebiasis, giardiasis, campylobacter
- Lactose intolerance
- Laxative abuse
- Ulcerative colitis
- Imbalanced intestinal flora
- Malabsorption conditions, such as celiac disease or pancreatic insufficiency

If you have irritable bowel syndrome (IBS), you are not alone. Once a relatively rare disorder, IBS now affects an estimated 20 to 30 percent of the U.S. population. Although women are two times more likely than men to seek treatment for IBS, it is thought that men and women are affected in equal numbers. It is the most common reason for a referral to a gastroenterologist. IBS is characterized by a malfunction in the digestive tract. Usually, waste material is delivered through the tract to the rectum by rhythmic contractions of the intestines. In IBS, those contractions become erratic and irregular. Bowel movements are unpredictable and painful, with attending constipation, diarrhea, or an alternation of both. The abdomen may be cramped or bloated, certain foods can no longer be tolerated, and other all-too-familiar signs of gastric distress develop. In some cases, waste matter is pushed through the tract with such force that stool incontinence results. Studies have also found that people with IBS have increased sensitivity to pain in the digestive tract.

There are really five main fundamental causes of IBS. The modern-day, fast-food diet is definitely one of them. Refined foods that are hard to digest contribute to many symptoms of poor digestion. Second, poor stress-coping mechanisms trigger nervous system reactions that contribute to IBS. Unresolved emotional traumas can have this negative effect as well. Third, chronic infections of the digestive tract with candida, parasites, and bacteria can be causative factors. Fourth, poorly functioning digestive organs contribute to IBS symptoms. These include dysbiosis, where there is a deficiency of the good bacteria that are involved with digestion and detoxification. The fifth cause, and the least common, is a structural abnormality of some type. Spinal misalignments, for example, impair nerve flow to the digestive tract, which contributes to digestive problems.

It is important that you consult with a doctor to find out whether you have IBS or some other condition that causes similar symptoms. However, in our opinion, natural therapies are the only sensible approach for the long-term control and the resolution of this condition, as they treat the underlying cause(s).

SYMPTOMS

- Constipation
- Diarrhea
- Alternating constipation and diarrhea
- Mucus in stools
- Abdominal pain and cramping, usually either relieved by going to the bathroom or brought on by it
- Flatulence and abdominal rumblings
- Nausea
- Headache
- Intolerance to certain foods
- Fatigue
- Gurgling and rumbling of the abdomen
- Burping
- Heartburn
- Occasional vomiting
- Unpleasant taste in the mouth

- Feeling full easily
- Depression
- Anxiety
- Mental "fog"
- Frequent urination

- Painful sexual intercourse (dyspareunia)
- Painful periods
- Irritation of the rectum
- Insomnia

ROOT CAUSES

- A diet that's high in refined, man-made foods and sugars and low in fiber
- Food allergies or sensitivities

- Candida overgrowth, parasite infection, and dysbiosis
- Poor stress-coping mechanisms

Testing Techniques

The following tests help assess possible reasons for irritable bowel syndrome:

Hormone testing (thyroid, DHEA, cortisol, testosterone, estrogen, progesterone)—saliva, blood, or urine

Intestinal permeability—urine

Detoxification profile—urine

Digestive function and microbe/parasite/candida testing—stool analysis

Food and environmental allergies/sensitivities—blood, electrodermal

---

TREATMENT

Diet

The most reliable way to calm an irritable bowel is to adhere to a good diet. You may find that the following suggestions advocate a drastic change from your present way of eating, but the difference in the way you feel will be worth it.

Even when eating the most healthful of foods, however, you must be careful not to eat just before going to bed.

Recommended Food

For IBS sufferers, a high-fiber diet is an absolute must. Although fiber may not sound appealing to you if you have diarrhea, it will actually regulate your bowels and soothe your digestive tract. Your diet should be based on high-fiber foods, especially whole grains, raw or lightly cooked vegetables, and legumes. You should slowly increase the amount of fiber-rich foods in your diet so that your body can adjust.

Drink a glass of clean water every two hours to ease the transit of waste matter and to keep your whole body functioning smoothly.

Irritable bowel syndrome can deplete your intestines of friendly bacteria. Eat a cultured product such as live yogurt, kefir, or sauerkraut every day.

Food to Avoid

The first step in treating IBS is to determine whether your problem is actually an allergy to food. See Food Allergies, and follow the elimination diet there. If you can trace your symptoms to a particular food or foods, make it a priority to avoid those allergens. Keep a close eye on how dairy products affect you; lactose is often a trigger for IBS-like symptoms.

Wheat and sugar products are common offenders as well.

Saturated, hydrogenated, and partially hydrogenated fats disturb the intestines and are hard to digest. Stay away from red meat, butter, margarine, and fried foods.

Avoid mucus-forming foods that encourage toxins to accumulate. Foods that promote mucus include all dairy products, fried and processed foods, refined flours, and chocolate.

Caffeine, alcohol, spicy foods, and tobacco all irritate the stomach lining, so eliminate them from your diet. Many of these items also contribute to stress.

Although a high intake of fiber is a necessity, steer clear of wheat bran. It often triggers allergies in IBS sufferers, and because the fiber is insoluble, it can propel waste matter through the intestines faster than is comfortable. Ground flaxseeds are a better choice.

Avoid ice-cold drinks, which inhibit digestion and may cause cramping.

Recent research shows that many people with IBS are sensitive to the sweetener fructose. It should be avoided or limited in the diet.

Detoxification

A vegetable juice fast lasting three days is a good way to eliminate toxins that have built up as a result of improper bowel functioning; do this fast once a month for three consecutive months.

℞ Super Seven Prescriptions—Irritable Bowel Syndrome

Super Prescription #1   Peppermint oil (*Mentha piperita*)
Take 1 to 2 enteric-coated peppermint oil capsules twice daily between meals. This herb reduces gas and cramping, and studies show that it is effective for IBS.

Super Prescription #2   Gentian root (*Gentiana lutea*)
This improves overall digestive function. Take 300 mg or 10 to 20 drops five to fifteen minutes before meals. It works well as part of a "bitters" herbal formula.

Super Prescription #3   Digestive enzymes
Take 1 to 2 capsules of a full-spectrum enzyme product with each meal. Enzymes help you to digest food more efficiently.

Super Prescription #4   Probiotic
Take a product containing at least 4 billion active organisms daily. Friendly bacteria such as *Lactobacillus acidophilus* and *bifidus* are involved with digestion and prevent the overgrowth of candida and other harmful microbes.

Super Prescription #5   Ginger root (*Zingiber officinale*)
Drink 1 cup of fresh tea or take 500 mg of the capsule form with each meal. Ginger reduces gas, bloating, and diarrhea and improves the functioning of the stomach.

Super Prescription #6   Skullcap (*Scutellaria lateriflora*)
Take 250 mg or 2 ml with each meal. It relaxes the nervous system and promotes digestion.

Super Prescription #7   Aloe vera juice
Drink ¼ cup twice daily or as directed on the container. Aloe is very soothing and healing to the digestive tract, and it fights intestinal infection.

General Recommendations

Peppermint (*Mentha piperita*) is a hallowed remedy for digestive troubles. Take peppermint tea after meals, instead of having dessert. Use it with caution if you have acid reflux.

A toxic liver can aggravate IBS, and IBS can put additional stress on the liver. Support yours with detoxifying milk thistle (*Silybum marianum*). For the best effect, you'll need to take this herb on a continuing basis. Take 250 mg daily of a product standardized for 80 to 85 percent silymarin content. Take it with each meal.

Slippery elm (*Ulmus fulva*) and pau d'arco (*Tabebuia avellanedae*) are both traditional soothers of an irritated bowel. Take 800 to 1,000 mg of slippery elm three or four times daily, or use 5 cc of a tincture three times daily. The dosage for pau d'arco is 100 mg of the powdered bark or 0.5 to 1.0 cc of a tincture three times a day.

Betaine hydrochloride supports stomach acid levels for better digestion. Take 1 to 2 capsules with each meal.

Homeopathy

Pick the remedy that best matches your symptoms in this section. Take a 6x, 12x, 6C, 12C, or 30C potency twice daily for two weeks to see if there are any positive results. After you notice improvement, stop taking the remedy, unless symptoms return. Consultation with a homeopathic practitioner is advised.

Argentum Nitricum is for bloating, gas, and diarrhea accompanied by anxiety and nervousness. Digestive upset comes on after eating sweets.

Arsenicum Album is for burning pains and diarrhea accompanied by great restlessness and anxiety. The person tends to be chilly and prefers sipping warm drinks. Symptoms are often worse from midnight to 2 A.M.

Colocynthis is a good remedy when one has constriction and cutting pains in the abdomen. Symptoms often come on after eating fruit or during diarrhea. Bending over, heat, and pressure make the symptoms better. Symptoms may come on after suppressed anger.

Lycopodium (*Lycopodium clavatum*) is the remedy when there are bloating, distension, and gurgling noises with abdominal pain. Symptoms are typically worse between 4 and 8 P.M. The person has a strong craving for sweets and feels better from warm drinks. The person has low self-confidence and is irritable.

Magnesia Phosphorica is for abdominal cramping and spasms that are better from warm drinks and warm applications to the abdomen.

Natrum Carbonicum is for people with multiple food allergies, who experience indigestion and heartburn. They crave milk, potatoes, and sweets but experience irritable bowels when ingesting them. They desire to be left alone.

Nux Vomica is helpful for people with abdominal pains and bowel problems caused by stress and a poor diet. Constipation is common, and they feel as if they never complete a bowel movement. Spasms may occur in their digestive tracts. Symptoms are worse from anger or excitement. They have a strong craving for spicy foods, alcohol, tobacco, coffee, and other stimulants, which worsen the digestive symptoms.

Sulphur is a good choice for people who experience diarrhea that wakes them up early in the morning to rush to the bathroom. Diarrhea may occur frequently throughout the day, although constipation can be present as well. Often, the gas has a foul smell like rotten eggs. The rectum is often irritated, itchy, and burning. There is a craving for sweets, spicy foods, and alcohol.

Acupressure

See pages 668–675 for information about pressure points and administering treatment.

- The point of choice for relieving abdominal pain is Conception Vessel 12; this point can also prevent indigestion when used before a meal.
- Conception Vessel 6 soothes abdominal pain, constipation, and gas.
- Pericardium 6 has a calming effect and soothes an upset stomach.
- Large Intestine 11 relaxes the colon if you are constipated.
- Stomach 36 is an overall toner and strengthens the digestive system in particular.

Bodywork

Massage

Some self-massage techniques are helpful for stimulating digestion and relaxing cramps.

Use your finger to massage your tongue and gums in the morning. This technique prepares the upper part of your digestive tract for the work of the day.

At night, or whenever you feel IBS pain or cramps, massage your abdomen. Lie down in bed, with your knees bent, and gently examine the area for regions of tension. When you find those regions, massage them with the flat of your hand, using firm but gentle pressure.

Reflexology

See pages 686–687 for information about reflexology areas and how to work them.

For diarrhea, work the areas that correspond to the liver, the ascending colon, the transverse colon, and the adrenal glands.

If you are constipated, massage the areas corresponding to the liver, the gall bladder, the colon, and the adrenal glands.

For flatulence, work the areas corresponding to the intestines, the liver, and the sigmoid colon.

Work the solar plexus to reduce tension.

Aromatherapy

Neroli, chamomile, and lavender will relax abdominal cramping and reduce pain. You can use them separately or together in a warm bath or a hot compress. You might also like to add one or more to a carrier oil to use in an abdominal self-massage.

Black pepper can relieve constipation and improve a sluggish digestion. Use it on a hot compress applied directly to the abdomen.

Stress Reduction

General Stress-Reduction Therapies

Any antistress technique can help, but positive mental imagery and deep breathing are particularly beneficial. It is helpful to work with a counselor who teaches stress-reduction techniques.

People with severe anxiety should consider EEG biofeedback, which will teach them how to control their brainwaves and relax their nervous system.

Bach Flower Remedies

Select the appropriate remedy, and place 10 drops of the liquid under your tongue. Hold the drops in place for thirty seconds and swallow. Use as often as needed.

Rescue Remedy is a reliable way to ease the effects of a crisis, whether physical or emotional. You can use it when you feel a strong attack of IBS coming on or during a period of emotional stress that you fear may result in an IBS episode.

Irritable bowel syndrome has been linked to perfectionist personalities who need to have a great deal of control. If this description suits you, try Beech to help balance these qualities.

If you are highly sensitive and inhibited, and if you suffer from a great degree of stress, Agrimony will help.

Other Recommendations

- When your intestines feel tight and cramped, lie down with a heating pad or a warm compress against your abdomen.
- Constitutional hydrotherapy is effective for reducing abdominal pain and bloating. You can do a treatment for acute symptoms, and regular treatments are effective for improving overall digestive function.

Kidney Stones

Kidney stones have become an increasingly common medical problem in Western society, mainly due to poor dietary habits. Although many kidney stones are so small that they pass unnoticed, they may sometimes become very large, up to the size of a marble. It is not hard to imagine that as these large stones move through the urinary tract, they cause great—and often excruciating—pain. Kidney stones are most likely to affect white men over the age of the thirty. People of any race or sex who live in the southern United States also have a higher risk, probably because of dietary habits in that region.

Complementary therapies offer effective, natural pain relief for more minor cases, as well as strategies for keeping the stones from growing any larger, but on the whole, it is far easier to prevent kidney stones in the first place. History holds a clue to their prevention: Back in the early 1900s, when Americans ate natural, wholesome foods, kidney stones were largely unheard of. As the century wore on, and as diets became lower in fiber and higher in fat, sugar, dairy, and junk, the disorder became much more common. Now a man living in America has a 10 percent chance of passing a kidney stone at least once in his life. If you suffer from kidney stones, take heart in the knowledge that you can prevent a recurrence of this painful condition with changes in diet and lifestyle and by using specific nutritional supplements.

There are different types of kidney stones, with 80 percent being composed of calcium salts, especially the oxalate type. Some stones are also composed of calcium phosphate, uric acid, struvite, cystine, or other materials. If your stones are mainly composed of uric acid, please follow the recommendations in the Gout section. This section focuses on the prevention and the treatment of calcium-oxalate stones.

If you have been diagnosed with or suspect that you have kidney stones, then you should be under the care of a professional. Your doctor will rule out other conditions or underlying causes and will check for infection. In cases of very large stones or severe pain, you may need to be hospitalized. This condition can be a medical emergency when stones block the urinary tract for a long time, causing urine to back up and distend the kidney (hydronephrosis). You are also at more risk for a urinary tract infection during an acute kidney stone crisis. Conventional treatment may involve breaking the stones up with sound waves (lithotripsy) or surgical removal.

Smaller stones that are not causing symptoms or an infection will usually pass through without any problems if you follow our recommendations. People with a chronic susceptibility to this condition should remember that an effective prevention program generally requires the nutritional approach outlined in this chapter.

SYMPTOMS

- Pain on one side of the lower back, in the belly, or down into the groin
- A frequent urge to urinate
- Blood and sediment in the urine
- Nausea and vomiting
- Chills and fever, if the stone causes a blockage and an infection

ROOT CAUSES

- A poor diet
- Dehydration
- Urinary pH balance
- Allergies and food sensitivities
- Infections that disturb the flow of fluids
- Obesity
- Inactivity
- A magnesium and potassium deficiency
- An inherited inability to absorb calcium properly or to excrete too much oxalic acid
- Metabolic disorders that increase the risk of kidney stone formation, such as hyperparathyroidism, Cushing's syndrome, sarcoidosis, cancer, and others

TREATMENT

Diet

Recommended Food

Many people with kidney stones suffer from dehydration. A lack of fluids increases the mineral concentration in the kidneys and, with it, the chance that stones will crystallize. While you have a kidney stone, drink $2\frac{1}{2}$ to 3 quarts of clean water every day. Once the stone has passed, resume a normal daily dose of 1 glass every two waking hours. Hydration is the single most important tactic in the treatment and the prevention of kidney stones.

Vegetarians have a much lower risk of getting kidney stones than meat eaters do. Follow a diet based on fresh, raw vegetables and whole grains; eat beans, nuts and seeds, and fish for protein. If you must eat animal products, stick to lean, high-quality sources of white meat.

Consume oat and wheat bran daily, as they reduce the risk of kidney stones being formed.

Lemon juice mixed with a little hot water is another remedy that will help acidify

---

Testing Techniques

The following tests help assess possible reasons for kidney stones:

Urine pH and type of crystals formed—urinalysis

X-rays, ultrasound, or CT scan

Detoxification profile—urine

Vitamin and mineral analysis (especially for magnesium, B6, vitamin D, calcium)—blood, urine

Food and environmental allergies/sensitivities—blood, electrodermal

Heavy metal toxicity (especially cadmium)—hair or urine

---

the urine and ease the passage of calcium-oxalate stones. Drink some at breakfast and throughout the day. Orange juice has been shown to be helpful as well.

Vitamin A is healing to the urinary tract, so be sure to eat lots of orange-yellow and green vegetables.

Consume ¼ cup of pumpkin seeds daily. Studies show that consuming these seeds reduces risk factors for kidney stone formation.

A magnesium deficiency has been linked to recurring kidney stones. Boost your levels of this nutrient by eating green leafy vegetables, kelp, soybeans, almonds, and apples.

Celery, parsley, and watermelon help cleanse the urinary tract, so add these foods to your regular meals.

Food to Avoid

Eliminate foods that contain high amounts of oxalic acid from your diet. By far the worst offenders are spinach, rhubarb, tomatoes, collards, eggplant, beets, celery, summer squash, sweet potatoes, peanuts, almonds, blueberries, blackberries, strawberries, Concord grapes, parsley, and cocoa.

Avoid grapefruit juice, which studies show increases the risk of kidney stones.

Animal fat causes the body to excrete calcium, creating a build-up in the kidneys. Avoid all red meat, and limit your consumption of other animal products.

Avoid calcium overload by eliminating dairy products from your diet. The calcium from milk, cheese, ice cream, and the like is not easily absorbed by the digestive system and ends up as extra waste matter in your kidneys.

When you eat too much sugar, the resulting high levels of insulin leach calcium from the bones and divert it into the urinary tract. Stay away from all products that contain refined sugar. Of particular importance are soft drinks that contain phosphoric acid. They should be completely avoided, as some studies show that they cause an increase risk in kidney stones.

Salt, caffeine, and alcohol all conspire to dehydrate your body and increase the concentration of minerals in the urine. Cut out caffeine and alcohol, and dramatically restrict your salt intake.

Detoxification

A three-day vegetable juice fast will cleanse your body of a mineral overload and will encourage the stone to pass as painlessly as possible. Drink a variety of vegetable and fruit juices: those made from green vegetables, carrots, lemons, parsley, celery, and watermelon are especially helpful for a kidney cleanse.

A study of 55 people with reoccurring kidney stones looked at the effect of supplementing 500 mg of magnesium daily for up to 4 years. The average number of recurrences of kidney stones dropped by 90 percent. Also, 85 percent of the people in the study remained stone free, as compared to 41 percent who did not supplement magnesium. Studies have also shown that the combination of magnesium and vitamin B6 supplementation is very effective in reducing kidney stone formation. One study of 149 people with recurrent kidney stones who supplemented B6 (10 mg) and magnesium (300 mg) had a 92.3 percent improvement in stone formation.

℞ Super Seven Prescriptions—Kidney Stone

Super Prescription #1   Magnesium
Take 250 mg twice daily with meals. Magnesium prevents the formation of calcium-oxalate crystals.

Super Prescription #2   Vitamin B6
Take 50 mg daily. Vitamin B6 has been shown to reduce calcium-oxalate levels, and studies show that people with kidney stones tend to be deficient in B6.

Super Prescription #3   IP-6 (inositol hexaphosphate)
Take 120 mg daily. Studies show that this supplement reduces calcium-oxalate crystals in the urine.

Super Prescription #4   Vitamin E
Take 400 IU daily. Vitamin E may be helpful for people who have a history of elevated calcium-oxalate levels.

Super Prescription #5   Cranberry extract (*Vaccinium macrocarpona*)
Take 400 mg twice daily of a standardized extract or as directed on the container. Studies have shown that cranberry reduces urinary calcium levels in people with a history of kidney stones. It also is used to prevent urinary tract infections.

Super Prescription #6   Aloe vera
Drink ¼ cup daily or as directed on the container, as it reduces urinary crystals.

Super Prescription #7   Vitamin A
Take 5,000 IU daily. A deficiency of this vitamin is considered a risk factor for kidney stone formation.

General Recommendations

Uva ursi is a traditional herbal treatment for kidney stones. It relieves pain, cleanses the urinary tract, and fights infection. Take 250 to 500 mg three times daily. Do not take uva ursi for more than fourteen days at a stretch.

Dandelion root (*Taraxacum officinale*) is an effective kidney cleanser. Take 500 mg two times daily. Do not take dandelion root for more than a month at a time.

Horsetail (*Equisetum arvense*) has beneficial diuretic qualities. To make a tea, macerate horsetail leaves and steep them in cold water for twelve hours. Heat the mixture and drink 3 to 4 cups daily. If you prefer capsules or tablets, take 2 grams three times a day.

Juniper berry (*Juniperus communis*) tea is another strong diuretic kidney cleanser. Drink 3 or 4 cups every day until the stone passes.

Vitamin C supplementation has been shown to lower the incidence of kidney stone formation, when the level is below 4,000 mg daily. However, in certain individuals it may accelerate stone formation; therefore, people with a history of kidney stones should have their urinary oxalate levels monitored by a doctor.

Homeopathy

Pick the remedy that best matches your symptoms in this section. Take a 6x, 12x, 6C, 12C, or 30C potency twice daily for two weeks to see if there are any positive results. After you notice improvement, stop taking the remedy, unless symptoms return. Consultation with a homeopathic practitioner is advised.

Belladonna (*Atropa belladonna*) is for sudden, excruciating pain in the right kidney. Symptoms are worse with any jarring. A high fever and a flushed face may be present.

Berberis Vulgaris is helpful when there are sharp, stitching, or shooting pains that radiate throughout the ureters, the bladder, the testes, or the thighs.

Dioscorea helps when the kidney stone pain causes one to stretch or arch backward for pain relief.

Lachesis is for left-sided kidney pain. Hemorrhaging may occur from the kidney stone.

Lycopodium (*Lycopodium clavatum*) is for kidney stones that cause pain on the right side of the back or the belly. Symptoms are often worse between 4 and 8 P.M.

Nux Vomica is for stone pain (colic), accompanied by cramping, nausea, or vomiting. People who benefit from this remedy may have futile urges to empty their bowels or bladders and may feel very irritable.

Acupressure

See pages 668–675 for information about pressure points and administering treatment.

- Work Large Intestine 4 to relieve kidney stone pain.

Bodywork

Acupuncture is recommended to help combat the pain of a kidney stone and to promote a more effective passage.

Reflexology

See pages 686–687 for information about reflexology areas and how to work them.

To help pass kidney stones and ease the pain, work the following points daily: ureters, kidneys, bladder, diaphragm, parathyroid, and lower back. If you want to prevent the recurrence of stones, work these areas on a weekly basis.

Hydrotherapy

A hot sitz bath helps to relieve the pain. You can drink water or herbal tea while sitting in the water to encourage faster elimination of the stone. For some people, a constitutional hydrotherapy feels even better.

Aromatherapy

To relieve abdominal pain, use any of the following, either alone or in a combination that pleases you: chamomile, lavender, and marjoram. You can add them to a sitz bath (or a regular bath, if you like), or mix them with a carrier oil and rub it directly on your abdomen.

Stress Reduction

General Stress-Reduction Therapies

Learn to meditate. When kidney stones are agonizing, you can use meditative breathing techniques to disengage yourself from the pain.

Bach Flower Remedies

Select the appropriate remedy, and place 10 drops of the liquid under your tongue. Hold the drops in place for thirty seconds and swallow. Use as often as needed.

Many people with kidney stones suffer from resentment and bitterness. If this is true for you, Willow will help you feel more forgiving and content.

Elm is for people who are overwhelmed and depressed by work and who feel inadequate to the tasks at hand.

Hornbeam is another remedy for overwork, especially when it leaves you too exhausted to care.

Other Recommendations

- Antacids that contain aluminum may cause kidney stones, especially when taken along with dairy products. Choose an antacid made without this metal, or, better yet, simply avoid foods that give you indigestion.

REFERENCES

Johnson, G., et al. 1982. Effects of magnesium hydroxide in renal stone disease. *Journal of the American College of Nutrition* 1:179–85.

Prien, E. L., and S. N. Gershoff. 1974. Magnesium oxide-pyridoxine therapy for recurrent calcium oxalate calculi. *Journal of Urology* 112:509–12.

Lupus

Lupus is an autoimmune disorder, in which antibodies mistakenly identify the body's tissues as foreign substances and attack them, causing inflammation and pain. The disease most often strikes women in their childbearing years; only 10 percent of people with lupus are men. For reasons that are as yet unknown, African American women are three times more likely to receive a diagnosis than are their Caucasian counterparts, and American women of Asian or Hispanic descent are also more susceptible. Lupus is a rare condition, but, as with other autoimmune disorders, the number of incidents has been on the rise in recent years.

Lupus takes two related but quite distinct forms: discoid lupus erythematosus (DLE) and systemic lupus erythematosus (SLE). In DLE, the only symptom is a scaly red rash that spreads across the cheeks and the nose, and sometimes the forehead and the scalp. We tend to think of this rash as butterfly-shaped, but in a different era, the pattern reminded doctors of a wolf's face—hence the name *lupus,* which means "wolf" in Latin. The red patches usually come and go in cycles, but sometimes they leave disfiguring scars. Scars that occur on the scalp may prevent hair from growing in the area they cover. DLE can be distressing, but it does not pose a serious health threat. Since the rash is often triggered by exposure to sunlight, the most effective treatment is to remain inside during peak daylight hours and to shade the face and the head when outdoors.

Sufferers of SLE may also experience a rash, and their disease, like DLE, goes through periods of remission and activation, but the similarity between the two disorders stops there. Systemic lupus, as the name implies, affects not just the skin but the entire body. The process that produces the red rash spreads to the joints and the muscles, creating pain and inflammation very similar to that of rheumatoid arthritis. People with SLE suffer from frequent low-grade fevers that may spike when the disease cycle is at its peak. Not surprisingly, the fever and the pain leave their victims exhausted and sometimes depressed. For some people, the symptoms never progress beyond this point. In other cases, the inflammation spreads to the kidneys, the liver, the heart, or the spleen, creating dangerous and even life-threatening problems.

No one knows the exact cause of lupus. Conventional medicine focuses on factors that often trigger flare-ups; certain medications, viral and bacterial illnesses, birth-control pills, pregnancy, and periods of extreme stress are all suspects, but it is likely that there is no single culprit. Holistic doctors such as ourselves take a close look at other factors; when these are addressed, it can be quite helpful to people with this disease. The factors include food allergies, hormone balance, digestive function ("leaky gut syndrome") and detoxification, heavy metal toxicity, and nutritional deficiencies.

Earlier in this century, lupus was fatal within a few years of its onset. Now almost all people with lupus live out a normal lifespan, provided that they and their doctors monitor the symptoms and control any threatening developments. Today, quality of life is the most pressing issue for the majority of lupus sufferers. Although some people experience very little inflammation and pain, others are nearly crippled by it. Doctors can help ease the worst flare-ups with medications for pain control and antibody suppression, but it's best to try to avoid the need for aggressive measures. An anti-inflammatory diet, adequate rest and stress control, and specific natural treatments can all help you to reduce the chance of flare-ups and minimize the symptoms when they do occur.

SYMPTOMS OF DLE

- A butterfly-shaped facial rash that may spread to the forehead or the scalp

SYMPTOMS OF SLE

- Facial rash
- Fever
- Fatigue and malaise
- Joint and muscle pain
- Weight loss
- Hair loss
- Sensitivity to the sun
- Mouth sores
- Vulnerability to illness
- Enlarged lymph nodes
- Nausea
- Constipation or diarrhea
- Recurring bladder infections
- Presence of lupus antibodies in the blood

ROOT CAUSES

The cause or causes of lupus are unknown. Following are some of the top suspects:

- An allergic reaction to medications or vaccines
- Viruses
- Bacteria, especially streptococcus
- Extreme and prolonged emotional or physical stress
- Estrogen disruption related to pregnancy or birth-control pills
- Use of synthetic hormones
- Deficiency of certain hormones (especially DHEA, progesterone, testosterone, and growth hormone)
- Food allergies
- Poor digestion and detoxification
- Heavy metal toxicity

Testing Techniques

The following tests help assess possible causes of lupus:

Hormone testing (thyroid, DHEA, cortisol, testosterone, IGF-1, estrogen, progesterone)—saliva, blood, or urine

Intestinal permeability—urine

Detoxification profile—urine

Vitamin and mineral analysis—blood

Essential fatty acid balance—blood or urine

Digestive function and microbe/parasite/candida testing—stool analysis

Food and environmental allergies/sensitivities—blood, electrodermal

Heavy metal toxicity—hair or urine

TREATMENT

Diet

Recommended Food

Give your body optimal support by eating well-rounded, varied meals of whole foods. Buy organic products whenever possible, to reduce your exposure to toxins and pesticides. If you must buy conventional produce, wash it thoroughly in clean water before eating.

Raw vegetables and citrus fruits will help return your body to an alkaline state. These foods are also high in fiber, which relieves digestive problems, and in antioxidants, which counteract inflammation.

For extra antioxidant protection, eat wheat germ and cold-pressed oils (like olive oil) for vitamin E.

Essential fatty acids are the "good" fats that actually help reduce inflammation. Eat cold-water fish from a clean water source several times a week, and add 1 to 2 tablespoons of ground flaxseeds or flaxseed oil to a daily salad.

During a flare-up of lupus, antibodies will attack your own joint cartilage. You can repair some of the damage by eating foods that are high in sulfur. Good sources include onions, garlic, and asparagus.

If you're prone to bladder infections, drink unsweetened natural cranberry juice every day.

Corticosteroid use is associated with bone loss and osteoporosis. If you must take these drugs, increase your intake of calcium by eating plenty of green leafy vegetables and soy products.

For good general health, drink a glass of clean water every two waking hours. You'll also keep your joints lubricated: water makes their cartilage soft and flexible and maintains proper levels of joint fluid.

Five Ways to Use Wheat Germ

Wheat germ may sound like a flavorless holdover from the hippie era, but it actually has a mild, nutty taste that's quite pleasant. Nevertheless, most people prefer not to eat wheat germ straight out of the jar. Here are some tips for incorporating it into your meals:

1. Add a few tablespoons to muffin batter or dough before baking.

2. Stir some into oatmeal or another hot cereal.

3. Use it as a topping for yogurt. Add some berries, and you have a healthful breakfast or a luncheon side dish.

4. When you're making juice, smoothies, or other drinks, add some wheat germ before you blend.

5. A tablespoon of wheat germ adds a light crunch and depth of flavor to salads.

Food to Avoid

Saturated fats, hydrogenated fats, and partially hydrogenated fats make inflammation worse; in fact, some people find that their pain goes away completely when they eliminate animal meats and fried or greasy foods from their diet.

An internal acidic environmental also promotes inflammation and pain. You already know to avoid saturated fats, but you'll also need to radically restrict your intake of eggs, sugar, refined carbohydrates, alcohol, and caffeine.

If you need another reason to avoid sugar and refined carbohydrates, here it is: these products damage the immune system and leave you even more susceptible to infection and illness.

Food allergies can mimic lupus symptoms or make them worse. Try the elimination diet on page 253 to determine whether there's a food or foods that you should avoid. Wheat, in particular, tends to cause problems in people with lupus.

You are highly vulnerable to microorganisms and toxins, so never drink tap water.

Be kind to your kidneys. Along with avoiding saturated fats and animal meats, restrict your salt intake.

Detoxification

Anyone with an autoimmune disorder should practice regular juice fasts to keep the body functioning at its peak. Try a three-day juice fast once a month. You can support the fast with plenty of green drinks and cleansing herbal teas.

R̻ Super Seven Prescriptions—Lupus

Super Prescription #1   Fish oil
Take up to 20 grams of fish oil daily and a minimum of 8 grams. High doses of fish oil were shown to be of help in a human study. *Note:* High-potency fish oil formulas are available, so that less capsules will need to be taken.

Super Prescription #2   Plant sterols and sterolins
Take 20 mg three times daily on an empty stomach. These naturally occurring plant chemicals were shown to have a balancing effect on the immune system for people with autoimmune diseases.

Super Prescription #3   DHEA
Take up to 200 mg daily, under the supervision of a doctor. Studies have shown DHEA to improve symptoms of systemic lupus in women.

Super Prescription #4   Gentian root (*Gentiana lutea*) and herbal bitters
Take 300 mg or 10 to 20 drops five to fifteen minutes before meals. Gentian root and herbal bitters formulas improve overall digestive function.

Super Prescription #5   Methylsulfonylmethane (MSM)
Take 2,000 to 8,000 mg daily. MSM has natural anti-inflammatory benefits and contains the mineral sulfur, an integral component of cartilage. Reduce the dosage if diarrhea occurs.

Super Prescription #6   Enzymes
Take 1 to 2 capsules of a full-spectrum enzyme product with each meal. Enzymes help you to digest food more efficiently. Protease enzymes can be taken between meals for an anti-inflammatory effect.

In a double-blind trial, the combination of 20 grams of fish oil daily and a low-fat diet led to improvement in 14 of 17 people with systemic lupus in 12 weeks.

Super Prescription #7   Bowsellia (*Boswellia serrata*)

Take 1,200 to 1,500 mg of a standardized extract containing 60 to 65 percent boswellic acids two to three times daily. This herb has powerful anti-inflammatory effects.

General Recommendations

Vitamin E may be helpful for people with discoid lupus. Take 800 to 2,000 IU daily.

Turmeric (*Curcuma longa*) has anti-inflammatory benefits. Take a product containing 450 mg of curcumin twice daily.

Take a super green food supplement, such as chlorella or spirulina, or a mixture of super green foods, each day. Take as directed on the container.

A high-potency multivitamin contains a strong base of the antioxidants and other nutrients that protect against tissue damage. Take as directed on the container.

A probiotic is a supplement that contains friendly bacteria, such as *Lactobacillus acidophilus* and *bifidus,* that aid in digestion and detoxification. Take a product containing at least 4 billion active organisms daily.

Evening primrose oil, black currant, or borage oil contain the essential fatty acid GLA, which reduces joint inflammation. Take up to 2.8 grams of GLA daily.

Green tea (*Camellia sinensis*) contains a rich source of antioxidants and substances that assist detoxification. Drink the organic tea regularly (2 cups or more daily) or take 500 to 1,500 mg of the capsule form.

Milk thistle (*Silybum marianum*) improves liver function and protects against the potential damage of pharmaceutical medications. Take 250 mg of a standardized extract of 80 to 85 percent silymarin three times daily.

Ginkgo biloba improves circulation through the kidneys and has anti-inflammatory benefits. Take 60 to 120 mg twice daily of a product standardized to 24 percent flavone glycosides.

You can often avoid harsh conventional painkillers by using analgesic herbs. White willow bark (*Salix alba*) will soothe joint pain. Find a white willow extract that is standardized for salicin content, and take 30 to 60 mg twice daily. A lotion or a cream made with capsicum will also reduce the pain.

Devil's claw (*Harpagophytum procumbens*) root is a potent herb that will control inflammation. Take 2.5 to 5.0 grams twice a day, or use 1 to 2 cc of a tincture three times a day. Expect to take devil's claw root at least two months before you see results.

Teas made with burdock root (*Articum lappa*) or red clover (*Trifolium pratense*) have a detoxifying effect. Drink them during a fast or any time you want a little extra housecleaning.

Lupus can send stress levels soaring. If you've lost weight and are very slender, however, a very strong relaxant might be too much for you. Instead, try tea made with a moderately potent herb, like skullcap or hops. If neither of these herbs works, or if you have a larger frame, move on to valerian (*Valeriana officinalis*) or kava kava (*Piper methysticum*).

Homeopathy

Pick the remedy that best matches your symptoms in this section. Take a 6x, 12x, 6C, 12C, or 30C potency twice daily for two weeks to see if there are any positive results. After you notice improvement, stop taking the remedy, unless symptoms return. Consultation with a homeopathic practitioner is advised.

Arsenicum Album will relieve burning joints that feel better with warm applications. The person tends to feel anxious and restless.

Belladonna (*Atropa belladonna*) works on joints that are hot, red, and burning and that feel worse with motion. Pain and swelling may come on suddenly.

Sepia is for women with lupus, who find that their symptoms flare up near their menstrual cycles. There are usually signs of hormone imbalance, such as PMS or extreme menopausal symptoms. There is a craving for sweet, salty, and sour foods. The person tends to be chilly, irritable, and depressed.

Pulsatilla (*Pulsatilla pratensis*) is helpful if your pains wander from joint to joint and if your symptoms improve in fresh, cool air or with cool applications.

Rhus Toxicodendron relieves lupus symptoms that are worse in the cold and the damp or with long periods of inactivity. Stiffness of the joints is the main symptom, which improves with some movement and warmth.

Sulphur is for burning pains that are better with cold applications. The person tends to get overheated easily and prefers a cool environment. There is a strong craving for spicy foods and ice-cold drinks.

Acupressure

Acupressure works wonders on rheumatic pains. As the following points are probably quite tender, don't massage them. Instead, use firm pressure. Plan to work the appropriate points two or three times a day for several months before you see results; it may take six months for the pain to subside completely. Once the pain has been significantly reduced, you can reduce your sessions to one a day. For more information about pressure points and administering treatment, see pages 668–675.

- Large Intestine 4 is used for relief of pain anywhere on the body, but it is especially effective for pain in the hands, the wrists, the elbows, the shoulders, or the neck.
- For elbow and shoulder pain, use Large Intestine 11.
- If your ankles are affected, work Spleen 5 and Kidney 3.
- To relieve stress, work Lung 1 on a regular basis.
- For acute anxiety and nervousness, add Pericardium 6 to your daily practice or use as needed.

Bodywork

Acupuncture is worth trying for people with this condition, to reduce inflammation and pain.

Reflexology

See pages 686–687 for information about reflexology areas and how to work them.

Lupus is a systemic disorder, so if you have time, it's best to work the whole foot. If that's not possible, concentrate on the adrenals to reduce swelling and on any specific areas that are causing you pain.

To relieve tension, also work the area corresponding to the solar plexus.

Hydrotherapy

A hot bath with Epsom salts will temporarily reduce pain and draw toxins away from your joints and muscles.

Constitutional hydrotherapy is an excellent long-term therapy to minimize lupus symptoms. See pages 676–677 for directions.

Aromatherapy

Find a few relaxing oils that you like and use them regularly in a bath or a room diffuser. Some good choices to start with are lavender, rose, jasmine, and geranium.

Black pepper and ginger encourage blood flow and will help revive tired joints and muscles. If you're constipated, you can add a few drops of either essence to a carrier oil and rub it onto your abdomen.

If you want to detoxify your body, use lemon balm or juniper in a hot bath.

Stress Reduction

General Stress-Reduction Therapies

It doesn't matter how you reduce stress—just find a technique that you like and use it regularly—on a daily basis, if possible. If you're not sure where to start, a basic yoga class will help you relax and will give you the gentle exercise you need.

If your pain is intense, consider thermal biofeedback. This therapy will teach you to send warming, nourishing blood to your joints.

Many people with lupus find that support groups are as essential to their health as regular check-ups are. Ask your doctor or local hospital for information about groups in your area.

Bach Flower Remedies

Consult the chart on pages 648–650 to determine the best remedy for your particular needs. Following are some suggestions. Once you've chosen a remedy, place 10 drops of the liquid under your tongue. Hold the drops in place for thirty seconds and swallow. Use as often as needed.

For deep fatigue, take Hornbeam, Olive, or a combination of both.

If you're convinced that you'll never feel better, use Gorse.

A diagnosis of lupus can be difficult to handle; if you feel great distress and cannot be consoled, Star of Bethlehem will help you feel better.

Other Recommendations

- Avoid the bright sunlight, especially in the warm months or when snow (which reflects the sun) is on the ground. When you do go outside, always wear a hat and protective clothing. Your skin may be sensitive to some sunscreens; if so, talk to your doctor about a nonirritating prescription sunblock.
- Although you may not feel like exercising, gentle movement is highly recommended to reduce pain and promote good general health. A daily walk in the early morning sunlight is an excellent idea.
- Birth-control pills and synthetic hormones may trigger flare-ups, so it's wise to avoid them.
- Women with lupus were once counseled to avoid pregnancy, but pregnancy can sometimes actually lead to a remission of the disease. For many women, it's the stressful months after the baby is born that cause a flare up. The decision regarding the safety of pregnancy must be made on a case-by-case basis, so talk to your doctor.
- Chinese herbal therapy can be helpful. See a qualified practitioner.

REFERENCES

Walton, A. J. E., M. L. Snaith, M. Locniskar, et al. 1991. Dietary fish oil and the severity of symptoms in patients with systemic lupus erythematosus. *Annals of Rheumatological Disease* 50:463–66.

Macular Degeneration

The macula is the part of the eye that allows us to see detail in the center of our vision field. When the macula breaks down or is damaged, fine work like reading, sewing, and painting becomes difficult or impossible. Small objects—stitches on fabric, for example, or type on a page—may look wavy or bent, and there may be dark spots over the item you're trying to see. This visual impairment begins at the center of the vision and, if not halted, will slowly expand toward the periphery. In the United States, macular degeneration is the leading cause of serious visual impairment in people over fifty-five, and in those sixty-five and older, it is the second-highest cause of blindness, next only to cataracts. There are two kinds of macular degeneration: atrophic (or "dry") and neovascular ("wet"). Atrophic is by far the more common of the two and accounts for 80 to 95 percent of all cases. Although its effects usually don't show until a relatively advanced age, atrophic macular degeneration happens over a lifetime, as cellular debris gradually accumulates under the retina. No one knows exactly why this debris builds up, but it is thought that damage by free radicals (the unbalanced molecules that damage cells), along with inadequate supplies of blood and oxygen to the macula, play a significant role. Although no conventional treatment exists, many alternative therapies can halt and possibly reverse the retinal damage by fighting free radicals and improving circulation.

Neovascular macular degeneration isn't actually degeneration at all. Instead, it is caused by an abnormal growth of blood vessels under the retina. If these blood vessels leak, the fluid can scar the macula and impair central, detailed vision. Unlike atrophic degeneration, this form of the disease can frequently be reversed with laser treatment, as long as it's caught early enough. It can often be prevented altogether, with the same alternative therapies used to treat atrophic degeneration.

Major conventional risk factors for macular degeneration include smoking, atherosclerosis, aging, and high blood pressure. Research in recent years has proven that diet is a critical element in the prevention of this disease. A diet that's high in cholesterol and saturated fat appears to increase susceptibility, while a diet that's rich in fruits, vegetables, and fish is protective. Carotenoids, found in fruits and particularly in vegetables, are quite protective antioxidants against macular damage from sunlight. A holistic approach also considers the role of inefficient digestion and absorption, which can contribute to mineral deficiencies that play a role in this disease. Also, toxic metals can increase free radical damage of the macula and the eye and should be dealt with, if a problem. Finally, several nutritional supplements, especially minerals and carotenoids, have proven to be effective in the prevention and the treatment of macular degeneration.

If you experience any kind of blurred vision, do not attempt to diagnose yourself. See a physician or an eye doctor to rule out an underlying disorder; if you do have macular degeneration, your doctor should run a test to discover whether you are affected by the atrophic or neovascular form. And since both kinds of macular degeneration—as well as many other eye problems—can be detected by a doctor long before the symptoms appear, you should always have regular eye exams, especially if you're age fifty-five or older.

SYMPTOMS

- Blurring, distortion, or dark spots at the center of the vision field, especially when looking at detail.

ROOT CAUSES

Anything that causes free radical damage or poor circulation can contribute to macular degeneration, including the following:

- Aging
- Smoking
- A diet that's low in antioxidants, which fight free radical damage
- Arteriosclerosis (hardening of arteries)

- High blood pressure
- Exposure to ultraviolet light
- Environmental toxins (particularly toxic metals)
- Poor digestion and detoxification
- Nutritional deficiencies

Testing Techniques

The following tests help assess possible reasons for macular degeneration:

Blood pressure

Hormone testing (thyroid, DHEA, cortisol, testosterone, IGF-1, estrogen, progesterone)—saliva, blood, or urine

Intestinal permeability—urine

Detoxification profile—urine

Vitamin and mineral analysis (especially zinc, carotenoids, vitamins E and C, selenium)—blood

Digestive function and microbe/parasite/candida testing—stool analysis

Blood-sugar balance—blood

Toxic metals (mercury, lead, arsenic, etc.)—hair or urine

TREATMENT

Diet

If you have arteriosclerosis or high blood pressure, see the relevant entry for additional dietary recommendations. Reducing the blockage or the pressure in your arteries will also improve the circulation of blood and oxygen to your eyes.

Recommended Food

Keep toxins moving quickly through your body by eating plenty of fiber, especially whole grains and beans.

Water will also help flush away toxins and keep the eye tissues supple. Drink a glass of clean water every two waking hours.

Consume your carotenoids, which are fruits and vegetables that fight free radicals. Good sources include dark leafy greens, spinach, collard greens, kale, bell peppers (all colors), yellow squash, carrots, tomatoes, celery, oranges, red grapes, mangoes, and melons.

Vitamin C and bioflavonoids work together against free radicals; they also strengthen the capillaries and the tissues of the eye. Eat red, blue, and purple fruits and vegetables—berries, cherries, tomatoes, and plums—for bioflavonoids, and enjoy citrus fruits as a source of vitamin C.

Food to Avoid

Stay far away from foods that contain free radicals. Fats that are saturated, hydrogenated, or partially hydrogenated are the worst offenders in the American diet, but caffeine, sugar, alcohol, and charred or grilled meats are also sources of these disease-causing molecules.

Detoxification

A three-day juice fast will help clear the build-up from your system. You'll eliminate many of the toxins that are linked to free radical damage; in addition, your blood will flow more freely, allowing for a better supply of oxygen and nutrients to your eyes. You can use a wide variety of juices for a fast, but be sure to include those made from several of the fruits and vegetables listed previously.

℞ Super Seven Prescriptions—Macular Degeneration

Super Prescription #1   Lutein
Take 15 mg daily with a meal. It prevents oxidative damage of the macula.

Super Prescription #2   Zeaxanthin
Take 3 mg daily with a meal. It prevents oxidative damage of the macula.

Super Prescription #3   Betaine hydrochloride
Take 1 to 3 capsules with each meal or as directed by a health-care professional. This supplement increases stomach acid for the improved absorption of nutrients, especially minerals.

Super Prescription #4   Zinc
Take 45 mg daily, along with 2 mg of copper. Zinc is required for proper vision and is an antioxidant, which was shown in studies to help macular degeneration.

Super Prescription #5   Ginkgo biloba
Take 120 mg twice daily of a product standardized to 24 percent flavone glycosides. Ginkgo improves circulation and has potent antioxidant effects. One study found it helpful for early-stage macular degeneration.

Super Prescription #6   Bilberry (*Vaccinium myrtillus*)
Take 240 to 600 mg a day of a standardized formula containing 25 percent anthocyanosides.
This herb contains flavonoids—phytochemicals that protect the eyes against oxidative damage. It also strengthens the capillaries and the connective tissues of the eye.

Super Prescription #7   High-potency multivitamin
Take a high-potency multivitamin. It provides a base of antioxidants and nutrients for eye health.

One study involved over 3,600 people, ages 55 to 80 years, who were at risk for age-related macular degeneration. Those who took antioxidants plus zinc were less likely than those who took only antioxidants or only zinc to lose their vision over the six-year study. Individuals who took a placebo were the most likely to develop advanced age-related macular degeneration and vision loss.

A survey of 876 elderly individuals found that people whose intake of lutein and zeaxanthin was in the top 20th percentile were 56 percent less likely to have age-related macular degeneration, as compared with people who had a low intake of these two carotenoids.

A double-blind trial found that supplementation with 45 mg of zinc daily for one to two years significantly slowed the rate of visual loss in people with macular degeneration.

General Recommendations

Fish oil contains DHA, which is concentrated in the retina of the eye. The consumption of fish has been shown to reduce the risk of macular degeneration. Take a fish oil product containing 1,000 mg of DHA daily.

Vitamin E-complex acts as an antioxidant and has been shown to improve vision in people with age-related macular degeneration. Take 400 IU daily with a meal.

A mixed carotenoid complex contains a blend of carotenoids that protects against ultraviolet light damage. Take 25,000 IU twice daily.

Digestive enzymes improve digestion and absorption. Take a full-spectrum complex with each meal.

Grapeseed extract or maritime pine bark extract scavenges free radicals from the eye and the brain and improves circulation. Take 150 to 300 mg daily.

Taurine is an amino acid that is believed to protect the retina from ultraviolet light damage. Take 500 mg twice daily on an empty stomach.

Homeopathy

Homeopathy may be helpful for macular degeneration. See a homeopathic practitioner for a constitutional remedy.

Acupressure

See pages 668–675 for information about pressure points and administering treatment.
Work Large Intestine 3 and 4 to improve circulation to your head.

Bodywork

An all-over massage will improve circulation and help deliver oxygen to all parts of the body, including the eyes.

Reflexology

See pages 686–687 for information about reflexology areas and how to work them.
Work the eye/ear area of the foot, which is located at the base of the toes.

Hydrotherapy

Alternating hot and cold cloths to the eyes will improve circulation.

Stress Reduction

General Stress-Reduction Therapies

Vision problems can be alarming and discouraging. Cope with the stress by setting aside time to relax every day.

Bach Flower Remedies

According to Bach remedy theory, eye disorders are caused by blindness to reality, but if none of the following remedies suit your needs, consult the chart on pages 648–650. Once you've selected the appropriate remedy, place 10 drops of the liquid under your tongue. Hold them in place for thirty seconds and swallow. Use as often as needed.
Clematis is for dreamy people who live a world of their own making.

If you prefer to relive days gone by instead of facing the present, Honeysuckle will help.

For vague fears that you can't or won't confront or face head-on, take Aspen.

Other Recommendations

- Smoking is a potent way to deliver free radicals to your body. If you smoke, stop. If you don't, protect yourself from secondhand smoke.
- Regular, moderate exercise will help keep your blood flowing properly to the eyes.
- Protect your eyes from the sun. In bright light, wear sunglasses that filter out 98 percent of the ultraviolet spectrum.
- For advanced cases of macular degeneration, consider a nutrition-oriented doctor who uses intravenous vitamin and mineral therapy.

REFERENCES

Archives of Ophthalmology. 2001. 119:1417–36, 1439–52, 1533–34.

Newsome, D. A., M. Swartz, N. C. Leone, et al. 1988. Oral zinc in macular degeneration. *Archives of Ophthalmology* 106:192–98.

Seddon, J. M., et al. 1994. Dietary carotenoids, vitamins A, C, and E, and advanced age-related macular degeneration. *Journal of the American Medical Association* 272:1413–20.

Memory Problems

Misplaced documents. Forgotten names. Missed appointments. More than two-thirds of people over sixty-five say that they have trouble recalling old details and absorbing new ones. To some people, memory problems are just part of what used to be called "senility," an unfortunate but natural part of old age. For others, periodic forgetfulness sets off alarm bells: Is this Alzheimer's? Stroke? Dementia?

Poor memory is a problem but not an inevitable part of the aging process. While it's true that nerve cells in the brain do shrink a little with advanced age and that it's harder for them to form connections with one another, most researchers now believe that memory loss is caused mainly by lifestyle factors. Most cases can be prevented or reversed with some simple changes in diet, exercise, and habits.

Many people with memory problems are actually suffering from a malnourished brain. The brain, like the rest of the body, needs to receive its supply of oxygen and nutrients from the blood if it is to function at its best. Chemicals called neurotransmitters, which enable the brain cells to communicate and create memory links, are especially dependent on good nutrition. The brain also needs high doses of nutrients to fight damage from free radicals. Of particular importance are essential fatty acids, which are required for the cell walls of brain cells. These essential fatty acids, particularly DHA, impact memory and concentration in a positive fashion. When the circulation is sluggish and blood is low in "brain food," memory disturbances may well be the result.

Other factors can contribute as well. Several medications, alone or in combination, can cause memory loss, as can underlying illnesses like depression, thyroid problems, and chronic fatigue. Sometimes even allergic reactions to food can impair memory. Poor digestion can be at the root of memory problems, as can a hormone imbalance. In particular, elevated levels of the stress hormone cortisol can impair memory. One must also consider hypoglycemia as a possibility of poor memory. This makes sense, considering that glucose is the primary fuel source for the brain. Systemic candidiasis frequently causes a foggy or poor memory. Also, toxic metals such as lead, mercury, and others can impair mental function and should be chelated out, if they're a problem.

If you try the suggestions here and your problems don't improve within a couple of weeks, see your doctor.

SYMPTOMS

- Difficulty recalling details

Caution: If you have trouble recalling the names of close friends and family members, or if your memory problems began after a head injury, see your doctor immediately.

ROOT CAUSES

- A poor diet, especially one that's high in fat and low in nutrients
- Free radicals
- Inactivity, both physical and mental
- Medications
- Abuse of alcohol or street drugs
- Underlying disorders, such as candidiasis, heavy-metal poisoning, depression, dementia, thyroid disorders, and hypoglycemia
- Nutritional deficiencies (especially of DHA, vitamin B12, folic acid)

TREATMENT

Diet

A good diet is crucial to brain health.

Recommended Food

Eat a wholesome diet of basic, unprocessed foods. Because conventionally grown foods often contain toxins, buy organic whenever possible. If organic food is unavailable or too expensive, wash your food thoroughly before eating.

The antioxidant vitamins A, C, and E will combat damage from free radicals. Fresh fruits and vegetables are among the best sources of antioxidants, so have a couple of servings at every meal. For vitamin E, add wheat germ to salads, cereals, or juices. Nuts and seeds are other good sources of this vital nutrient.

A deficiency of the B-complex vitamins can cause memory problems. Brewer's yeast is a potent source of B vitamins, as are wheat germ, eggs, and spirulina.

To improve circulation, increase energy levels, and detoxify your body, drink a glass of clean water every two waking hours.

Eat plenty of fiber to keep toxins moving through your digestive tract and to prevent them from taking up residence in your body. Whole grains, oats, and raw or lightly cooked vegetables are good sources of fiber that are also nutritionally dense.

Consume fish, such as salmon, mackerel, and other clean fish, three times weekly for their essential fatty acids.

Testing Techniques

Toxic metal testing—for elements toxic to brain tissue, such as aluminum, mercury, lead, arsenic, and others. The best test is a toxic element challenge urinalysis. The patient takes a chelating agent such as DMSA or DMPS, which pulls toxic metals out of tissue storage. Urine is then collected, usually for twenty-four hours. Hair analysis can also be used as a screening test.

Oxidative stress analysis—urine or blood testing

Antioxidant testing (urine, blood, or skin scanning)

Digestive function and microbe/parasite/candida testing—stool analysis

Anemia—blood test (CBC, iron, ferritin, % saturation)

Hormone analysis by saliva, urine, or blood (estrogens, progesterone, testosterone, DHEA, cortisol, melatonin, IGF-1, thyroid panel)

If you're older, your digestive system may not be able to absorb nutrients as well as it used to. Fresh fruit and vegetable juices are easily absorbable and packed with the vitamins you need, so have several glasses daily.

Food to Avoid

Determine whether your memory problems are caused or aggravated by food allergies. See the Food Allergies section and try the elimination diet on page 253; you may want to focus on cutting out wheat and dairy, as allergic responses to these items are most likely to lead to memory problems. If your memory improves when a food or foods are removed from your diet and worsens when they are reintroduced, banish those products from your diet.

Drastically reduce your intake of foods that are high in cholesterol or saturated fat. They impede blood flow.

Avoid sugar and processed foods, which add nothing or very little in the way of vitamins or minerals and actually deplete much-needed nutrients from your brain cells.

Alcohol destroys brain cells, causes dehydration, and clouds the mind. Stay away from it.

Detoxification

If your memory problems persist, you may want to determine whether you suffer from heavy metal poisoning. Consult an expert for a test.

A three-day juice fast once a month will help flush toxins out of your body. Support your fast with a wide variety of juices so that you get the nutrition you need.

℞ Super Seven Prescriptions—Poor Memory

Super Prescription # 1   Phosphatidylserine
Take 300 mg daily. This naturally occurring phospholipid improves brain cell communication and memory.

Super Prescription #2   Bacopa (*Bacopa monniera*)
This nutrient has been shown to improve memory and recall. Take 300 mg daily.

> ### Super Prescription #3   Ginkgo biloba (24 percent)
> Take 120 mg two to three times daily. It improves circulation to the brain, improves memory, and has antioxidant benefits.
>
> ### Super Prescription #4   Vitamin B12
> Take 800 to 1600 mcg daily. Consider using a sublingual form at 400 mcg. A vitamin B12 deficiency contributes to poor memory.
>
> ### Super Prescription #5   Club moss (*Huperzia serrata*)
> Take a product standardized to contain 0.2 mg of huperizine A daily. This compound has been shown to increase acetylcholine levels in the brain and to improve memory in people with Alzheimer's disease.
>
> ### Super Prescription #6   Essential fatty acids
> Take 1 to 2 tablespoons of flaxseed oil or 2 to 5 grams of fish oil daily. It supplies essential fatty acids for proper brain function.
>
> ### Super Prescription #7   Acetyl-L-carnitine
> Take 500 mg three times daily. It improves brain cell communication and memory.

General Recommendations

Ashwagandha (*Withania somniferum*) is used as a brain tonic in Ayurvedic medicine. It reduces stress hormone levels. Take 100 to 3,000 mg daily.

Phosphatidylcholine is a nutrient that increases acetylcholine levels to improve memory. Take 1,000 to 1,500 mg daily.

Panax ginseng improves memory and balances stress hormone levels. Take a standardized product containing 4 to 7 percent ginsenosides at 100 to 250 mg twice daily. Do not use it if you have high blood pressure.

DHEA is an important hormone for cognitive function. If your level of DHEA is low, talk with your doctor about starting at a dosage of 15 mg.

Cordyceps sinensis is used in Chinese medicine for poor memory. Take 2 to 4 capsules daily.

DMAE helps the body produce acetylcholine for memory and has antioxidant properties. Take 100 mg daily.

Gotu kola is an Ayurvedic herb that historically has been used as a brain tonic. Take 120 mg daily.

B-complex contains the B vitamins that are involved with brain function. Take 100 mg daily.

Antioxidant formula: choose a formula that contains a wide range of antioxidants, such as selenium, carotenoids, vitamin C, and others.

Reishi (*Ganoderma lucidum*) extract improves mental alertness. Take 800 mg twice daily.

Chlorella improves the detoxification of toxic metals that may be causing free radical damage. Take as directed on the container.

A high-potency multivitamin supplies most of the vitamins and the minerals involved with memory. Take as directed on the container.

Homeopathy

Pick the remedy that best matches your symptoms in this section. Take a 6x, 12x, 6C, 12C, or 30C potency twice daily for two weeks to see if there are any positive results. After you notice improvement, stop taking the remedy, unless symptoms return. Consultation with a homeopathic practitioner is advised.

Alumina can clear confusion and reduce memory impairment. Constipation is often present in people who can benefit from Alumina.

Calcarea Carbonica is for a shortened attention span, confusion, childish behavior, and difficulty recalling words (not just names). The person tends to be flabby and chilly and perspires easily on the back of the head and the feet.

Kali Phosphoricum is for poor memory and mental fatigue.

Lycopodium (*Lycopodium clavatum*) is helpful if you're fearful and have trouble recalling words. You often have digestive problems, such as gas and bloating.

Sulfur will help people who have problems remembering names and who generally have better recall after resting during the day. They tend to be very warm and crave spicy foods and ice-cold drinks.

Acupressure

See pages 668–675 for information about pressure points and administering treatment.

- If you're getting older and need an all-around tune-up, set aside a few minutes each day to work Stomach 36. It benefits all the systems of the body and also helps you absorb nutrients from your food.
- If you're under stress, work Lung 1 to encourage deep, calming breaths.
- Work Large Intestine 4 to encourage circulation to the brain.

Bodywork

Massage

An all-over massage will stimulate blood flow to each part of the body, including the brain. Add one of the essential oils listed under Aromatherapy in this section for an even more potent effect.

Reflexology

See pages 686–687 for information about reflexology areas and how to work them.

To clear out mental cobwebs and stimulate brain function, work the areas corresponding to the head and the neck.

The liver point will aid in detoxification of the blood.

Hydrotherapy

Constitutional hydrotherapy is effective in promoting circulation to the brain. See pages 676–677 for directions.

Aromatherapy

Basil promotes mental clarity and concentration. In addition, it has an uplifting effect. Use it in a diffuser, a steam inhalation, a bath, or a massage.

Rosemary is refreshing to both the brain and the body. It increases alertness and improves circulation; try it in any preparation you like.

Add juniper oil to a massage to encourage the breakdown of fatty deposits and other toxins.

Stress Reduction

General Stress-Reduction Therapies

Set aside time every morning to meditate. Meditation helps you weed out mental distractions so that you begin your day with focus and clarity.

Bach Flower Remedies

Consult the chart on pages 648–650 to determine the best remedy for your particular needs. Following are some suggestions. Once you've chosen a remedy, place 10 drops of the liquid under your tongue. Hold the drops in place for thirty seconds and swallow. Use as often as needed.

If you have difficulty learning or concentrating, try Chestnut Bud to improve your memory skills.

When memory problems are caused by a lack of attention, Impatiens will help.

Clematis is for people who are dreamy, absent-minded, and unable to concentrate. They may also have a strong desire to nap or sleep.

Other Recommendations

- When it comes to brain function, more and more evidence shows that the old adage "Use it or lose it" is good advice. If you don't work your brain, it will grow lazy and bored. By contrast, people who continue to engage in intellectual and social activities throughout old age retain their brain power and general health much longer than people who retire to the easy chair. Crosswords, chess, checkers, and reading are all examples of daily mind-exercising events.
- Regular, moderate exercise will keep the blood circulating to your brain. Consider taking up a sport, such as tennis or golf, that has a social component; that way, you'll stimulate your mind as well as your body.

Menopause

Menopause is a good example of Western medicine's focus on disease, rather than on health and wellness. In this case, a natural state—the end of menstruation—is defined by many conventional doctors as a disease that must be treated with medication. Women who don't take their estrogen pills, Western medicine implies, will lose their femininity and their value to society. Luckily, many women instinctively know better, and studies have proven that there are extreme health risks with synthetic hormone replacement. To these wise women, menopause is a time of freedom from the menstrual cycle and the onset of wisdom and power. And it's no coincidence that these women, who refuse to view themselves as "diseased," experience far fewer (and sometimes none) of the problems usually associated with this change of life.

Since attitude plays a significant role in the physical response to menopause, it helps to understand the changes that are taking place. These changes can start several years before menopause proper actually sets in, with erratic periods or unusually heavy or light bleeding. This phase is called perimenopause or premenopause and provides an opportunity to prepare emotionally and physically for the larger transition to come. During premenopause, the ovaries no longer ovulate on a regular basis. This is the basis for the cycle changes and the beginning of symptoms such as hot flashes. Menopause itself usually begins in the mid-forties to early fifties. When the ovaries stop producing significant amounts of estrogen and progesterone, the menstrual cycle ceases; a woman who has had no periods for a year is said to be menopausal.

Women's reactions to menopause vary widely. Some enjoy the change, while others suffer from problems like hot flashes, vaginal dryness, heart palpitations, and mood swings, often for years. But if a woman is healthy, active, and well nourished, her adrenal glands will usually respond to menopause by creating precursor hormones such as pregnenolone and DHEA, which are then converted into estrogen, progesterone, and testosterone. And if she takes natural steps to encourage this process, it is likely that she can avoid harsh and possibly dangerous medications altogether.

The days of routinely prescribing synthetic estrogen, synthetic progesterone, or both, should be over. Several studies, including the well-publicized Women's Health Initiative Study, which involved over 16,000 women, concluded that the "benefits did not outweigh the risks" of using the combination of synthetic estrogen (Premarin) and synthetic progesterone (Provera). A significant increased incidence of breast cancer and cardiovascular disease stopped this study short of its completion.

There are also times when menopause really is a disorder or a serious problem. If menopause arrives for unnatural reasons, such as from anorexia, bulimia, or extremely intense exercise, the root cause must be treated so that the cycle returns. When menopause is brought about by a hysterectomy or removal of the ovaries, natural hormonal replacement therapy may be necessary to counter the sudden depletion of estrogen and progesterone and the resulting bone loss.

We believe that every woman must be addressed individually. Optimally, it is best to get a hormone test done to find out which hormone imbalances you may have. Saliva testing is a good option. For women with mild to moderate symptoms of menopause, we generally recommend the use of diet, exercise, and nutritional supplements, especially herbal and homeopathic remedies. The beauty of this approach is that these natural supplements balance the hormones that are already present in the body. In addition, the use of natural progesterone appears to be very safe and effective when a stronger approach is needed. Likewise, precursor hormones, such as pregnenolone and DHEA, may be helpful.

For women with extreme symptoms that are unresponsive to nutritional supplements, the use of natural hormone replacement may be required. This is particularly true of women who had their ovaries removed at an early age or for others with moderate to severe osteoporosis. This is, of course, best done with a doctor who is knowledgeable in natural hormones.

SYMPTOMS

- Cessation of periods
- Hot flashes
- Vaginal dryness and thinning
- Night sweats
- Insomnia
- Dizziness
- Heart palpitations
- Headaches
- Memory problems and difficulty concentrating
- Cold hands and feet
- Reduced libido
- Bladder problems, including incontinence
- Mood swings
- Depression and anxiety
- Fatigue
- Joint pain
- Skin changes (acne, facial hair, hair loss on scalp)

ROOT CAUSES OF EARLY MENOPAUSE

- Eating disorders
- Extraordinarily intense exercise or physical training
- Ovarian disease
- Surgical removal of the ovaries, usually as part of a hysterectomy
- Hypofunctioning adrenal glands

> ## Testing Techniques
>
> The following tests help assess hormone balance and other issues related to menopause:
>
> Hormone testing (thyroid, DHEA, cortisol, testosterone, IGF-1, estrogen, progesterone, FSH)—saliva, blood, or urine
>
> Complete blood count and chemistry profile—blood
>
> Thyroid panel—blood or saliva or urine
>
> Cardiovascular profile—blood (see Cardiovascular Disease section for more detail)
>
> Bone resorption assessment—urine
>
> Bone density—DEXA scan (X-ray)

TREATMENT

Diet

If you begin to incorporate these suggestions into your diet at the onset of peri-menopause, you will likely experience far fewer problems when menopause begins in earnest.

Recommended Food

Eat a diet loaded with plant foods, especially whole grains, legumes, fresh vegetables, and fruits. These contain phytosterols, naturally occurring nutrients that have a hormone-balancing effect. You'll also get the fiber you need to keep your heart healthy and the nutrients that will encourage a strong, vibrant response to menopause.

Japanese women have significantly fewer problems during menopause, thanks to their consumption of soybeans, tofu, miso, and flaxseeds, all of which are excellent sources of phytoestrogens. Add these to your diet, unless you have a soy allergy.

Essential fatty acids protect the heart and promote smooth, radiant skin. Good sources are cold-water fish like salmon, cod, and tuna, as well as flaxseeds.

Vitamin E regulates estrogen production. Make sure to include cold-pressed nut and seed oils in your diet, perhaps as a dressing for a green salad.

Consume 1 to 2 tablespoons of ground flaxseeds daily. They contain lignans, which are phytonutrients that have estrogen-balancing properties and that lower cholesterol. Take each serving with 10 ounces of water.

Drink a glass of clean water every two waking hours. You'll flush out toxins and replace fluid you may have lost during hot flashes.

Food to Avoid

To protect yourself against heart disease, reduce red meat and other sources of saturated fat from your diet. Eat hormone-free animal products to avoid causing a hormone imbalance.

Carbonated drinks also deplete calcium from your body, so you should avoid them.

Caffeine and alcohol aggravate hot flashes, so eliminate them from your diet.

Detoxification

Keep your system clear of artery-clogging toxins by doing a three-day juice fast once every three months. Regular fasting is especially beneficial for women on hormone-replacement therapy, whose livers may be taxed with extra waste.

℞ Super Seven Prescriptions—Menopause

Super Prescription #1   Black cohosh (*Cimicifuga racemosa*)
Take 80 mg one to two times daily. This herb has been shown in numerous studies to alleviate a multitude of menopausal symptoms, including hot flashes.

Super Prescription #2   Natural progesterone cream
Perimenopausal women should apply ¼ teaspoon (20 mg) to the skin on the inside of their wrists and forearms one to two times daily, from days 14 to 25 of the menstrual cycle or as directed by their health-care practitioner.

Menopausal women should apply ¼ teaspoon (20 mg) to the skin on the inside of their wrists and forearms two times daily, three to four weeks of the month or as directed by their health-care practitioner.

Postmenopausal should women apply ⅛ teaspoon (10 mg) to the skin on the inside of their wrists and forearms once daily, three weeks of the month.

Natural progesterone alleviates a multitude of menopausal symptoms and may help bone density.

Super Prescription #3   Vitex (chasteberry)
Take 160 to 240 mg of an 0.6 percent aucubin extract daily. Vitex relieves hot flashes and prevents a heavy menses for perimenopausal women. Do not use it if you are taking the birth control pill.

Super Prescription #4   American ginseng (*Panax quinquefolius*)
Take 600 to 1,200 mg daily. This herb supports adrenal function, improves energy, relaxes the nervous system, and has a cooling effect.

Super Prescription #5   Hops (*Humulus lupulus*)
Take 250 mg two to three times daily. Hops reduces anxiety and tension and has mild hormone-balancing properties.

Super Prescription #6   Rehmania (*Rehmania glutinosa*)
Take 25 to 100 mg daily. This Chinese herb has a cooling effect and reduces hot flashes, night sweats, heart palpitations, and other common menopause symptoms.

Super Prescription #7   Soy protein powder (preferably fermented)
Take up to 60 grams a day, as studies show that it reduces hot flashes. Do not use it if you have a soy allergy.

A study involving 131 doctors and 629 female patients revealed that black cohosh (*Cimicifuga racemosa*) alleviated several menopausal symptoms in 80 percent of women within six to eight weeks. Symptoms that were improved included hot flashes, headaches, vertigo, heart palpitations, nervousness, ringing in the ears, anxiety, insomnia, and depression. Another study of 80 women going through menopause found that black cohosh (*Cimicifuga racemosa*) had the best results in alleviating symptoms, as compared to Premarin or a placebo.

General Recommendations

DHEA supports memory, libido, and mood. If your level of DHEA is low, take 5 to 15 mg as a starting dosage, under the guidance of your doctor.

Pregnenolone is a precursor hormone to make estrogen and progesterone. Take 30 mg twice daily, under the guidance of your doctor.

Adrenal glandular extract supports the hormone-producing adrenal glands. Take 1 to 2 capsules twice daily on an empty stomach.

For memory and concentration problems, take Gingko biloba. It increases blood

For every synthetic hormone prescription, there exists a natural version that is identical to what is found in your body. If you need hormone-replacement therapy, consult a doctor who is knowledgeable in natural hormone replacement. These hormones are available from a compounding pharmacy in your area. *Note:* Most hormones require a prescription.

A double-blind trial found that transdermal natural progesterone cream reduced hot flashes in 83 percent of women, compared with improvement in only 19 percent of those given a placebo. Transdermal natural progesterone has also been shown to prevent the build-up of the endometrium (lining of uterus) among postmenopausal women who take synthetic estrogen (Premarin).

flow to the brain. Take 120 to 240 mg daily of an extract standardized to 24 percent flavone glycosides.

Hormone-replacement therapy puts a great stress on the liver. If you choose to take this medication, detoxify with milk thistle (*Silybum marianum*). Find a formula that's standardized to 70 to 80 percent silymarin content, and take 250 mg twice a day.

Saint-John's-wort (*Hypericum perforatum*) has been shown to fight depression that comes on with menopause. Take 900 mg daily of a 0.3 percent hypericin extract.

If you have heart palpitations, take motherwort (*Leonurus cardiaca*) at a dosage of 200 mg or 2 ml three times daily.

Sage (*Salvia officinalis*) helps control the sweating associated with hot flashes. Take a daily dose of 4 to 6 grams.

Red clover (*Trifolium pratense*) has been shown in some studies to reduce the symptoms of menopause. Take 40 mg one to two times daily.

If you need to unwind and destress, find a quiet moment to drink a cup of tea made from chamomile, peppermint, or passion flower. Each of these herbs is relaxing and calming.

Vitamin E-complex may help reduce the symptoms of menopause. Take 800 to 1,200 IU daily. Do not use this high of a dosage if you're on blood-thinning medications.

For mild vaginal dryness, use a lubricant from your health food store or pharmacy. For severe vaginal dryness, have your doctor prescribe vaginal estriol cream. Insert 1 gram nightly, containing 0.5 mg, for two weeks and then as needed.

A high-potency multivitamin provides a base of vitamins and minerals for overall health.

Take a daily total of 1,000 mg of calcium and 500 mg of magnesium, or a bone formula for bone health.

For a more powerful relaxing effect, especially if you need to sleep, drink valerian tea.

Homeopathy

Pick the remedy that best matches your symptoms in this section. Take a 6x, 12x, 6C, 12C, or 30C potency twice daily for two weeks to see if there are any positive results. After you notice improvement, stop taking the remedy, unless symptoms return. Consultation with a homeopathic practitioner is advised.

Belladonna (*Atropa belladonna*) is a remedy for sudden hot flashes that cause a flushing of the face. Throbbing symptoms may occur in the head or other areas of the body, accompanied by heat. Heart palpitations, restlessness, and right-sided headaches are common symptoms.

Calcarea Carbonica will help menopausal symptoms such as night sweats, heavy flow, and hot flashes even though the woman is chilly. There is often a sense of anxiety, fatigue, and a feeling of being overwhelmed. Women may also experience leg cramps and crave both eggs and sweets. There is weight gain with the menopausal transition.

Lachesis will ease a variety of menopausal complaints, including hot flashes, anxiety, headaches, insomnia, memory problems, and lack of concentration. It is a specific remedy for heart palpitations that are worse from lying on the left side. The woman is often very talkative and may have strong emotions such as jealousy, suspiciousness, or anger. Tight clothing around the neck is avoided. The libido often increases with menopause.

Natrum Muriaticum is for women who experience backaches and migraines, along with a craving for salt and cold drinks. It is also used for hot flashes and vaginal dryness. Symptoms are worse in the sun. Depression and aversion to people may be present. The woman cries easily.

Oophorinum is a specific remedy for hot flashes in women who have had their ovaries removed.

Pulsatilla (*Pulsatilla pratensis*) is for women who feel much worse in a warm room and who strongly desire fresh air. Mood swings and weepiness are characteristic symptoms. They may have a strong craving for sweets, pastries, and chocolate.

Sepia is for menopausal women who experience pain or anxiety during intercourse, usually because of vaginal dryness. If periods still occur, there may be heavy bleeding. This remedy may help uterine prolapse and incontinence. Women who benefit from this remedy usually feel irritable and exhausted. They have a strong craving for chocolate, sweets, or sour foods and have an aversion to sex.

Sulphur is a good remedy for hot flashes and night sweats. The woman perspires easily and throws the covers off at night. She has a strong thirst for ice-cold drinks.

Acupressure

See pages 668–675 for information about pressure points and administering treatment.

- Governing Vessel 24.5 regulates glands and will minimize headaches and hot flashes.
- Work Governing Vessel 20 for improved concentration and memory, as well as for relief from headache pain.
- Conception Vessel 17 will soothe tension and help you sleep. It also helps reduce hot flashes.
- If you suffer from anxiety that leads to heart palpitations, work Pericardium 6. You can use this point as part of a daily practice, or you can press it whenever you feel tension coming on.
- To strengthen the urinary tract, work Bladder 60.

Bodywork

Massage
Massage therapy is a terrific stress reliever. If you don't already receive regular massage treatments, this is a good time in your life to start.

If you're feeling less sexual desire than you used to, you may be suffering from touch deprivation. Keep up physical contact with your partner by learning a few simple massage techniques for the head, the shoulder, or the back.

Reflexology
See pages 686–687 for information about reflexology areas and how to work them.

If you have only a short amount of time, concentrate on the area corresponding to the uterus. You can also work the ovaries, the fallopian tubes, and all glands.

For stress relief, work the solar plexus.

The chest and lung area will strengthen your heart.

Hydrotherapy
A warm sitz bath will increase circulation to the pelvic area and will improve vaginal dryness and decreased libido.

Aromatherapy

Geranium and rose oils have a gentle balancing effect on hormone levels. They have the additional benefit of reducing stress. Add these oils to a bath or use them in a massage.

If you want to lift your spirits, you can try several oils. Bergamot, rose, and jasmine are some of the best; use them in any preparation you like.

Patchouli and ylang ylang instill a sense of calm, while arousing sexual desire. Try a few drops in the bath or a room diffuser, or use in a massage.

Add chamomile to a lotion, and apply to dry skin for a softening, smoothing effect.

Stress Reduction

General Stress-Reduction Therapies

For some women, menopause is difficult. Any of the techniques in the Exercise and Stress Reduction chapter can help you relieve stress. The key is to pick one or a couple and do them regularly. Walking has been shown in studies to alleviate hot flashes.

Bach Flower Remedies

Select the appropriate remedy and place 10 drops of the liquid under your tongue. Hold the drops in place for thirty seconds and swallow. Use as often as needed.

Walnut is the remedy for anxiety about a new phase of life. Take it if you need help adjusting to the transition.

If menopause brings on specific fears—of aging or loss, for example—Mimulus will help.

If your fear is more general, one that you can't exactly name, take Aspen.

Mustard will relieve sadness that seems to have no obvious cause.

Other Recommendations

- Remember that one year without a single period must pass before menopause can officially be declared. If a full year has not passed since your last cycle, it's possible that you could still get pregnant. Take appropriate precautions.
- Don't smoke. Smoking is linked to premature menopause, as well as to heart disease.
- Regular exercise improves general health, as well as many symptoms of menopause. Nonimpact workouts like swimming and cycling are good for your cardiovascular system, but to prevent bone loss you'll need to include weight-bearing exercise as well. Walking is one of the best all-over conditioners, and weight lifting has been shown to increase bone density and vitality even for people in their nineties.
- Acupuncture can be helpful for alleviating a variety of menopausal symptoms, as can Chinese herbal therapy. See a qualified practitioner.

REFERENCES

Anasti, J. N., H. B. Leonetti, and K. J. Wilson. 2001. Topical progesterone cream has antiproliferative effect on estrogen-stimulated endometrium. *Obstetrics and Gynecology* (4 Suppl 1): S10.

Leonetti, H. B., S. Long, and J. M. Anasti. 1999. Transdermal progesterone cream for vasomotor symptoms and postmenopausal bone loss. *Obstetrics and Gynecology* 94:225–28.

Stoll, W. 1987. Phytopharmacon influences atrophic vaginal epithelium: Double-blind study—Cimicifuga vs. estrogenic substances. *Therapeutikon* 1:2–30.

Stolze, H. 1982. An alternative to treat menopausal complaints. *Gyne* 2:4–16.

Motion Sickness

Whether on air, land, or sea, some people are immune to motion sickness, and others just aren't. These are the unhappy people who spend entire vacations green-faced and prostrate; while their travel companions enjoy the view, people with motion sickness hope for nothing more than to avoid another debilitating round of vomiting. Even after the trip is over, they may feel ill for several days. If you're a member of this unfortunate segment of the population, you may be tempted to avoid travel altogether. Before you give up your vacations, however, give these suggestions a try. They might not completely eliminate motion sickness, but often they will significantly reduce the symptoms.

Motion sickness occurs when the mechanism that controls internal equilibrium is disturbed. One of the most important body structures for maintaining balance is the vestibular apparatus, located in the inner ear. Rolling or bumpy movements can cause the ear's fluid to slosh around, and sometimes the flow of liquid pushes against the vestibular apparatus, which in turn sends alarm messages along the nerve pathways. These messages are translated in the brain as the familiar feelings of nausea, dizziness, cold sweats, or rapid breathing, and they're probably meant as a kind of warning system, telling you in no uncertain terms that the body is facing a grave danger. The problem, of course, is that there is no danger—just a road, perhaps, with an unusual number of hills and sharp turns.

The eyes also contribute to the body's sense of balance, or lack thereof. When you're sitting in a train during a smooth ride over flat land, for example, your ear fluid remains stable, which tells your brain that the body is still and unmoving. But your eyes are sending a completely different message: they report that the landscape is whipping by at seventy miles per hour. These conflicting transmissions can upset your equilibrium, which explains how some people can get sick just from watching a movie about riding in a hot-air balloon.

Neither of these explanations helps us understand why some people develop motion sickness and others actually enjoy riding the waves. We do know, however, that anxiety, stress, poor dietary habits, low air quality, and dehydration all contribute to the condition, and this information gives us a good place to start for treatment. If you're prone to motion sickness, plan ahead so that you can avoid these aggravating factors. You can also use several techniques to reduce your chances of feeling nauseated, but in most cases, you must employ them before you travel. By the time you're really sick, you may not be able to hold down any therapeutic foods or herbs.

SYMPTOMS

- Queasiness
- Nausea
- Cold sweats
- Dizziness
- Rapid breathing
- Fatigue
- Vomiting
- Loss of coordination

ROOT CAUSES

- Disturbance of inner ear
- Conflicting messages sent to the brain from the eyes and the inner ears
- Anxiety and stress
- Overeating
- Eating heavy foods before or during travel
- Dehydration
- Poor ventilation

Testing Techniques

The following tests help assess possible reasons for motion sickness:

Inner ear or vision testing by your doctor

Food and environmental allergies/sensitivities—blood, electrodermal

---

TREATMENT

Diet

Recommended Food

Eat lightly before your trip and while traveling. Soups and steamed vegetables will help your stomach stay calm. If you're taking a trip on a commercial airliner, a train, or a ship, phone ahead and explain that you'll need special meals. Most companies are happy to provide vegetarian or healthier dishes for their customers.

Incorporate wheat germ or brown rice into your meals. These foods are high in B vitamins, which prevent stomach upset and relieve stress. Whole-grain crackers are another good source of this nutrient, so bring some along with you and make a snack of them. You may also want to nibble on a few if you feel queasy.

Chew on parsley, or add it to your meals, as it relieves nausea.

Stay hydrated. Drink at least one glass of clean water every two waking hours, more if you're going to be in the dry atmosphere of an airplane cabin. Liquids in general will feel more soothing if you drink them at room temperature or slightly heated.

If you feel queasiness coming on, suck on a slice of lemon or lime.

Food to Avoid

Beginning a day or two before your trip, avoid heavy foods—nothing fried, greasy, or fatty. Fats only contribute to nausea and stomach upset.

If you're going on vacation, you may be in a celebratory mood. Resist the temptation to drink even a little alcohol, which is dehydrating and can negatively affect the inner ear.

Many people change their diets when they travel, but if you're subject to motion sickness, this is not the best time to try new foods or to indulge yourself with treats.

℞ **Super Seven Prescriptions—Motion Sickness**

Super Prescription #1   Ginger (*Zingiber officinale*)
Sip on a cup of fresh ginger tea, or take 500 mg of the capsule form or 2 ml of ginger extract three to four times daily.

Super Prescription #2   Homeopathic Combination Motion Sickness/Nausea formula
This contains a mixture of the most common remedies used for motion sickness. Take as directed on the container.

Super Prescription #3   Peppermint (*Mentha piperita*)
Sip on a cup of peppermint tea, or take 500 mg of the capsule form or 2 ml of peppermint extract three to four times daily.

Super Prescription #4   Vitamin B6
Take 50 mg daily to prevent nausea.

Super Prescription #5   Magnesium
Take 250 mg twice daily to prevent stomach acidity and cramping.

Super Prescription #6   Black horehound (*Ballota nigra*)
Sip on a cup of tea, or take 2 ml of the tincture extract three to four times daily.

Super Prescription #7   Cinnamon (*Cinnamomum zeylanicum*)
Sip on a cup of tea, or take 1 ml of the tincture extract three to four times daily.

Several studies have found that ginger is an effective remedy for motion sickness. A study in 1982 revealed that ginger was more effective than the drug Dramamine for reducing motion sickness. A later study completed in 1994, which involved 1,741 people, confirmed that ginger was very effective for motion sickness.

Homeopathy

Borax is helpful for downward motions, such as those from an airplane, that make a person nauseous. The person may also be sensitive to noise, warm temperatures, and smoke.

Cocculus is a great remedy for nausea and dizziness that occur while riding in a vehicle like a car or a boat. The smell or the thought of food makes the nausea worse, while the symptoms are improved from fresh air. The motion sickness is worse from not getting enough sleep.

Petroleum is for nausea and dizziness that happens from rising. There is a sinking sensation in the stomach. The person feels better from eating and worse from fresh air.

Tabacum is helpful when violent nausea, dizziness, cold sweating, and faintness occur from the least motion. The person feels much better in the cool air or from vomiting.

Acupressure

Acupressure offers quick, effective relief of motion sickness. For more information about pressure points and administering treatment, see pages 668–675.

- If you can massage only one point, make that point Pericardium 6. It will greatly reduce nausea and even stop vomiting. Many health-food stores carry inexpensive acupressure bracelets that are made to provide constant steady pressure against this point; consider buying one before your next trip.
- Pericardium 5 is another good point for nausea relief. You can alternate between the two Pericardium wrist points if you have a few moments.
- Stomach 36 will help you properly digest the food you've eaten.

Bodywork

Reflexology

See pages 686–687 for information about reflexology areas and how to work them.
    Work the area corresponding to the ear to improve your sense of balance.

To reduce tension and increase circulation to the head, work the neck and the cervicals.

Aromatherapy

Essential oils of ginger and peppermint are quite helpful when the herbs can't be taken orally. Bring along a vial of either oil; if you begin to feel sick, place the container under your nose and inhale deeply. For a more subtle but longer-lasting effect, rub some ginger or peppermint cream onto your skin before and during your trip.

Stress Reduction

Deep breathing relieves tension and also helps prevent the onset of nausea. Spend some quiet time before your trip relaxing and consciously attending to your breathing. While you're traveling, take a few minutes every hour to relax with deep breaths.

Beginning a few days before your trip—give yourself more time if you're very anxious about motion sickness—and spend some time each day visualizing a successful, sickness-free journey. Imagine yourself as you begin the trip, and see yourself healthy and calm as you go through the details of your travels.

Other Recommendations

- Be wary of over-the-counter motion sickness pills. They make most people very drowsy and often have other unwanted side effects.
- Stuffy rooms and cars can make nausea worse. If it's at all possible, try to open a window or stop at regular intervals for fresh air. If you're on a ship, try to think of sea air as a tonic, and go above deck as often as you can.
- Again, where possible, keep your eyes open and focused on a stationary object. This will help reduce conflicting signals from your eyes and ears.
- If you're traveling by car or bus, sit up front, where there's less likely to be jarring movement.
- Some people are so susceptible to motion sickness that it threatens to confine them to their homes. If this describes you, talk to your doctor. He or she can usually prescribe medication that will help.

REFERENCES

Grontved, A., T. Brask, J. Kambskard, et al. 1988. Ginger root against seasickness. *Acta Oto-Laryngologica* 105:45–49.

Mowrey, D. B., and D. E. Clayson. 1982. Motion sickness, ginger, and psychophysics. *Lancet* 1:655–57.

Multiple Sclerosis

Multiple sclerosis (MS) is a chronic, progressive degenerative disease of the central nervous system. Because nerves are delicate, highly sensitive structures, they are sheathed in a protective material known as myelin. In a person with MS, the myelin degenerates, leaving sections of the nerves bare and vulnerable. If nerves are damaged and scarred over, the areas of the body that are controlled by the affected nerves will malfunction. Although MS is not a common disorder, it does strike more frequently than most other neurological diseases, and in recent years, the percentage of cases has increased. It's estimated that between 250,000 and 350,000 Americans currently suffer from MS. Multiple sclerosis can develop at any age, but onset usually occurs between the ages of twenty and forty. About two-thirds of MS victims are women.

The course of MS is highly individual and depends mainly on which nerves are affected and on the extent of the damage. Nevertheless, the disease does exhibit some general symptom patterns. Multiple sclerosis always occurs in cycles of flare-ups, called exacerbations, and remissions. The first attack and the exacerbations that follow may consist of nothing more than some blurred vision or unexplained fatigue. Because the symptoms are vague and disappear after a short time—sometimes after just days—and because a person may spend years in remission, MS often goes undiagnosed in these extremely early stages. Exacerbations get progressively worse, however, and when a person experiences more obviously alarming symptoms like facial paralysis, weak or numb limbs, or slurred speech, it's likely that a doctor will investigate the possibility of MS.

How the disease moves on from this stage varies from person to person. Some people will go into complete, lifelong remission. Just as rare is the case in which the disease hits with more force, causing significant, lasting damage after the very first attack. The vast majority of sufferers fall somewhere in-between these two extremes. Many will recover from the first major exacerbation and will experience only mild recurrences every ten years or so. Some will suffer from more frequent relapses that slowly become more severe and leave permanent disability in their wake. As the decades go on, a person may have trouble with movement, balance, and coordination and eventually develop the classic staggering gait. In the advanced stages, there may be blindness, incontinence, paralysis, or difficulty breathing. Because MS affects the brain's functions, many sufferers also experience mood alterations, swinging up to euphoria and then plunging down into a deep depression.

Why the sheaths of myelin degenerate in some people remains a mystery, but there's no shortage of theories. The prevailing hypothesis is that MS is an autoimmune disorder in which white blood cells mistake myelin for an invader and attack it. Another popular theory is that MS is caused by a virus or another latent infection, and indeed, the symptoms of MS are similar to those of some viral infections—so similar that doctors are often not able to distinguish a viral attack from MS in its early stages. Possibly, MS is caused by a combination of these factors, and the virus somehow causes the formation of antibodies that attack myelin.

Although multiple sclerosis is appearing with increasing frequency in the United States, the disease is rare in Eastern and developing countries and in the tropics. Any time this kind of geographical discrepancy occurs, it makes sense to investigate lifestyle and environmental factors as potential causes. Also, MS occurs more frequently in higher latitudes. High-risk areas include the northern United States, Canada, Great Britain, Scandinavia, Tasmania, and northern Europe, as examples. The reason for this is unclear, although studies show that people who had a higher sun exposure between the ages of six and fifteen have a significantly reduced risk of the disease. This may have something to do with vitamin D from sun exposure.

It's well known that extreme stress and poor nutrition can bring on an exacerbation, so it's quite possible that they also contribute to the onset of the disease. Environmental toxins, especially heavy metals, can produce symptoms similar to those of MS and may damage both DNA and myelin. And in the case of allergies, food allergies or sensitivities appear to be a factor for some people with this condition. Many researchers are currently looking into the relationship between an allergy to wheat or dairy and the incidence of MS. One must also look at the possibility of toxic metal accumulation, such as mercury, as a causative or aggravating factor. Good digestion is important, as there is a link between autoimmune diseases and malabsorption. Several nutritional deficiencies, especially of essential fatty acids and vitamin B12, are critical, as they are involved with a healthy myelin sheath.

Compounding the frightening symptoms of MS is the inability of many patients to receive a definitive diagnosis, especially in early stages of the disease. Doctors can perform spinal taps, testing the cerebrospinal fluid, or do MRI scans to look for abnormal antibodies and myelin damage, but because MS may cause damage much like that from a virus or other autoimmune disorders, the tests are often inclusive. In most cases, a diagnosis is made only when all other possibilities are ruled out.

If you have MS or MS-like symptoms, it's critical that you find a good specialist and work closely with him or her. Despite the common perception, many people with MS live long, productive lives. Disabilities caused by severe attacks, when they happen at all, often occur several decades after a diagnosis and can often be managed quite well. It is crucial that you also work with a holistic doctor to address the underlying reasons for your illness. We have had several patients with MS remain relatively symptom-free by following a comprehensive natural approach, as described in this section.

SYMPTOMS

Multiple sclerosis occurs in cycles of remission and exacerbation. Symptoms may occur singly at first, but later on, they usually appear in groups of two or more.

- Deep fatigue
- Blurred vision
- Dizziness
- Impaired speech
- Facial paralysis
- Numbness or weakness in the limbs
- Loss of balance

- Poor coordination
- Nausea and vomiting
- Constipation
- Staggering gait
- Tremors
- Bowel and bladder incontinence
- Blindness
- Paralysis

ROOT CAUSES

Doctors aren't sure what causes MS, but the leading theories are listed here.

- Chronic infection (viral, bacterial, candida)
- Long periods of extreme stress
- Stress hormone imbalance
- Poor nutrition (especially vitamin D deficiency

- Environmental toxins
- Toxic metals
- Food allergies
- Free radical damage
- Immunizations

TREATMENT

Diet

Recommended Food

Eat meals and snacks made with whole, unprocessed foods. Try to prepare meals yourself so you know what goes into them. Buy organic products as often as possible.

Testing Techniques

The following tests help assess possible reasons for multiple sclerosis:

Immune system imbalance or disease—blood

Hormone testing (thyroid, DHEA, cortisol, testosterone, IGF-1, estrogen, progesterone)—saliva, blood, or urine

Intestinal permeability—urine

Detoxification profile—urine

Vitamin and mineral analysis (especially magnesium, B12)—blood

Essential fatty-acid balance—blood or urine

Amino acid balance—blood or urine

Digestive function and microbe/parasite/candida testing—stool analysis

Food and environmental allergies/sensitivities—blood, electrodermal

---

Have several helpings of deeply colored fresh fruits and vegetables every day. These foods are high in antioxidants, which fight free radical damage to your cells. They're also high in fiber, which will keep your colon free of wastes and will help you avoid constipation.

Essential fatty acids reduce inflammation of the nerve fibers and strengthen myelin. Eat fish from a clean water source three or more times a week, and have a tablespoon of flaxseeds or flaxseed oil every day.

Lecithin may also help to strengthen the myelin sheath. Good sources include tofu and other soy products, bean sprouts, and cabbage.

To reduce stress, add whole grains, wheat germ, and brewer's yeast to your meals. The B vitamins in these foods are calming to the nervous system.

Food to Avoid

Reduce your exposure to chemicals and pesticides by eating organic foods. Do not eat junk food or packaged food that contains artificial flavoring, colorings, or preservatives.

If you're allergic to any food, you need to find out now. Read the Food Allergies section in this book and follow the elimination diet presented there. You should make it a priority to look for allergies to gluten (wheat and other grains) or dairy, but corn, yeast, sugar, peanuts, soy, and eggs are also common sensitivities.

Eliminate inflammatory foods from your diet that may make your nerve damage and muscle problems worse. If you've stopped eating red meat and dairy, you've already made great strides toward this goal. You should also avoid other foods that are fatty, fried, or greasy.

Keep up your resistance to infection by restricting your sugar consumption. If you're feeling well, the occasional treat is fine, but for the most part, you should avoid colas, sweet baked goods, candies, cakes, and other items made with refined sugar.

Roy Swank, M.D., a professor of neurology at the University of Oregon Medical School, prescribed a special diet for 150 patients with MS. This included the elimination of margarine, hydrogenated oils, and shortenings. Saturated fat was limited to 20 grams per day or less. The diet included vegetable oils that are rich in polyunsaturated fatty acids and 5 grams per day of cod liver oil. Patients were to eat fish three or more times a week and consume a normal amount of protein. Results showed that 95 percent of the people who started this regimen and had minimal disability to begin with showed very little or no progression of the disease over a thirty-year period. Also, people who followed the diet had a death rate significantly lower than a study group with MS who didn't follow the diet (31 percent versus 80 percent).

If you want to fight MS, you need all the nutritional support you can get. Avoid alcohol and caffeine, which deplete vitamins and minerals from your body and worsen inflammation.

Detoxification

Frequent short-term fasts will help you cleanse your body of toxins and will give you a lighter, more energetic feeling. During periods of remission, try a juice fast once a month. Be sure to supplement the fast with a wide variety of fruit and vegetable juices and broths.

Fasting during exacerbations is not recommended, as you need to keep up optimum nutrition at those times. Instead, supplement your regular healthful diet with lots of vegetable juices.

℞ **Super Seven Prescriptions—Multiple Sclerosis**

Super Prescription #1   Fish oil
Take a minimum of 5 grams daily and up to 20 grams daily. Omega-3 fatty acids reduce inflammation and are required for healthy nerve functioning. Dr. Swank used 5 grams of cod liver oil in his thirty-year study, while other studies have used up to 20 grams.

Super Prescription #2   Vitamin B12
Take 400 to 800 mcg of the sublingual form daily or receive the injectable form from your doctor. Vitamin B12 is involved in the formation of the myelin sheath, and nutrition-oriented doctors such as ourselves find B12 helpful for people with this condition.

Super Prescription #3   High-potency multivitamin
Take as directed on the container. It contains a base of the nutrients needed for healthy immune and nervous systems.

Super Prescription #4   Plant sterols and sterolins
Take 20 mg three times daily on an empty stomach. These naturally occurring plant chemicals have been shown to have a balancing effect on the immune systems of people with autoimmune diseases.

Super Prescription #5   Digestive enzymes
Take 1 to 2 capsules of a full-spectrum enzyme product with each meal. Enzymes help you to digest food more efficiently and lessen autoimmune reactions. Protease enzymes can be taken between meals to reduce autoimmune complexes and inflammation.

Super Prescription #6   Gamma linoleic acid (GLA)
Take 300 to 500 mg daily. It is found in evening primrose and borage oil. GLA is a fatty acid that has an anti-inflammatory effect.

Super Prescription #7   Vitamin E-complex
Take 400 IU of a mixed complex daily. Vitamin E is a potent antioxidant.

General Recommendations

Gingko biloba has potent antioxidant activity for the nerves and improves circulation. Take 60 to 120 mg twice daily of a standardized product containing 24 percent flavone glycosides and 6 percent terpene lactones.

Ashwagandha (*Withania somniferum*) balances the stress hormones. Take 1,000 to 3,000 mg daily.

Take a super green food supplement, such as chlorella or spirulina, or a mixture of super green foods, each day for detoxification and pH balance. Take as directed on the container.

DHEA is a stress hormone that is helpful for many autoimmune diseases. Have your levels tested, and if they are low, start with 15 mg daily under the supervision of a doctor. Higher doses of up to 100 mg are sometimes necessary.

It's important to avoid stress, so keep a stash of calming herbal teas on hand. skull-cap, hops (*Humulus lupulus*), and passionflower are all good choices.

Homeopathy

Pick the remedy that best matches your symptoms in this section. Take a 6x, 12x, 6C, 12C, or 30C potency twice daily for two weeks to see if there are any positive results. After you notice improvement, stop taking the remedy, unless symptoms return. Consultation with a homeopathic practitioner is advised.

Agaricus is helpful when there are symptoms of twitching, muscle spasms, poor coordination, and uncontrolled eye movement.

Alumina is for symptoms of progressive paralysis and confusion and the legs feel very heavy. Weakness and paralysis of the lower extremities may occur. There is delayed nerve conduction. Constipation is common.

Argentum Nitricum is for loss of balance and poor coordination that is progressing to paralysis.

Arsenicum Album is for progressive paralysis and burning sensations. The person tends to be anxious and restless.

Causticum is indicated when there is slow, progressive paralysis of the limbs, as well as of muscles that control speech, swallowing, and respiration. There may be numbness of the hands and the feet. Incontinence is common.

Cocculus is helpful when there is progressive paralysis, as well as dizziness when looking at moving objects. The vision is slow to accommodate.

Conium is for ascending paralysis that begins with weakness in the thighs. There is heaviness in the lower limbs. The person drops things easily.

Gelsemium (*Gelsemium sempervirens*) is helpful when there is great weakness and trembling of the muscles. There may also be numbness of the face and the tongue and double vision. The eyelids feel heavy. The symptoms are better after urination.

Ignatia (*Ignatia amara*) will help when multiple sclerosis, especially paralysis, comes on after grief. There is twitching and muscle spasms.

Lachesis is for left-sided symptoms, such as numbness or paralysis. Jealousy or anger worsens symptoms.

Natrum Muriaticum helps when there are symptoms of awkwardness, such as dropping things. Optic neuritis is usually present, as well as numbness throughout the body. The person wants to be alone and feels depressed. The symptoms may come on after grief. The symptoms are worse in the sun.

Nux Vomica is helpful when there is paralysis, along with muscle spasms, cramps, and twitching. The person is highly driven and irritable and craves alcohol and stimulants.

Phosphorous is for numbness in the hands and the feet. The person has problems with incontinence and vision. There is a craving for ice-cold drinks.

Plumbum is for progressive paralysis and wasting of the muscles. There is a tremendous heaviness of the legs.

Acupressure

See pages 668–675 for information about pressure points and administering treatment.

- Governing Vessel 26 can reduce muscle spasms and strengthen you when you feel faint or dizzy.
- If you feel anxious or depressed, work Lung 1.
- Stomach 36 improves your ability to digest foods and receive the maximum amount of nutrition from them. It also stimulates a general sense of well-being.

Bodywork

Massage

Regular massage is highly recommended for MS sufferers. It will help keep the muscles functioning and may hasten recovery time after an exacerbation, and it will also improve circulation and reduce stress.

Reflexology

See pages 686–687 for information about reflexology areas and how to work them.

To stimulate blood supply to the nerves, work the entire spinal area.

Work the diaphragm and the solar plexus to reduce tension and support the central nervous system.

It's also a good idea to work the area corresponding to any part of the body affected by MS.

Acupuncture from a qualified practitioner can be helpful for many of the symptoms of MS.

Hydrotherapy

Avoid saunas and hot baths. They may sound relaxing, but high heat often aggravates the symptoms of MS. A cool or cold bath or shower, however, will stimulate your blood flow and even lift your spirits.

Aromatherapy

Experiment with relaxing oils until you find a few you like, and then rotate them so that you don't become immune to the effects of any single oil. Lavender, jasmine, geranium, ylang ylang, and rose are all good choices to start with. Use them in any preparation you like.

Stress Reduction

Make stress reduction a priority. Biofeedback, deep breathing, prayer, and yoga are all good choices.

A diagnosis of MS, or an attack of MS-like symptoms, can be a shock. Professional counseling can assist you as you try to understand your disorder and make sense of its place in your life.

Bach Flower Remedies

Consult the chart on pages 648–650 to determine the best remedy for your particular needs. Following are some suggestions. Once you've chosen a remedy, place 10 drops of the liquid under your tongue. Hold the drops in place for thirty seconds and swallow. Use as often as needed.

Keep a bottle of Rescue Remedy in your medicine cabinet, and take some whenever you feel stressed or when you sense that an exacerbation might be starting.

Other Recommendations

- Gentle exercise will keep your muscles in good shape, improve circulation, keep your digestive system regular, and help you release stress. Swimming and walking are especially helpful for MS patients, as are stretching exercises.
- Rest whenever you feel the need. If you think you might be getting ill or experiencing the beginning of an exacerbation, get to bed right away and stay there for a few days. You might be able to head off the worst of the symptoms.
- Don't forget that tobacco smoke is an environmental toxin best avoided.
- Consult with a holistic dentist to make sure there are no chronic root canal infections, mercury-filling problems, or other dental issues that may be triggering the immune system.
- Get 15 minutes of sunlight exposure daily.

REFERENCES

Swank, R. L. 1991. Multiple sclerosis: Fat-oil relationship. *Nutrition* 7:368–76.

Swank, R. L., et al. 1990. Effect of low saturated fat diet in early and late cases of multiple sclerosis. *Lancet* Jul 7; 336:37–39.

Muscle Aches and Cramps

You might experience back soreness after a long day playing with the kids, have aching shoulders after overdoing it in the swimming pool, or feel calf pains during the night. Occasional muscle aches and cramps often just accompany the rigors of life. They are rarely a cause to worry.

Muscle aches can affect an active child, as well as a sedentary child who sits in front of the television playing video games and watching programs. The pain often occurs when muscles are overused and pulled or strained, particularly after a vigorous workout that didn't follow a warm-up or stretching session. The pain can range from

---

Testing Techniques

The following tests help assess possible reasons for chronic muscle cramps and aches:

Hormone testing (thyroid, DHEA, cortisol, testosterone, IGF-1, estrogen, progesterone)—saliva, blood, or urine

Intestinal permeability—urine

Vitamin and mineral analysis (especially magnesium, calcium, potassium, zinc)—blood, hair

Digestive function and microbe/parasite/candida testing—stool analysis

Food and environmental allergies/sensitivities—blood, electrodermal

Toxic metals—hair or urine

mild to severe and usually dissipates after a few restful days. Lingering or recurrent pain, especially when accompanied by a fever, decreased muscular strength, or joint swelling, could suggest a severe strain, possibly injury.

The feeling of a muscle turning into a knot indicates a muscle cramp. Muscle cramps could afflict any child, regardless of fitness or diet. Heat cramps, which are common to the calves, the thighs, and the abdomen, can strike a person who exercises in hot weather or a hot gymnasium and who needs water. Night cramps often knot up the muscles of the calves, the feet, and the thighs, causing sharp pains and tightened muscles, which commonly awaken people from a sound sleep.

Nutritional deficiencies of calcium, magnesium, potassium, and the B vitamins are often the root cause of muscle aches and cramps. Lack of sleep can also contribute to this problem.

TREATMENT

Diet

Recommended Food

Eat foods that are high in calcium: kelp, cheese, collards, kale, turnip greens, almonds, yogurt, milk, broccoli, and calcium-enriched rice and soymilk.

Also eat foods that are high in magnesium: whole grains, nuts, legumes, soy, and green leafy vegetables.

Foods that are high in potassium are beneficial as well: fruits and vegetables, especially apples, bananas, carrots, oranges, potatoes, tomatoes, cantaloupes, peaches, plums, strawberries, meat, and fish.

Electrolyte drinks can help you quickly restore lost minerals. We recommend these drinks only on a short-term basis, though. Many contain artificial colorings and large amounts of sugar, although more healthful alternatives are available.

Drinking water on hot days or after physical activity is important.

Food to Avoid

Avoid products that lead to the loss of minerals, such as soda pop, candy, and refined breads and pastas.

℞ Super Seven Prescriptions—Muscle Aches and Cramps

Super Prescription #1   Magnesium
Take 250 mg twice daily. Magnesium is a muscle relaxer, and a deficiency contributes to cramping, aching, and tightness.

Super Prescription #2   Calcium
Take 500 mg twice daily. Calcium is required for muscle and nerve relaxation. It works in tandem with magnesium to relax muscles.

Super Prescription #3   Potassium
Take up to 300 mg daily. A potassium deficiency can lead to muscle cramping. *Note:* If you are on blood pressure medication, use under the guidance of your doctor.

Super Prescription #4   Homeopathic Magnesia Phosphorica
Take 3 pellets of a 6x potency three to five times daily. This remedy is specific for muscle cramping.

Super Prescription #5   High-potency multivitamin

Take a high-potency multivitamin and mineral formula daily, as it will contain a strong base of the nutrients that protect against muscle cramping.

Super Prescription #6   Super green food supplement

Take an organic super green food, such as chlorella or spirulina, or a mixture of "supergreen foods" each day. Take as directed on the container. It contains a variety of minerals for muscle relaxation.

Super Prescription #7   Methylsulfonylmethane (MSM)

Take 500 mg three times daily. This nutrient has natural antispasmodic properties. It is especially good for muscle cramps and aches related to an injury. Reduce the dosage if diarrhea occurs.

General Recommendations

B vitamins can become depleted, due to the effect of stress, thus causing muscle cramps and aches. Take a 50 mg complex twice daily.

Protease enzymes reduce muscle aching and inflammation. Take 1 capsule three times daily between meals.

Black cohosh (*Cimicifuga racemosa*) reduces spasms of the muscles. Take 40 mg of a 2.5 percent triterpene glycoside extract twice daily.

Arnica (*Arnica montana*) oil relieves muscle pain and tenderness. Apply the oil to painful areas twice daily.

Horse chestnut (*Aesculus hippocastanum*) is helpful for spasms in the legs due to poor circulation. Take 300 mg twice daily.

Homeopathy

Pick the remedy that best matches your symptoms in this section. Take a 6x, 12x, 6C, or 30C potency twice daily for two weeks to see if there are any positive results. After you notice improvement, stop taking the remedy, unless symptoms return. Consultation with a homeopathic practitioner is advised.

Arnica (*Arnica montana*) is the top choice for pain that feels deep and bruised and for all-over tenderness. The symptoms are worse after exertion.

Calcarea Carbonica is for people who get muscle cramps and soreness from exertion and from cold, damp climates. They are usually chilly, with clammy hands and feet. They crave sweets and eggs. They often feel anxious, overwhelmed, and easily fatigued.

Causticum is helpful when the muscles and the joints become stiff and sore from overuse and from the cold or in dry weather. The symptoms are improved with warm applications. The muscles and the joints feel contracted.

Cimicifuga is for muscles that feel sore, bruised, and worse in the cold. The back of the neck is sore and stiff. The person is prone to depression and hormone imbalance.

Ignatia Amara is for tight, spasmodic, or cramping muscles or for muscle spasms and cramps that begin after an emotional upset or stress.

Magnesia Phosphorica is for cramping or spasming muscles that feel better from warm applications.

Nux vomica (*Strychnos nux vomica*) is for tight muscles that spasm. The person is chilly, and the symptoms are worse in cold weather and better with warm applications. Digestive problems, such as stomach ache or heartburn, are often present. The person is irritable and fatigued.

Rhus Toxicodendron is for pain and stiffness that are worse in the early morning or after resting and in cold, rainy weather. The symptoms ease with continued movement and warm applications. The person feels restless.

Acupressure

See pages 668–675 for information about pressure points and administering treatment.

- To relax cramped muscles and soothe your nerves, use Liver 3.

Bodywork

Massage

Massage is excellent to work the cramps out by improving the circulation.

Aromatherapy

Add 1 drop of lavender and 1 drop of peppermint to a carrier oil and massage onto the muscle. If the muscle aches or cramps occur at night, use black pepper, instead of peppermint.

Other Bodywork Recommendations

Stretching is important to relax the muscles and prevent overtightening.

Spinal alignment by a chiropractor, an osteopath, or a naturopathic doctor can be helpful for cases of chronic muscle spasm and aches.

Obesity

Obesity is the single most common problem that doctors see in their practices. Unfortunately, it's also a risk factor for a host of disorders. People who are more than 20 percent over the recommended weight for their height and sex are more vulnerable to degenerative diseases—heart problems, certain cancers, diabetes, arthritis, and so on—than the rest of the population is. High blood pressure, strokes, hemorrhoids, hiatal hernias, varicose veins, kidney problems, infertility, gallstones, and liver disease are all more likely to strike the overweight. And since heavy people are likely to consume high quantities of toxic food, their immune systems are depressed, leaving them susceptible to any virus or bug that happens to be going around at home or in the office.

But most people with weight problems already know all that. Weight loss is probably the most written-about subject in America, but despite all the diets, pills, spas, and programs, only a small percentage of people are able to lose weight and keep it off. In fact, the rising occurrence of obesity can be traced in part to our attempts to fight it. Take the low-protein, high-carbohydrate diet that in the early 1990s was universally espoused as healthful: People filled up their plates with so much pasta, bread, and fat-free sweets that they actually ended up eating more calories—and, of course, gaining more weight. Other strategies, such as appetite suppressants, and extreme diets, do indeed help people lose weight in the short term. But they're also too dangerous to use for long, so at some point those people have to return to a lifestyle that is healthful. Because many "diet gurus" haven't taught people how to put healthful eating in the context of their daily routines, they soon put the weight right back on.

There are several reasons why a person is susceptible to obesity. Genetics is an obvious factor that makes it more difficult for some people to lose weight. One example is people who have syndrome X (see pages 498–502). This inherited condition makes some people more likely to put on weight from simple carbohydrate consumption than others are. Insulin levels spike upward and result in fat deposition. This problem is compounded by the fact that the average American consumes 150 pounds of sugar each year! In addition, some researchers feel that the body has a genetically programmed "set point." This refers to the theory that the body tries to maintain a set metabolic rate at which calories are burned, especially the fat cells. For people with a genetic susceptibility, it is even more important to be diligent with the diet and lifestyle recommendations we make. Also, nutritional supplements can help to lessen genetic tendencies.

The amount of calories someone consumes is an obvious reason for weight gain. Consuming too many calories without burning them results in a simple mathematical reality—weight gain. To stay within a certain parameter for your metabolism, it is helpful to grasp the concept of general calorie amounts of commonly consumed foods.

The second important concept, after calorie consumption, is the calories expended through movement and exercise. The more calories are utilized for energy, the less will go toward fat accumulation. In this technologically advanced and television-addicted society, people are expending many less calories than they used to.

Hormone balance is also important for the prevention and the treatment of obesity. Many hormones in the body have an effect on metabolism. The most notable are thyroid hormones, which greatly influence the metabolic rate in our cells. However, several others hormones, such as DHEA, testosterone, and growth hormones, have powerful effects as well. We have also found that an estrogen and progesterone imbalance contributes to fat deposition and water retention, and thus to weight gain. This seems to be particularly true for women who use synthetic hormones. A hormone balance also includes the level of the brain hormone serotonin. Low levels of this neurotransmitter contribute to feelings of hunger and to sugar/carbohydrate cravings. There are natural ways to optimize this neurotransmitter, as discussed in this section and in the section on Depression. Further research in this field will shed more light on the role of neurotransmitters and obesity.

Toxins in the body also pose a problem for people who are overweight. Many of the chemicals that people are exposed to interfere with normal cell function, including metabolism. Pesticides, heavy metals such as mercury, and others are a part of our polluted world. Interestingly, many of these toxins are stored in fat tissue in order to prevent damage to vital body organs, such as the brain and the heart.

In addition, a diet that is devoid of nutrients leads to nutritional deficiencies. The body does not burn fat by magic but requires several vitamins, minerals, and enzymes. It appears that certain nutrients can help in the prevention and the treatment of obesity. While none should be considered "magic bullets," they can in some cases be quite helpful as part of a comprehensive weight or fat reduction protocol.

The mental and the emotional, as well as the spiritual, well-being of a person cannot be ignored in regard to obesity. Imbalances in these areas often supersede genetic and physical reasons for weight gain. For example, many people with depression and anxiety consume comfort foods as a way to feel a false sense of love or worth. Some patients with obesity first began to have problems with weight after experiencing an unresolved emotional trauma. Treating the whole person is of paramount importance with obesity.

Test #1: Body Mass Index (BMI)

The body mass index, or BMI, helps you determine the appropriate weight for your frame. For most people, the BMI test is more reliable than scales or height/weight charts are, but you should know that people with very muscular physiques may come up with a misleading reading. Because muscle weighs more than fat, many professional athletes have high BMIs—although, clearly, they don't need to lose weight.

Here's how to calculate your BMI. After each step are sample calculations, made for a person who is 5'8" and 150 pounds:

1. Write down your height in inches:

   _____

   (5'8" = 68 inches)

2. Multiply the number in Line 1 by .025:

   _____

   (68 × .025 = 1.70)

3. Square the number in Line 2: _____
   (1.70 × 1.70 = 2.89)

4. Write down your weight in pounds:

   _____

   (150)

5. Multiply the number in Line 4 by .45:

   _____

   (150 × .45 = 67.50)

6. Divide the number in Line 5 by the number in Line 3: _____
   (67.50/2.89 = 23.36)

Interpreting the Results

If your BMI is between 18.9 and 24.9, you are considered to be of a healthy weight. Like everyone else, you need to eat well and exercise, but if you take the second test here and it doesn't indicate a health risk, you don't need to lose pounds.

If your BMI is 25 or higher, there's a good chance that you need to lose weight. If you have any weight-related health problems like heart disease, high blood pressure, high cholesterol, joint or back pain, or diabetes, you should make a concerted effort to burn more calories than you take in. People who smoke, who drink heavily, or who have a family history of the diseases listed previously would also be wise to lose weight. If you don't have any of these concerns, it's possible that you are simply a large but healthy person. Take the second test to further assess your health risk.

If your BMI is below 18.9, you may be underweight. If you're an otherwise healthy adolescent who does not have an eating disorder, you're probably just going through a phase. When you get a little older, your metabolism will likely right itself. Adults, however, should talk to a doctor about what a low BMI means for them as individuals. And anyone who suffers from an eating disorder should get professional help right away.

Test #2: Waist Circumference

Measure your waist circumference, using your navel as the defining point of your waist. For men, a waist circumference of more than forty inches is considered a health risk. Women should not have a waist circumference of more than thirty-five inches.

No one is quite sure why, but large waists are an indicator of possible future health problems, especially of cardiovascular conditions like heart disease and high blood pressure. If you have a large waist circumference, you should read these pages for advice about losing weight.

If you have a high BMI but have a normal waist circumference, are healthy, have no family history of weight-related disease, and don't drink excessively or smoke, your weight is probably just fine. If it bothers you, or if you sense that your weight is slowing you down or affecting your health, see your doctor for an individual assessment. And remember: Even if you don't need to lose weight, you should still eat well and exercise on a regular basis.

SYMPTOMS

- Weight gain and fat deposition
- Increased sweating
- Difficulty breathing

ROOT CAUSES

Obesity is almost always caused by a combination of the first two items listed here: taking in more calories than are expended. But, as we described, there can be many factors at work.

- Poor diet (high in calories and simple carbohydrates)
- Inactivity
- Hormone imbalance (particularly thyroid)
- Toxins
- Neurotransmitter imbalance (serotonin)
- Mental, emotional, or spiritual issues
- Preexisting medical conditions (e.g., hypothyroidism)
- Genetics
- Side effects of pharmaceutical medications (e.g., antidepressants)

TREATMENT

Diet

Instead of counting calories or fat grams, your best bet for health and weight loss is to focus on eating foods that are fresh, whole, and nutritionally dense.

Recommended Food

Don't rely on someone else: start cooking for yourself. Shop for a variety of basic, whole foods. You can eat vegetables, fruits, nuts, and seeds raw for their fiber and digestive enzymes; the rest of the time, use light cooking methods like broiling, steaming, roasting, or grilling.

Make sure you get enough protein every day. Otherwise, you'll feel deprived and downright hungry. Fish is an excellent source of protein, but few of us can eat it every

---

Testing Techniques

The following tests help assess possible reasons for weight gain:

Hormone testing (thyroid, DHEA, cortisol, testosterone, IGF-1, estrogen, insulin, progesterone)—saliva, blood, or urine

Intestinal permeability—urine

Detoxification profile—urine

Vitamin and mineral analysis (especially magnesium, l-carnitine, chromium, and CoQ10)—blood

Digestive function and microbe/parasite/candida testing—stool analysis

Food and environmental allergies/sensitivities—blood, electrodermal

Blood-sugar balance—blood

Toxic metals—hair or urine

---

single day. Plan on having beans, lean poultry, soy products, nuts, or yogurt with every meal. High-quality protein drinks from whey, eggs, or rice are good choices.

Whole, complex carbohydrates like brown rice, whole-grain bread, and oats are necessary for a healthful eating plan. They're also high in fiber, which helps you feel full and keeps you free of toxins. Use common sense, though; carbohydrates are meant to be one part of your diet, not all of it. Have a small or moderately sized serving at each meal—no more.

Essential fatty acids are just what their name implies: fats that are good for you. Cold-water fish, flaxseeds, and cold-pressed oils like olive oil are necessary for proper functioning of almost every body system, and they help you feel satisfied after a meal. As with everything else, however, use EFAs in moderation. Extra helpings of anything, even of salmon fillets, contribute to your waistline but not to your health. Sauté your vegetables in a tablespoon, not a cup, of olive oil.

Low levels of serotonin, a neurotransmitter, may increase your desire for refined and complex carbohydrates, including for sugar. Eat foods that are high in trypto-phan—turkey, chicken, tuna, soymilk, and live unsweetened yogurt. This chemical encourages the production of serotonin and may stave off cravings.

Vegetable juice is healthful and filling. Drink a glass a half hour before meals to keep your appetite in check.

Water also takes the edge off your hunger. Plan on drinking a glass of clean water every two waking hours.

Eat a balanced ratio of the major food groups. Many people do well on a diet that is 40 to 50 percent carbohydrates (mainly, complex carbs), 30 percent fats (mainly, good fats), and 30 percent protein. This is just a sample percentage. Some people do better with a slightly higher protein intake.

Eat more small, regular meals throughout the day to quench your appetite and balance blood-sugar levels.

Do not skip meals, particularly breakfast. This puts the body into a starvation mode that can increase fat accumulation.

Food to Avoid

Americans are addicted to sugar. Sugar is high in calories and causes mood swings and blood-sugar crashes that may only increase your cravings. If you're trying to lose weight, your first priority should be to reduce or, in some cases, eliminate refined sugar from your diet. No cookies, cakes, candy, ice cream, sodas, white breads, pastas, and crackers, and especially no low-fat sweets, which contain extra sugar to make up for the missing richness. It's also wise to limit your intake of natural sugars. Fruit sugars, honey, and molasses are less damaging to your body than refined products are, but in large quantities, they can still lead to weight gain. Eat them only in moderation.

Avoid processed and junk food. Food made with artificial flavors, colors, and preservatives offers you little in the way of real sustenance. Their toxins are also highly addictive. As most of us know, even one fast-food cheeseburger or a handful of greasy, salty potato chips is enough to derail your body from its natural sense of what's healthful.

Refined flours are another example of the proverbial "empty calories." Pasta, white bread, and white rice are stripped of most of their nutrients, leaving you with nothing but a plate full of calories.

You've heard it a thousand times, and it's still true: you must radically cut back on your consumption of "bad" fats. If you stop eating processed food (including margarine and shortening), you'll go a long way toward this goal. Naturally sweetened baked goods are also high in saturated fats. If you enjoy any of these items, reserve them for the occasional treat.

Detoxification

If you're overweight, chances are that you've been eating food that's highly toxic. A short juice fast will encourage your fat cells to release their waste products and toxins. A few days without solid food will also help you break your addictions, so that your body "remembers" the healthful foods it needs and begins to crave those instead of junk. Consider beginning your diet with a one- to three-day juice fast.

People who are overweight may also suffer from frequent constipation. The best course of action is to follow the eating plan given here; with less fat and more fiber, you'll soon find that you're regular again.

Identify your food sensitivities. Food sensitivities or allergies can contribute to weight gain. See the Food Allergies/Sensitivities section.

℞ Super Seven Prescriptions—Obesity

Super Prescription #1   Conjugated linoleic acid (CLA)
Take 3.4 grams daily. Studies show that this fatty acid reduces body fat composition.

Super Prescription #2   Green tea (*Camellia sinensis*) **extract**
Take 1,500 mg of green tea extract standardized to 80 to 90 percent polyphenols and 35 to 55 percent epigallocatechin gallate. Studies have shown that green tea extract increases thermogenesis, the body's ability to burn energy. *Note:* Green tea contains caffeine, which may account for some of this benefit.

Super Prescription #3   5-hydroxytryptophan (5-HTP)
Take 100 to 300 mg three times daily; 5-HTP reduces carbohydrate cravings and improves satiety. *Note:* Do not take 5-HTP if you are currently using pharmaceutical antidepressants or antianxiety medications.

Super Prescription #4   Chromium
Take 500 mcg twice daily. Chromium helps with blood-sugar balance and sweet cravings.

Super Prescription #5   Pyruvate (pyruvate acid)
Take 25 grams daily. Studies show that pyruvate may aid weight loss when combined with a low fat diet and/or exercise.

Super Prescription #6   L-carnitine
Take 500 to 1,000 mg three times daily. L-carnitine is involved with burning fat as a fuel source for the cells.

Super Prescription #7   Essential fatty acids
Take 1 tablespoon of flaxseed oil or 3 grams of fish oil daily, along with 100 mg of GLA (gamma linoleic acid). Essential fatty acids are required to burn fat as fuel.

General Recommendations

A high-potency multivitamin provides a base of vitamins and minerals required for people on a restricted diet.

A randomized, double-blind study involving sixty overweight and obese people demonstrated that people supplementing conjugated linoleic acid (CLA) had a significantly higher reduction in body fat mass, as compared to people taking a placebo.

A double-blind study by the University of Rome included twenty obese people for two phases of time. The first phase involved a nonrestrictive diet, and the second phase focused on a calorie-restricted diet. During both phases, people receiving 900 mg of 5-HTP had a reduction in carbohydrate intake and the consistent presence of an early sensation of fullness.

Supplementing 7-KETO (3-acetyl-7-oxo-dehydroepiandrosterone) has been shown in a study of overweight people to help with weight and fat loss. Take 100 mg twice daily.

Dandelion root (*Taraxacum officinale*) improves liver metabolism and detoxification, which may support weight loss. Take 300 mg or 2 ml with each meal.

Bladderwrack (*Fucus vesiculosus*) supports thyroid function. Use it if you have suboptimal thyroid activity. Take 100 mg or 1 ml twice daily.

Homeopathy

Pick the remedy that best matches your symptoms in this section. Take a 6x, 12x, 6C, 12C, or 30C potency twice daily for two weeks to see if there are any positive results. After you notice improvement, stop taking the remedy, unless symptoms return. Consultation with a homeopathic practitioner is advised.

Calcarea Carbonica for people who tend to be flabby and chilly. The palms, the feet, and the back of the head sweat easily. They have a strong craving for eggs, sweets, and dairy products. They tend to feel easily overwhelmed.

Ignatia (*Ignatia amara*) is for highly sensitive people who use food to make themselves feel better. There is often a recent history of acute grief or an emotional trauma.

Pulsatilla (*Pulsatilla pratensis*) is helpful when there is a strong craving for sweets. The person gets warm easily and strongly desires the windows to be open or wants to be outside. There is a sense of sadness, with a desire to be consoled.

Staphysagria is for people with a history of abuse, leading to overeating as a way to deal with suppressed anger. The anger tends to build over time. They have a craving for sweets.

Acupressure

See pages 668–675 for information about pressure points and administering treatment.

- Conception Vessel 6 stimulates digestion and increases your metabolism.
- Use Spleen 16 to return an out-of-control appetite to a more normal state.

Bodywork

Reflexology

See pages 686–687 for information about reflexology areas and how to work them.

Work the liver to increase metabolism and stimulate detoxification. For additional cleansing, work the colon.

Instead of eating when you're nervous, work the diaphragm and the solar plexus areas to calm down.

Aromatherapy

Bergamot blunts hunger pangs. For an immediate effect, hold the vial of oil directly under your nose and inhale.

Support a cleansing fast by adding juniper oil to a bath. Juniper promotes the release of toxins from fatty tissue.

Try using essential oils, instead of sugar, to lift your mood. Lavender, rose, geranium, and orange will make you feel more cheerful.

Stress Reduction

General Stress-Reduction Therapies

Every day, take some time out for deep breathing and visualization. Imagine yourself making healthful food choices and turning down less-nutritious offers. See yourself doing the things you'd like to do but can't because of your excess weight: running a mile, playing with your grandkids, even climbing a mountain.

Yoga, a technique that encourages control of the senses, will help you learn to handle stress without turning to the refrigerator. It's also a good gentle exercise for people who haven't been active for a while.

Stress can make you eat, but sticking to a weight-loss plan can be stressful itself. Find a couple of friends who will lend a sympathetic ear; it helps if they're also trying to lose weight. Or you could join a support group.

Bach Flower Remedies

Consult the chart on pages 648–650 to determine the best remedy for your particular needs. Following are some suggestions. Once you've chosen a remedy, place 10 drops of the liquid under your tongue. Hold the drops in place for thirty seconds and swallow. Use as often as needed.

If you think about food constantly, take White Chestnut to stop obsessive thoughts.

Heather is for people who find it hard to be alone, even for a short length of time.

People who are good-humored on the surface but who overeat as a means of handling inner tension should take Agrimony.

Crab Apple, the cleansing remedy, will help people who feel ashamed about their weight.

Other Recommendations

- Exercise. It's more effective than dieting alone. But you don't have to run a marathon to reap the benefits of activity; in fact, it's far better for you to take a brisk walk every day than to engage in more strenuous activity once or twice a week. Overall, it is best to pick an exercise that you really enjoy. If you're very out of shape or have heart problems, contact your doctor before starting an exercise program. And whatever you're doing, ease into it gradually.

REFERENCES

Blankson, H., J. A. Stakkestad, H. Fagertun, E. Thom, J. Wadstein, and O. J. Gudmundsen. 2000. Conjugated linoleic acid reduces body fat mass in overweight and obese humans. *Journal of Nutrition* 130(12):2943–48.

Cangiano, C., F. Ceci, A. Cascino, M. Del Ben, A. Laviano, M. Muscaritoli, F. Antonucci, and F. Rossi-Fanelli. 1992. Eating behavior and adherence to dietary supplements in obese adult subjects treated with 5-hydroxytryptophan. *American Journal of Clinical Nutrition* 56(5):863–67.

Osteoporosis

In the United States, nearly 50 percent of all women between the ages of forty-five and seventy suffer from some degree of osteoporosis. This disorder, which translates literally as "porous bones," is so common that we tend to think of its effects—frailty, broken bones, back pain, a stooped posture, and the so-called dowager's hump—as the normal results of aging. In reality, osteoporosis is a condition brought on by faulty dietary and lifestyle habits. Studies of cultures that have more healthful lifestyles than Americans do find that its occurrence is much more rare.

Childhood, adolescence, and early adulthood are the prime opportunities for building healthy bones. Bones reach their greatest mass and density at around age thirty; after that, they begin to weaken. Some bone loss is entirely normal and not terribly worrisome, but when the process is accelerated, the bones turn frail and brittle. Unfortunately, the disorder rarely rings any warning bells until serious damage is already done. The first sign may be a minor fall or an accident that results in a broken bone or back pain caused by a collapsed vertebra.

Researchers have found that there is a connection between a dysfunctional immune system and osteoporosis. A group of immune cells known as cytokines can initiate a type of inflammatory response that leads to bone breakdown. Fortunately, a healthful diet and lifestyle, hormone balance, and specific nutritional supplements, as described in this chapter, contribute to normal cytokine activity.

Hormone balance is critical for good bone density. A good example is a premenopausal woman who has her ovaries removed. Studies show that this can lead to a sudden drop in bone density, due to low estrogen and progesterone levels. Many hormones are important for bone cell (osteoblast) activity, including estrogen, progesterone, testosterone, DHEA, growth hormone, and calcitonin. On the other hand, excessive levels of cortisol, thyroid, and parathyroid hormones can lead to bone loss.

Diet is important for strong bones. This should include foods that are rich in bone-building minerals, such as green leafy vegetables, nuts and seeds, flax, soy, and fish. On the other hand, soda pop, caffeine, salt, and alcohol all contribute to bone breakdown when consumed in excess.

One of the best ways to prevent bone loss or halt its progress is to engage in a weight-bearing exercise. This stimulates bone cell formation.

Many vitamins and minerals are required for healthy bones. Calcium is the obvious one, but several others, such as magnesium, vitamin D, boron, silicon, vitamin C, strontium, vitamin K, and others, play important roles in bone metabolism.

A combination of a good diet, exercise, and nutritional supplements is important for healthy bones. Exposure to sunlight is important as well. More severe cases of osteoporosis may require natural hormone therapy and, in some cases, drug therapy.

SYMPTOMS

Osteoporosis is largely asymptomatic, but watch out for the following danger signs:

- A stooped posture
- Dowager's hump
- Sleeves and hems that used to fit but that now are too long
- Backache
- Easily broken bones

ROOT CAUSES

- Inactivity
- Poor diet
- Hormones
- Long-term use of certain medications (anticonvulsants, prednisone, heparin, methotrexate, lithium, isoniazid, furosemide (Lasix), antacids, chemotherapy, thyroid, and others)
- Smoking
- Hormone deficiencies and imbalances
- Nutritional deficiencies
- Lack of sun exposure
- Eating disorders
- Prolonged stress
- Toxic metals
- Medical conditions (diabetes, Cushing's disease, kidney and liver disease, homocystinemia, hyperthyroidism, malabsorption, and others)
- Heredity
- Acidic pH balance

TREATMENT

Diet

Recommended Food

Eat foods that are high in calcium and the other nutrients needed for its assimilation. Sea vegetables, green leafy vegetables (except spinach), soybeans, nuts, molasses, salmon, oysters, sardines (with the bones), broccoli, and unsweetened cultured yogurt are all good sources.

Green vegetables such as collard greens, kale, romaine lettuce, and others are important for their vitamin K content. Vitamin K1 is the form of vitamin K found in plants that is important for bone formation.

Fermented soy products, such as tofu and miso, are good for the bones.

Essential fatty acids found in walnuts, almonds, flaxseeds, and fish are important for healthy bones.

The gold standard for testing your bone density is an X-ray known as the DEXA (dual energy X-ray absorptiometry) scan. Yet by the time this test shows a decrease in bone density, you may have had a significant loss of bone. A good test to monitor current bone metabolism is a urine test that measures bone breakdown. When bone (and cartilage) breaks down, it releases two substances known as deoxypyridinium and pyridinium, which are excreted in the urine. The rate of excretion parallels the degree of bone turnover. A high level signifies that there is likely too much bone breakdown, which is imbalanced with bone building. This test is helpful as a way to assess the protocol currently being used to prevent or treat your osteoporosis.

Testing Techniques

The following tests help assess possible reasons for osteoporosis:

Immune system imbalance or disease—blood

Hormone testing (thyroid, DHEA, cortisol, testosterone, IGF-1, estrogen, progesterone)—saliva, blood, or urine

Intestinal permeability—urine

Vitamin and mineral analysis (especially magnesium, calcium, vitamin K, vitamin D)—blood, hair

Toxic metals—urine or hair

Digestive function and microbe/parasite/candida testing—stool analysis

Food and environmental allergies/sensitivities—blood, electrodermal

Bone resorption (pyridinium and deoxypyridinium)—urine

Calcium Content

Wakame (sea vegetable), $^1/_2$ cup—1,700 mg

Agar (sea vegetable), $^1/_4$ cup—1,000 mg

Nori (sea vegetable), $^1/_2$ cup—600 mg

Kombu (sea vegetable), $^1/_4$ cup—500 mg

Sardines with bones, $^1/_2$ cup—500 mg

Tempeh, 1 cup—340 mg

Collard greens, 1 cup—355 mg

Milk, 1 cup—300 mg

Calcium-enriched rice milk or soymilk, 1 cup—300 mg

Almonds, 1 cup—300 mg

Spinach, 1 cup—280 mg

Yogurt, 1 cup—270 mg

Sesame seeds, $^1/_2$ cup—250 mg

Kale, 1 cup—200 mg

Broccoli, 1 cup—180 mg

Tofu, 1 cup—150 mg

Walnuts, $^1/_4$ cup—70 mg

Black beans, 1 cup—60 mg

Lentils, 1 cup—50 mg

A 12-year study of more than 77,000 women found that those who drank more than 14 glasses of milk a week had 45 percent more hip fractures, as compared to women who consumed 1 glass a week or less.

Food to Avoid

One reason Westerners have such a high rate of osteoporosis is their consumption of foods that are high in sugar. Eliminate sugar, refined grains, and soda pop drinks from your diet.

Reduce your intake of red meat. A high intake may contribute to bone loss in some individuals.

A high salt intake is linked to bone loss. Do not eat processed foods, which are usually loaded with salt, and never add conventional table salt to your meals.

Moderate your use of caffeine and alcohol, as they contribute to bone loss.

It may surprise you to learn that countries where people drink the most milk are also those with the highest rates of osteoporosis. This may be due to the fact that lactose intolerance and casein (protein found in cow's milk) allergy are very common and lead to malabsorption. Also, calcium from cow's milk is not well absorbed, at a rate of 25 percent. Milk products lead to other health problems as well, so don't rely on them as a source of calcium. Unsweetened, cultured yogurt is an exception.

℞ Super Seven Prescriptions—Osteoporosis

Super Prescription #1   Calcium
Take 500 to 600 mg twice daily in divided doses of well-absorbed calcium complexes, such as citrate, citrate-malate, chelate, or hydroxyappatite. Calcium is the main mineral that composes bone.

Super Prescription #2   Magnesium
Take 250 to 350 mg twice daily in divided doses. Magnesium is required for proper calcium metabolism, through parathyroid hormone production and vitamin D activation. Some researchers feel that it is as important as calcium. *Note:* Reduce the dosage if loose stools occur.

Super Prescription #3   Vitamin D
Take 800 to 1,200 IU daily if you have osteoporosis and 400 IU daily if you are supplementing vitamin D for prevention. This vitamin improves intestinal calcium absorption and reduces the urinary excretion of calcium.

Super Prescription #4   Vitamin K

Take 2 to 10 mg daily and up to 500 mcg daily for preventative purposes. vitamin K is needed to form the protein osteocalcin, a substance that attracts calcium into the bone matrix. Low levels of vitamin K are associated with osteoporosis and fractures. *Note:* Do not use if you are taking blood-thinning medications.

Super Prescription #5   Ipriflavone

Take 600 mg daily with food. Some, but not all, studies have shown this supplement to increase bone density when combined with calcium, vitamin D, or hormone replacement. *Note:* Have your lymphocyte (a type of white blood cell) levels monitored by your doctor when using this supplement, as one study found that it lowered the levels in 29 out of 132 women.

Super Prescription #6   Essential fatty acids

Take 4 grams of fish oil daily, along with 3,000 mg of evening primrose oil (*Oenothera biennis*). Studies show that these essential fatty acids improve calcium absorption and deposition into the bone.

Super Prescription #7   Strontium

Take 680 mg daily. Studies show strontium improves bone density.

A study in the *American Journal of Clinical Nutrition* reported that a low intake of vitamin K was associated with an increased risk of hip fracture. The data from the study came from reviewing the diets of over 72,000 women. Studies have also shown that vitamin K supplementation improves bone density.

General Recommendations

High-potency multivitamin provides a base of nutrients required for healthy bones. Take as directed on the container.

Boron is a mineral that activates vitamin D and supports estrogen levels for effective calcium metabolism. Take 3 to 5 mg daily.

Vitamin C is used to manufacture collagen, an important component of bones. Take 500 to 1,000 mg twice daily.

Silicon is a mineral that is involved in collagen and calcification. Take 50 to 20 mg daily.

Zinc is required for enzymatic reactions that build bone. Take a daily total of 30 mg, along with 2 to 3 mg of copper.

Manganese is involved with bone calcification. Take 15 to 30 mg daily.

Vitamins B12, B6, and folic acid prevent the buildup of homocysteine, a by-product of protein metabolism that can cause osteoporosis. See the Cardiovascular Disease section.

Betaine hydrochloric acid improves stomach acid levels for digestion and absorption. Take 1 to 3 capsules with each meal. *Note:* Do not use if you have an active ulcer.

A greens formula that contains super green foods, such as chlorella, spirulina, and others, has an alkalinizing effect and is rich in minerals. Take as directed on the container.

Soy protein powder has been shown to protect against bone loss. Take 40 grams daily, containing 90 mg of isoflavones.

Strontium is a nutrient shown to be helpful in increasing bone density when combined with calcium. Take 340 to 680 mg daily.

A study in the *Journal of Aging* found that the combination of the essential fatty acids EPA (fish oil) and GLA (evening primrose oil [*Oenothera biennis*]), along with 600 mg of calcium, improved bone density in senior women. During the first 18 months, the lumbar spine density remained the same with the treatment group but decreased 3.2 percent overall in the placebo group. Thigh bone density increased 1.3 percent in the treatment group, but decreased 2.1 percent in the placebo group. During the second period of 18 months, with all patients receiving the essential fatty-acid combination, lumbar spine density increased 3.1 percent in patients who remained on active treatment, and 2.3 percent in patients who switched from placebo to active treatment. Thigh bone density in the latter group showed an increase of 4.7 percent.

Homeopathy

Pick the remedy that best matches your symptoms in this section. Take a 6x, 12x, 6C, 12C, or 30C potency twice daily for four weeks to see if there are any positive results.

After you notice improvement, stop giving the remedy, unless symptoms return. Homeopathy is best used in conjunction with the diet, lifestyle changes, and other areas covered in this chapter. Although you cannot "feel" bone density improvement, symptoms such as bone aching or pain or the healing of fractures can be observed. Consultation with a homeopathic practitioner is advised.

Calcarea Carbonica is a remedy for people with signs of calcium imbalance, such as osteoporosis, aching bones, muscle cramps, and swollen joints. People who require this remedy are generally chilly and flabby and feel worse in the cold and the dampness. They are easily fatigued and get overwhelmed. They crave sweets, milk, and eggs.

Calcarea Phosphorica is a good remedy for osteoporosis or fractures. This remedy stimulates bone building. Symptoms of neck and back pain and stiffness, which feel worse from cold drafts, are often present. Calcium deposits may occur, even with bone loss. People who require this remedy often have a feeling of discontent and a strong desire for travel or a change. Calcarea Phosphorica is a remedy that can be used for bone support even if you don't have any particular symptoms.

Phosphorus is a remedy for weak bones or fractures that heal slowly. People who require this remedy tend to be tall, thin, and very social and suggestible. They have a strong craving for ice-cold drinks.

Silica (Silicea) is for people who have poor bone density and tend to be very thin. People who need this remedy are often nervous, easily fatigued, and chilly and have a low resistance to infection.

Symphytum is a specific remedy for healing fractures and reducing their pain more quickly.

Acupressure

See pages 668–675 for information about pressure points and administering treatment.

- To increase your ability to absorb nutrients (including calcium), work Stomach 36. With regular practice, your digestion will improve, and you'll find that you have more energy than before.
- To reduce stress, work Lung 1 on a daily basis.
- If you have pain, work Large Intestine 4. Do not use this point if you are pregnant.
- For pain in the ankles, use Spleen 5 and Kidney 3.
- Governing Vessel 24.5 will help bring about hormonal balance.

Bodywork

Massage

Massage is a good wellness measure, especially for the elderly. Don't let fear of pain or injury prevent you from receiving massage treatment; instead, find a reputable therapist with experience in degenerative diseases.

Reflexology

See pages 686–687 for information about reflexology areas and how to work them.

If you have osteoporosis, reflexology can help ease pain. Be careful, however. Do not treat the foot or the hand roughly or with too much pressure.

Work the areas corresponding to the vertebrae; the hip, the back, and the sciatic areas; and the lower back.

Aromatherapy

Black pepper and rosemary both have warming qualities that soothe aching bones and joints. Use them in a massage, a lotion, or a bath.

If bone loss leads to stress, try any of several oils that have a relaxing, uplifting effect. You may want to start with lavender, geranium, or rose; use them in any preparation that suits you.

Stress Reduction

General Stress-Reduction Therapies

It can be difficult to handle the restricted motion and the fear that often accompany osteoporosis. If you're in the early or middle stages of the disorder, try taking a yoga or Pilates class from an experienced instructor. In addition to relieving your stress, you'll strengthen your bone and muscle mass. You'll also improve your balance, which reduces your chances of falling and breaking a bone.

Bach Flower Remedies

Bach remedy philosophy holds that osteoporosis, in which the spine compresses and the shoulders hunch, may be connected to an inability or unwillingness to "stand tall" emotionally. If you do not face the world with your chin up, either choose the most appropriate of the following remedies or select another from the chart on pages 648–650. Once you've selected a remedy, place 10 drops of the liquid under your tongue. Hold the drops in place for thirty seconds and swallow. Use as often as needed.

Larch will instill self-confidence in people who lack it.

If you are timid and shy, take Mimulus.

If you often feel exploited, or if other people tend to take advantage of you, Centaury will help.

Other Recommendations

- Undertake a regular weight-bearing exercise. Although swimming and cycling are excellent for cardiovascular toning, they are not as aggressive for building bone mass. Instead, try an aerobic workout with gentle impact (walking is a good idea). Then supplement that exercise with weightlifting. You don't have to join a gym and pump heavy iron—even very small hand weights can make a real difference in bone strength. If you've never lifted weights before, you should make an appointment with a trainer to get yourself started.
- Don't smoke or expose yourself to secondhand smoke. Smoking makes bones brittle and weak and is also a cause of many other "age-related" diseases.
- Natural hormone replacement should be considered if you have moderate to severe osteoporosis, especially if testing shows your levels to be deficient. Work with a doctor who is knowledgeable in natural hormones. Important ones include estrogen, progesterone, testosterone, DHEA, and growth hormone.

REFERENCES

Feskanich, D. et al. 1997. Milk, dietary calcium, and bone fractures in women: A 12 year prospective study. *American Journal of Public Health* 87:992–97.

Feskanich, D., P. Weber, W. C. Willett, H. Rockett, S. L. Booth, and G. A. Colditz. 1999. Vitamin K intake and hip fractures in women: A prospective study. *American Journal of Clinical Nutrition* 69(1):74–79.

Iwamoto, I., S. Kosha, S. Noguchi, et al. 1999. A longitudinal study of the effect of vitamin K2 on bone mineral density in postmenopausal women: A comparative study with vitamin D3 and estrogen-progestin therapy. *Maturitas* 31:161–64.

Kruger, M. C., H. Coetzer, R. de Winter, G. Gericke, and D. H. van Papendorp. 1998. Calcium, gamma-linolenic acid and eicosapentaenoic acid supplementation in senile osteoporosis. *Aging* (Milano) 10(5):385–94.

Shiraki, M., Y. Shiraki, C. Aoki, and M. Miura. 2000. Vitamin K2 (menadione) effectively prevents fractures and sustains lumbar bone mineral density in osteoporosis. *Journal of Bone and Mineral Research* 15:515–21.

Parasites (Intestinal)

Microorganisms naturally inhabit and move through the body. Some are harmless, while others cause sickness. Infections can occur when parasites make their homes in your skin, gastrointestinal tract, lungs, liver, and other organs. Parasites require a host (e.g., human cells) to live and thrive.

Parasitic infections were once thought of as a problem that existed mainly in underdeveloped countries. After all, diarrheal disease (from parasites and bacteria) is the greatest worldwide cause of death. Global travel has been a major contributor to the spread of parasitic infections in North America. Contaminated water and food are also major contributors. In addition, better diagnostic techniques have provided a more accurate identification of parasites and have led researchers to conclude that parasitic infections are much more common than previously thought. One laboratory that specializes in stool analysis states "almost 30 percent of specimens examined are positive for a parasite."

Diarrhea and abdominal pain are the most common symptoms of a parasitic infection. However, in many cases of a parasite infection, these symptoms may not be present. A whole list of symptoms and conditions could be related to a parasitic infection. Examples include loss of appetite, fatigue, constipation, depressed immunity, food allergy, fever, chills, heartburn, stomach pain, inflammatory bowel disease, lower back pain, itchy anus, rash and skin itching, hives, weight loss, arthritis, bloody stools, mucus in the stool, colitis, Crohn's disease, flatulence, foul-smelling stools, malabsorption, rectal bleeding, mood changes (depression, irritability), and vomiting.

Parasites interfere with the normal activities of the cells they infect, which may lead to symptoms and disease. The secretions released by a parasite can trigger a bodily response in which the immune system attacks its own tissues. This is known as an autoimmune reaction. Examples include rheumatoid arthritis and Crohn's disease. Not all parasites are necessarily harmful. Some parasites live symbiotically in the digestive tract. It is thought that certain parasites become a problem only when the environment of the body changes. For example, dysbiosis—the imbalance between friendly and potentially harmful bacteria in the digestive tract—can lead to certain parasites becoming pathogenic (disease causing). The nutritional status of a person, as well as a compromised immune system, dictates whether a parasite can become a problem.

Parasites are commonly transmitted through food that is contaminated with fecal matter (e.g., from food preparers who do not wash their hands after going to the restroom), waste, and the water supply.

There are many different types of parasites. Following are some of the more common ones in North America.

Blastocystis hominis. This parasite is detected in a high number of stool tests. Researchers are unclear whether it is a pathogen, because many people carry it but do not have symptoms. However, it can cause various digestive symptoms, such as cramps, nausea, weight loss, bloating, and others. It is also associated with conditions like irritable bowel syndrome, chronic fatigue, and arthritis.

Dientamoeba fragilis. Symptoms of this parasite, which resides in the large intestine, include diarrhea and abdominal pain.

E. histolytica. This amoeba is linked to diarrhea and a variety of digestive symptoms.

Giardia. This is one of the most common parasites found in humans. It is transmitted through water, in food, between children in day-care centers, via a fecal-oral route, or through sexual intercourse. Epidemics from contaminated streams and community water systems occur every year in the United States.

Cryptosporidium. This is transmitted through contaminated food and water and from person-to-person contact. Explosive diarrhea is a common symptom. This parasite is of particular concern for children who are HIV-positive, as their immune systems may not be able to fight off the parasite, making it a life-threatening condition.

Ascaris lumbroides. This parasite causes the most common human worm infection in the world. Infection is common in the southeastern United States. In children, it can cause abdominal cramps and malnutrition. Fecal-oral transmission often occurs via uncooked or unwashed vegetables.

Hookworm. Hookworm is not as common in the United States as in other parts of the world, yet cases do occur. It usually causes no symptoms, although a skin itch may be present. Acute symptoms can include abdominal pain, diarrhea, weight loss, anemia, and many others. These worms can live up to ten years. They are transmitted via direct contact with soil containing the eggs of hookworms.

Strongyloides. The eggs of these worms can penetrate the skin and migrate to the lungs and the intestines. Most infections occur via the fecal-oral route. Infected people may be asymptomatic or may have various digestive problems. Liver and nervous system infection can also be serious problems.

Trichinosis. Infection occurs from eating undercooked or processed meat. There may be no symptoms, or else nausea, abdominal cramps, fever, and muscle pain (larvae can invade muscle tissue) can occur.

The conventional treatment focuses on antiparasitic medications to eradicate the infection. Toxicity and side effects vary for each medication.

The first step in treating a parasitic infection is to get a proper diagnosis. This is mainly dependent on a stool analysis. We highly recommend using a laboratory that specializes in comprehensive parasitology testing. Many of the stool tests done by clinics are not sensitive enough to pick up all of the different forms of parasites. Certain blood tests by your doctor can also help to pinpoint a diagnosis. In some cases, we treat patients for a parasite infection when they have the symptoms and the history that match a parasite infection, even though lab testing does not show a positive result. Some parasitic infections are hard to detect, but when diagnosis is uncertain, they should be treated. Natural therapies work well and should be used for a minimum of two months. One standard that many natural health practitioners follow is to treat for

Surprising Fact: Approximately 25 percent of the world's population is infected with hookworms.

Surprising Fact: It is estimated that more than 1 billion people are infected with ascariasis worldwide, of whom 20,000 die each year.

one additional month after the symptoms of a parasite infection have cleared. In some cases, conventional antiparasitic medication may also be required. Please note that natural treatment of parasitic infections should be done under the guidance of a knowledgeable health-care practitioner or doctor. Pregnant women should not follow the parasitic protocol in this section.

SYMPTOMS

- Loss of appetite
- Fatigue
- Constipation
- Depressed immunity
- Food allergy
- Fever
- Chills
- Heartburn
- Stomach pain
- Inflammatory bowel disease
- Lower back pain
- Itchy anus
- Rash and skin itching
- Hives
- Weight loss
- Arthritis
- Bloody stools
- Mucus in stool
- Colitis
- Crohn's disease
- Flatulence
- Foul-smelling stools
- Malabsorption
- Rectal bleeding
- Mood changes (depression, irritability)
- Vomiting

ROOT CAUSES

- Contaminated food or water
- A weakened immune system
- Dysbiosis (imbalanced gut flora)

Testing Techniques

The following tests help assess a parasite infection:

Immune system imbalance or disease—blood

Parasite testing—stool analysis and blood work

TREATMENT

Diet

Recommended Food

Fresh garlic, ginger, and onions are excellent as prepared foods, because they have been shown to have antiparasitic effects.

Raw pumpkin seeds kill worms and parasites. They can be ground up if desired. Consume ¼ cup to ½ cup daily with 8 oz of water.

Papaya juice has antiworm effects.

Food to Avoid

Sugar products should be reduced or avoided to optimize the health of your immune system.

Make sure that all fruits and vegetables are washed and cleaned properly. Meat and seafood products need to be thoroughly cooked. Avoid giving raw seafood to children.

℞ Super Seven Prescriptions—Parasites

Super Prescription #1 Black walnut (*Juglans nigra*)
Adults should take 30 drops or 250 mg three times daily. This herb has a long history of use by herbalists and naturopathic doctors for the treatment of parasites.

Super Prescription #2 Wormwood (*Artemisia absinthium*)
Take 20 drops or 200 mg three times daily with meals. Wormwood is a common herbal therapy for parasites and is generally used in a combination formula.

Super Prescription #3 Coptis (gold thread)
Take 20 drops or 200 mg three times daily with meals. This Chinese herb has antiparasitic effects.

Super Prescription #4 Oregano oil (*Origanum vulgare*)
Take 500 mg of the capsule form four times daily or as directed on the container. Oregano oil has powerful antibacterial and antiparasitic effects.

Super Prescription #5 Grapefruit seed extract
Take as directed on the container for a powerful antiparasitic effect.

Super Prescription #6 Goldenseal (*Hydrastis canadensis*)
Take 30 drops or 300 mg four times daily. Goldenseal helps fight infections in the digestive tract.

Super Prescription #7 Ginger (*Zingiber officinale*) **root**
Take 500 mg, 20 drops of the tincture, or 1 cup of fresh tea four times daily. Ginger has antiparasitic effects and reduces intestinal bloating and cramping.

General Recommendations

Peppermint (*Mentha piperita*) has been shown to be effective against some parasites. Take 2 ml or drink a fresh cup of tea four times daily.

Take a probiotic containing at least 4 billion active organisms twice daily, thirty minutes after meals. It supplies friendly bacteria such as *Lactobacillus acidophilus* and *bifidus*.

A combination parasitic homeopathic remedy helps stimulate the immune system to fight off an infection. Take as directed on the container.

Propolis has been shown to fight certain parasitic infections, such as giardia. Take 500 mg or 30 drops four times daily.

Rhubarb (*Rheum officinale*) is often used in parasite formulas as a stimulating laxative to help clear the intestines of a parasite. Take as directed on the container.

Homeopathy

Pick the remedy that best matches your symptoms in this section. For acute parasitic infections, take a 30C potency four times daily. For chronic infection, take a 6x, 12x, 6C, 12C, or 30C twice daily for two weeks to see if there are any positive results. After you notice improvement, stop taking the remedy, unless symptoms return. Consultation with a homeopathic practitioner is advised.

Cina is a specific remedy for pinworm or threadworm infections. The child is very irritable, does not want to be touched, and picks at the nose and the rectum. The child's appetite is very great. There may be pale, dark circles under the eyes. The child grinds his or her teeth at night.

Filix Mas is a specific remedy for tapeworms. The person has swollen glands, an itchy nose, and dark circles around the eyes and feels irritable and anxious.

Natrum Phosphoricum is a remedy that can be used for all types of worms. The person has signs of overacidity, such as belching and heartburn. There is often a yellow, creamy coating on the tongue.

Sabadilla is for a person with pinworms or tapeworms, characterized by itching of the rectum that alternates with itching of the nose or the ears.

Spigelia is a homeopathic remedy for worms. The person has an itchy rectum and pain around the navel. Bad breath is common.

Teucrium is a good remedy for pinworms, threadworms, and round worms. The child has itching and a crawling sensation in the nose and the rectum and feels very irritable and nervous.

Bodywork

Chinese herbal therapy and moxibustion treatments from a qualified practitioner can be helpful in the treatment of parasites.

REFERENCES

Great Smokies Diagnostic Laboratory Functional Assessment Resource Manual. 1998. Asheville, N.C.

Parkinson's Disease

Parkinson's disease is a chronic, degenerative disorder of the nervous system, in which voluntary movement is impaired or lost. Although the disease may come to affect your entire body, it most noticeably weakens your ability to control motions categorized as semivoluntary: keeping your jaw in place so that the mouth stays closed; swinging your arms as you walk; moving your tongue so that your speech is clear and precise. Parkinson's disease rarely affects people under sixty years of age, and men are about 30 percent more likely to develop it than women are.

Although muscle movement is an extraordinarily complex process that involves millions of nerve cells, this disease pinpoints relatively small sections of the brain, called the basal cell ganglia. When the nerve cells there begin to deteriorate, they create a chemical upset that can ultimately render the whole body disabled. In a healthy brain, two neurotransmitters, called acetylcholine and dopamine, work in tandem to regulate muscle actions. Acetylcholine helps muscles contract—without it, we'd be limp, unable to stand or even sit down—while dopamine tempers acetylcholine's effect. But the brain deterioration of Parkinson's throws this chemical duo off balance, reducing the quantities of dopamine and resulting in muscles that are too tightly contracted.

The symptoms of Parkinson's develop gradually, usually over a period of ten or fifteen years. The first sign is usually a tremor in one hand, which disappears when you move the hand or go to sleep. As the disorder progresses, the trembling is more pronounced and spreads to other parts of the body, usually the arms, the legs, and the head. The arms and the legs, in addition to shaking, may feel heavy and rigid, and you gradually lose the ability to write smoothly and speak clearly. As your muscles tighten, you may have trouble moving your bowels regularly. You may shuffle as you walk, with your head, neck, and shoulders hunched over and your arms held to your sides. One or both hands develop the characteristic "pill-rolling" movement, in which the thumb and the forefinger rub against each other, one making a clockwise circular motion, the other moving counterclockwise. Parkinson's often keeps the facial muscles in a nearly constant state of contraction; the face may take on a masklike appearance, with staring, unblinking eyes and a drooling mouth. Eventually, everyday tasks become difficult to manage. Simply getting out of a chair or speaking a clear sentence may be impossible. Although the muscular debility in these advanced stages is overwhelming, the person's mind is unaffected, and the affected body parts usually don't hurt or even feel numb.

Scientists still haven't determined exactly what causes the nerve cells of the basal cell ganglia to deteriorate, resulting in low dopamine levels, but we can base some tentative theories on several clues. For one, the incidence of Parkinson's is rising at an extraordinary rate: the percentage of cases in the United States has increased tenfold since the 1970s. This soaring rate suggests that the disease is strongly influenced by environmental factors. Finally, medications—both prescription and illicit—and environmental toxins are known to induce tremors in individuals. Given these facts, it seems likely that a poisoned body system greatly increases the risk of incurring Parkinson's. Bodies can be made toxic from exposure to heavy metals, carbon monoxide, pesticides, insecticides, and drugs; they can also be poisoned by a poor diet or allergic responses to food. Finally, free radicals, which destroy or damage cells, are a suspect in any degenerative disease.

The most common therapy for this disease is levodopa (L-dopa), which is sold in the United States under the brand name Sinemet. Levodopa is taken up by the brain and changed into dopamine. For some patients, it significantly improves mobility and allows them to function more normally. As Parkinson's disease worsens over time, larger doses must be taken. The drug can have debilitating side effects for some patients, such as involuntary movements, tics, and hallucinations. Also carbidopa, the other active ingredient (besides levodopa) in the drug Sinemet, works to prolong the effects of levodopa and help reduce its side effects. Carbidopa works by slowing the conversion of levodopa to dopamine in the bloodstream so that more of it reaches the brain. Another common drug is Comtan (entacapone), which has the same effect as carbidopa when taken along with levodopa. It blocks a key enzyme that is responsible for breaking down levodopa before it reaches the brain. Similarly, the drug deprenyl (Eldepryl) can enhance and prolong the levodopa response by delaying the breakdown of levodopa-formed dopamine. Other medications such as Parlodel (bromocriptine), Requip (ropinirole), Permax (pergolide), and Mirapex (pramipexole dihydrocholoride) work directly on cells of the substantia nigra in the brain in a way that imitates dopamine. Still other drugs like Artane (trihexyphenidyl), Symmetrel (amantadine), and Cogentin (benztropine) are used to help improve tremors. The most common side effects of drugs for Parkinson's disease are hallucinations, mental confusion, and dyskinesia. Surgery is generally used as a last resort. This involves destroying certain parts of the brain that are overactive in this disease. A less invasive option than destroying certain brain tissues is deep brain stimulation, where a thin electrode is implanted into the brain to block signals that cause symptoms of Parkinson's disease, especially tremors.

If you've been diagnosed with Parkinson's, you should be under the care of an experienced neurologist. He or she will usually want to place you on medications that reduce the symptoms of the disease. Sometimes these drugs are highly effective, but they almost always have strong side effects, so it's important to choose a doctor who listens to your concerns and helps you make informed decisions about the medications

A study published in the *International Journal of Epidemiology* that analyzed data concerning pesticide use in California counties reported that there was an increased mortality rate from Parkinson's disease in counties that used agricultural pesticides. The same study also reported that California growers use approximately 250 million pounds of pesticides annually, accounting for a quarter of all pesticides used in the United States.

or the procedures you try. You should also support your body with good nutrition and take up a cleansing regime to rid yourself of possible toxins. Specific supplements, such as coenzyme Q10, should also be highly considered. In addition, holistic doctors report impressive results with intravenous glutathione therapy.

SYMPTOMS

- Tremors
- Rigid or heavy-feeling arms and legs
- A "pill-rolling" motion of the hand and the thumb
- Constipation
- Difficulty speaking
- A shuffling gait, with the arms close to the body

- A stooped posture
- A masklike facial expression
- Drooling
- Eventually, an inability to perform most voluntary and semivoluntary movements

ROOT CAUSES

There are no definitive causes known for Parkinson's disease. Suspect causes or aggravating factors may include

- Insecticides, pesticides, and herbicides
- Heavy metals
- Carbon-monoxide poisoning

- Inflammatory brain disorder
- Free radicals
- Poor nutrition
- Food allergies

TREATMENT

Diet

Recommended Food

Studies have found that eating most of the day's protein intake at dinner and keeping protein levels low earlier in the day is helpful. This type of diet should be supervised by a health-care professional.

Raw foods (fruits, vegetables, nuts, and seeds) are high in fiber, which will keep you regular, and contain antioxidants that fight free radical damage. Follow a diet that is composed of 50 to 75 percent raw, organic foods. If you can't find or afford organic products, make sure to wash everything in clean water before eating.

When you do eat protein, focus on beans, legumes, soy products, or fish (from a clean water source). *Note:* The consumption of beans has been found to lower the risk of Parkinson's disease.

Use cold-pressed oils in salad dressings. They're high in vitamin E, a powerful antioxidant that's important in the prevention and the treatment of Parkinson's disease.

Fresh vegetable juices are excellent for their mineral content.

Eat live unsweetened yogurt or another cultured product every day. The "friendly" bacteria in cultured foods will help your digestive system to work smoothly.

Drink a glass of clean water every two waking hours. Clean—not tap—water will flush toxins and other impurities from your body and will also lend general support to every body system.

Testing Techniques

The following tests help assess possible reasons for Parkinson's disease:

   Hormone testing (thyroid, DHEA, cortisol, testosterone, IGF-1, estrogen, progesterone)—saliva, blood, or urine

   Intestinal permeability—urine

   Detoxification profile—urine

   Vitamin and mineral analysis (especially CoQ10)—blood

   Digestive function and microbe/parasite/candida testing—stool analysis

   Food and environmental allergies/sensitivities—blood, electrodermal

   Toxic metals—hair or urine analysis

   Pesticides and other environmental toxins—urine or blood

Food to Avoid

It has been observed that a high percentage of people with Parkinson's have an over-abundance of protein in their diets. Many patients who stop eating animal meats have noted an improvement in muscle control and coordination.

Do not eat processed or junk food, which contains high levels of chemicals and other toxins.

Avoid artificial sweeteners and preservatives that are known as "excitotoxins." These include aspartame and monosodium glutamate.

Avoid alcohol, caffeine, and sugar, as they can disrupt neurological function.

Overeating leads to a dangerous number of free radicals in your body. It's never a good idea to stuff yourself at mealtimes, but people with Parkinson's should try to keep caloric intake low, while maintaining an excellent nutritional status. Following the recommendations to avoid animal meats and processed food will go a long way toward keeping your calorie count down.

Food allergies are a possible aggravator of Parkinson's disease. Read the Food Allergies section, and follow the elimination diet there. If you feel better after abstaining from certain foods, keep them out of your diet.

Detoxification

Every month, do a raw foods fast for two to three days (under a doctor's supervision), meaning that you eat nothing but raw foods and juices (although you can have hot herbal teas). This will help move toxins out of your body and will help step up your digestive process so that you absorb nutrients more efficiently.

Regularly consume fresh vegetable and fruit juices, water, broths, and herbal teas.

℞ Super Seven Prescriptions—Parkinson's Disease

Note: These supplements should be used under the supervision of a doctor.

Super Prescription #1   Coenzyme Q10
   Take 1,200 mg daily. Coenzyme Q10 is an antioxidant that has been shown in one preliminary study to reduce the progression of early-stage Parkinson's disease.

In a trial of people with early Parkinson's disease, the combination of vitamins C (750 mg four times daily) and E (800 IU four times daily) was able to delay the need for drug therapy (i.e., L-dopa) by an average of about two and a half years, when compared with people not taking the vitamins.

Super Prescription #2   Vitamin C

Take 750 mg four times daily. Vitamin C is an important antioxidant that prevents free radical damage.

Super Prescription #3   Vitamin E-complex

Take 800 IU four times daily. Vitamin E is an important antioxidant that prevents free radical damage.

Super Prescription #4   Greens formula

Take an organic greens formula containing one or more of the super green foods, such as spirulina, chlorella, and wheatgrass. This approach supports detoxification.

Super Prescription #5   Essential fatty acids

Take a fish oil product that will provide at least 1 gram of DHA and EPA daily. Flaxseed oil and evening primrose oil (*Oenothera biennis*) are additional options.

Super Prescription #6   Nicotinamide adenine dinucleotide (NADH)

Take 5 mg twice daily. Preliminary research has found that this supplement improves brain function and reduces symptoms in people with Parkinson's disease.

Super Prescription #7   N-acetylcysteine (NAC)

Take 500 mg three times daily. NAC increases levels of glutathione, an important antioxidant.

A placebo-controlled, multicenter clinical trial led by Clifford Shults, M.D., of the University of California, San Diego School of Medicine, looked at a total of eighty people with Parkinson's disease at ten centers across the country to determine whether coenzyme Q10 is safe and whether it can slow the rate of functional decline. During the study period, the group that received the largest dose of coenzyme Q10 (1,200 mg/day) had 44 percent less decline in mental function, motor (movement) function, and ability to carry out activities of daily living, such as feeding or dressing themselves. The greatest effect was on activities of daily living. The side effects of supplementing CoQ10 were mild, and no one had to reduce his or her dosage. Researchers believe that coenzyme Q10 (CoQ10) works by improving the mitochondria, the energy production unit of cells. Mitochondria function is impaired in people with this disease. Coenzyme Q10 also has potent antioxidant effects.

General Recommendations

Ginkgo biloba improves blood flow and has potent antioxidant properties. Take a standardized extract containing 24 percent flavone glycosides, and take 60 to 80 mg twice daily.

Milk thistle (*Silybum marianum*) is another detoxifying herb that allows your liver to throw off accumulated toxins and prevents damage from pharmaceutical treatment. Take 250 mg three times daily of an 80 to 85 percent silymarin extract.

Green tea (*Camellia sinensis*) contains a rich source of antioxidants and substances that assist detoxification. Drink the organic tea regularly (2 cups or more daily), or take 500 to 1,500 mg of the capsule form.

Calcium and magnesium are important for nervous system function. Take 1,000 mg of calcium and 500 mg of magnesium.

Calming teas can help you deal with the stress produced by a degenerative disorder. Try passionflower (*Passiflora incarnata*), skullcap, or valerian.

Consult with a holistic doctor for intravenous glutathione treatment. Glutathione is one of the body's most potent antioxidants, and some doctors report benefit for people with Parkinson's disease from this nontoxic therapy.

Homeopathy

Pick the remedy that best matches your symptoms in this section. Take a 6x, 12x, 6C, or 12C potency twice daily for two weeks to see if there are any positive results. After you notice improvement, stop taking the remedy, unless symptoms return. Consultation with a homeopathic practitioner is advised.

Argentum Nitricum is for people who lose their balance and have uncoordinated movement as early symptoms. Tremors of the hands may prevent them from writing. It is also helpful for tremors that appear periodically.

Causticum is for slow paralysis, with the right side being more affected, and hand tremors that are worse when writing.

Gelsemium (*Gelsemium sempervirens*) is for tremors, difficulty controlling the tongue and the eyes, and a staggering walk.

Helleborus is for very slow speech. The patient appears to be in a deep fog.

Mercurius Solubilis or Vivus is helpful if your hands are trembling so much that it is difficult to eat or drink. You have slow or stammering speech.

Natrum Muriaticum is for hand tremors that occur when you write. You constantly nod your head and drop things easily. You suppress your emotions.

Plumbum is for progressive paralysis and muscle wasting. Cramping accompanies the paralysis.

Rhus Toxicodendron will ease muscle stiffness (usually accompanied by little or no trembling) that feels better when the affected body part is in motion. You find it hard to walk on first attempt but are successful once motion is started.

Acupressure

Acupressure or acupuncture from a qualified practitioner is highly advised for improved nerve function.

- Gallbladder 20 will stimulate better coordination of the nerves and the muscles.
- Stomach 36 helps you digest and absorb food properly.

Bodywork

Massage

Enjoy a lymphatic massage on a daily basis. It will drain toxic build-up from fatty deposits; better still, a massage can keep you in touch with your body during a time when you may feel estranged from it.

Reflexology

See pages 686–687 for information about reflexology areas and how to work them.

As with most body-wide disorders, it's best to work the entire foot for Parkinson's treatment. If you have limited time or want to concentrate on a few specific areas, work the brain and the spine regions to stimulate blood flow and strengthen the central nervous system.

Aromatherapy

Lavender, jasmine, rose, and geranium all help reduce stress. Use them in baths, diffusers, massages, or any way you like.

Stress Reduction

General Stress-Reduction Therapies

In the early stages of Parkinson's, yoga is a good choice for stress reduction, because it offers the additional benefit of stretching your muscles and improving coordination.

Meditation is a perfect technique for people who are more sedentary.

Current research is underway for the use of the macuna bean. Macuna beans (*Mucana pruriens*) have been used in Brazil and India by traditional healers for people with Parkinson's disease. These beans are a natural source of L-dopa, as well as a rich source of vitamin E. They appear to have similar benefits to L-dopa pharmaceutical treatment, but further research will clarify their effectiveness.

After a diagnosis of Parkinson's, you may feel like withdrawing. Although some quiet, private time may be helpful for a while, try to stay engaged with your usual activities. If that becomes impossible, at least try to keep meeting with friends and family members. Their support is crucial to your health.

Bach Flower Remedies

Following are some suggestions, but you should consult the chart on pages 648–650 to determine the best remedy for your particular needs. Once you've chosen a remedy, place 10 drops of the liquid under your tongue. Hold the drops in place for thirty seconds and swallow. Use as often as needed.

Take Rescue Remedy to see you calmly through the shock of a Parkinson's diagnosis or through any crisis periods of the illness.

If fear of the future causes you to dwell excessively on past good times, to the extent that you neglect your current life, take Honeysuckle.

Oak is for people who are usually brave in the face of adversity but who feel that they can no longer put up a fight against their illness.

Other Recommendations

- Some form of regular movement is quite beneficial during all the stages of Parkinson's. Walking is appropriate for the early and the middle stages; for a more advanced case, passive stretching and movements, usually carried out by a physical therapist, keep the body in the best shape possible.
- Plan ahead. Install guardrails and banisters in your house, and invest in a few chairs with high arms to help keep yourself mobile as long as possible.

REFERENCES

Fahn, S. 1992. A pilot trial of high-dose alpha-tocopherol and ascorbate in early Parkinson's disease. *Annals of Neurology* 32:S128–32.

Ritz, B., and F. Yu. 2000. Parkinson's disease mortality and pesticide exposure in California 1984–1994. *International Journal of Epidemiology* 29:323–29.

Shults, C. W., D. Oakes, K. Kieburtz, F. Beal, R. Haas, S. Plumb, J. L. Juncos, J. Nutt, I. Shoulson, J. Carter, K. Kompoliti, J. S. Perlmutter, S. Reich, M. Stern, R. L. Watts, R. Kurlan, E. Molho, M. Harrison, M. Lew, and the Parkinson Study Group. 2002. Effects of coenzyme Q10 in early Parkinson disease: Evidence of slowing of the functional decline. *Archives of Neurology* 59:(10); 1541–50.

Poisoning

Poisoning can occur a number of ways. It can occur because of a dangerous mixture of medications, from an overdose, from swallowing dangerous household chemicals or insecticides, and from ingesting poisonous plants, food, or nicotine.

A person's reaction can vary, dependent on the type and the amount of toxins ingested, with possible emergency and fatal outcomes. Reactions can include inflammation or burning around the lips, if the substance was taken orally; difficulty swallowing; nausea; sudden behavior changes; extreme thirst; breathing difficulties; unconsciousness; headaches; convulsions; vomiting; and death.

Among children ages five and under, 60 percent of poisoning exposures are by nonpharmaceutical products, such as cosmetics, cleaning substances, plants, foreign bodies and toys, pesticides, art supplies, and alcohol. The remaining 40 percent are from pharmaceuticals.

Millions of poisoning exposures occur each year in the United States, resulting in nearly 900,000 visits to emergency rooms. About 90 percent of poisonings happen in the home, and more than half of these involve children under age six.

Prevention is the key. Following are recommendations from the American Association of Poison Control Centers that can help you protect children from poisons:

- Post the telephone number for your poison control center near your phone, in a place where all family members will be able to find it quickly in an emergency.

- Remove all nonessential drugs and household products from your home. Discard them according to the manufacturer's instructions.

- If you have small children, avoid keeping highly toxic products, such as drain cleaners, in the home, the garage, the shed, or any other place that children can access.

- Buy medicines and household products in child-resistant packaging, and be sure that caps are always on tight. Do not remove child-safety caps. Avoid keeping medicines, vitamins, or household products in anything but their original packaging.

- Store all of your medicines and household products in a locked closet or cabinet—including products and medicines with child-resistant containers.

- Crawl around your house, including inside your closets, to inspect it from a child's point of view. You'll likely find a poisoning hazard that you hadn't noticed before.

- Never refer to medicine or vitamins as "candy."

- Make sure that visiting grandparents, family members, friends, or other caregivers keep their medications away from children. For example, if Grandma keeps pills in her purse, make sure the purse is out of the children's reach.

- Keep a bottle of syrup of ipecac in your home—this can be used to induce vomiting. Use it only when the poison control center tells you to.

- Avoid products such as cough syrup or mouthwash that contain alcohol—these are hazardous for young children. Look for alcohol-free alternatives.

- Keep cosmetics and beauty products out of children's reach. Remember that hair permanents and relaxers are toxins as well.

Carbon monoxide (CO) is an invisible, odorless, poisonous gas that can also cause sickness and death. The incomplete burning of fuels such as natural gas, oil, kerosene, propane, coal, and wood produce carbon monoxide. Also, fuel-burning appliances that are not working properly or are installed incorrectly can produce fatal concentrations of carbon monoxide in your home. Other hazards include burning charcoal indoors and running a car in the garage, both of which can lead to dangerous levels of CO in your home.

The following simple tips from the Centers for Disease Control will prevent carbon monoxide poisoning.

- Install carbon monoxide alarms near the bedrooms and on each floor of your home. If your alarm sounds, the U.S. Consumer Product Safety Commission suggests that you press the reset button, call emergency services (911 or your local fire department), and immediately move to fresh air (either outdoors or near an open door or window). If you learn that fuel-burning appliances were the most likely cause of the poisoning, have a serviceperson check them for malfunction before turning them back on. Refer to the instructions on your CO alarm for more specific information about what to do if your alarm goes off.

- Symptoms of CO poisoning are similar to those of the flu, only without a fever (headache, fatigue, nausea, dizziness, shortness of breath). If you experience any of these symptoms, get fresh air immediately and contact a physician for a proper diagnosis. Also, open windows and doors, turn off combustion appliances, contact emergency services, and take the steps listed previously to ensure your home's safety.

- To keep carbon monoxide from collecting in your home, make sure that any fuel-burning equipment, such as a furnace, a stove, or a heater, works properly, and never use charcoal or other grills indoors or in the garage. Do not leave your car's engine running while it's in the garage, and consider putting weather stripping around the door between the garage and the house.

Iron Poisoning from Supplements or Medicines

From 1986 through 1997, more than 218,000 children, ages five and under, ingested iron preparations, and 46 died. Again, make sure that medicines and supplements are out of the reach of children.

Lead

The ingestion of dust from deteriorating lead-based paint is the most common cause of lead poisoning among children. Currently, more than 80 percent of public and privately owned housing units built before 1980 contain some lead-based paint.

Improper use of medications, such as an overdose or the mixture of one medication with another without the doctor's recommendation, can trigger an adverse reaction. Many prescription medications can have negative effects when combined with others. Also, some people unknowingly harbor allergies to medications, which could lead to poisonous predicaments.

Children with access to household chemicals, detergents, and cleaners that are poorly capped and stored are vulnerable to sampling these poisons. The immediate response could include vomiting or gagging. Also, children may accidentally lick, chew, or swallow poisonous plants or nicotine patches, which could induce dizziness or possibly only transitory distress.

Another more common form of poisoning comes from the ingestion of tainted food that was improperly cleaned, cooked, or refrigerated. These foods can contain dangerous bacteria and contaminants that create a feeling of pain, bloating, and nausea for three to six hours after consumption, as well as diarrhea, stomach cramps, and vomiting (see the Food Poisoning section).

The most serious type of food poisoning, particularly with improperly canned foods and seafood, is a potentially fatal form known as botulism. Generally, the longer it takes for the symptoms of food poisoning to appear, the more serious the poisoning.

SYMPTOMS

- Difficulty swallowing
- Nausea
- Sudden behavior changes
- Extreme thirst
- Breathing difficulties
- Unconsciousness
- Headaches
- Convulsions
- Vomiting

ROOT CAUSES

- Ingestion of a toxic substance

TREATMENT

Basic Plan

Acute Poisoning (Internal)

If you suspect that your child has ingested a poison, first get the poisonous substance away from your child. If there is still some in his or her mouth, have the child spit it out into a bowl, so that you have the substance if a doctor needs to examine it. Next, check your child for these signs:

- Severe throat pain or discomfort
- Excessive drooling
- Trouble breathing
- Convulsions
- Drowsiness

If your child has any of these signs, call an ambulance or get the child to an emergency room immediately. If there is no sign of these serious symptoms, call your local poison control center. The number is usually listed on the inside cover of your phone book (it's best to have it on a sheet near your phone for emergency use). If you cannot find the number, call 911 and ask for poison control. You can also call your pediatrician. Do not make your child vomit unless instructed to do so by the poison control center or your doctor.

Poison on the Skin

If a chemical is spilled on your skin, remove your clothes and rinse the skin with lukewarm water for fifteen minutes. Then call the poison control center for further advice. Do not apply any topical treatment unless instructed to do so.

Poison in the Eye

Immediately flush your eye with lukewarm water. Aim for the inner corner of the eye. Flush for fifteen minutes, and call the poison control center for further directions.

Testing Techniques

The following tests help assess poisons that have accumulated in the body:

Variety of different poisons, as ordered by your doctor—blood

Digestive function and microbe/parasite/candida testing—stool analysis

Toxic metals—hair or urine

℞ Super Seven Prescriptions—Poisoning

Note: These recommendations are not to be used instead of conventional/emergency therapy for poisoning.

Super Prescription #1   Activated charcoal capsules
Take 3 capsules three times daily for two days. Charcoal binds toxins in the digestive tract so that they can be excreted out with the stool.

Super Prescription #2   Homeopathic Nux Vomica (*Strychnos nux vomica*)
Take a 30C potency four times daily. It is specific for poisoning from foods, medications, recreational drugs, or alcohol. The person is irritable and constipated.

Super Prescription #3   Homeopathic Arsenicum Album
Take a 30C potency four times daily. It is specific for the symptoms of food poisoning, such as vomiting and diarrhea.

Super Prescription #4   Milk thistle (*Silybum marianum*)
Take 250 mg of an 85 percent silymarin extract three times daily. It protects the liver and the kidneys from being damaged and improves detoxification.

Super Prescription #5   Alpha lipoic acid
Take 100 mg three times daily to prevent liver damage, especially from a medication overdosage.

Super Prescription #6   Vitamin C
Take 1,000 mg three times daily, or request the intravenous form from your doctor. Vitamin C aids in detoxification and prevents organ damage.

> **Super Prescription #7   N-acetylcysteine (NAC)**
> Take 500 mg three times daily. NAC improves detoxification and increases the level of the antioxidant glutathione.

General Recommendations

Reishi (*Ganoderma lucidum*) extract supports liver and kidney detoxification. Take 800 mg twice daily.

Bodywork

Acupuncture

Acupuncture is recommended to reduce the side effects of poisoning. See a qualified practitioner.

Other Bodywork Recommendations

Talk with your doctor about using these complementary therapies along with conventional therapy to recover from poisoning.

Pregnancy-Related Problems

Pregnancy is a joyful time, but it's rarely a comfortable one. There are probably as many different combinations of pregnancy-related problems as there are pregnant women. Nevertheless, most uncomfortable conditions are caused by one of three factors: hormonal changes; nutritional deficiencies, whether preexisting or brought on by the additional needs of the baby; and the pressure placed on bones and internal organs by the weight of the growing child.

If you're pregnant, it's essential to have regular check-ups. Your doctor should monitor your health, as well as your baby's, and should remain vigilant for any signs of trouble. Good conventional care has saved the lives of many women and their developing babies, and serious problems can often be successfully treated when caught early

---

When to Call the Doctor

During pregnancy, your body goes through an astounding number of changes. Some will seem normal to you, but you may worry about others. It's wise to develop a good relationship with your doctor long before you get pregnant, so that you are well-informed and comfortable with asking questions. No matter how often you see or talk to a doctor, however, you should always call a medical professional right away if you experience any of the following:

- Vaginal bleeding

- Persistent abdominal pain or cramping

- Continuous or intense morning sickness during the first trimester

- Nausea and vomiting that occur after the first trimester is over

In rare cases, water retention and swelling are signs of a potentially dangerous condition. While most women do experience these symptoms during the course of a normal, healthy pregnancy, it's always a good idea to have them checked out by your doctor, just to be on the safe side.

enough. But as valuable as conventional medicine can be for pregnant women, it rarely offers ways to handle the daily discomfort. During this time, a woman may come to fully appreciate the gentle power of natural therapies. Although some highly potent herbs and other treatments are too strong for the baby, there are still many complementary strategies that will minimize the less-serious problems that accompany pregnancy. Each of the following recommendations is safe to use during pregnancy, but always alert your doctor or midwife to what you are using as nutritional supplements.

ANEMIA

During pregnancy, your body needs more iron than usual. A deficiency can result in anemia, a disorder in which the body's cells don't receive enough oxygen. As a result, you feel tired and drained, and you may be more vulnerable to illness.

TREATMENT

Diet

Recommended Food

To overcome pregnancy-induced anemia, consume foods that are high in iron. Organic calf's liver is far and away the best source, but if you're a vegetarian or just can't hold organ meats down right now, you do have some other options. Molasses, green leafy vegetables (with the exception of spinach), leeks, cashews, cherries, strawberries, dried fruits, figs, and eggs are all rich in iron.

Food to Avoid

- Spinach, rhubarb, tomatoes, and chocolate are high in oxalic acid, a substance that blocks the absorption of iron.
- If you're pregnant, you've already been advised to stay away from caffeine, which can harm the baby. Caffeine also inhibits iron absorption, as do carbonated sodas and dairy products.
- Do not take iron pills with meals that are high in fiber. The fiber will sweep the iron out of your system before you've had a chance to digest it.

℞ Super Seven Prescriptions—Anemia

Super Prescription #1   Iron
If you have been diagnosed with iron-deficiency anemia by your doctor, take 50 to 200 mg (or the amount recommended by your doctor, depending on the severity) of an easily absorbed form of iron, such as iron citrate, gluconate, glycinate, or fumarate, one to two times daily. Also, iron chelate is generally well absorbed. Avoid the use of iron sulfate (ferrous sulfate), which is poorly absorbed and can cause digestive upset.

Super Prescription #2   Prenatal multivitamin
Take as directed on the container. It supplies a wide range of nutrients for healthy red blood cells.

Super Prescription #3   Ferrum Phosphoricum
Take 5 pellets of the 3x or 6x potency three times daily. This homeopathic remedy improves iron utilization in the cells.

Super Prescription #4   Yellow dock (*Rumex crispis*)
Take 1 (300 mg) capsule or 20 drops of the tincture with each meal. It contains iron and improves iron absorption.

Super Prescription #5   Nettles (*Urtica diocia*)
Take 2 ml of the tincture twice daily or 300 mg of the capsule form, or drink 1 cup of the tea twice daily (organic source). This herb is a source of iron and other blood-building minerals.

Super Prescription #6   Chlorella
Take as directed on the container for a host of iron-building nutrients, including chlorophyll.

Super Prescription #7   Vitamin C
Take 100 mg with each dose of iron. It provides an acidic environment for enhanced iron absorption.

General Recommendations

See the Anemia section for further details.

BACK PAIN

Most pregnant women experience some degree of back pain, thanks to the extra weight and the shifting center of gravity.

TREATMENT

Diet

Constipation, to which pregnant women are especially vulnerable, makes back pain worse. See the recommendations for Constipation listed on pages 167–171.

When back pain strikes, try drinking a glass or two of water immediately. If the pain is caused by dehydration, water will help.

℞ **Super Seven Prescriptions—Back Pain**

Super Prescription #1   Calcium and magnesium
Take a complex of these two minerals that contains 500 mg of calcium and 250 mg of magnesium. Take it twice daily. These minerals reduce muscle spasms.

Super Prescriptions #2–#7   (see the Homeopathic remedies listed next)
Pick the remedy that best matches your symptoms in this section. For acute back pain, take a 30C potency four times daily. For chronic back pain, take it twice daily for two weeks to see if there are any positive results. After you notice improvement, stop taking the remedy, unless symptoms return. Consultation with a homeopathic practitioner is advised.

Aesculus Hippocastanum is for lower back or sacral pain that is worse when you are sitting. The pain often radiates into the right hip.

Arnica (*Arnica montana*) is for an injury that leaves your back feeling bruised and sore and when you have difficulty moving around.

Bryonia (*Bryonia alba*) is for lower back pain and stiffness that feel worse with any movement and in cold, dry weather and that feel better when the area is rubbed.

Calcarea Carbonica is for chronic lower back pain and weakness in overweight individuals who also are chilly. Symptoms are worse in the cold and the dampness.

Cimicifuga Racemosa is for a stiff, aching neck and back. Muscles feel bruised but feel better with warmth. Also, it's used for menstrual cramps, with lower back pain radiating to the thighs.

Ignatia (*Ignatia amara*) is for back spasms and cramping, as the result of emotional stress.

Magnesia Phosphorica is for muscle spasms in the back that feel better from warmth.

Nux Vomica is for back spasms and cramping, especially of the lower back. The person may also have constipation and may feel chilly and irritable. Symptoms are worse from cold and better with warmth.

Rhus Toxicodendron is for a stiff lower back that is worse in the cold and the damp and better with movement. It is specific for sprained back muscles or ligaments.

Ruta Graveolens is for pain near the neck or in the lower back. The area of the injury feels lame, and the pain is worse at night. It's useful for back sprains and strains.

Bodywork

Massage
A pregnancy massage can provide temporary but welcome relief from back pain. Make an appointment with a therapist who is experienced in working with pregnant women.

Other Bodywork Recommendations
Acupressure and acupuncture can be helpful, when performed by an experienced practitioner.

Reflexology
See pages 686–687 for information about reflexology areas and how to work them.

Work the base of the heel, which corresponds to the spine, the hips, and the tailbone.

Hydrotherapy
Floating in water makes you feel weightless and takes the pressure off your back (at least, for the duration of your swim). You don't need much in the way of special equipment, just a pool or, in good weather, a lake or other body of clean water.

Alternating hot and cold towels over the back or the use of a hot pack for five minutes or less can be helpful.

Other Recommendations

- Prenatal yoga or stretching classes can be effective.
- At night, support your back and belly with pillows.
- When you're pregnant, the last thing you may think about is your posture. Make an extra effort to check that your back is straight, even when you're sitting down.
- Use common sense: don't wear high heels, and don't lift heavy objects.

BLEEDING GUMS IN PREGNANCY

Increased estrogen production can make your gums soft, swollen, and prone to bleeding. Proper diet and supplements will reduce the severity of bleeding gums.

TREATMENT

Diet

Recommended Food

Good sources of calcium include sea vegetables, green leafy vegetables (with the exception of spinach), soybeans, and unsweetened cultured yogurt.

Enjoy citrus fruits and green vegetables for vitamin C

Food to Avoid

Spinach, rhubarb, tomatoes, and chocolate inhibit your body's ability to absorb calcium.

℞ Super Seven Prescriptions—Bleeding Gums

Super Prescription #1   Vitamin C
Take 200 mg twice daily. Try a nonacidic vitamin C to prevent digestive upset.

Super Prescription #2   Homeopathic Ferrum Phosphoricum
Take 3 pellets of a 6x potency twice daily. This homeopathic remedy safely reduces bleeding and inflammation. Take until the bleeding stops, then discontinue.

Super Prescription #3   Bioflavonoid complex
Take 250 mg twice daily. Bioflavonoids reduce inflammation of the gums.

Super Prescription #4   Prenatal multivitamin
Take as directed on the container. It supplies a variety of nutrients that are required for gum health.

Super Prescription #5   Calendula (*Calendula officinalis*)
Put 15 drops of calendula tincture in 2 ounces of water. Swish it in your mouth, and spit it out. Calendula is healing to the mucosa of the gums.

Super Prescription #6   Homeopathic Mercurius Solubilis
Take a low potency (6x, 12x, 6C, 12C, or 30C) twice daily for swollen, bleeding gums that are accompanied by heavy salivation and bad breath. Stop using it when the bleeding stops.

Super Prescription #7   *Myrrh cerifera*
Put 15 drops of myrrh tincture in 2 ounces of water. Swish it in your mouth, and spit it out. Myrrh is healing to the mucosa of the gums.

Bodywork

Massage

In the morning and before you go to bed, use your finger to massage your gums lightly.

CONSTIPATION

The hormonal changes of pregnancy, along with the positioning of the baby and fiber and fluid intake, make pregnant women more susceptible to constipation. Iron pills (ferrous sulfate) can also lead to constipation.

TREATMENT

Diet

Recommended Food

Eat plenty of fiber—fresh fruits and vegetables, whole grains, and beans—to encourage regularity. Dried fruits—especially that old standby, prunes—are another good choice.

Drink a glass of clean water every two waking hours. You will keep food moving through your digestive system.

A hot beverage at breakfast will often wake up a sluggish digestive system. Try herbal tea or hot water with a little lemon juice.

Food to Avoid

Do not eat fatty, greasy, or fried foods, which travel slowly through the intestines.

℞ Super Seven Prescription—Constipation

Super Prescription #1   Psyllium
Take 1 teaspoon or 5 grams of psyllium husks twice daily or as directed on the container. Take it with 10 ounces of water. Psyllium acts as a bulk-forming laxative.

Super Prescription #2   Probiotic
Take a product containing at least 4 billion active organisms daily. Friendly bacteria such as *Lactobacillus acidophilus* and *bifidus* help with digestion and elimination.

Super Prescription #3   Chlorella
Take 1,500 mg of organic chlorella daily. This algae supplement provides a healthy source of fiber.

Super Prescription #4   Homeopathic Sepia
Take a 6x, 12x, 6C, 12C, or 30C potency twice daily for three days to see if there are any positive results. After you notice improvement, stop taking the remedy, unless symptoms return. Consultation with a homeopathic practitioner is advised.

Sepia is indicated for pregnant women who feel irritable and chilly and have stools that are hard to pass. A heavy sensation in the rectum and the lower abdomen is present. There is a strong craving for chocolate.

Super Prescription #5   Homeopathic Nux Vomica
Take a 6x, 12x, 6C, 12C, or 30C potency twice daily for three days to see if there are any positive results. After you notice improvement, stop taking the remedy, unless symptoms return. Consultation with a homeopathic practitioner is advised.

Nux Vomica is indicated when one has an urgent feeling but can't pass stools or stools are never completed. The person feels irritable and overstressed. Nux Vomica works well for people who work too hard, exercise too little, and eat and drink too much.

> **Super Prescription #6   Homeopathic Natrum Muriaticum**
> Take a 6x, 12x, 6C, 12C, or 30C potency twice daily for three days to see if there are any positive results. After you notice improvement, stop taking the remedy, unless symptoms return. Consultation with a homeopathic practitioner is advised.
>
> This is a remedy for women with constipation who have strong cravings for salt and water. They may suffer from depression and are often sensitive to the sun or to light.
>
> **Super Prescription #7   Homeopathic Lycopodium** (*Lycopodium clavatum*)
> Take a 6x, 12x, 6C, 12C, or 30C potency twice daily for three days to see if there are any positive results. After you notice improvement, stop taking the remedy, unless symptoms return. Consultation with a homeopathic practitioner is advised.
>
> This remedy is for a woman who has constipation and problems with gas and bloating. She craves sweets, and her symptoms are worse in the late afternoon. Her digestive system feels better with warm drinks.

Bodywork

Reflexology

See pages 686–687 for information about reflexology areas and how to work them. Work with a knowledgeable therapist.

Exercise can stimulate bowel contractions. If you're feeling sluggish, go out and take a brisk walk.

FLUID RETENTION (EDEMA)

Hormonal changes and increased fluids can cause your hands, legs, and feet to swell, especially in the later months of pregnancy. Although many women experience fluid retention, you should always have it checked out by a doctor, as it's sometimes a symptom of a serious disorder.

TREATMENT

Diet

Recommended Food

As you lower your intake of salt, you must also increase your consumption of potassium. A combination of excess sodium and a deficiency in potassium has been found in many people with hypertension. Good sources of potassium include apples, asparagus, cabbage, oranges, tomatoes, bananas, kelp, and alfalfa.

Food to Avoid

Restrict your intake of salt. Obviously, you should avoid table salt, but you should also stay away from processed or junk food, both of which contain alarming amounts of sodium.

℞ Super Seven Prescriptions—Fluid Retention

> **Super Prescription #1   Dandelion leaf** (*Taraxacum officinale*)
> With your doctor's supervision, take 3 ml or 300 mg twice daily. Dandelion leaf is a gentle diuretic.

Super Prescription #2   B-complex vitamins
Vitamin B6 and other B-complex vitamins may help reduce edema. Take 50 mg twice daily.

Super Prescription #3   Homeopathic Natrum Muriaticum
Take 3 pellets of a 6x potency three times daily. It is particularly indicated if you have a strong desire for salt and the fluid retention is worse from being in the sun or from heat.

Super Prescription #4   Vitamin C
Take 500 mg twice daily. Vitamin C improves the lymph flow.

Super Prescription #5   Vitamin B6
Take 50 mg daily under the guidance of a doctor. Vitamin B6 has been found to reduce water retention, most likely due to its function in helping liver metabolism.

Super Prescription #6   Quercitin
Take 500 mg twice daily. Quercitin is a flavonoid that improves circulation.

Super Prescription #7   Garlic
Take 200 mg twice daily. Garlic has mild anti-edema properties.

Bodywork

Reflexology

See pages 686–687 for information about reflexology areas and how to work them.
Work the lymph areas to reduce swelling.

Other Recommendations

- Regular exercise will minimize swelling. A daily walk or swim is a good idea.
- Swollen feet are uncomfortable, but tight shoes are even worse. For the duration of your pregnancy, you may want to wear shoes that are larger than your usual size.

GAS

Even women with normally hardy digestive systems may find themselves suffering from gas and flatulence when pregnant. This bothersome condition is usually due to the slower movement of food through your intestines. Sometimes women also find that they are upset by certain foods for the duration of the pregnancy.

TREATMENT

Diet

Recommended Food

Papaya soothes the intestinal tract and is high in enzymes that help you digest food properly.

Instead of taxing your digestive system with large meals, eat several small ones throughout the day.

If your digestion is not as efficient as usual, try incorporating more easily digestible foods into your diet, such as soups, broths, and steamed vegetables.

Food to Avoid

If you suspect that a particular food is giving you gas, your body is trying to tell you something. Avoid that food until after you've delivered your child and finished nursing. Common offenders include beans, cow's milk, sugar, and spicy foods.

Keep a record of the food you eat during the day, and take note of when gas occurs. (Do not, however, try an elimination diet. It's too severe for you right now.) If you can isolate the food that irritates you, avoid it until the baby arrives and is weaned.

℞ Super Seven Prescriptions—Gas

Super Prescription #1   Ginger (*Zingiber officinale*)
Drink a cup of ginger tea when you feel bloated or after meals. You can also use 300 mg of the capsule form or 2 ml of the tincture.

Super Prescription #2   Chamomile (*Matricaria chamomilla*)
Drink a cup of chamomile tea when you feel bloated or after meals. If you prefer to use an extract, take 500 mg twice a day, or use 2 ml of a tincture twice daily.

Super Prescription #3   Homeopathic Magnesia Phosphorica
Take 3 pellets of a 6x potency up to three times daily for gas and cramping.

Super Prescription #4   Homeopathic Carbo Vegetabilis
Take a low potency (6x, 12x, 30x, 6C, or 30C) as needed, for gas and bloating that are accompanied by belching.

Super Prescription #5   Homeopathic Pulsatilla (*Pulsatilla pratensis*)
Take a low potency (6x, 12x, 30x, 6C, or 30C) as needed, for gas and bloating that occur from eating rich or fatty foods.

Super Prescription #6   Homeopathic Lycopodium (*Lycopodium clavatum*)
Take a low potency (6x, 12x, 30x, 6C, or 30C) as needed, for gas and bloating that occur in the evening. Warm drinks improve the symptoms as well.

Super Prescription #7   Homeopathic Nux Vomica
Take a low potency (6x, 12x, 30x, 6C, or 30C) as needed, for gas and bloating that occur from stress and spicy foods. Heartburn is also a common symptom treated by this remedy.

General Recommendations

Take a probiotic supplement that contains at least 4 billion organisms, thirty minutes after breakfast and dinner. These good bacteria reside in the digestive tract and aid digestion.

HEARTBURN

The position of the baby may cause stomach acid to back up into the esophagus, leaving you with a burning pain in your chest. You may also experience some regurgitation of acid into your throat and mouth.

TREATMENT

Diet

Recommended Food

Whenever you feel heartburn pain, drink a glass of clean water to flush the gastric acids back down into your stomach.

Eat papaya for its healing qualities, or drink its juice.

Eat small meals throughout the day, instead of three large ones. If your stomach isn't completely full, there's less of a chance that its contents will back up.

Food to Avoid

Some foods are more challenging to digest than others are. If you stay away from fried and greasy foods, spicy foods, and heavy sauces, you may find that your problem resolves itself.

Avoid minty foods, such as peppermint, which can aggravate heartburn.

Allow a few hours between your last meal or snack and bedtime. You'll give your stomach a chance to process its contents before you lie down.

Food allergies are linked to heartburn. If a food causes you trouble, eliminate it from your diet. You may find that your symptoms improve significantly or even disappear.

℞ Super Seven Prescriptions—Heartburn

Super Prescription #1   Licorice root (DGL)
Chew one 400 mg tablet (or take it in powder form) for the relief of heartburn. DGL is a special type of licorice extract that soothes and heals the stomach and the esophagus. It does not cause high blood pressure.

Super Prescription #2   Homeopathic Nux Vomica
Take a low potency (6x, 12x, 30x, 6C, or 30C) as needed, for heartburn that occurs from stress and spicy foods.

Super Prescription #3   Slippery elm (*Ulmus fulva*)
Take 1 teaspoon, 300 mg of the capsule form, or 3 ml of tincture three times daily. This herb is used to soothe and reduce inflammation of the lining of the esophagus and the stomach.

Super Prescription #4   Marshmallow root (*Althea officinalis*)
Take 300 mg of the capsule or 3 ml of tincture three times daily. Marshmallow root soothes and reduces inflammation of the lining of the esophagus and the stomach.

Super Prescription #5   Digestive enzymes
Take 1 to 2 capsules of a full-spectrum blend with each meal. Enzymes help you to digest foods more effectively so that they are less likely to cause irritation *Note:* Some people may need to use a formula that contains no protease, as this protein digestive enzyme may irritate the stomachs of some individuals.

Super Prescription #6   Probiotic
Take a product containing at least 4 billion active organisms daily. It contains friendly bacteria, such as *Lactobacillus acidophilus* and *bifidus,* that improve digestive function.

> **Super Prescription #7   Calcium**
>
> Liquid calcium is soothing to the stomach. Take a formula containing 500 mg of calcium and 250 mg of magnesium twice daily. Magnesium helps to relax tightened muscles of the esophagus and the stomach.

General Recommendations

A super green food supplement, such as chlorella or spirulina, or a mixture of super green foods in a drink, helps to neutralize acidity. Take as directed on the container.

Chamomile tea is soothing to the digestive tract. Drink 1 to 2 cups daily.

Homeopathy

Pick the remedy that best matches your symptoms in this section. For chronic acid reflux, take a 6x, 12x, 6C, 12C, or 30C twice daily for two weeks to see if there are any positive results. After you notice improvement, stop taking the remedy, unless symptoms return. Consultation with a homeopathic practitioner is advised.

Arsenicum Album is for a burning sensation in the esophagus or the stomach that is alleviated by drinking milk or by frequently sipping warm water and sitting up. The person feels anxious and restless

Carbo Vegetabilis will help people whose sluggish digestion leads to flatulence, belching, and bloating in the upper abdomen. People who benefit from this remedy are often pale and cold. Despite their chilliness, they feel better with cool air and drinks.

Lycopodium (*Lycopodium clavatum*) is also for gas and bloating, but in this case the symptoms are usually brought on by anxiety and lack of confidence. The person feels worse when wearing tight clothes and better when sipping warm drinks. There may be a sour taste in the mouth. Symptoms are often worse in the late afternoon and the evening.

Natrum Carbonicum is for people who have trouble digesting most foods, especially milk.

Nux Vomica is for people with heartburn and reflux that occur from stress, spicy foods, and alcohol. They generally feel chilly, irritable, and oversensitive to stimuli (noise, light). Constipation is often a problem as well.

Pulsatilla (*Pulsatilla pratensis*) is helpful if you feel worse after eating rich and fatty foods. Symptoms are worse in a warm room and better with fresh air. You also tend to feel tearful when ill, and you greatly desire to be comforted.

Phosphorous helps when you have a burning pain in the stomach that feels better from cold drinks. However, soon after drinking, you are nauseous and may vomit.

Sulphur is for burning pain and belching, accompanied by diarrhea. You tend to be very warm and get relief from ice-cold drinks.

Other Recommendations

Structure your day so that you don't have to bend over, lie down, or perform any strenuous activity within a couple of hours after eating.

HEMORRHOIDS

During pregnancy, both constipation and pressure on the lower part of the body can produce hemorrhoids.

TREATMENT

Diet

Recommended Food

Fiber will soften your stool and make it easier to pass. Eat whole grains, fresh or dried fruits and vegetables, or beans with every meal.

Another way to soften stools is to drink a glass of clean water every two waking hours.

Food to Avoid

Don't eat foods that are difficult for your body to process. Greasy, fried, and junk foods are all off-limits; so are any other items that are high in saturated fat.

Cow's milk is constipating for some pregnant women.

℞ Super Seven Prescriptions—Hemorrhoids

Super Prescription #1   Psyllium
Psyllium is a good fiber supplement and has been shown to reduce the pain and the bleeding associated with hemorrhoids. Take 5 to 7 grams daily, along with 10 ounces of water.

Super Prescription #2   Flaxseed oil
Take 1 to 2 tablespoons daily. Flaxseed oil improves regularity and reduces straining. It also contains essential fatty acids that promote tissue healing. *Note:* Reduce the dosage if diarrhea occurs.

Super Prescription #3   Bilberry (*Vaccinium myrtillus*)
Take a standardized extract containing 25 percent anthocyanosides at 160 mg twice daily. Bilberry improves circulation and strengthens capillary walls.

Super Prescription #4   Witch hazel (*Hamamelis virginiana*)
Apply it as a gel or a cream to external hemorrhoids, or add 1 ounce to a sitz bath daily.

Super Prescription #5   Probiotic
This contains friendly bacteria, such as lactobacillus and bifido bacterium, which improve digestion and constipation. Take a product that contains at least 4 billion active organisms daily.

Super Prescription #6   Bioflavonoid complex
Take 1,000 mg two to three times daily. Various flavonoids, such as rutin and hesperidin, have been shown to be effective in treating hemorrhoids. They reduce swelling and prevent bleeding.

Super Prescription #7   Greens drink
Consume a greens drink that contains a blend of super green foods, such as chlorella, spirulina, and so on. It provides fiber. Take as directed on the container.

A study of fifty-one pregnant women found that supplementation of bilberry significantly improved the pain, the burning, and the itching associated with their hemorrhoids.

Homeopathy

Pick the remedy that best matches your symptoms in this section. Take a 6x, 12x, 6C, 12C, or 30C potency twice daily for two weeks to see if there are any positive results. After you notice improvement, stop taking the remedy, unless symptoms return. Consultation with a homeopathic practitioner is advised.

Aesculus Hippocastanum is for a pain that feels as if the rectum is being poked with sticks. The pain extends to the back.

Aloe Vera is for large, painful hemorrhoids. Your doctor states that the hemorrhoids look like a "bunch of grapes." They feel better with cold compresses. You may be prone to diarrhea.

Calcarea Fluorica is helpful when bleeding and itching occur with the hemorrhoids. Often, lower back pain is present. You may have problems with flatulence and constipation.

Ignatia (*Ignatia amara*) is for hemorrhoids that cause a stabbing or sticking pain, along with rectal spasms. Symptoms feel worse from emotional upset.

Nux Vomica is for painful hemorrhoids that come on as a result of chronic constipation and straining with bowel movements. The woman feels irritable.

Ratanhia helps when one experiences a lot of pain after a bowel movement. There is a cutting pain that feels as if one is sitting on broken glass.

Sulphur is for large, itching, burning hemorrhoids that tend to be worse at night. The anal area is red and inflamed, and there is often flatulence with a foul odor.

Bodywork

Hydrotherapy

A sitz bath, if it's comfortable for you, offers temporary relief of pain and swelling.

Other Recommendations

Keep moving. A daily walk will improve your circulation and keep you regular.

INSOMNIA

In the last trimester, it may be difficult to find a comfortable position to sleep in. Changing moods can also make it hard to get a good night's sleep.

TREATMENT

Diet

Recommended Food

Pregnant women are often deficient in B vitamins, which are healing to the nerves and necessary for good sleep. Incorporate whole grains, green leafy vegetables, and wheat germ into each meal.

Try to have at least one of the following at dinner: turkey, chicken, tuna, tofu, soymilk, and live unsweetened yogurt. Each of these foods stimulates serotonin, a neurotransmitter that helps you get to sleep. They're also low in sugar.

For a bedtime snack, have some turkey or chicken on a whole-grain cracker.

Pregnant women are often low in calcium and magnesium, two nutrients that encourage restful sleep. Eat lots of leafy greens, sesame and sunflower seeds, oats, almonds, and walnuts.

Food to Avoid

You should already be avoiding caffeinated beverages, a common cause of insomnia, but now you need to add refined-sugar products to your list of foods to eliminate. Chocolate, which contains both sugar and caffeine, should be at the top of that list.

℞ Super Seven Prescriptions—Insomnia

Super Prescription #1   Calcium/magnesium
Take 500 mg of calcium and 250 mg of magnesium each evening. Both minerals help relax the nervous system. Some people have better results taking one of the minerals alone in the evening and the other earlier in the day. Experiment to see what works better for you.

Super Prescription #2   Chamomile (*Matricaria chamomilla*)
This relaxes the nervous system. Drink a fresh cup of tea in the evening, or take 300 mg of the capsule form.

Super Prescription #3   Homeopathic Coffea Cruda
Take a low potency (6x, 12x, 30x, 6C, or 30C), as needed, for insomnia. This homeopathic remedy is very specific for people with insomnia caused from overstimulation. You find yourself wide-awake at 3 A.M., with a racing mind.

Super Prescription #4   Homeopathic Ignatia (*Ignatia amara*)
Take a low potency (6x, 12x, 30x, 6C, or 30C), as needed, for insomnia. This is a remedy for insomnia caused by emotional upset—usually grief or a loss. There can be uncontrollable crying, loss of appetite, and mood swings. The person often sighs a lot during the day, and the muscles may twitch during sleep.

Super Prescription #5   Homeopathic Kali Phosphoricum
Take a low potency (6x, 12x, 30x, 6C, or 30C), as needed, for insomnia. It is helpful for insomnia that results from nervous exhaustion caused by overwork or mental strain.

Super Prescription #6   Homeopathic Arsenicum Album
Take a low potency (6x, 12x, 30x, 6C, or 30C), as needed, for insomnia. This remedy is for pregnant women who have tremendous anxiety and restlessness. They often wake up between the hours of midnight and 2 A.M. They tend to be perfectionists and have many insecurities and fears.

Super Prescription #7   Sulphur
Take a low potency (6x, 12x, 30x, 6C, or 30C), as needed, for insomnia. This remedy is for insomnia that comes on from itching at night or from feeling too hot at night. One throws the covers off or sticks one's feet out. There is a strong craving for ice-cold drinks and spicy foods.

Bodywork

Reflexology
See pages 686–687 for information about reflexology areas and how to work them.
If nervous tension is keeping you up, work the diaphragm and the solar plexus.

Hydrotherapy
About twenty minutes before bedtime, soak your feet in a hot bath. Not only will your burdened soles appreciate the attention, but you'll also draw blood away from your head and promote sleepiness.

Stress Reduction

Change, even when it comes in the welcome form of a new child, is always stressful. Spend twenty minutes before bedtime with positive mental imagery and prayer. You'll unwind, destress, and prepare yourself for deep sleep.

Other Recommendations

Use pillows under your back and belly or between your knees to get more comfortable at night.

If you simply can't sleep, lying in bed will only make you frustrated and angry. Instead, have some light reading or another easy activity on hand that you can enjoy during the night. (When the baby comes, you may look back on these idle hours as a gift.)

LEG AND FOOT CRAMPS

Poor circulation, due to hormonal changes and mineral deficiency (usually, calcium and/or magnesium), can cause painful cramps in the leg and the foot. As the baby grows and the pressure on the lower half of your body increases, the cramps may get worse.

TREATMENT

Diet

Recommended Food

Eat sea vegetables, green leafy vegetables (except spinach), soy products, and live unsweetened yogurt for calcium.

Food to Avoid

Avoid caffeine, alcohol, and high-sugar products that deplete the body of minerals.

℞ Super Seven Prescriptions—Leg and Foot Cramps

Super Prescription #1   Calcium and magnesium
Take a complex of these two minerals that contains 500 mg of calcium and 250 mg of magnesium, twice daily. These minerals reduce muscle spasms and cramps.

Super Prescription #2   Homeopathic Magnesia Phosphorica
Take 3 pellets of a 6x potency three times daily. This homeopathic remedy is very helpful and safe in the treatment of cramps and spasms.

Super Prescription #3   Prenatal multivitamin
Take as directed on the container. It provides a base of nutrients involved in relaxing the muscles.

Super Prescription #4   Super green foods
Take a single super green food, such as chlorella or spirulina, or try a blended mixture. These foods provide minerals that prevent cramping and spasms.

Super Prescription #5   B-complex vitamins
Take a 50 mg B-complex to ensure proper nerve and muscle function.

Super Prescription #6   Fish oil
Take 4,000 mg of fish oil daily, for essential fatty acids that support proper blood flow.

Super Prescription #7   Essential fatty acids
Take 1,000 mg of borage, evening primrose oil (*Oenothera biennis*), or black currant oil for essential fatty acids that support proper blood flow.

Bodywork

Massage

Rubbing the legs and the feet will stimulate blood flow and reduce cramping. A regular full-body massage will improve circulation throughout the entire body.

Other Recommendations

- Exercise daily to keep your blood moving. Walking and water aerobics are good, gentle choices.
- A hot compress on the cramped area will relax the muscles.
- Elevate your legs as often as possible, so that blood can flow back up to the heart.

MORNING SICKNESS

Many pregnant women experience nausea and vomiting in their first trimester, as a result of hormone changes. *Morning sickness,* the traditional term, is a misnomer, as the symptoms may occur at any time of the day or the night. If the nausea and the vomiting are continuous or severe, talk to your doctor; you need to be sure that you stay hydrated and that you and the baby are receiving adequate nutrition. While morning sickness during your first trimester is generally considered normal, nausea and vomiting after the twelfth or thirteenth week may be indicative of a serious problem.

TREATMENT

Diet

Your body is telling you what to eat and what not to eat, so it's probably best to follow its advice. Following are some additional dietary suggestions.

Recommended Food

B vitamins ward off queasiness, so start your day with whole-grain toast or crackers. Brown rice, oats, and wheat germ are other good options.

Although it's important to take in lots of nutrients during pregnancy, don't try to force yourself to eat large meals. Instead, plan on several small meals throughout the day.

Leafy greens are rich in vitamin K, which helps prevent nausea.

If you feel nauseated, try chewing a piece of fresh ginger or sucking on a slice of lemon or lime.

℞ Super Seven Prescriptions—Morning Sickness

Super Prescription #1   Ginger root (*Zingiber officinale*)
Drink a fresh cup of tea two to three times daily, or take 300 mg of the capsule form three times daily.

Super Prescription #2   Vitamin B6
Take 25 mg three times daily. Double-blind studies have found this to be effective. Vitamin B6 injections or intravenous administration by your doctor may be even more effective.

A study in the *Journal of Obstetrics and Gynecology* reported that 28 of 32 pregnant women supplementing ginger had improvement in nausea symptoms, compared with 10 of 35 in the placebo group. Researchers found no adverse effects of ginger on pregnancy outcome.

Super Prescription #3   Homeopathic Ipecacuanha

Take a low potency (6x, 12x, 30x, 6C, or 30C), as needed, for relief of nausea and vomiting. A characteristic symptom for this remedy is constant nausea that is not relieved by vomiting.

Super Prescription #4   Homeopathic Nux Vomica

Take a low potency (6x, 12x, 30x, 6C, or 30C), as needed, for relief of nausea and vomiting. Women who require this remedy feel irritable. Along with the nauseousness and the vomiting may be constipation and heartburn.

Super Prescription #5   Homeopathic Colchicum

Take a low potency (6x, 12x, 30x, 6C, or 30C), as needed, for relief of nausea and vomiting. Women who benefit from this remedy feel nauseous from the smell or the sight of food, especially eggs and fish.

Super Prescription #6   Homeopathic Tabacum

Take a low potency (6x, 12x , 30x, 6C, or 30C), as needed, for relief of nausea and vomiting. Women who benefit from this remedy have tremendous nausea and a sinking feeling in their stomachs. Any movement makes them nauseous.

Super Prescription #7   Vitamin K

Take 5 mg daily or receive injections or intravenous administration from your doctor. Vitamin K has been shown to relieve morning sickness.

General Recommendations

Chamomile (*Matricaria chamomilla*) and red raspberry (*Rubus idaeus*) tea help some women with morning sickness. Drink the tea throughout the day.

Homeopathy

Homeopathic Lacticum Acidum is for women who feel morning sickness as soon as they wake up. There is increased salivation and a burning sensation in the stomach. They feel better after eating.

Homeopathic Pulsatilla (*Pulsatilla pratensis*) is for women who crave sweets and creamy foods but get digestive upset from them. They tend to be weepy and easily upset. They should take a low potency (6x, 12x, 30x, 6C, or 30C), as needed, for relief of nausea and vomiting.

Homeopathic sepia is helpful when odors trigger morning sickness. The woman craves sweets, vinegar, and sour foods. Emotionally, she is irritable and feels worn out.

Other Recommendations

Acupuncture and acupressure have been found to be effective for morning sickness. Commercial acupressure wristbands that relieve nausea are available.

PREECLAMPSIA

Preeclampsia, also referred to as toxemia, is a problem that occurs in some women during pregnancy. It can happen during the second half of pregnancy and involves the combination of high blood pressure, swelling, and large amounts of protein in their urine. Preeclampsia is more common in a woman's first pregnancy and in women whose mothers or sisters had preeclampsia. The risk of preeclampsia is higher in women carrying multiple babies, in teenage mothers, and in women older than age forty. Other women at risk include those who had high blood pressure or kidney disease before they became pregnant. The cause of preeclampsia isn't known, although nutritional deficiencies appear to be a major factor.

TREATMENT

Diet

Recommended Food
Plenty of water is important, as is adequate protein.

Essential fatty acids, as found in fish, nuts and seeds, and ground flaxseeds, are recommended.

Food to Avoid
Avoid foods that are high in trans-fatty acids, as found in fried food (cooked vegetable oils), margarine, and some packaged foods.

℞ Super Seven Prescriptions—Preeclampsia

Super Prescription #1   Calcium
Take 500 mg three times daily. Several studies have found that calcium supplementation reduces the risk of developing preeclampsia, especially in women who are at high risk.

Super Prescription #2   Magnesium
Take 500 mg twice daily. Some studies have shown magnesium to reduce the risk of developing preeclampsia, plus it helps to lower blood pressure.

Super Prescription #3   Homeopathic Apis (*Apis mellifica*)
Take a 30C potency twice daily if you have swelling of the lower limbs or protein in your urine.

Super Prescription #4   Homeopathic Natrum Muriaticum
Take a 30C potency twice daily if you have swelling and water retention, as well as a strong craving for salt and an intolerance of warm rooms.

Super Prescription #5   Homeopathic Sepia
Take a 30C potency twice daily if you have preeclampsia, feelings of chilliness, and irritability. You have a strong craving for chocolate.

Super Prescription #6   Homeopathic Lachesis
Take a 30C potency twice daily if you have very high blood pressure, accompanied by great heat and flushing of the skin.

Super Prescription #7   Prenatal multivitamin
A high-quality prenatal multivitamin is recommended to provide a base of nutrients that promote good health. Particularly important are vitamins B2 and B6.

General Recommendations

Vitamins E-complex and C may be helpful as antioxidants. Take 400 IU daily of vitamin E and 500 mg of vitamin C.

STRETCH MARKS

When your body expands to accommodate the baby, the fibers of the skin can tear, leaving thin, red lines that eventually turn white or silver. There are a few ways to prevent stretch marks, but once you have them, they won't go away (although with time, they do fade significantly.)

TREATMENT

Diet

Recommended Food

Eat wheat germ and use cold-pressed oils in your salad dressings and cooking. The vitamin E in these products promotes skin elasticity.

Essential fatty acids (EFAs) also keep the skin healthy and pliant. Fish, flaxseeds, and flaxseed oil are all high in EFAs, as are the cold-pressed oils mentioned earlier.

℞ Super Prescription—Stretch Marks

Super Prescription #1　Vitamin E oil
Apply the oil to the stretch marks each morning and evening.

VARICOSE VEINS

These enlarged veins on the surface of the leg are caused by the weight of the baby and by hormonal changes. Straining to have bowel movements also places pressure on the veins. If you're having trouble passing stools, consult the recommendations for constipation during pregnancy. See the Varicose Veins section (pages 518–523).

TREATMENT

Diet

Recommended Food

Vitamin E will prevent blood clots, a possible side effect of varicose veins. Wheat germ and cold-pressed oils are good sources of this nutrient.

Red- or blue-colored berries are an ideal dessert or snack for you. They fortify vein walls and improve their elasticity.

Buckwheat strengthens capillaries.

℞ Super Seven Prescriptions—Varicose Veins

Super Prescription #1　Bilberry (*Vaccinium myrtillus*)
Take a standardized extract containing 25 percent anthocyanosides at 160 mg twice daily. Bilberry improves circulation and strengthens capillary walls.

Super Prescription #2　Flaxseed oil
Take 1 to 2 tablespoons daily. Flaxseed oil improves regularity and reduces straining. It also contains essential fatty acids that promote tissue healing. *Note:* Reduce the dosage if diarrhea occurs.

Super Prescription #3   Witch hazel (*Hamamelis virginiana*)
Apply it as a gel or a cream to external varicose veins.

Super Prescription #4   Bioflavonoid complex
Take 1,000 mg two to three times daily. Bioflavonoids reduce swelling and inflammation.

Super Prescription #5   Homeopathic Hamamelis
Take a low potency (6x, 12x, 30x, 6C, or 30C) twice daily for varicose veins that are large, sore, and easily irritated and that sting.

Super Prescription #6   Homeopathic Arnica (*Arnica montana*)
Take a low potency (6x, 12x, 30x, 6C, or 30C) twice daily for varicose veins that are large, sore, and easily irritated and that sting. It's also helpful for varicose veins that are swollen and look bruised.

Super Prescription #7   Homeopathic Pulsatilla Nigrans
Take a low potency (6x, 12x, 30x, 6C, or 30C) twice daily for varicose veins in the legs that are hot and painful at nighttime. The legs feel better out of the covers and with the windows open.

Bodywork

Massage
Although a regular massage is usually an excellent tonic for pregnant women, do not rub varicose veins directly. Instead, ask your therapist to work around the affected area.

Reflexology
See pages 686–687 for information about reflexology areas and how to work them.
Work the colon, the liver, and the kidneys to keep your points of elimination open and to reduce the pressure on your legs.

Hydrotherapy
To minimize inflammation, make a wet compress using witch hazel, and apply it to the affected area.

Other Bodywork Recommendations
Make time every day to lie down with your feet higher than your head. Even if you don't suffer from varicose veins, this will improve other pregnancy-related discomforts and will reduce the chances that varicose veins will develop later.

Other Recommendations

- Bicycling is usually recommended to improve circulation, but if you're pregnant, you may find it uncomfortable to ride a bike. Instead, try swimming or aqua-aerobics, which are good nonimpact exercises.
- Maternity support hose are available in many department and specialty stores. It's best to put them on first thing in the morning or after a period of rest, when your legs aren't already swollen. Make sure to get a good fit—anything that's too tight will make varicose veins worse.

REFERENCES

Sahakian, V., D. Rouse, S. Sipes, et al. 1991. Vitamin B6 is effective therapy for nausea and vomiting of pregnancy: A randomized, double-blind placebo-controlled study. *Obstetrics and Gynecology* 78:33–36.

Teglio, L., et al. 1987. Vaccinium myrtillus anthocyanosides (Tegens) in the treatment of venous insufficiency of lower limbs and acute piles in pregnancy. *Quadeni di Clinica Osterica e Ginecologica* 42(3):221–31.

Vutyavanich, T., S. Wongtra-ngan, and R. Ruangsri. 1995. Pyridoxine for nausea and vomiting of pregnancy: A randomized, double blind, placebo-controlled trial. *American Journal of Obstetrics and Gynecology* 173:881–84.

Premenstrual Syndrome (PMS)

Premenstrual syndrome, more commonly known as PMS, is a disorder that affects high numbers—almost 75 percent—of menstruating women. It usually occurs a week or two before bleeding begins and is characterized by a wide range of symptoms, including (but not limited to) bloating, breast tenderness, emotional changes, cramps, and fatigue. Some women with PMS experience just one or two of these symptoms and find them quite mild and tolerable; others are hit with several symptoms, each so intense as to be incapacitating. Most women's symptoms exist somewhere between the two extremes, producing a moderate level of discomfort and at least some disruption of daily activities.

Because so many women experience PMS, Western medicine long considered most PMS symptoms a normal part of womanhood. If a woman had debilitating PMS, she was likely to be dismissed—to a Western doctor, her symptoms were clearly "all in her head." We now know that PMS is a physical disorder—and a highly treatable one, at that.

Each month, a woman's hormones follow a predictable cycle of change. Some fluctuation is absolutely normal and necessary, but when the ups and downs become severe, or when the different kinds of hormones needed to regulate body functions are knocked out of balance, the result is water retention, cramps, fatigue, or any of the other symptoms of PMS. Hormone imbalance is a common problem with PMS. While excessive estrogen and progesterone deficiency (or an imbalanced ratio between the two) are believed by many practitioners and researchers to be the key imbalance, there can also be issues with elevated prolactin (pituitary hormone), increased aldosterone (adrenal gland dysfunction), serotonin deficiency, and thyroid abnormality (usually, low thyroid). One must also consider the role of the liver with PMS, as it is responsible for metabolizing hormones. Improving liver function with natural therapies often helps to lessen the symptoms of PMS.

Poor diet and nutritional deficiencies can be root problems of PMS as well. One must also consider the role of "hormone disrupters" in the environment, such as pesticides and herbicides.

In addition, PMS can be caused or aggravated by food allergies, seasonal affective disorder, stress, and depression; a wise course of treatment will address each of these potential triggers. If you have severe PMS that is not resolved by using the home treatments suggested here, consult with a holistic doctor. You may have an underlying disorder, such as hypoglycemia or an underactive thyroid.

SYMPTOMS

Psychological

- Irritability
- Tension
- Anxiety
- Mood swings
- Aggression
- Loss of concentration
- Depression
- Forgetfulness
- Mental confusion and fatigue
- Insomnia
- Change in libido
- Crying spells

Physiological

- Bloating
- Weight gain (fluid)
- Breast tenderness
- Headache
- Pelvic discomfort and pain
- Change in bowel habits
- Increased appetite
- Sugar cravings
- Generalized aches and pains
- Physical tiredness
- Weakness
- Clumsiness

ROOT CAUSES

- Hormonal imbalances
- Poor diet
- Food allergies
- Seasonal affective disorder
- Stress
- Depression

- Hypoglycemia
- Thyroid problems
- Environmental toxins (e.g., pesticides)
- Poor liver function
- Nutritional deficiencies

Testing Techniques

The following tests help assess possible reasons for PMS:

Hormone testing (thyroid, DHEA, cortisol, testosterone, IGF-1, estrogen, progesterone, prolactin)—saliva, blood, or urine

Detoxification profile—urine

Vitamin and mineral analysis (especially magnesium, calcium, B6, B12)—blood

Food and environmental allergies/sensitivities—blood, electrodermal

Blood-sugar balance—blood

TREATMENT

Diet

A diet that's high in meat, fat, sugar, and salt will make hormones fluctuate out of control and will intensify the symptoms of PMS. It has been shown that vegetarian women have much less circulating free estrogen in their blood than nonvegetarian women do. This does not mean you have to become totally vegetarian. However, it does suggest that a diet that focuses on plant foods leads to less circulating estrogen, thus decreasing one's susceptibility to PMS. A good, wholesome diet can significantly reduce or even eliminate problems altogether.

Recommended Food

Meals based on whole, high-fiber foods will balance your blood sugar, ease digestive problems, and reduce stress on your liver. Vegetables, fruits, whole grains, legumes, herbs, nuts, and seeds should be plentiful in the diet.

Fermented soy products, such as tofu, tempeh, and miso, can also help prevent PMS, due to their hormone-balancing phytonutrients.

Make sure your animal products (meat, poultry, etc.) are hormone free.

Eat at least two servings of green leafy vegetables every day. They're a good source of calcium, which supports and calms the nervous system, and they also have a diuretic effect.

Essential fatty acids, found in cold-water fish, flaxseeds, and flaxseed oil, will reduce inflammation.

Consume 1 tablespoon of ground flaxseeds daily, along with 10 ounces of water, to promote healthy estrogen metabolism.

Vitamin B6 has been shown to significantly reduce the symptoms of PMS. Add wheat germ or brewer's yeast to one of your meals every day.

Food to Avoid

A diet that's low in saturated fat (the type found in red meat and dairy products) helps reduce excess estrogen levels. It is also important to avoid harmful fats, such as trans-fatty acids, which occur in margarine and partially hydrogenated oils. Studies have shown that women who follow a low-fat diet experience a reduction in PMS symptoms.

Food allergies often mimic the symptoms of PMS or make existing symptoms worse. Consult the Food Allergies section, and use the elimination diet on page 253. If you can identify foods that give you trouble, eliminate them from your diet completely.

Sugar throws blood-sugar levels off balance, promoting mood swings and tension. Excessive consumption of highly refined sugar can deplete valuable reserves of chromium, magnesium, zinc, manganese, and B vitamins. These nutrients are necessary for the metabolism of sugar. Sugar also worsens symptoms of hypoglycemia (low blood sugar), especially premenstrually, resulting in symptoms of irritability, poor concentration, sugar cravings, and headaches. Restrict your intake of sugary food throughout the month, and eliminate it during the two weeks before your period.

If you retain water, drastically restrict your consumption of sodium. Processed and junk foods are the highest sources of salt in the American diet.

Restrict caffeine-containing products, such as coffee, soft drinks, chocolate, and some pain relievers. Caffeine worsens PMS symptoms, such as anxiety, depression, and breast tenderness. Instead of coffee, we recommend that you focus on herbal teas, such as peppermint and chamomile.

Alcohol has a dehydrating effect, which only makes many PMS symptoms worse. It also wreaks havoc on your blood-sugar levels. Avoid it during the two weeks before your period.

Detoxification

Every month, plan a vegetable juice fast for one to two days before your symptoms usually begin. If they don't begin at a predictable time, do the fast two weeks before your period starts. This fast will help eliminate the toxins, especially the environmental estrogens, that make PMS worse, and it also gives your liver a break from processing hormonal imbalances.

Studies show that women who consume more sugar also suffer from more severe PMS symptoms. A study in the *Journal of Reproductive Medicine* that included 853 female university students investigated the impact of a high-sugar diet. Researchers found a strong correlation between high sugar consumption and PMS.

℞ Super Seven Prescriptions—PMS

Super Prescription #1   Vitex (chasteberry)

Take 40 drops of tincture or 180 to 240 mg in capsule form of a standardized extract of 0.6 percent aucubine or 0.5 percent agnuside. Take it daily for four to six months. Vitex is the most well-studied herbal treatment for PMS. Improvements are usually noted within two cycles. Do not take it if you are using the birth control pill.

Super Prescription #2   Homeopathic Combination PMS Formula

Take as directed on the container. It contains a blend of the most common homeopathic remedies for PMS. It's very effective for acute relief or can be used preventatively.

Super Prescription #3   Vitamin B6

Take 50 mg daily. Numerous studies have found vitamin B6 to help PMS. It works synergistically with magnesium as a cofactor for estrogen metabolism by the liver.

Super Prescription #4   Magnesium

Take 250 mg twice daily. Magnesium is a cofactor required for the metabolism of estrogen, and it relieves cramping.

Super Prescription #5   Natural progesterone cream

Apply 1/4 teaspoon (10 mg) twice daily to areas of thin skin, such as the insides of your forearms and your wrists, beginning after ovulation (approximately Day 15 if you have a regular 28-day cycle) until one day before your period begins. Natural progesterone is a stronger therapy for women with severe PMS.

Super Prescription #6   Calcium

Take 500 mg twice daily. Studies have shown that this mineral prevents PMS.

Super Prescription #7   Dong quai (*Angelica sinensis*)

Take 300 to 500 mg twice daily, on the last seven days of your cycle. Dong quai reduces the painful cramps and the breast tenderness that are associated with menses. It is thought to relax the smooth muscles of the uterus, thereby relieving cramps.

General Recommendations

Passionflower (*Passiflora incarnata*) gently relaxes the nervous system and improves symptoms of restlessness, irritability, and insomnia. Take 2 ml or 300 mg three times daily for anxiety and irritability.

Dandelion leaf (*Taraxacum officinale*) lessens the water retention that is associated with PMS. Take 3 ml or 300 mg three times daily for the one to two weeks before your cycle when you experience water retention.

Zinc has been shown to be low in women with PMS. Take 15 to 30 mg daily as part of a multivitamin.

Vitamin E-complex helps to effectively reduce the breast tenderness that is associated with PMS. It has also been shown to significantly reduce other PMS symptoms. We recommend 400 to 800 IU daily. Natural vitamin E (d-alpha-tocopherol), with a blend of mixed tocopherols and tocotrienols, is best.

Evening primrose oil (*Oenothera biennis*) is an excellent dietary source of GLA. This essential fatty acid is a precursor to prostaglandins, which have a regulating effect on hormones and other systems of the body. Some studies have shown the benefits of evening primrose oil supplementation for PMS-related depression, irritability, breast pain and tenderness, and fluid retention. Take 2,000 mg (200 mg of GLA) to

Vitex has a balancing effect on progesterone levels, as well as on the hormone prolactin. A two-month study compared the effects of Vitex to those of the pharmaceutical antidepressant Prozac. Both were found to be beneficial overall. Researchers noted that Vitex was more helpful for physical complaints and Prozac more beneficial for psychological symptoms.

Numerous double-blind, clinical trials on vitamin B6 have been conducted over the last twenty years. In one six-month, double-blind, crossover trial, 84 percent of the women undergoing vitamin B6 treatment reported greater improvement than they did during treatment with a placebo. Another study found that vitamin B6 supplementation improved premenstrual acne flare-ups in approximately 75 percent of women.

One double-blind study looked at 497 women who were given either 1,200 mg of calcium or a placebo for three menstrual cycles. By the third month, a significant improvement in four PMS symptoms (negative mood, water retention, food cravings, and pain) was experienced by the group taking calcium.

3,000 mg (300 mg of GLA), along with an oil blend that includes omega-3 fatty acids (flaxseed oil and fish oil).

D-glucarate is a phytonutrient that assists the liver in metabolizing estrogen. Take 500 mg twice daily.

Indole-3 carbinole assists the liver in metabolizing estrogen. Take 300 mg daily.

Milk thistle (*Silybum marianum*) improves liver detoxification. Take 250 mg of a 80 to 85 percent silymarin extract three times daily.

Dandelion root (*Taraxacum officinale*) also promotes good liver detoxification. Take 300 mg three times daily.

Crampbark (*Viburnum opulus*) is an herb that alleviates menstrual cramps. Take 3 ml or 500 mg every thirty to sixty minutes for acute menstrual cramps.

A high-potency multivitamin provides a base of nutrients that promotes hormonal health. Take as directed on the container.

The supplement 5-HTP reduces depression and anxiety associated with PMS. Take 50 to 100 mg three times daily for relief of symptoms. Do not use it if you are taking a pharmaceutical antidepressant or an antianxiety medication.

Homeopathy

Pick the remedy that best matches your symptoms in this section. Take a 6x, 12x, 6C, 12C, or 30C potency three times daily for acute symptoms or two weeks before the menses to prevent reoccurring symptoms. Consultation with a homeopathic practitioner is advised.

Bovista is a good choice when there is PMS accompanied by puffiness in the extremities and swelling. Another peculiar symptom is diarrhea that occurs before or during menses. The woman may feel very awkward and clumsy and have a tendency to drop things.

Calcarea Carbonica is indicated when a woman experiences fatigue, anxiety, and a feeling of being overwhelmed, along with PMS. Other common symptoms include water retention and breast tenderness. The period often comes early and lasts a long time. These women are usually chilly and have clammy feet and hands. They have a strong desire for eggs, dairy products, and sweets.

Chamomilla (*Matricaria chamomilla*) is a great remedy to relieve unbearable, painful menses. The woman feels irritable, angry, and very sensitive to pain. The symptoms are better with motion and worse with warm applications.

Cimicifuga (*Actaea racemosa*) is a remedy for a painful menses that gets worse as the flow increases. The woman experiences cramping and shooting pains that go across the legs or the thighs. Headache stiffness in the neck and the back are common.

Lachesis is specific for the emotional symptoms of PMS, which include jealousy, irritability, suspiciousness, and rage. The symptoms improve once the menstrual flow starts. The woman feels hot and is intolerant of anything touching her throat.

Lilium Tigrinum is a remedy for a premenstrual syndrome that's characterized by great irritability, along with a sensation that the woman's internal organs will prolapse through her pelvis. She crosses her legs to get relief from this sensation. Fresh air brings relief.

Lycopodium (*Lycopodium clavatum*) is for women who experience digestive upset, such as gas and bloating, especially in the late afternoon. They feel irritable and want to boss others around, although they lack self-confidence. They crave sweets and have a large appetite.

Natrum Muriaticum is for a woman who feels depressed and lonely. She feels worse when given consolation or sympathy. Migraine headaches or lower back pain that accompany the menses are common symptoms. There is a strong craving for salt and an aversion to being in the sun.

Nux Vomica is for emotional symptoms of PMS that include impatience, anger, and irritability. Constipation becomes worse with the period. There is a craving for alcohol, coffee, spicy, or fatty foods. The woman often feels chilly and improves from warmth and rest.

Pulsatilla (*Pulsatilla pratensis*) is a great hormone balancer for women with PMS who experience mood swings, weepiness, and irritability. Their symptoms improve when they receive consolation and attention. They desire to be in the fresh air and feel worse in warm rooms. They have a strong craving for chocolate and sweets.

Sepia is for symptoms of irritability and fatigue that accompany PMS. There is a bearing-down sensation in the uterus, as if it is going to fall out, and painful breast tenderness that occurs before or with the menses. Exercise improves the symptoms. There is a strong craving for chocolate and sweets.

Acupressure

See pages 668–675 for information about pressure points and administering treatment.

- Conception Vessel 4 and 6 will reduce the pain of menstrual cramps.
- Conception Vessel 6 also relieves diarrhea and constipation.
- For lower back pain, work Bladder 25, 31, and 40.
- Liver 3 eases tension and stress.

Bodywork

Massage

For back pain and cramps, have a massage that incorporates deep kneading. It will relax your muscles and improve blood flow.

If you have cramps or digestive problems, try this self-massage: Lie down with your knees bent, and press the surface of your abdomen until you find the spots that are most tender. Massage these points with the flat of your hand, using firm but gentle pressure.

Reflexology

See pages 686–687 for information about reflexology areas and how to work them.

Work the areas corresponding to the uterus, the fallopian tubes, the endocrine glands, and the lower spine.

Hydrotherapy

To improve circulation to the pelvic region and to ease cramps, you can use the constitutional hydrotherapy method. See pages 676–677 for directions.

Aromatherapy

Black pepper and rosemary have a warming, soothing effect on cramped abdominal muscles. Use either of these oils in a bath or a massage for best results.

Geranium and rose oils are known to balance female hormones. They also have an uplifting emotional effect. Add them to a massage oil or use them in a bath.

If you want to reduce stress, use geranium or rose oils, as mentioned earlier, or try lavender, bergamot, or jasmine. Use these oils in any preparation you like.

Patchouli and ylang ylang are traditionally used to ignite sexual desire. If PMS has depressed your sex drive, add a few drops of these oils to a bath or a room diffuser. You could also add them to a massage.

Stress Reduction

Although PMS is largely a physical problem, the techniques here will help you address any emotional components of your disorder.

General Stress-Reduction Therapies

Yoga serves a triple purpose for women with PMS: It relieves cramps, improves digestion, and releases stress.

Bach Flower Remedies

If none of the following suggestions suits your individual needs, consult the chart on pages 648–650 to find the remedy that's right for you. Once you've chosen a remedy, place 10 drops of the liquid under your tongue. Hold the drops in place for thirty seconds and swallow. Use as often as needed.

If, in the weeks before your period, you find yourself feeling lonely, obsessed with personal problems, and unusually talkative, Heather will restore your sense of independence.

Olive will relieve the deep fatigue and the exhaustion brought on by PMS.

Scleranthus is for women whose mood swings render them incapable of making a decision and sticking to it.

If PMS turns you into a fast-moving, hyperkinetic workaholic, with no patience for others, take Impatiens. It will encourage greater tolerance and a healthier pace.

Some women experience barely controllable, violent rage as a symptom of PMS. If this happens to you, Cherry Plum will help you resolve your tension.

Other Recommendations

- Women who exercise regularly experience fewer PMS symptoms than their sedentary counterparts do. A daily half-hour walk, even on days when you feel at your worst, can do wonders to both reduce symptoms and prevent them in the first place.
- Place a hot compress on your abdomen to relieve menstrual cramps and gastrointestinal troubles.
- Seasonal affective disorder has been linked to PMS. If your symptoms are worse in the winter, take walks in the morning sunshine, as suggested earlier, and try to spend your daylight hours near a sunny window. See Seasonal Affective Disorder on pages 466–472 for more information and suggestions.

REFERENCES

Atmaca, M., S. Kumru, and E. Tezcan. 2003. Fluoxetine versus Vitex agnus castus extract in the treatment of premenstrual dysphoric disorder. *Human Psychopharmacology* 18(3):191–95.

Rossignol, A. M., et al. 1991. Prevalence and severity of the premenstrual syndrome: Effects of foods and beverages that are sweet or high in sugar content. *Journal of Reproductive Medicine* 36(2):131–36.

Snider, B. L., and D. F. Dieteman. 1974. Letter: Pyridoxine therapy for premenstrual acne flare. *Archives of Dermatology* 110(1):130–31.

Thys-Jacobs, S., P. Starkey, D. Bernstein, and J. Tian. 1998. Calcium carbonate and the premenstrual syndrome: Effects on premenstrual and menstrual symptoms. Premenstrual Syndrome Study Group. *American Journal of Obstetrics and Gynecology* 179(2):444–52.

Prostate Enlargement (Benign Prostatic Hyperplasia)

The prostate is a male reproductive gland that sits at the outlet of the urinary bladder and surrounds the urethra (the channel that carries urine away from the bladder). Normally, the prostate is about the size of a walnut. In many men, however, especially those who are middle-aged or older, the gland becomes inflamed or enlarged. When this happens, the prostate compresses the urethra, obstructing the flow of urine and causing other problems (i.e., infection, bladder stones, etc.).

Benign prostatic hyperplasia (BPH) is the medical term, but the disorder is more commonly known as enlarged prostate. When a man reaches middle age, the prostate often starts growing. There can be several reasons why this growth occurs, but it appears to be mainly caused by hormonal changes associated with aging.

Almost half of all men over forty-five suffer from at least some degree of prostate enlargement. At first, an enlarged prostate produces no symptoms, but as it grows and puts increased pressure on the urethra, urinary problems develop. It may be difficult to start urinating, and once the flow has begun, it may be hard to stop. There may be dribbling in-between urination, along with a sense that the bladder isn't completely empty. Many men find that they awaken several times a night to urinate. Although the symptoms are uncomfortable and disruptive, benign enlargement is usually not a sign of a more serious disease. In some cases, however, the prostate can become so enlarged that the bladder can rarely empty itself completely. This urine retention can lead to an infection of the bladder or the kidneys; in severe cases, a constantly full bladder can place a dangerous level of pressure on the kidneys and even cause them to fail. A poor diet, especially one that's low in fiber and high in saturated fat, likely contributes to prostate enlargement as well.

As men age, their hormone balance changes. Testosterone levels decline, while the estrogen class of hormones increases. One prevailing theory as to why the prostate enlarges centers around the increased conversion of testosterone to one of its metabolites, known as dihydrotestosterone (DHT). The enzyme responsible for this conversion of testosterone to DHT is 5-alpha reductase. It is believed that the activity of this enzyme increases as men age, so that DHT levels increase. DHT is implicated in prostate growth. Recent studies show that there is more to the story than just DHT. In recent years, there has been growing evidence that estrogen plays a role in prostate enlargement. A man's body contains the hormone estrogen, albeit in lesser amounts than in women. Some research shows that the balance between estrogen, testosterone, and DHT is the main issue with prostate cell growth. It is interesting to note that the enzyme aromatase converts testosterone to a potent form of estrogen known as estradiol. Estradiol causes prostate cells to grow and multiply. Keep in mind that pesticides, herbicides, and other environmental pollutants mimic estrogen in the body. It is also postulated that a rise in the estrogen-to-testosterone ratio amplifies the effects of DHT on the cell receptors of the prostate, which leads to cell growth. This relative increase in estrogen also reduces the ability of the prostate cells to clear out DHT. It makes some sense that DHT may not be the major villain in prostate enlargement. Rather, it is the balance between estrogen, testosterone, and DHT—and, likely, even progesterone—that really matters. The point is that proper hormone balance through diet, exercise, nutritional supplements, and detoxification is the key to helping this condition.

Prostatic enlargement responds well to natural treatment. Dietary and herbal therapies are especially effective at reducing the swelling and balancing the hormones. It's wise, however, to have any urinary or prostate problems checked out by a doctor, preferably a urologist, just to rule out any underlying cause. And if you experience weight loss, bone pain, or bloody urine, call your doctor right away.

SYMPTOMS

- Frequent urination
- Urination that is hard to start or stop
- Dribbling
- The sensation of an incompletely emptied bladder
- Increased nighttime urination
- Burning pain with urination
- Reoccurring bladder infections

ROOT CAUSES

- Hormonal changes
- A diet that's high in fat and low in fiber
- Nutritional deficiencies

TREATMENT

Diet

Recommended Food

A diet of basic, whole foods will provide plenty of fiber and will regulate hormone levels. Eat lots of whole grains and fresh vegetables, and get your protein from beans, fish, and soy products. To keep chemicals and pesticides out of your system, buy organic whenever possible.

Tomatoes are an excellent source of lycopene, a phytochemical that has an important protective effect on the prostate. This book usually recommends fresh food, but when it comes to lycopene, there's an important exception: cooked tomato products are actually a more potent source of this phytochemical than fresh ones are. Incorporate both into your meals daily.

Pumpkin seeds are a traditional remedy for prostate problems, and for good reason. They're full of zinc, a nutrient that's necessary for good prostate health. You can snack on raw pumpkin seeds throughout the day, but resist the urge to toast and salt them. You'll just add unwanted fat and sodium.

To reduce swelling, eat cold-water fish, flaxseeds (1 to 2 tablespoons daily, along with 10 ounces of water), and flaxseed oil. These foods are high in essential fatty acids, which are known for their anti-inflammatory properties.

Whirl a cup of pumpkin seeds in the food processor for a few minutes, and you'll have pumpkin butter. It makes a delicious spread for sandwiches or crackers.

Testing Techniques

The following tests help assess possible reasons for prostate enlargement:

Hormone testing (thyroid, DHEA, cortisol, testosterone, DHT, estrogen, progesterone)—saliva, blood, or urine

Intestinal permeability—urine

Detoxification profile—urine

Vitamin and mineral analysis—blood

Digestive function and microbe/parasite/candida testing—stool analysis

Food and environmental allergies/sensitivities—blood, electrodermal

Toxic metals—hair or urine

Essential fatty acid balance—blood or urine

Drink green tea (decaffeinated) instead of coffee, as it promotes healthy detoxification.

Take the aforementioned flaxseeds daily, along with 10 ounces of water. Flaxseeds contain a phytonutrient known as lignans, which balance estrogen levels.

Drink a glass of clean water every two waking hours to keep fluid moving through the urinary tract.

Food to Avoid

Eliminate all fats that are saturated, hydrogenated, or partially hydrogenated. These fats lead to inflammation and have been closely linked with several prostate disorders.

Sugar wreaks havoc on hormone levels and worsens inflammation. Radically restrict your consumption of refined sugar, or, better yet, banish it from your diet altogether.

Processed food is full of chemicals that may cause or contribute to prostate problems. Stay away from it.

Avoid alcohol and caffeine. They are irritants to the prostate gland.

Detoxification

The prostate gland is highly sensitive to environmental and dietary toxins. To flush waste out of the prostate, do a one- to three-day juice fast. Focus on vegetable juices and broths—too much fruit juice will throw your hormone levels out of balance.

℞ Super Seven Prescriptions—Prostate Enlargement

Super Prescription #1   Saw palmetto (*Serenoa repens*)

Take 320 mg daily of a product standardized to 80 to 95 percent fatty acids. Saw palmetto has been shown in numerous studies to improve the symptoms of this condition. It appears to reduce hormone stimulation of the prostate tissue.

Super Prescription #2   *Pygeum africanum*

Take 160 to 200 mg daily of a product standardized to 13 percent total sterols. Pygeum is an extract from the bark of an African tree that has a long history of use, as well as scientific validation, for reducing prostate enlargement.

A study involving three urology centers looked at the effects of *Pygeum africanum* extract (50 mg twice daily) on the symptoms of BPH. Researchers concluded through urine-flow measurements that pygeum induced significant improvements, including with nighttime urination.

> ### Super Prescription #3   Rye pollen extract
> Take as directed on the container (generally, 3 tablets twice daily). Several studies have shown that this extract lessens the symptoms of BPH.
>
> ### Super Prescription #4   Nettle (*Urtica diocia*) root
> Take 120 mg twice daily. Nettles are commonly used in prostate formulas, along with other nutrients. Studies have shown that they lessen BPH symptoms.
>
> ### Super Prescription #5   Beta-sitosterol
> Take 60 to 130 mg daily. Studies show that this phytonutrient improves the symptoms of benign prostatic hyperplasia.
>
> ### Super Prescription #6   Zinc
> Take 100 mg daily for two months and then 50 mg as a maintenance dosage, and take 3 mg of copper, along with the zinc.
>
> ### Super Prescription #7   Essential fatty acids
> Take 1 tablespoon of flaxseed oil or 3,000 mg of fish oil daily. Essential fatty acids reduce inflammation.

Saw palmetto (*Serenoa repens*) has been found to have many favorable effects on the prostate, including

- Inhibiting the activity of the enzyme 5-alpha reductase, which reduces the conversion of testosterone to DHT
- Blocking DHT from binding to prostate cells
- Reducing the effects of estrogen and progesterone on the prostate cells
- Causing smooth muscle relaxation (theoretically allowing the urethra to open more effectively and preventing the back-up of urine)
- Reducing inflammation and edema by inhibiting the effects of inflammation-producing chemicals called prostaglandins
- Altering cholesterol metabolism in the prostate
- Modifying the levels of sex hormone–binding globulin (SHBG)

The *Journal of the American Medical Association* reported a review on the therapeutic efficacy and the safety of saw palmetto extract in men with symptomatic BPH. The authors reviewed 18 randomized controlled trials, involving 2,939 men with BPH. They concluded that saw palmetto was as effective as Proscar (finasteride), a commonly prescribed pharmaceutical medication for BPH. The benefit of saw palmetto, compared to that of a pharmaceutical treatment, was the absence of side effects, such as impotence or loss of libido.

Another study, using before- and after-treatment ultrasound images, demonstrated that the combination of saw palmetto and nettle root reduced the size of prostate swelling in men with BPH.

General Recommendations

Amino acids relieve urinary symptoms of BPH. Take glycine, alanine, and glutamic acid, as this was the combination used in one successful study. Take 750 mg three times daily for two weeks and then 375 mg three times daily as a maintenance dose.

Pumpkin seed oil is often used in combination with saw palmetto (*Serenoa repens*) for the relief of BPH symptoms. Take 160 mg three times daily with meals.

A high-potency multivitamin provides a base of nutrients for prostate health. Take as directed on the container.

D-glucarate is a phytonutrient that assists the liver in metabolizing estrogen. Take 500 mg twice daily.

Indole-3 carbinole assists the liver in metabolizing estrogen. Take 300 mg daily.

Milk thistle (*Silybum marianum*) improves liver detoxification and, indirectly, hormone balance. Take 250 mg of an 80 to 85 percent silymarin extract three times daily.

Homeopathy

Apis mellifica is for prostate enlargement when stinging pain accompanies urination. There may also be urinary retention present.

Causticum is indicated when one loses urine from coughing or sneezing. There can be a pressure sensation extending from the prostate to the bladder. Causticum is also indicated when sexual pleasure during orgasm has diminished.

Chimaphilla Umbellate is a remedy that helps with urine retention. There is often a sensation that one is sitting on a ball. The person may feel as if a ball is lodged in the pelvic floor or may experience pressure, swelling, and soreness that feel worse when sitting down.

Clematis is a specific remedy for swelling of the prostate that leads to slow urine passage or a dribbling of urine.

Lycopodium (*Lycopodium clavatum*) may be helpful for prostate enlargement accompanied by sexual dysfunction, such as impotence. Men who need this remedy often have digestive problems, such as gas and bloating. They tend to feel chilly and crave sweets.

Pulsatilla (*Pulsatilla pratensis*) is for prostate problems with bladder pain at the end of urination. Men who require this remedy tend to get warm easily and feel better in the fresh air.

Sabal Serrulata is a good remedy for urine retention, especially in elderly men. There may be a cold sensation in the prostate or the bladder. It is useful for men with prostate enlargement who are prone to bladder infections.

Selenium is for an enlarged prostate and the involuntary dribbling of urine or prostatic fluid. Symptoms are worse after walking or urination. Impotence is another indication for this remedy.

Staphysagria is for urinary retention and the chronic dribbling of urine. There can be a burning sensation in the urinary tract and the prostate. Men who require this remedy may have suppressed emotions, as well as impotence.

Thuja (*Thuja occidentalis*) is for an enlarged prostate and a frequent urge to urinate. Sometimes a forked stream of urine is seen.

Acupressure

See pages 668–675 for information about pressure points and administering treatment.

- All the bladder points along the groin (Bladder 27–34) regulate the reproductive organs and increase circulation to the prostate. With regular work, they will help reduce inflammation, as well as lower back pain.

Bodywork

Reflexology

See pages 686–687 for information about reflexology areas and how to work them.

Work the areas corresponding to the prostate, the lower back/bladder, and the lymph/groin area.

Hydrotherapy

Hot and cold hydrotherapy in the pelvic region stimulates circulation to the genitals and the urinary tract. Splash first hot water, then cold, onto your lower abdomen. Repeat three times.

Constitutional hydrotherapy is a good long-term treatment for this condition. See the directions on pages 676–677.

Aromatherapy

Bergamot and chamomile reduce inflammation. Add them to a bath, or use them in a full-body massage.

If you have prostatitis, use a few drops of tea tree oil in a bath to fight the infection. This oil can sometimes be irritating, so start by adding just 2 or 3 drops under the tap. If you do not have a reaction, you can add a few more drops the next time around.

For a constant urge to empty the bladder, use sandalwood for its diuretic effect. A bath or a full-body massage is the best means of delivering this treatment.

Stress Reduction

General Stress-Reduction Therapies

Excess unresolved stress can alter your hormones, so keep tension in check by practicing any of the therapies discussed in the Exercise and Stress Reduction chapter on a regular basis.

Bach Flower Remedies

Consult the chart on pages 648–650 to determine the best remedy for your particular needs. Once you've chosen a remedy, place 10 drops of the liquid under your tongue. Hold the drops in place for thirty seconds and swallow. Use as often as needed.

If prostate problems make you feel ashamed, take Crab Apple for a more positive attitude.

Other Recommendations

Exercise to keep your cholesterol down and to work off stress. Low-impact workouts are best, as a jarring exercise like jogging may be painful if you have an enlarged prostate. Avoid bicycling, which puts too much pressure on the prostate.

REFERENCES

Breza, J., O. Dzurny, A. Borowka, T. Hanus, R. Petrik, G. Blane, and H. Chadha-Boreham. 1998. Efficacy and acceptability of tadenan (*Pygeum africanum* extract) in the treatment of benign prostatic hyperplasia (BPH): A multicentre trial in central Europe. *Current Medical Research and Opinion* 14(3):127–39.

Overmyer, M. 1999. Saw palmetto shown to shrink prostatic epithelium. *Urology Times* 27(6):1, 42.

Wilt, J., et al. 1998. Saw palmetto extracts for treatment of benign prostatic hyperplasia: A systematic review. *Journal of the American Medical Association* 280(18):1604–9.

Prostatitis

Prostatitis is an infection or a chronic inflammation of the prostate gland. Unlike an enlarged prostate, it strikes men of all ages. The most common form is chronic non-bacterial prostatitis (NBP), also called chronic abacterial prostatitis. This condition is caused by a fungus, a virus, or mycoplasma infections and often cannot be resolved by antibiotics (especially for the fungal and viral infections). An acute bacterial infection, usually by *E. coli*, is another cause. An enlarged prostate gland predisposes one to this condition, since urine flow is not as efficient and microbes are more likely to accumulate. In addition, pain in the pelvic floor muscles can cause pain in the prostate region.

When infected, the prostate becomes inflamed and tender, and the man has difficulty producing a constant flow of urine. The infection produces other symptoms as well, which may include a fever, chills, a pain in the lower back, and bloody urine. The greatest danger of prostatitis is that it will become a chronic problem, in which the bladder cannot empty itself. As with benign enlargement, this constant urine retention can cause an infection or kidney disorders. We have successfully treated several men who had chronic prostatitis who were unresponsive to previous doctors' treatments with antibiotics. Many of the natural therapies mentioned in this chapter work at the root causes of prostatitis, which include nonbacterial infections and prostate enlargement. Homeopathy can be particularly effective for this condition, as can certain nutritional therapies, such as rye pollen extract.

SYMPTOMS

- Urination problems, as with an enlarged prostate
- Fever
- Chills
- Lower back pain
- Urine with blood or pus
- Pain in the region between the genitals and the anus
- Impotence

ROOT CAUSES

- Infection
- Food allergies
- Dehydration
- Prostate enlargement (contributing to infection)

TREATMENT

Diet

Recommended Food

Eat lots of whole grains and fresh vegetables, and get your protein from beans, fish, and soy products. To keep chemicals and pesticides out of your system, buy organic produce whenever possible.

Pumpkin seeds are a traditional remedy for prostate problems, and for good reason. They're full of zinc, a nutrient that's necessary for good prostate health. You can snack on raw pumpkin seeds throughout the day, but resist the urge to toast and salt them. You'll just add unwanted fat and sodium.

To reduce swelling, eat cold-water fish, flaxseeds (1 to 2 tablespoons daily, along with 10 ounces of water), and flaxseed oil. These foods are high in essential fatty acids, which are known for their anti-inflammatory properties.

Drink green tea (decaffeinated) instead of coffee, as it promotes healthy detoxification.

Take the aforementioned flaxseeds daily, along with 10 ounces of water. Flaxseeds contain a phytonutrient known as lignans, which balance estrogen levels.

Drink a glass of clean water every two waking hours to keep fluid moving through the urinary tract.

Testing Techniques

The following tests help assess possible reasons for prostatitis:

Urine culture—determine whether there is a fungal or bacterial growth

Intestinal permeability—urine

Detoxification profile—urine

Vitamin and mineral analysis—blood

Digestive function and microbe/parasite/candida testing—stool analysis

Food and environmental allergies/sensitivities—blood, electrodermal

Toxic metals—hair or urine

Essential fatty acid balance—blood or urine

Several studies have demonstrated that rye pollen extract improves the symptoms of chronic prostatitis, including prostate pain. One study published in the British Journal of Urology looked at the effects of a commercial rye pollen extract and ninety men with chronic prostatitis. These men were given 1 tablet three times daily for six months. Patients' symptoms, as well as laboratory tests and doctor evaluations after three and six months, found favorable results in 78 percent of the men; 36 percent were reported cured and 42 percent improved.

Food to Avoid

Eliminate all fats that are saturated, hydrogenated, or partially hydrogenated. These fats lead to inflammation and have been closely linked with several prostate disorders.

Sugar wreaks havoc on hormone levels and worsens inflammation. Radically restrict your consumption of refined sugar, or, better yet, banish it from your diet altogether.

Processed food is full of chemicals that may cause or contribute to prostate problems. Stay away from it.

Avoid alcohol and caffeine. They are irritants to the prostate gland.

Detoxification

The prostate glands are highly sensitive to environmental and dietary toxins. To flush waste out of the prostate, do a one- to three-day juice fast. Focus on vegetable juices and broths—too much fruit juice will throw your hormone levels out of balance.

℞ Super Seven Prescriptions—Prostatitis

Super Prescription #1   Rye pollen extract
Take as directed on the container (generally, 2 tablets twice daily). Several studies have shown that this extract improves the symptoms of prostatitis.

Super Prescription #2   Quercitin
Take 500 mg twice daily. Quercitin is a type of flavonoid that reduces inflammation.

Super Prescription #3   Echinacea (*Echinacea purpurea*) and **goldenseal** (*Hydrastis canadensis*)
Take 500 mg of the capsule form or 4 ml of the tincture four times daily. These herbs enhance immune function to combat infection.

Super Prescription #4   Oregano oil (*Origanum vulgare*)
Take 500 mg of the capsule form four times daily for acute prostatitis and twice daily for chronic problems. Oregano oil has powerful antifungal, antibacterial, and antiviral effects.

Super Prescription #5   *Pygeum africanum*
Take 160 to 200 mg daily of a product standardized to 13 percent total sterols. It has been shown to be helpful for this condition.

Super Prescription #6   Zinc

Take 100 mg daily for two months and then 50 mg as a maintenance dosage. Take 3 mg of copper, along with the zinc. Zinc improves immune function and reduces prostate congestion.

Super Prescription #7   Saw palmetto (*Serenoa repens*)

Take 320 mg daily of a product standardized to 80 to 95 percent fatty acids. Saw palmetto reduces the prostate enlargement that often underlies chronic prostatitis.

General Recommendations

Thuja (*Thuja occidentalis*) is a great herb for nonbacterial prostatitis, since it has antiviral and antifungal properties. Take 10 drops three times daily of the herbal tincture form.

Vitamin A enhances immune function. Take 25,000 to 50,000 IU daily for one week.

D-mannose is a special type of sugar that prevents bacteria from being able to attach to the urinary tract and the bladder wall. Take 500 mg four times daily.

Uva ursi can be helpful for bacterial prostatitis. Take a standardized capsule containing 250 mg of arbutin or 5 ml of the tincture four times daily.

A probiotic should be taken in the form of a product containing at least 4 billion organisms daily. It contains friendly bacteria that prevent the overgrowth of harmful bacteria and yeast, which contributes to prostatitis. It is especially important to take if you are using antibiotics. Take it at a separate time during the day, and continue use for two months.

Vitamin C enhances immune function, inhibits the growth of *E. coli,* and makes the urine more acidic so that bacteria cannot grow as easily. It also has anti-inflammatory properties that may benefit men with prostatitis. Take 1,000 mg four to five times daily.

Bromelain has a natural anti-inflammatory effect and has been shown to be helpful for prostatitis when combined with vitamin C. Protease enzyme products also have this benefit. Take 500 mg three times daily between meals. Look for products standardized to 2,000 M.C.U. (milk-clotting units) per 1,000 mg or 1,200 G.D.U. (gelatin-dissolving units) per 1,000 mg.

Cranberries (*Vaccinium macrocarpona*) prevent bacteria from adhering to the bladder wall. This plant is best used for the prevention of urinary tract infections but can be used as part of a comprehensive protocol for acute infection. Take 400 to 500 mg twice daily of cranberry extract capsules.

Homeopathy

Apis Mellifica is for prostatitis accompanied by stinging or burning pain during urination. Urinary retention may also be present.

Causticum is indicated when one loses urine from coughing or sneezing. There can be a pressure sensation extending from the prostate to the bladder. Causticum is also indicated when sexual pleasure during orgasm has diminished.

Chimaphilla Umbellate is a remedy that helps acute prostatitis and urinary retention. There is often a sensation that one is sitting on a ball. The person may feel as if a ball is lodged in the pelvic floor or may experience pressure, swelling, and soreness that feel worse when sitting down.

Quercitin has been shown to be helpful for nonbacterial prostatitis, as well as for prostate pain (prostadynia). One study found that 500 mg taken twice daily for two weeks significantly improved symptoms in 59 percent of men with chronic prostatitis. A separate double-blind study showed that quercitin supplementation for one month improved symptoms in 67 percent of men with nonbacterial prostatitis. The effects of quercitin may be improved with the supplementation of bromelain and papain, two protease enzymes.

Clematis is a specific remedy for swelling of the prostate that leads to slow urine passage or a dribbling of urine.

Lycopodium (*Lycopodium clavatum*) may be helpful for men who have a painful stream of urine. Symptoms are worse after urination. There can also be sexual dysfunction, such as impotence. Men who need this remedy often have digestive problems, such as gas and bloating. They tend to feel chilly and crave sweets.

Medorrhinum is for men with prostatitis that occurs after having gonorrhea or a new sexual partner.

Pulsatilla (*Pulsatilla pratensis*) is for prostate problems accompanied by bladder pain at the end of urination. Men who require this remedy tend to get warm easily and feel better in the fresh air.

Sabal Serrulata is a good remedy for urine retention, especially in elderly men. There may be a cold sensation in the prostate or the bladder. It's useful for men with prostatitis who are prone to bladder infections.

Selenium is for an enlarged prostate and the involuntary dribbling of urine or prostatic fluid. Symptoms feel worse after walking or urination. Impotence is another indication for this remedy.

Staphysagria is for urinary retention and the chronic dribbling of urine. There can be a burning sensation in the urinary tract and the prostate. Men who require this remedy may have suppressed emotions, as well as impotence.

Sulphur is for prostatitis characterized by burning in the urethra or the prostate. Lower back pain is common. Symptoms are worse while standing and after sexual activity.

Thuja (*Thuja occidentalis*) is for prostatitis that develops after being treated for gonorrhea or other sexually transmitted diseases. Sometimes a forked stream of urine is seen.

Acupressure

See pages 668–675 for information about pressure points and administering treatment.

All the bladder points along the groin (Bladder 27–34) regulate the reproductive organs and increase circulation to the prostate. With regular work, they will help reduce inflammation, as well as lower back pain.

Bodywork

Acupuncture and Chinese herbal therapy offered by a qualified practitioner can be helpful for chronic prostatitis.

Reflexology

See pages 686–687 for information about reflexology areas and how to work them.

Work the areas corresponding to the prostate, the lower back/bladder, and the lymph/groin area.

Hydrotherapy

Hot and cold hydrotherapy in the pelvic region stimulates circulation and reduces inflammation. First sit in a warm tub for two minutes, then sit in cool water for thirty seconds. Repeat three times.

Constitutional hydrotherapy is a good long-term treatment for this condition. See the directions on pages 676–677.

Aromatherapy

Bergamot and chamomile reduce inflammation. Add them to a bath or use them in a full-body massage.

If you have prostatitis, use a few drops of tea tree oil in a bath to fight the infection. This oil can sometimes be irritating, so start by adding just 2 or 3 drops under the tap. If you do not have a reaction, you can add a few more drops the next time around.

For a constant urge to empty the bladder, use sandalwood for its diuretic effect. A bath or a full-body massage is the best means of delivering this treatment.

Stress Reduction

General Stress-Reduction Therapies

Excess unresolved stress can alter your hormones, so keep tension in check by practicing any of therapies in the Exercise and Stress Reduction chapter on a regular basis.

Bach Flower Remedies

Consult the chart on pages 648–650 to determine the best remedy for your particular needs. Once you've chosen a remedy, place 10 drops of the liquid under your tongue. Hold the drops in place for thirty seconds and swallow. Use as often as needed.

If prostate problems make you feel ashamed, take Crab Apple for a more positive attitude.

Other Recommendations

Avoid bicycling, which puts too much pressure on the prostate.

REFERENCES

Rugendorff, E. W., W. Weidner, L. Ebeling, and A. C. Buck. 1993. Results of treatment with pollen extract (Cernilton N) in chronic prostatitis and prostatodynia. *British Journal of Urology* 71:433–38.

Shoskes, D. A., S. I. Zeitlin, A. Shahed, and J. Rajfer. 1999. Quercetin in men with category III chronic prostatitis: A preliminary prospective, double-blind, placebo-controlled trial. *Urology* 54:960–63.

Psoriasis

Psoriasis, a common skin disorder, occurs when skin cells replicate too quickly. The skin produces new cells at about ten times its normal rate, but also it continues to slough off old ones at its usual, slower pace. With nowhere else to go, the new cells pile up under the surface, creating patches of red, swollen skin covered with silvery or whitish scales. Psoriasis can appear anywhere on the body, but it most often surfaces on the scalp, the knees, the elbows, the buttocks, and the backs of the wrists. The rash usually doesn't itch, but if you scratch, it may bleed. Psoriasis comes and goes in cycles and leaves no scars, although the area may be thick and dry even in times of remission. The nails may also be affected and may develop stipples and pitted areas.

Occasionally, in a condition known as pustular psoriasis, blisters will rise on the palms of the hands or the soles of the feet. Psoriasis has also been linked to inflammatory arthritis of the fingers and the toes.

Psoriasis can cause a type of arthritis that resembles rheumatoid arthritis in some individuals. The nails are affected in 30 to 50 percent of people with psoriasis, resulting in a pitting, a discoloration, and a thickening of the nails' plates.

The exact cause of psoriasis remains unknown, but the prevailing theory connects the high rate of cell replication to a genetic flaw. This theory is backed up by the large number of cases that run in families. As with most genetic disorders, however, it's also likely that people simply inherit a predisposition to psoriasis. Lifestyle choices play an important part in determining the severity and the frequency of the condition or whether you'll even experience it at all. A poor diet, for example, often worsens this condition. The identification and the treatment of food allergies is the key for some individuals. The digestive tract is a focal point for many people with psoriasis. Poor digestion, especially incomplete protein digestion, leads to the creation of toxins known as polyamines, which contribute to excessive skin proliferation. Also, the overgrowth of *Candida albicans* and various bacteria by-products is thought to worsen this condition. Along with the overgrowth of these microbes is often an imbalance or a deficiency of friendly flora, the good bacteria that help detoxify the body. Liver function is of critical importance, as it is the body's main filtering system. Optimizing liver function with sound nutrition and nutritional supplements can be helpful.

We have also found a connection between psoriasis and a low intake of essential fatty acids (EFAs). Finally, stress, fluctuating hormones, sunburn, and other environmental factors can also contribute to flare-ups.

SYMPTOMS

- Red, inflamed patches of skin, covered with silvery or white scales
- Thick, dry skin in times of remission
- Dull, distorted nails
- Blisters on the palms of the hands or the soles of the feet (in cases of pustular psoriasis)

ROOT CAUSES

- Genetics
- A poor diet, especially one that's low in fiber and EFAs
- Difficulty digesting protein
- Overgrowth of *Candida albicans* and other microbes
- Poor liver function
- Stress
- Hormonal changes
- Sunburn
- Illness or infection
- Certain medications

TREATMENT

Diet

As with all skin disorders, psoriasis is best treated by encouraging the body to eliminate toxins through the bowels and the urinary tract, rather than through the skin.

Recommended Food

Get your protein from fish and vegetarian sources like tofu and beans. These foods are much easier to digest than animal proteins are.

Testing Techniques

The following tests help assess possible reasons for psoriasis:

Hormone testing (thyroid, DHEA, cortisol, testosterone, IGF-1, estrogen, progesterone)—saliva, blood, or urine

Intestinal permeability—urine

Detoxification profile—urine

Vitamin and mineral analysis—blood

Digestive function and microbe/parasite/candida testing—stool analysis

Food and environmental allergies/sensitivities—blood, electrodermal

Toxic metals—urine or hair

Increase your intake of fiber. Eat fresh, whole foods and include whole grains, raw fruits and vegetables, or beans at every meal.

Essential fatty acids reduce inflammation and have been shown to greatly improve psoriasis. Cold-water fish like mackerel and salmon are excellent sources of EFAs, and so are both flaxseeds and flaxseed oil. (Flaxseeds are also a concentrated source of the fiber you need. Take 1 to 2 tablespoons daily, along with 10 ounces of water.)

Many psoriasis sufferers are deficient in zinc and vitamin A. Eat pumpkin seeds for zinc; for vitamin A, eat orange, yellow, or green vegetables.

Drink a glass of clean water every two waking hours to improve digestion, flush away toxins, and reduce inflammation.

Food to Avoid

Avoid red meat, poultry, and milk. People with psoriasis often have difficulty digesting protein, and these foods are the hardest on your intestines. In addition, both red meat and milk contain arachidonic acid, which aggravates inflammation.

Do not eat other foods that are difficult to digest. Fatty, fried, and junk foods all fall into this category, as do products that are high in refined sugar.

Alcohol causes inflammation and triggers psoriasis in many people. Drink only in moderation and monitor your intake; if alcohol leads to a flare-up, you should stop drinking altogether.

In some people, psoriasis is brought on by allergic reactions to food. Read the Food Allergies section, and follow the elimination diet there. If a certain food triggers an episode of psoriasis or makes an existing one worse, remove it from your diet. Gluten, cow's milk, sugar, and citrus fruits are common offenders.

Make sure to avoid caffeine.

Detoxification

A detoxification program will reduce toxic waste and return your digestive system to a more efficient working order. You may discover that detoxification, especially fasting, brings on an episode of psoriasis or makes an existing flare-up worse, but that's because you're shedding toxins at an increased rate. Once your body system is clean again, you may find a dramatic improvement in your skin.

Fast on juices for two to three days. Green drinks and detoxifying herbal teas are good choices for extra cleansing power.

℞ Super Seven Prescriptions—Psoriasis

Super Prescription #1 Hydrochloric acid

Take 1 to 3 capsules with each meal. Reduce if a warm or burning sensation occurs. It improves protein digestion.

Super Prescription #2 Fish oil

Take 10 grams daily of a high-quality fish oil. Fish oil contains a substance known as EPA that has anti-inflammatory effects.

Super Prescription #3 Sarsaparilla

Take 500 mg or 4 ml three times daily. This herb reduces the effects of bacterial toxins that aggravate psoriasis.

Super Prescription #4 Milk thistle (*Silybum marianum*)

Take 250 mg three times daily of an 80 to 85 percent silymarin extract. Milk thistle improves liver detoxification and reduces cellular proliferation.

Super Prescription #5 Vitamin B12

Get a 1 cc injection from your doctor daily for ten days and then twice weekly. Some patients notice an improvement in their psoriasis after six weeks of treatments. Sublingual B12 may also be helpful, at 400 to 800 mcg daily.

Super Prescription #6 Super green food supplement

Take an organic super green food, such as chlorella or spirulina, or a mixture of super green foods, each day. Take as directed on the container.

Super Prescription #7 Digestive enzymes

Take 1 to 2 capsules of a full-spectrum enzyme product with each meal. Enzymes help you to digest food more efficiently.

In a double-blind study, researchers examined the effect of people with psoriasis supplementing 10 grams of fish oil daily for eight weeks versus the results in another group taking a placebo. The fish oil group had a significant lessening of itching, redness, and scaling.

General Recommendations

Flaxseed oil contains omega-3 fatty acids that reduce inflammation of the skin. Take 1 to 2 tablespoons daily.

Reishi (*Ganoderma lucidum*) extract improves liver detoxification. Take 800 mg twice daily.

A probiotic supplement provides friendly bacteria, such as *Lactobacillus acidophilus* and *bifidus,* which are important for detoxification and skin health. Take a product containing at least 4 billion active organisms daily.

Gentian root (*Gentiana lutea*) improves overall digestive function. Take 300 mg or 10 to 20 drops five to fifteen minutes before meals.

A high-potency multivitamin provides a base of nutrients for skin health. Take as directed on the container.

Drink a quarter cup of aloe vera juice for its cooling, anti-inflammatory effect, or apply aloe vera gel directly to the affected area.

Homeopathy

Arsenicum Album is for psoriasis characterized by dry, scaly, itching, and burning skin. Symptoms are better with warm applications. People who require this remedy are usually restless and anxious.

Calcarea Carbonica is recommended when there are dry, scaly plaques that often crack open. People who are helped by this remedy are usually overweight and chilly and have clammy hands and feet. They crave sweets, dairy products, and eggs. They have a sensation of being overwhelmed, anxious, and easily fatigued.

Graphites is for psoriasis that has lesions that ooze, often in a yellow-brown color. Lesions mainly occur on the backs of the hands and the ears, on the head and the scalp, and on the genitalia. Symptoms are usually worse at night.

Mercurius Solubilis may benefit people who seem introverted and formal but are very intense internally, with strong emotions and impulses. They tend to have swollen lymph nodes and moist or greasy-looking skin and are very sensitive to changes in temperature. The areas affected by psoriasis may become infected easily.

Mezereum is for a person who has fine, white, scaly plaques that cover large areas. The skin may itch intensely and crust easily and feels better with cold applications.

Petroleum is a remedy for psoriasis characterized by extreme dryness of the skin all over the body. People who benefit from this remedy usually have very dry skin in general. Itching will be worse at night and from getting warm in bed. Symptoms are much worse in the winter and in cold, dry weather.

Rhus Toxicodendron is for psoriasis characterized by dry, red, chapped, raw skin that itches intensely. Symptoms are better from hot applications or baths. The person is restless and often has a craving for cold milk.

Sepia is one of the most common homeopathic remedies for psoriasis. There is a thickening of the skin, with circular eruptions and dryness. This remedy is recommended for women with a hormonal imbalance. They feel chilly and irritable.

Staphysagria is for persistent psoriasis that erupts after suppressed grief or emotions. The scalp is most commonly affected.

Sulphur is a good choice for intense itching and burning and inflamed eruptions that are worse from warmth and bathing. The lesions are often moist and oozing. It is also commonly used for psoriatic arthritis.

Acupressure

See pages 668–675 for information about pressure points and administering treatment.

- Work Stomach 36 to strengthen your digestive tract.
- For psoriasis related to stress, use Bladder 10.
- If hormonal changes trigger your psoriasis, use Triple Warmer.

Bodywork

Reflexology

See pages 686–687 for information about reflexology areas and how to work them.

The thyroid, which controls the rate of skin-cell replacement, is the most important area of the foot to work.

Work the kidneys and the liver to purify the blood.

For hormone regulation, stimulate the endocrine glands.

Hydrotherapy

Constitutional hydrotherapy is a good long-term therapy for psoriasis, as it promotes detoxification. See pages 676–677 for details.

Aromatherapy

Lavender oil reduces inflammation and relieves stress. Add a few drops to a lotion or a cream, and rub it gently into the affected areas of skin, while breathing deeply to inhale the scent.

Stress Reduction

General Stress-Reduction Therapies

If stress brings on your psoriasis, you may actually be lucky: People with stress-induced psoriasis have a much greater chance of controlling their condition than do people with other triggers. Any stress-reduction technique will help; choose one you are comfortable with.

Bach Flower Remedies

If psoriasis makes you feel ashamed, Crab Apple will help you feel clean again.
Gorse is for people who've given up hope of finding a cure.
If you tend to be indecisive and doubt your own judgment, use Cirato.

Other Recommendations

- Many people find that mild sunlight greatly improves psoriasis. Try taking a walk in the morning sun; the exercise will reduce stress and improve your digestion.
- If you have patches of psoriasis on your scalp, do not use a blow dryer. Let your hair dry naturally instead.
- Your doctor may prescribe a topical agent for psoriasis. Although these drugs improve the condition temporarily, the problem will return when you stop using them. It's better to rely on measures that address the root of the problem.
- Sometimes other medications can trigger psoriasis. If you're taking non-steroidal anti-inflammatories, lithium, chloroquine, or beta-blockers, talk to your doctor about possible substitutions.
- See the Candidiasis section. Treatment of underlying candida problems can be helpful.
- We have seen low thyroid function be an aggravator of this condition. See the Hypothyroidism section for more information. In addition, the use of synthetic hormone replacement in menopausal women may be an irritant to the skin. See the Menopause section for natural ways to balance your hormones.

REFERENCES

Bittiner, S. B., W. F. G. Tucker, I. Cartwright, and S. S. Bleehen. 1988. A double-blind, randomised, placebo-controlled trial of fish oil in psoriasis. *Lancet* i:378–80.

Rosacea

Rosacea is an inflammatory skin disorder in which the nose, the cheeks, the forehead, or the chin are chronically reddened and prone to breaking out in acne-like welts. Unlike acne, however, rosacea never produces blackheads or whiteheads, and it rarely appears during adolescence. Instead, rosacea generally sets in during a person's thirties or forties, beginning with a mild pink blush that doesn't go away. If treated early, the condition may never progress any further or may even recede a bit. But in advanced cases, it can cause permanent thickening and redness, especially on the nose.

Although women are more likely to have rosacea than men are, men who do have rosacea tend to have more severe cases.

Anything that dilates blood vessels in the face can lead to a flare-up of rosacea. Specific triggers differ from person to person, but the most common are alcohol, hot liquids, coffee, spicy or fatty foods, extreme temperatures, sun exposure, harsh wind, and stress. It's important to minimize the exposure to triggers, because each time the blood vessels expand, they lose some elasticity. Over time, they become incapable of constricting properly and they remain in a dilated state—hence the redness. A person who already has the early flushing of rosacea will find that triggers make his or her face even redder, or that they lead to pimples that may or may not disappear when the trigger is removed.

Although we understand the elements that make rosacea worse, there is no one underlying cause of this. Skin conditions generally point to some kind of digestive problem, and rosacea is no exception. Many rosacea sufferers have been found to have low levels of stomach acid, which prevents proper digestion of trace minerals and possibly the overgrowth of bacteria that aggravates the skin. Sluggish bowels and constipation may have a similar effect on digestion. And whenever pimples or red spots appear, it's likely that the skin is pushing out toxins that an impaired digestive tract is unable to process. Leaky gut syndrome, which is characterized by malabsorption, may be an issue for people with rosacea. Also, B-vitamin deficiencies, especially of B12, are common with this condition. Friendly flora that are involved with detoxification and that prevent the overgrowth of infectious bacteria are often depleted. We have also found that rosacea becomes a problem as the result of a hormone imbalance. Premenopausal and menopausal woman often find that rosacea starts to act up until they get their hormones balanced with natural therapies. On the other hand, synthetic hormone replacements and birth control pill use initiate or worsen this condition for some women. Finally, hidden food allergies may cause flushing that is mistaken for rosacea.

Conventional treatment for rosacea involves antibiotics, either oral or topical, which have a minimal effect and which must be taken continuously. While people with severe cases that may lead to disfigurement might want to consider medication, most people will be better off making an effort to avoid their personal triggers and improve their digestion.

SYMPTOMS

- Redness across the nose, the cheeks, the forehead, or the chin
- Red pimples or welts

ROOT CAUSES

- Repeated exposure to rosacea triggers (alcohol, wind, sun, etc.)
- Low levels of stomach acid
- Constipation
- A diet that's high in fat and low in fiber
- Food allergies
- Nutritional deficiencies (especially of B vitamins)
- Dysbiosis (imbalance of the gut bacteria)
- Hormone imbalance
- Reaction to synthetic hormones

Testing Techniques

The following tests help assess possible reasons for rosacea:

Hormone testing (thyroid, DHEA, cortisol, testosterone, IGF-1, estrogen, progesterone)—saliva, blood, or urine

Intestinal permeability—urine

Detoxification profile—urine

Vitamin and mineral analysis (especially B12)—blood

Digestive function and microbe/parasite/candida testing—stool analysis

Food and environmental allergies/sensitivities—blood, electrodermal

---

TREATMENT

Diet

Recommended Food

Eat lots of raw foods. In their natural state, vegetables, fruits, nuts, sprouts, and seeds all possess enzymes that help you convert food into the nutrients that are needed for skin and circulatory health. Green leafy vegetables are especially good for rosacea patients, as they're an excellent source of trace minerals.

Drink several glasses of fresh vegetable juices a day. If you have rosacea, it's likely that your digestive system isn't processing food thoroughly, and juices are a potent way to deliver nutrients directly to your bloodstream.

Make sure your diet includes plenty of fiber. If you're eating a couple of servings of raw foods at every meal, you're probably getting almost as much fiber as you need to keep toxins moving through your digestive tract, instead of erupting from your skin. Add whole grains and beans to round out your meals.

Essential fatty acids reduce inflammation. Have cold-water fish from a clean source several times a week, and eat flaxseeds (1 to 2 tablespoons, with 10 ounces of water) each day.

A deficiency of B vitamins has been found in many people who have rosacea. Brown rice, oats, wheat germ, nutritional brewer's yeast, and whole-grain bread and crackers are all good sources. If you tend to be anxious, B vitamins will also help you feel calmer.

It's generally inadvisable to take antibiotics for most cosmetic disorders (save them for the more severe infections), but if you feel you must take them, be sure to eat some live unsweetened yogurt or another cultured product every day. Cultured foods replace the "friendly" intestinal bacteria that antibiotics strip away.

Food to Avoid

Avoid food items that make you flush. Spicy food, caffeine, and alcohol are tripwires for most rosacea sufferers. Sugar and iodized salt may also dilate your blood vessels. Learn which foods bother your skin, and eliminate them from your diet.

Be careful of food and drinks that are hot in temperature. Allow hot beverages and soups to cool before you eat them.

Saturated fat has an inflammatory effect on many body systems, including the skin. If you stay away from red meat and fried, greasy foods, you'll also improve your digestion.

Food allergies may mimic the symptoms of rosacea or make an existing problem worse. Read the Food Allergies section on pages 251–256, and follow the elimination diet there.

Detoxification

Follow a one- to three-day juice fast to clean toxins and irritants from your body and to put your digestive system in optimum working order. You should drink a variety of liquids during your fast, but green drinks and cleansing herbal preparations are especially supportive of detoxification.

℞ Super Seven Prescriptions—Rosacea

Super Prescription #1   Gentian root (*Gentiana lutea*)
Gentian root improves overall digestive function. Take 300 mg or 10 to 20 drops five to fifteen minutes before meals. It also works well as part of a bitters digestion formula.

Super Prescription #2   Betaine hydrochloride
Take 1 to 3 capsules with each meal. Reduce the dose if you feel a warming or burning sensation. This supplement improves stomach acidity and digestion, especially of proteins. It also prevents the overgrowth of bacteria in the digestive tract that may influence rosacea.

Super Prescription #3   B-complex vitamins
Take a 50 mg B-complex twice daily. It supplies B vitamins that improve rosacea.

Super Prescription #4   Vitamin B12
Take 400 to 800 mcg sublingually or 1 cc injection by your doctor weekly. This B vitamin works to reduce flare-ups of rosacea.

Super Prescription #5   Burdock root (*Articum lappa*)
Take 300 mg or 3 ml three times daily. Burdock has historically been prescribed for rosacea and other chronic skin disorders. It appears to improve detoxification, as well as hormone balance.

Super Prescription #6   Natural progesterone
See the Menopause section for proper usage, which depends on where you are with your menopausal transition. This hormone has anti-inflammatory benefits and improves skin conditions if it is deficient and then supplemented correctly.

Super Prescription #7   Probiotic
Take a product containing at least 4 billion active organisms twice daily, thirty minutes after meals. It supplies friendly bacteria, such as *Lactobacillus acidophilus* and *bifidus,* that improve skin health.

General Recommendations

Milk thistle (*Silybum marianum*) improves liver function and detoxification for optimal skin health. Take 250 mg three times daily of a 80 to 85 percent silymarin extract.

Digestive enzymes help you to digest food more efficiently. Take 1 to 2 capsules of a full-spectrum enzyme product with each meal. Lipase enzymes that digest fat appear to be particularly important for people with this condition.

Black cohosh (*Cimicifuga racemosa*) improves hormone balance for premenopausal and menopausal women affected by rosacea. Take 80 mg of a 2.5 percent triterpene glycoside extract daily.

Studies completed during the early part of the twentieth century found that a significant percentage of people with rosacea had low stomach acid (hypochlorhydria). Supplementation with hydrochloric acid resulted in an improvement of their skin.

A study of ninety-six people with rosacea found that supplementation with six tablets of brewer's yeast plus iron resulted in an improvement of their skin lesions.

Green tea (*Camellia sinensis*) contains a rich source of antioxidants and substances that assist detoxification. Drink the organic tea regularly (2 cups or more daily) or take 500 to 1,500 mg of the capsule form.

Essential fatty acids reduce inflammation of the skin. Take 1 to 2 tablespoons of flaxseed oil or 5 grams of fish oil daily, or a formulation that contains a mixture of omega-3, 6, and 9 fatty acids.

Reishi (*Ganoderma lucidum*) extract improves liver function, which is important for healthy skin. Take 800 mg twice daily.

A super green food supplement supplies phytonutrients that improve skin health. Take an organic super green food such as chlorella, spirulina, alfalfa, or a mixture of super green foods each day. Take as directed on the container.

Aloe vera gel is soothing and anti-inflammatory. Apply it directly to the affected area. Test it out on a small patch of your skin first, as you may be highly sensitive to many preparations, even gentle herbal ones.

Homeopathy

Choose the appropriate remedy from the following list, and take 6C three times daily for up to three weeks.

Use a combination acne formula or one of the following if it matches your symptoms. Use a 6x, 12x, 6C, 12C, or a 30C potency for two weeks. If there is improvement, discontinue using unless symptoms return.

Arsenicum Album is for hot, dry, and flaky skin. The person tends to be anxious and restless, gets cold easily, and prefers warm drinks.

Hepar Sulfuris may provide relief if you have several pus-filled spots that are painful when touched, and if the skin lesions feel better with a warm compress.

Pulsatilla (*Pulsatilla pratensis*) is for rosacea associated with the hormonal changes of puberty, menstrual onset, or menopause. Women tend to be sensitive and weepy. They crave sweets. They feel better in the fresh air and worse in warm rooms.

Sepia is for rosacea associated with the hormonal changes of puberty, menstrual onset, or menopause. Great irritability and fatigue are present. The woman craves chocolate and salty and sour foods. She tends to get chilly easily.

Sulphur is for chronic redness and inflammation that is worsened by the sun, hot baths or showers, and warm climates. The person has a high thirst for cold drinks and prefers a cool climate.

Acupressure

See pages 668–675 for information about pressure points and administering treatment.
- Stomach 36 improves digestion and the absorption of nutrients.
- Spleen 10 clears excess heat from the blood.
- Stomach 3 will clear up rosacea blemishes.
- Use Bladder 10 if rosacea is aggravated by stress.

Bodywork

Reflexology
See pages 686–687 for information about reflexology areas and how to work them.
To cleanse your blood, work the liver and the kidneys.
If you need to reduce stress, work the solar plexus and the diaphragm.

Hydrotherapy

Some people find that a warm foot bath pulls heat away from the face; for others, this treatment simply makes their faces even more inflamed. In no case you should use hot water for the foot bath, nor should you take hot baths, showers, or saunas.

Aromatherapy

Try placing a cool—not cold—compress made with lavender oil on your skin to reduce heat and swelling. Take advantage of the relaxing scent, and breathe deeply.

Stress Reduction

It's helpful if you can minimize stress before it brings on a flare-up (which usually leads to even more stress). As soon as you feel any anxiety, take a moment to breathe deeply. If you have five or ten minutes, try a brief meditation session.

Bach Flower Remedies

If rosacea redness or breakouts make you feel embarrassed or ashamed, take Crab Apple.

People who are highly efficient but find it frustrating to be around others who are slower should take Impatiens to develop their tolerance.

Gorse will brighten the outlook of people who despair of ever finding a cure for their disorder.

Other Recommendations

Bright sunlight is one of the most common rosacea triggers. Stay out of the midday sun, and when you do go outside, wear protective clothing and sunscreen. If over-the-counter sunscreens irritate your skin, ask your doctor about a gentle prescription formula.

Avoid intense exercise. You should still participate in some activity for thirty minutes a day, but you might want to stay in the lower range of your target heart rate. Don't go to gyms that lack proper ventilation and cooling systems.

Beauticians who see rosacea acne and dry skin may want to sell you facial treatments, but resist the temptation. The skin manipulation and the steam of facials will only make your condition much worse. If you want a relaxing, indulgent experience, have a body massage instead.

Limit the time you spend in cold and windy weather. When you must go outside, cover your face with a soft scarf or even a ski mask made from hypoallergenic material.

If you want to wear makeup, use gentle, hypoallergenic cosmetics and makeup-removal products.

If you are taking a synthetic hormone replacement, consult with a holistic doctor for a more natural approach, as these hormones can contribute to your acne rosacea.

REFERENCES

Ryle, J. A., et al. 1920. Gastric analysis in acne rosacea. *Lancet* 2:1195–96.

Tulipan, L. 1947. Acne rosacea: A vitamin B complex deficiency. *Archives of Dermatology* 56:589–91.

Seasonal Affective Disorder (SAD)

Seasonal affective disorder (SAD) is characterized by symptoms of depression that develop in the dark winter months and that lift with the onset of spring and summer. Although many of us feel a little less energetic in the winter, people with SAD suffer from more than just a prolonged bad mood. They have a medical condition typified by fatigue, poor concentration, and an intense craving for carbohydrates. They may also feel an overwhelming need for sleep, although the sleep itself is rarely refreshing. This general slowdown of the body, combined with an excessive intake of carbohydrates, may lead to weight gain and a suppressed immune system. Seasonal affective disorder should not be confused with the depression that afflicts some people during the holidays, when unresolved conflicts or problems tend to rise to the surface.

The most compelling theory regarding the cause of SAD has to do with the decreased amount of light that is available in the winter. A U.S. winter's day can have fewer than eight hours of sunlight, compared to sixteen hours of sun in the summer. In the last few years, we've learned that there's a reason that people feel more exuberant in the summer: Natural sunlight affects a substance in our bodies called melatonin, by acting as a control mechanism for it. As the sun sets, our pineal glands (located in our brains) sense the decrease in light and begin to secrete the sleep-inducing hormone melatonin. Melatonin secretion can be magnified by increasing our exposure to sunlight during the day. But when we're deprived of sunlight, there's nothing to keep melatonin levels in check, and it takes all our effort just to get out of our warm beds in the morning. Also, our stress hormone cortisol may rise, which contributes to fatigue, insomnia, depression, and decreased immunity. In addition, low levels of the neurotransmitter serotonin may occur, which contributes to depression. Researchers have found that serotonin production is directly affected by the duration of bright sunlight.

It is unclear why some people are affected by a lack of sunlight more than others. What has been demonstrated time and time again, however, is that light therapy is the most effective way to alleviate the symptoms of SAD. If you suffer from winter depression, there's a very good chance that you'll benefit greatly from just a few simple changes: utilizing specific light therapy, installing full-spectrum lights that imitate the effects of the sun, spending time outdoors every day, and arranging your life so that you're near a window as often as possible. Other natural treatments, including dietary changes and some herbal supplements, will round out an effective course of action for lifting the "winter blues."

SYMPTOMS

- Fatigue and lethargy
- Increased desire to sleep
- Fitful, unrestful sleep
- Inability to concentrate
- Cravings for sweets and other carbohydrates
- Weight gain
- Reduced sex drive

ROOT CAUSE

- Lack of natural sunlight

Testing Techniques

The following tests help assess possible causes of SAD:

Hormone testing (thyroid, DHEA, cortisol, testosterone, IGF-1, estrogen, progesterone)—saliva, blood, or urine

Intestinal permeability—urine

Detoxification profile—urine

Vitamin and mineral analysis (especially magnesium, B12, folic acid, B1)—blood

Digestive function and microbe/parasite/candida testing—stool analysis

Food and environmental allergies/sensitivities—blood, electrodermal

Blood-sugar balance—blood

Toxic metals—hair or urine analysis

Amino acid analysis—blood or urine

TREATMENT

Diet

Recommended Food

One way to maintain a good mood is to keep your blood-sugar levels steady. Vegetables and lean protein will stabilize blood sugar. Make a small meal or a snack of them every few hours to ward off the urge for bread or sweets. When you do eat carbohydrates, make sure they're complex carbohydrates, like oats, brown rice, or whole wheat. These foods are high in fiber, which slows the release of sugars into your bloodstream.

Put turkey, chicken, tuna, or salmon on your daily menu. These foods are high in protein, which you need for energy, and tryptophan, which stimulates the "feel-good" hormone in your brain.

B vitamins act as a tonic on the nervous system. Include brewer's yeast, green leafy vegetables, and live unsweetened yogurt in your meals or snacks.

Brussels sprouts are a perfect food for SAD sufferers. Brussels sprouts are a concentrated source of vitamin C, which fights fatigue and has a stimulating effect on your mood. Unlike citrus fruits, brussels sprouts are also low in sugar. Cooking destroys vitamin C, so eat brussels sprouts raw, perhaps in a salad or served with a dip.

Food to Avoid

Try to resist your cravings for sugar, bread, and other simple carbohydrates. Although these foods may temporarily lift your mood, your blood sugar will soon crash, leaving you feeling even worse than before. And the weight gain that often results from overindulging in carbohydrates will aggravate your fatigue and leave you susceptible to colds, the flu, and other winter ailments. If you must treat yourself to simple carbohydrates, make sure to have them as part of a complete meal—have an occasional sweet dessert, say, after eating a meal that consists of protein, vegetables, and some whole grains. That way, the sugar won't deliver as potent a punch to your bloodstream.

People with SAD also tend to rely on caffeine to rouse them in the morning and keep them alert during the day. But caffeine works much like sugar does, in that once the rush peaks and declines, you're left feeling exhausted and crabby. Caffeine also depletes your body of several nutrients that are essential for a healthy nervous system. Limit yourself to one cup of coffee or tea a day.

Junk food probably isn't a direct cause of SAD, but it can certainly exacerbate the symptoms: Weight gain, a suppressed immune system, and fatigue have all been linked to the consumption of additives and artificial ingredients. Avoid food that's had all the life processed out of it.

Alcohol is a depressant, so avoid wine, beer, and liquor. If you are so unhappy that you feel as if you need alcohol, talk to a doctor or a therapist. You may have a drinking problem—or you might be headed for one.

Detoxification

If you've been turning to carbohydrates and junk food for comfort, you could benefit from a detoxification plan. To remove excess sugar and toxic build-up from your system, go on a three-day juice fast. Green drinks will be especially stabilizing to your body at this time. At the end of your fast, you'll feel much lighter and more energetic.

℞ Super Seven Prescriptions—Seasonal Affective Disorder

Super Prescription #1   Saint-John's-wort (*Hypericum perforatum*)
Take 300 mg of a product standardized to 0.3 percent hypericin three times daily (a total of 900 mg). Saint-John's-wort (*Hypericum perforatum*) has been shown to be helpful for SAD, when combined with light therapy.

Super Prescription #2   S-Adenosylmethionine (SAMe)
For two weeks, take 200 mg twice daily of an enteric-coated form on an empty stomach. If you notice improvement, stay on this dosage. If there is little improvement, increase to 400 mg two to three times daily. SAMe increases the concentration of brain neurotransmitters that are responsible for your mood. Take a 50 mg B-complex, because B6, folic acid, and B12 are involved with proper SAMe metabolism. *Note:* People with bipolar disorder should use this supplement only with medical supervision.

Super Prescription #3   5-hydroxytryptophan (5-HTP)
Start with 50 mg taken three times daily on an empty stomach. The dosage can be increased to 100 mg three times daily, if necessary. The supplement 5-HTP is a precursor to the neurotransmitter serotonin. Take a 50 mg B-complex, as B6 is required for the proper metabolism of 5-HTP. *Note:* Do not take in conjunction with pharmaceutical antidepressants or antianxiety medications.

Super Prescription #4   B-complex vitamins
Take a 50 mg B-complex one to two times daily. B vitamins such as B12, folic acid, and B6 are intricately involved with neurotransmitter metabolism. Sublingual B12 and folic acid supplements are useful for seniors or people with absorption difficulties.

Super Prescription #5   Fish oil
Take a product containing a daily dosage of 500 to 1,000 mg of EPA/DHA. Essential fatty acids such as DHA improve neurotransmitter function.

Super Prescription #6   Ginkgo biloba
Take 60 to 120 mg twice daily of a standardized product containing 24 percent flavone glycosides and 6 percent terpene lactones. Ginkgo improves blood flow to the brain and enhances neurotransmitter activity.

Super Prescription #7   High-potency multivitamin
This provides a base of nutrients that are involved with brain function.

General Recommendations

DL-phenylalanine (DLPA) is an amino acid used by the brain to manufacture neurotransmitters. Take 500 to 1,000 mg on an empty stomach each morning. It should be avoided by people with anxiety, high blood pressure, or insomnia. Do not take it in combination with pharmaceutical antidepressants or antianxiety medications.

L-tyrosine is an amino acid that also helps depression. Take 100 to 500 twice daily on an empty stomach. Do not take it in combination with pharmaceutical antidepressants or antianxiety medications.

L-tryptophan has been a historic favorite of nutrition-oriented doctors for the treatment of depression. It acts as a precursor for the neurotransmitter serotonin. Take 500 to 1,000 mg three times daily on an empty stomach. This amino acid requires a prescription from your doctor and is available from compounding pharmacies.

Ashwagandha (*Withania somniferum*) improves stress hormone balance and relaxes the nervous system. Take 1,000 mg two to three times daily.

If you are low in the hormone DHEA, work with a doctor to normalize your levels. A good starting dosage is 5 to 15 mg.

Phosphatidylserine improves memory, and studies show that it's helpful for depression. Take up to 300 mg daily.

Vitamin D has been found in studies to help improve mood. It is particularly important for people who do not get regular sunlight, especially seniors. Take up to 1,000 IU daily.

Acetyl-L-carnitine has been shown to be helpful for seniors with depression. Take 500 mg three times daily.

If you feel tense and on edge, several herbal teas can help you calm down. Peppermint and chamomile have mild relaxing properties, but if you need something a little stronger, try hops (*Humulus lupulus*) or passionflower (*Passiflora incarnata*).

Oatstraw (*Avena sativa*) tea is a good tonic for the nerves. Drink a cup as needed.

For insomnia that accompanies or causes depression, valerian or kava kava tea, taken before bedtime, can be quite helpful.

Homeopathy

Pick the remedy that best matches your symptoms in this section. Take a 6x, 12x, 6C, or 30C potency twice daily for two weeks to see if there are any positive results. After you notice improvement, stop taking the remedy, unless symptoms return. Consultation with a homeopathic practitioner is advised.

Arsenicum Album is for people who are susceptible to depression and who also suffer from anxiety and insecurity. They are often perfectionists who may have severe phobias. Restlessness and insomnia between 12 and 2 A.M. are common.

Aurum Metallicum is for deep depression, in which there are thoughts of suicide. The person feels no joy and is in despair. There is relief from being in the sun. *Note:* Suicidal tendencies should always be discussed with a doctor.

Ignatia (*Ignatia amara*) eases depression that is brought on by grief or emotional trauma and that is characterized by rapid mood swings. Frequent sighing and a sensation of a lump in the throat are characteristics of people who benefit from this remedy.

Kali Phosphoricum is for depression as a result of overwork. Mental fatigue is a common symptom that this remedy will help.

Natrum Muriaticum is for depressed people who do not reveal their emotions and who hold their feelings inside. They feel emotionally reserved and withdrawn. They feel a deep need for the company of others but are then aggravated when people console them. They often have a strong craving for salt and an aversion to sunlight.

Pulsatilla (*Pulsatilla pratensis*) is for people who burst into tears at little or no provocation. They may also be driven to seek constant comfort and reassurance. They are very sensitive and feel better from crying, attention, sweets, and being in the open air. Their symptoms are worse in a warm environment. In women depression is often worse around the menstrual cycle or with menopause.

Sepia is for women who feel indifferent to their families. They have feelings of depression, fatigue, and irritability, as well as a low sex drive. They feel worse when others console them and better when they exercise. They are usually chilly. They have a strong craving for sweets (chocolate) and salty or sour foods. Depression that is associated with a hormone imbalance, as seen with PMS and menopause, is a strong indication for this remedy.

Staphysagria is for people who have suppressed emotions (such as anger) that contribute to depression. They usually are quiet and do not stand up for themselves, which results in their shame and resentment. Headaches and insomnia are also common.

Acupressure

See pages 668–675 for information about pressure points and administering treatment.

- Lung 1 relieves fatigue and depression. It also improves concentration.
- Other points that stimulate energy are Bladder 23, Gallbladder 20, and Stomach 36.

Bodywork

Massage

A circulatory massage will get your blood flowing and will increase your energy levels.

If you don't have the time or the money for a professional massage, ask a loved one to give you a head massage. This therapy stimulates blood flow to the brain.

Reflexology

See pages 686–687 for information about reflexology areas and how to work them.

To improve brain function, work the big toe, which controls the head.

Work the solar plexus and the diaphragm to balance the nervous system.

Hydrotherapy

Hot and cold hydrotherapy is an invigorating way to increase circulation and energy.

Aromatherapy

Lemon balm, melissa, and geranium will each rouse your spirits. Use them in any preparation you like.

If you have trouble sleeping, place a lavender-scented sachet under your pillow. This relaxing oil encourages a satisfying rest.

Stress Reduction

General Stress-Reduction Therapies

If you're depressed, you're experiencing powerful and probably continuous levels of stress. It is vital for your emotional and physical health that you find at least one way to control anxiety, fear, or tension. Prayer, counseling, and positive mental imagery are all helpful.

If you sense that your depression is more than you can handle, don't hesitate to seek help from a psychotherapist, a religious adviser, or a support group. It helps a great deal to talk to people who work with others' emotional pain.

Make an effort to stay in contact with beauty. If you have a garden or live near a nice park, spend as much time there as possible. And try to bring some of that beauty indoors: Buy yourself a bouquet of flowers, listen to a favorite CD, or hang a water-color of a nature scene on the wall in your office.

Regular exercise has been shown to be effective in improving depression. Try to get some physical activity every day for thirty minutes.

It may sound simplistic, but one quick way to feel better, at least temporarily, is to go dancing. Dancing releases endorphins, powerful hormones that will raise your spirits, and you'll benefit from the touch of other people, not to mention from the pleasure of losing yourself in the music.

Helping others with their problems is a great way to relieve depression.

Bach Flower Remedies

Consult the chart on pages 648–650 to determine the best remedy for your particular needs. Once you've chosen a remedy, place 10 drops of the liquid under your tongue. Hold the drops in place for thirty seconds and swallow. Use as often as needed.

Olive is the remedy for people who feel completely drained of energy and who have lost any interest in social or other activities.

If you have a strong sense of duty that forces you to carry on, despite severe exhaustion, and if you tend to neglect your personal needs and desires, take Oak.

If you have trouble making decisions and suffer from frequent mood swings, take Scleranthus.

Other Recommendations

The very best way to reduce the effects of SAD is to work with a doctor who can help with the proper use of light therapy. This can be done by getting outdoors between 5 and 7 A.M. and being exposed to light or using a bright light box (especially in northern climates, where the sun doesn't rise until later in the morning during short winter days, and frequent overcast skies dim the sunlight). Several different companies make bright light boxes. The most important thing to look for is a brightness rating of at least 10,000 lux. (In comparison, at a distance of two feet a standard 60-watt light bulb gives off only 300 lux.) Make sure the light box is equipped with a UV filter to protect the skin and the eyes. Also, use full-spectrum fluorescent lights in your home and workplace.

- Exercise is a proven mood-booster, and exercise in the sunlight does double duty for SAD sufferers. Take frequent walks outside, or participate in outdoor winter sports like ice-skating or cross-country skiing.

- Human beings weren't meant to spend their days in windowless offices. If changing jobs is not an option—and for most of us, it isn't—take your breaks outdoors. When the weather is good, pack a salad or another healthful lunch and dine al fresco. If it's too cold where you live to eat outdoors, then at least use your breaks to bundle up and take a quick stroll around the block. Even on cloudy, snowy, or rainy days, enough sunlight comes through to make a difference in your melatonin production.

Shingles (Herpes Zoster)

Shingles is a painful condition caused by herpes zoster, the same virus that causes chickenpox. Once you've had chickenpox (and most adults have had the disease at some point in their lives), the virus doesn't leave your body. Instead, it takes up residence in the nerves near the spine, where it lies dormant, usually for the rest of your life. Sometimes, however, herpes zoster is triggered back into activity. This time around, the symptoms are different and more severe. At the beginning of the illness, the area along one branch of nerves, usually one side of your trunk or face, is more sensitive than usual; you may also develop a fever or chills. The sensitive area then becomes acutely painful, and a rash of small blisters develops. After two or three weeks, these clear, water-filled blisters will turn yellow and form scabs. Eventually, they fall off, and sometimes they leave scars.

The nerve pain caused by shingles can be agonizing. You may not be able to bear even the lightest touch, and simple activities like shaving and showering may be out of the question. Even the weight of clothes or bed sheets may be too much. But this pain usually disappears when the blisters drop off. In a few cases, though, the blisters fade but the pain remains for months or even years. This condition, which usually strikes people over fifty, is known as postherpetic neuralgia. No single trigger will always cause herpes zoster to reactivate in the body, but the virus seems to thrive when the immune system is weakened. People undergoing aggressive treatment for cancer or other illnesses are at a greater risk for shingles, as are those who are under extreme emotional stress. Immune-compromising diseases like AIDS or lupus can also leave a body vulnerable to shingles.

Most people will be healthy and pain-free once the disease has run its course. Nevertheless, your doctor should monitor you frequently to make sure the virus doesn't spread to your eyes or your internal organs, where it can have a devastating effect. Sometimes the virus can lead to pneumonia or other secondary infections, which can be deadly to older people or those who suffer from severely compromised immune systems. Between visits to your doctor, you'll find that a wide range of complementary therapies can bolster your immune system and reduce your need for aggressive conventional pain medication.

SYMPTOMS

The symptoms usually appear in the following order:

- Sensitivity in one side of the chest, the back, or the face
- Fever, chills, or other flulike symptoms
- Extreme pain in the sensitive area
- Clear blisters that break out in the affected area
- Blisters turn yellow and scab over, then fall off

ROOT CAUSES

- Herpes zoster virus
- A weakened immune system

Testing Techniques

The following tests help assess possible causes of chronic shingles:

Immune system imbalance or disease—blood

Hormone testing (thyroid, DHEA, cortisol, testosterone, IGF-1, estrogen, progesterone)—saliva, blood, or urine

Intestinal permeability—urine

Detoxification profile—urine

Vitamin and mineral analysis—blood

Food and environmental allergies/sensitivities—blood, electrodermal

Blood-sugar balance—blood

Toxic metals—hair or urine

Amino acid analysis—blood or urine

TREATMENT

Diet

Recommended Food

During a case of shingles, the nervous system is under attack. Heal the damage by eating foods that are high in B vitamins, including wheat germ, brewer's yeast, eggs, and whole grains.

Eat green, orange, and yellow vegetables at every meal. These foods are packed with vitamins A and C, which will speed your skin's recovery from the inflammation and the blisters. Green leafy vegetables are also good sources of calcium and magnesium, which will help heal your nerve endings.

Food to Avoid

Avoid foods that encourage an overly acidic body system. Do not eat red meat, fried foods, or chocolate, and do not drink carbonated beverages (not even fizzy water) or drinks containing caffeine.

Sugar suppresses the activity of white blood cells, the immune system's foot soldiers in the war on illness. Stay away from refined sugar products, including cookies, cakes, sweet baked goods, and sodas, and eat naturally occurring sugars, such as those found in fruit, in moderation.

Detoxification

Follow a two- to three-day juice fast to remove any toxic build-up that may be depressing your immune system. Green drinks, fresh unsweetened cranberry juice (available at health food stores), and miso broth are nutritious and will alkalinize your body system.

℞ **Super Seven Prescriptions—Shingles**

Super Prescription #1   Homeopathic Rhus Toxicodendron
Take a 30C potency three times daily. This remedy is effective if you have burning pain that feels better from warm applications. The rash is itchy, with blisters. See the Homeopathic section for a complete listing of homeopathic remedies for shingles.

Super Prescription #2   Vitamin B12
Have your doctor give you a 1 cc injection daily for five days and then twice weekly. This helps the body recover more quickly and reduces the pain associated with shingles.

Super Prescription #3   Vitamin C
Take 1,000 mg four times daily for immune support. Reduce the dosage if diarrhea occurs.

Super Prescription #4   Capsaicin cream
Apply a cream with an 0.025 to 0.075 percent capsaicin extract two to four times daily to the affected area. This herbal extract blocks pain. *Note:* When this cream is first applied, you may feel a burning, stinging sensation during the first few days, but the pain will subside.

Super Prescription #5   Olive leaf extract (*Olea europa*)
Take 500 mg four times daily, to benefit from olive leaf's potent antiviral benefits.

Super Prescription #6   Echinacea (*Echinacea purpurea*)
Take 4 ml or 500 mg four times daily for immune support and antiviral effects.

Super Prescription #7   Vitamin E-complex
Take 1,200 to 1,600 IU daily for the treatment of postherpetic neuralgia and 400 IU daily to prevent neuralgia. You can also apply vitamin E oil topically.

In a double-blind study, thirty-two elderly patients with chronic postherpetic neuralgia were treated with either capsaicin cream or a placebo for a six-week period. After six weeks, almost 80 percent of capsaicin-treated patients experienced some relief from their pain.

General Recommendations

Lomatium root (*Lomatium dissectum*) is used for its immune support and antiviral effects. Take 4 ml or 500 mg four times daily.

Saint-John's-wort (*Hypericum perforatum*) has antiviral properties. Take 300 mg or 4 ml of the tincture three times daily.

Licorice root (*Glycyrrhiza glabra*) has antiviral properties. Take 500 mg in capsule form or 4 ml of the tincture three times daily. *Note:* Do not use it if you have high blood pressure.

Cat's claw (*Una de gato*) works against viruses and inflammation. Take 500 to 1,000 mg two or three times daily, until the inflammation is gone.

Zinc supports the immune system. Take 30 mg daily, along with 2 mg of copper.

Vitamin A supports immune function. Take 50,000 IU daily for two weeks.

A high-potency multivitamin provides a base of nutrients for immune support. It should include 200 mcg of selenium, a mineral that helps with viral infections.

Homeopathy

Pick the remedy that best matches your symptoms in this section. For acute shingles pain, take a 30C potency three times daily. For chronic shingles discomfort, take a 6x, 12x, 6C, 12C, or 30C twice daily for two weeks to see if there are any positive results. After you notice improvement, stop taking the remedy, unless symptoms return. Consultation with a homeopathic practitioner is advised.

Arsenicum Album is a good remedy when there is a burning, itching pain that is relieved by warm applications. Symptoms are often worse between midnight and 2 A.M. The person is restless, anxious, and chilly.

Apis Mellifica is for people who experience stinging and burning pain that feels better from cold applications and worse from warmth.

Iris Versicolor is indicated when the shingles are accompanied by stomach problems, with burning sensations and nausea. Eruptions tend to appear on the right side of the abdomen.

Mezereum is for people who feel burning that is followed by bright-red eruptions that itch intolerably. The pain is relieved from cold applications and is worse from warmth.

Ranunculus Bulbosus is a specific remedy for when the shingles affect the front or the back of the ribcage.

Rhus Toxicodendron is a great remedy if you have burning pain that feels better from warm applications. The rash is itchy, with blisters.

Sulphur is a good choice for burning pains that feel better from cold applications and worse from warmth. The person is usually very warm and prefers ice-cold drinks.

Variolinum is a remedy that stimulates the immune system to combat the shingles virus more effectively. It can be used in addition to any of the remedies described here for quicker healing.

Acupressure

See pages 668–675 for information about pressure points and administering treatment.

Large Intestine 4 is the point for effective relief of general pain. For more specific treatment of this complex condition, it's best to turn to an acupressure professional.

Bodywork

Reflexology

See pages 686–687 for information about reflexology areas and how to work them.
   To reduce pain and fight the virus, work the spine, in addition to the painful area.
   To heal nerves and reduce stress, work the solar plexus and the diaphragm.
   Stimulate the lower thoracic area to promote healing of the skin.

Other Bodywork Recommendations

Acupressure and acupuncture (especially electroacupuncture) have a good track record of successfully treating many painful conditions, including shingles and post-herpetic neuralgia. Chinese herbal therapy can be very helpful as well.

Hydrotherapy

Constitutional hydrotherapy stimulates the immune system and relieves pain. See pages 676–677 for directions.

Aromatherapy

Tea tree oil is a powerful antiviral agent that will help dry up blisters. Combine it with lavender or bergamot, two oils that have milder antiviral properties but that also reduce pain and stress. You can use a cotton swab to apply the oils directly to the blisters or the painful area, or you can add them to a bath. No matter what preparation you choose, use just a little at first, as tea tree oil is extremely potent and can be irritating in large quantities.

Stress Reduction

General Stress-Reduction Therapies

Constant pain is terribly stressful and can result in further depression of your immune system, so it's essential to find an activity that thoroughly engages your mind and takes you away from your pain, if only for a little while.

Bach Flower Remedies

Consult the chart on pages 648–650 to determine the best remedy for your particular needs. Once you've chosen a remedy, place 10 drops of the liquid under your tongue. Hold the drops in place for thirty seconds and swallow. Use as often as needed.

If you are overworked to the point of burnout, take Hornbeam.

Elm is for people who are depressed and overwhelmed by the tasks of everyday life. This remedy is often combined with Hornbeam.

People with postherpetic neuralgia may come to feel that nothing will ever relieve their pain and suffering. Gorse will help revive their hope and confidence.

If the rash of blisters makes you feel unclean, take Crab Apple.

If you have recently suffered a severe shock, such as a frightening diagnosis, the death of someone close to you, or an accident, take Star of Bethlehem. It will speed your emotional recovery.

Other Recommendations

Seek the consultation of a naturopathic or holistic doctor who can help you with a specific therapy for quicker improvement. Severe cases may also require pharmaceutical therapy.

REFERENCES

Bernstein, J. E., N. J. Korman, D. R. Bickers, M. V. Dahl, and L. E. Millikan. 1989. Topical capsaicin treatment of chronic postherpetic neuralgia. *Journal of the American Academy of Dermatology* (2 Pt 1):265–70.

Sinusitis

The sinuses are cavities in the bones around the nose, the cheeks, and the eyes. These cavities are lined with membranes that produce mucus, and when the sinuses are functioning normally, this mucus serves a protective purpose: It warms and moistens incoming air and filters it for germs. When sinuses can't drain properly, however, the mucus accumulates and becomes stagnant, making the area ripe for infection.

Sinusitis, which is the name for an infection of the sinus cavities, can be quite unpleasant and often painful. The mucus build-up leads to clogged nasal passages, thick drainage, and a general feeling of weariness and discomfort. The swollen membranes feel even worse, because they can fill up the tiny sinus cavities and press against the bones of the face. If you are unsure whether your head congestion is sinusitis, bend forward from the waist. If you feel heavy pressure or pain against your cheekbones or your eyes, you probably have sinusitis.

Sinusitis may be either acute or chronic. Acute sinusitis is usually caused by a complication from another respiratory infection, such as a cold, the flu, or bronchitis. Any of these infections can lead to blocked drainage, which in turn causes sinusitis. If the sinus membranes don't have a chance to heal fully, an acute case can easily turn into a chronic one.

Recurring colds and flus—warning signs of a suppressed immune system—may lead to chronic sinusitis, as can other factors that consistently cause an obstruction of the sinus cavities. Repeated exposure to environmental allergens and irritants, such as mold spores or tobacco, is a common cause, as are food allergies or a diet that's high in mucus-forming foods.

Research has shown that chronic sinusitis is most often related to an immune response to a fungal infection in the sinus cavity. This research was first released in 1999 by a Mayo Clinic study, and the results have since been duplicated in subsequent studies. Natural practitioners often treat people who have chronic sinusitis for a systemic fungal infection, and this condition is helped by such an approach.

Sinusitis is an all-too-familiar ailment, but it can often be treated and prevented with simple home care and immune-boosting strategies. If your symptoms don't disappear within a few weeks, however, or if you have intense sinus pain, consult your doctor. In severe and prolonged cases, sinusitis can lead to serious diseases like pneumonia or even meningitis.

SYMPTOMS

- Pressure and pain around the cheekbones and the eyes
- Clogged nasal passages
- Thick, greenish-yellow nasal discharge
- Diminished sense of smell or taste
- Toothache
- Fatigue
- Fever (more often in acute cases; rarely in chronic)

ROOT CAUSES

Anything that blocks the sinus cavities or causes the mucus membranes to swell can lead to sinusitis.

- A respiratory infection
- Environmental allergies, especially hay fever
- Environmental irritants, including tobacco and pollution
- Food allergies or sensitivities, especially to milk
- A diet that's high in mucus-forming foods
- A dental infection
- Any activity that places pressure on the sinuses: swimming, scuba diving, flying in planes
- An immune system reaction to a fungal infection in the sinus cavity
- Systemic candidiasis

TREATMENT

If allergies or recurring colds are the cause of your sinusitis, the following recommendations will help, but you should also see the appropriate section in this book. The suggestions there will help you resolve the root of your problem.

A Mayo Clinic study looked at the ability to test for sinus fungal infections in fifty-four patients who had a history of chronic sinusitis. Researchers found that with one of the testing methods, 100 percent of the patients tested positive for fungus, while another testing method showed that 76 percent had signs of fungus.

Testing Techniques

The following tests help assess possible reasons for chronic sinusitis:

Nasal swab—check for yeast or bacteria

Immune system imbalance or disease—blood

Blood pressure

Hormone testing (thyroid, DHEA, cortisol, testosterone, IGF-1, estrogen, progesterone)—saliva, blood, or urine

Intestinal permeability—urine

Detoxification profile—urine

Vitamin and mineral analysis (especially magnesium, B12, iron, and CoQ10)—blood

Digestive function and candida testing—stool analysis

Anemia—blood test (CBC, iron, ferritin, % saturation)

Food and environmental allergies/sensitivities—blood, electrodermal

Blood-sugar balance—blood

Diet

Recommended Food

During an acute infection, eat lightly. In addition to 1 glass of clean water every two waking hours, drink plenty of herbal teas, vegetable juices, and broths. Chicken soup—especially with lots of vegetables—is still one of the best therapies for any respiratory infection.

Once the worst stage of an infection has passed, focus on foods that produce little or no mucus: whole grains, fresh vegetables and fruits, cold-pressed oils, and raw seeds and nuts.

Several foods will aid mucus drainage and ease the pressure in your sinuses. Add cayenne, garlic, onions, or horseradish to your soups or meals. For a powerful sinus drainage remedy, eat a small spoonful of crushed horseradish mixed with lemon juice. (You may want to be near a sink or have a towel handy after taking this potent combination.)

Flaxseeds and flaxseed oil will reduce inflammation. Take a teaspoon of oil every day during the infection, or add some flaxseeds to cereals or salads.

If you must take an antibiotic for a sinus infection, be sure to consume a nondairy source of friendly bacteria, such as kefir or sauerkraut.

Food to Avoid

People who suffer from chronic sinusitis must banish all mucus-forming foods from their diet. Dairy products are the worst culprit, but refined flours, chocolate, eggs, and fried and processed food cause high levels of mucus as well. If your case is acute, avoid these products for the duration of your illness. When you feel better, restrict your consumption of them to prevent a recurrence.

Sugar and fruit juices should be reduced or eliminated because they feed yeast, which is often present in people who have chronic sinusitis.

See the Food Allergies section, especially the elimination diet on page 253, to see whether a certain food is triggering your sinus blockage. Examine your reaction to dairy and wheat very closely; these foods often cause coldlike symptoms.

Salt and alcohol both have dehydrating effect on the sinuses and result in further inflammation. Avoid alcohol and severely restrict salt intake.

Detoxification

During an acute infection, reduce your intake of solid foods and focus on water, broths, and juices. This will help your body focus on healing, rather than on digestion.

If you have a chronic case of sinusitis, go on a two- to three-day juice fast to rid your body of allergens, environmental irritants, and mucus. Green drinks will encourage mucus expulsion.

℞ Super Seven Prescriptions—Sinusitis

Super Prescription #1   Homeopathic Combination Sinusitis Formula
Take as directed on the container four times daily. These types of formulas contain the most common homeopathic remedies that are used for acute sinusitis.

Super Prescription #2   Echinacea (*Echinacea purpurea*) and **goldenseal** (*Hydrastis canadensis*)
Take 5 ml or 500 mg four times daily. This combination of herbs works well for acute sinusitis by enhancing immune function and reducing mucus congestion.

Super Prescription #3   Oregano oil (*Origanum vulgare*)
Take 500 mg or 0.5 ml four times daily, or take as directed on the container. Oregano oil has potent antibacterial and antifungal properties.

Super Prescription #4   N-acetylcysteine
Take 500 mg three times daily. This nutrient thins mucus secretions so that the sinuses can drain more effectively.

Super Prescription #5   Bromelain
Take 500 mg three times daily between meals. Look for products standardized to 2,000 M.C.U. (milk-clotting units) per 1,000 mg or 1,200 G.D.U. (gelatin-dissolving units) per 1,000 mg. Bromelain has a natural anti-inflammatory effect and has been shown in studies to improve acute sinusitis. Protease enzyme products also have this benefit.

Super Prescription #6   Grapefruit seed extract
This is available as a nasal spray for sinusitis. Use the spray four times daily for acute sinusitis and twice daily for chronic sinusitis.

Super Prescription #7   Collodial silver
Use it as a nasal spray, or dilute it in a saline solution. Use the spray four times daily for acute sinusitis and twice daily for chronic sinusitis.

General Recommendations

Vitamin C has anti-allergy and immune-enhancing effects. Take 1,000 mg four times daily. *Note:* Reduce the dosage if diarrhea occurs.

Bioflavonoids are helpful for people with allergies. Take 500 mg three times daily of a mixed bioflavonoid formula.

Grape seed extract or maritime pine bark extract reduces inflammation of the sinus. Take up to 300 mg daily for chronic sinusitis.

Garlic (*Allium sativum*) also fights infection and also helps to drain sinuses. Take 250 to 500 mg twice daily.

Elderflower tea is another traditional remedy that thins mucus. It also increases circulation to the sinus area.

Turmeric (*Curcuma longa*) is an anti-inflammatory herb—as well as a cooking spice—which will reduce sinus pressure. Find an extract standardized for 400 to 600 mg of curcumin (the active ingredient in turmeric) and take 400 to 600 mg three times a day, or use 1 to 2 cc of a tincture three times a day.

Homeopathy

Pick the remedy that best matches your symptoms in this section. For acute sinusitis, take a 30C potency four times daily. For chronic sinusitis, take a 6x, 12x, 6C, 12C, or 30C twice daily for two weeks to see if there are any positive results. After you notice improvement, stop taking the remedy, unless symptoms return. Consultation with a homeopathic practitioner is advised.

Belladonna (*Atropa belladonna*) is helpful for the first stage of a sinus infection. The person experiences a high fever and throbbing pain, especially on the right side of the sinus. The pain is made worse by bending the head forward.

Bryonia (*Bryonia alba*) is a remedy for when movement of the head, especially bending the head downward, causes sinus pain. The person has a great thirst and feels irritable.

Hepar Sulphuris is for a blocked, sore nose that's made worse by even the slightest draft. People who benefit from this remedy tend to be irritable while ill.

Kali Bichromium is indicated when there is thick, stringy, yellow and/or green mucus that causes pain at the root of the nose.

Mercurius Solubilis or Vivus is needed for people who are feverish and have pain around the nose and the cheekbones. They salivate excessively and have thick white- or yellowish-coated tongues. Their nasal discharge is foul smelling and so is their breath.

Pulsatilla (*Pulsatilla pratensis*) is for people with a thick yellow/green mucus discharge. They feel better in the open air or with a window open. Their symptoms are worse in a warm room. They have little thirst.

Silica (*Silicea*) is good remedy for chronic sinusitis where the nasal cavities will not drain. The person feels worse in the cold air, but the sinuses feel better with cold applications.

Acupressure

See pages 668–675 for information about pressure points and administering treatment.

- To relieve sinus congestion and headaches, work Bladder 2.
- Large Intestine 4 eases pain anywhere in the body but is particularly effective at treating pain in the front of the head, including in the sinus cavities.

Bodywork

Massage

To drain mucus and carry it away from the body, get a facial lymphatic drainage massage. You can also try this home technique: Lean over a sink or a towel and gently rub the areas over and below your eye sockets, then extend out from beneath your eye sockets in a straight line across your cheeks. This will allow your sinuses to drain.

Reflexology

See pages 686–687 for information about reflexology areas and how to work them.

The toes correspond to the sinuses. Work all of them.

Work the lymph area to encourage the production of antibodies and to fight infection.

Hydrotherapy

Hot baths, showers, and steams are all relaxing, effective ways to relieve sinus pressure. Add any of the essential oils listed in this entry for extra benefits.

Alternating hot (two minutes) and cold (thirty seconds) over the sinus area helps to reduce pain and inflammation of the sinuses.

Aromatherapy

Eucalyptus oil will clear out sinuses quickly. Use it in a massage, a steam inhalation, or a bath, or simply inhale deeply over an open bottle of oil.

Tea tree oil will fight both bacterial and viral infections. It's a powerful oil, so use just a few drops in a bath or a steam. You can also diffuse a little in your bedroom for nighttime sinus relief.

Lavender is a gentle oil that stimulates your immune system and helps you get to sleep. Use it in any preparation you like, or add it to any of the previous oils.

Stress Reduction

General Stress-Reduction Techniques

Stress isn't a direct cause of sinusitis, but constant unresolved tension can leave you less able to fight off infections. Use stress-reduction techniques to create a healthy immune system. You'll relieve stress, and the deep breathing will encourage good air flow through your nasal passages.

Other Recommendations

- Regular exercise will help keep your nasal passages clear. Try to work out daily, but use some common-sense precautions: don't exercise if you have a fever, and don't go outside if seasonal allergies are likely to strike.
- Saline rinses for the sinus are helpful, to reduce the effect of allergens that contribute to sinusitis. Saline nasal sprays are available; look for those that also contain xylitol, a natural extract that prevents bacteria from adhering to the nasal cavity.
- If you have chronic sinusitis, you may well have problems with candida overgrowth. See the Candidiasis section for more information.

REFERENCES

Taylor, M. J., J. U. Ponikau, D. A. Sherris, E. B. Kern, T. A. Gaffey, G. Kephart, and H. Kita. 2002. Detection of fungal organisms in eosinophilic mucin using a fluorescein-labeled chitin-specific binding protein. *Otolaryngology: Head and Neck Surgery* 127(5):377–83.

Sprains and Strains

Although most of us will experience a sprain or a strain at some point in our lives, very few people know the difference between the two kinds of injuries. A strain is what's commonly referred to as a "pulled muscle." As its name implies, a strain occurs when a muscle is overstressed by too much weight or by overuse. The injured muscle fibers may go into spasm, form knots, or swell up. If you have a strained muscle, you may feel a sharp pain when you try to use it, or you may experience a dull throb in the affected area. When muscles knot or spasm, the pain can be constant and severe. The worst symptoms of a strain will usually subside after a week, but they may leave behind an ache that lingers as long as a month.

Sprains, contrary to what most people believe, are not the result of muscle injury. In this case, the damage is done to a ligament, which is a band of fibrous connective tissue that holds bones together at the joints. When a ligament is overstressed, it may tear or stretch out of its normal position. You may even hear a snapping or popping sound at the time of injury. Not surprisingly, sprains cause immediate, acute pain. Once the first shock of pain passes, it is replaced by swelling and extreme soreness and sensitivity. In most cases, putting weight on the affected joint is out of the question. With proper treatment, the swelling goes away after about a week, but you may have pain for several weeks longer. The joint will usually feel stiff for months to come.

Most strains and sprains respond well to rest and home care, but you should be alert for signs that your injury needs a doctor's attention. If the pain is unbearable and if you can't move the joint, you may have a broken or fractured bone. Instead of going to bed, visit a doctor's office or the emergency room. Other red flags are discolored joints or severe swelling that doesn't go down after a few days.

Although sprains and strains are quite common, you can reduce your chances of injuring a muscle or a ligament. First, get some exercise on a regular basis. People who don't use their muscles and bones regularly are far more prone to damaging them. Second, always warm up your muscles before engaging in an activity. Stretch gently and ease into the movement. Finally, use common sense: Don't lift objects that are too heavy for you, and don't participate in activities that are painful.

SYMPTOMS OF STRAINS

- Acute pain when the muscle is in use
- A dull throb at other times
- Muscle spasms or knots
- Swelling

SYMPTOMS OF SPRAINS

- Severe pain at time of injury, subsiding into soreness
- Swelling
- Joint discoloration (indicative of a serious sprain)

ROOT CAUSES

- Overstressing muscles or ligaments, usually through lifting, exercise, or by accident
- Imbalance in oppositional muscles
- Nutritional deficiencies, making one more susceptible to injury

---

Emergency Care for Sprains and Strains

When you suspect that you've experienced a strain or a sprain, it helps to take quick action. The following simple techniques, if used immediately after the injury, will promote faster healing and can greatly reduce the amount and the duration of pain.

1. If you experience severe pain, significant swelling, discoloration at the site, or any of the following symptoms, get to a doctor as soon as possible. Be especially careful with injuries to the wrist or the ankle; these body parts are relatively delicate and vulnerable to fractures.

2. To reduce swelling and pain, apply an ice pack or a cold compress to the injured area. In a pinch, you can place some ice cubes in a plastic bag and then wrap the package up in a clean towel. You can even use a box of frozen vegetables. Just be sure that the ice doesn't touch your skin directly; otherwise, you'll have a sprain or a strain and frostbite. Keep the cold pack on for twenty minutes, then take a ten-minute break before reapplying.

3. To the extent possible, elevate the injured area so that it's higher than your heart. This allows blood to flow away from the site and decreases swelling.

4. Continue elevation and cold applications for the next day or two, and then alternate cold and warm applications. You no longer need to apply cold as often as in the first hour and a half after the injury; simply apply it intermittently as needed. If the swelling has not gone down significantly after this time, see a doctor.

TREATMENT

Diet

You might not think of diet as an important part of healing an injury, but good nutritional choices in the weeks following a sprain or a strain can speed your recovery and reduce your pain.

Recommended Food

You need lean protein to rebuild strong, elastic muscles and ligaments. Eat reasonable amounts of high-quality chicken, turkey, and fish, and incorporate beans into your meals.

An injury can result in the formation of free radicals, the unbalanced molecules that are thought to be responsible for many diseases. Combat free radicals with the antioxidants found in deeply colored fruits and vegetables.

Vitamin C will help to reduce swelling and repair tissues. Eat citrus fruits as a light dessert.

Testing Techniques

The following tests help assess possible reasons for the slow repair of sprains/strains:

Intestinal permeability—urine

Detoxification profile—urine

Vitamin and mineral analysis (especially magnesium, vitamin C, iron)—
  blood

Food to Avoid

You may be housebound and depressed following a sprain or a strain, but resist the temptation to console yourself with junk food. Fast food, processed food, fried food, and food that's high in salt and sugar will only make inflammation and swelling worse.

Double-blind trials have shown that proteolytic enzymes, such as bromelain, papain, and trypsin/chymotrypsin, speed the recovery of athletic injuries.

℞ Super Seven Prescriptions—Sprains/Strains

Super Prescription #1   Bromelain
Take 500 mg three times daily between meals. Look for products standardized to 2,000 M.C.U. (milk-clotting units) per 1,000 mg or 1,200 G.D.U. (gelatin-dissolving units) per 1,000 mg. Bromelain has a natural anti-inflammatory effect. Protease enzyme products also have this benefit (chymotrypsin, trypsin, fungal-derived protease).

Super Prescription #2   Methylsulfonylmethane (MSM)
Take 1,000 mg three to four times daily. This supplement has potent anti-inflammatory effects and is a natural source of the mineral sulfur, which promotes ligament and tendon health.

Super Prescription #3   Vitamin C
Take 1,000 mg two to three times daily. Vitamin C is required for the formation of connective tissue and has anti-inflammatory benefits.

Super Prescription #4   DMSO
Consult with a doctor to use this pain-relieving substance topically for pain relief.

Super Prescription #5   Boswellia (*Boswellia serrata*)
Take 1,200 to 1,500 mg of standardized extract containing 60 to 65 percent boswellic acids two to three times daily. This herb has a strong anti-inflammatory effect.

Super Prescription #6   Arnica (*Arnica montana*) **oil**
Apply to the injured site twice daily. This herbal oil reduces pain, bruising, and swelling. Do not use on broken skin.

Super Prescription #7   Essential fatty acids
Take 1 to 2 tablespoons of flaxseed oil or 5 grams of fish oil daily, or take a formulation that contains a mixture of omega-3, 6, and 9 fatty acids. Essential fatty acids reduce inflammation and promote tissue healing.

General Recommendations

A high-potency multivitamin supplies a host of vitamins and minerals required for ligament and tendon healing. Take as directed on the container.

A cool compress made with comfrey will ease pain and swelling.

White willow bark (*Salix alba*) is a natural pain reliever that doesn't have the side effects of aspirin and other over-the-counter drugs. Find an extract standardized for salicin content, and take 30 to 60 mg twice a day. If you prefer to use a tincture, take 1 to 2 cc three times daily.

Silica (*Silicea*) extract is important for connective tissue healing. Take 500 mg three times daily.

Glucosamine sulfate provides the raw materials known as glycosaminoglycans that are required by the body to manufacture ligaments and tendons. Take 1,500 mg daily.

Hyaluronic acid supplies substances that are required for ligament and tendon healing. Take 150 mg daily or as directed on the container.

Homeopathy

Pick the remedy that best matches your symptoms in this section. For acute sprain/strains, take a 30C potency four times daily. For chronic sprains/strains that have not healed, take a 6x, 12x, 6C, 12C, or 30C twice daily for two weeks to see if there are any positive results. After you notice improvement, stop taking the remedy, unless symptoms return. Consultation with a homeopathic practitioner is advised.

Arnica (*Arnica montana*) is helpful at the beginning of an injury, when there is bruising and swelling.

Bryonia Alba should be used when there is pain from any movement. The person feels irritable from the pain.

Calcarea Fluorica is indicated for chronic sprains and strains that do not heal, or for people who are susceptible to getting these types of injuries due to weak ligaments or tendons.

Ledum Palustre is for sprained ankles or knees that are swollen and that feel better with ice applications.

Rhus Toxicodendron should be used for injuries that cause stiffness, especially during the first movement, but that loosen up later in the day. The injury feels better from warm applications.

Ruta (*Ruta graveolens*) is for overused ligaments and sprains that result in swelling and a lame feeling in the joint.

Acupressure

See pages 668–675 for information about pressure points and administering treatment.

- To relieve pain and relax your muscles, use Gallbladder 20.
- Kidney 3 will reduce pain in either ankle.
- If you've strained your lower back, use Bladder 60.

Bodywork

Reflexology

See pages 686–687 for information about reflexology areas and how to work them.

Work the area that corresponds to the injured body part. Obviously, you should not practice reflexology on a hand or a foot that has been injured.

Hydrotherapy

Once the swelling has gone down, you can soak the injured part in warm water to relieve pain.

Other Bodywork Recommendations

Avoid putting weight on an injured joint or muscle, but do keep mobile. After the swelling is down and any acute pain has passed, try to work the body part through its range of motion. You'll help prevent stiffness.

Aromatherapy

After the swelling has subsided, try a combination of eucalyptus, peppermint, and lavender to stimulate a nourishing flow of blood to the area and reduce pain. You can use these oils in a warm bath or a compress.

Stress Reduction

General Stress-Reduction Therapies

If you're usually an active person, it can be terribly frustrating to spend days or even weeks laid up with an injury. Keep your stress levels down by meditating on a regular basis.

Bach Flower Remedies

Select the appropriate remedy, and place 10 drops of the liquid under your tongue. Hold the drops in place for thirty seconds and swallow. Use as often as needed.

When you're confronted with a physical crisis like a sprain or strain, take Rescue Remedy. It's calming to the body and the mind and allows healing to begin.

If an injury has left you feeling irritable and impatient with other people, take Impatiens.

Gentian will help if you are easily depressed when faced with a setback.

REFERENCES

Blonstein, J. L. 1967. Oral enzyme tablets in the treatment of boxing injuries. *Practitioner* 198:547.

Buck, J. E., and N. Phillips. 1970. Trial of Chymoral in professional footballers. *British Journal of Clinical Practice* 24:375–77.

Deitrick, R. E. 1965. Oral proteolytic enzymes in the treatment of athletic injuries: A double-blind study. *Pennsylvania Medical Journal* 35–37.

Holt, H. T. 1969. Carica papaya as ancillary therapy for athletic injuries. *Current Therapeutics Research* 11:621–24.

Rathgeber, W. F. 1971. The use of proteolytic enzymes (Chymoral) in sporting injuries. *South African Medical Journal* 45:181–83.

Tsomides, J., and R. I. Goldberg. 1969. Controlled evaluation of oral chymotrypsin-trypsin treatment of injuries to the head and face. *Clinical Medicine* 76(11):40.

Stroke

Like all parts of the body, the brain needs a continuous supply of oxygen to function properly. When that oxygen supply is cut off, brain tissues begin to die within minutes, never to regenerate. This tissue death is what happens during a stroke. A stroke occurs when blood carrying oxygen and other nutrients to the brain is blocked or interrupted; the extent of the damage to the brain usually depends upon the length of the interruption and the speed with which treatment is received. As most of us know, strokes are extremely serious and often fatal. They are the third leading cause of death in the United States, behind only heart disease and cancer.

An overwhelming percentage of strokes are caused by arteriosclerosis, a condition in which fatty deposits build up inside the arterial walls and obstruct blood flow. An artery leading to the brain may become so thick with plaque that the passage of blood is effectively blocked. The blood supply may also be shut off if a clot lodges itself in an artery that's already damaged and narrow. In a few cases, a cerebral blood vessel will actually rupture. High blood pressure is also a major predisposition to strokes, which damage the arteries and may cause a rupture; it, too, can often be managed with proper diet, exercise, supplementation, and stress management (see Blood Pressure, High).

Although we've been conditioned to think of strokes as tragic but unpreventable accidents that occur in old age, the truth is that arteriosclerosis is often a condition caused or made more probable by controllable lifestyle factors. Although arteries do tend to weaken, as we get older, poor diet and lack of exercise, along with uncontrolled stress, are reasons that plaque builds up in the arteries in the first place. Genetic cardiovascular risk factors also play a role for many people. See the Cardiovascular Disease section for a more in-depth discussion of these risk factors.

A few other factors also increase the risk for stroke. If you have an irregular heartbeat or a damaged heart valve or have suffered a recent heart attack, you should be especially vigilant about your health and should be monitored regularly by a doctor. Women who take oral contraceptives and who smoke also have a greater chance of developing blood clots, as so women on certain types of synthetic hormone replacement.

If you have a stroke, you have a significantly greater chance of surviving and even fully recovering when you receive medical treatment within three hours after the symptoms begin—the earlier, the better. Call an ambulance or get to an emergency room immediately if you experience any of the following symptoms: weakness or numbness along one side of the body; difficulty talking or understanding speech; blurred vision; confusion; a sudden, intense headache; unexplained dizziness or loss of balance; or loss of consciousness. These symptoms may come on suddenly, within a matter of seconds or minutes, or they may develop over the course of a day or two. If you have arteriosclerosis or are over fifty, you should be aware of these stroke warning signs so that you know when to get help, should it ever be necessary.

It's difficult to say exactly what the consequences of a stroke will be. The damage largely depends upon which brain tissues are deprived of oxygen and how long the interruption of blood flow lasts. If the blood flow is suspended for only a few seconds, you may experience visual and speech problems, weakness, trembling, or confusion, but it's likely that you'll soon return to normal. People who survive longer periods of oxygen deprivation may suffer lasting damage to their vision, speech, coordination, or movement, although physical therapy may restore some or even total functioning.

SYMPTOMS

- Paralysis or numbness on one side of the face or the body
- Dizziness
- A sudden, severe headache
- Blurred vision or blindness
- Confusion
- Impaired speech
- An inability to understand others' speech
- Loss of balance
- Loss of consciousness

ROOT CAUSES

- Poor diet
- Genetic cardiovascular risk factors (elevated fibrinogen, homocysteine, etc.)
- High blood pressure
- Smoking
- Diabetes
- Obesity
- Blood that clots too easily
- Irregular heartbeat
- Damaged heart valve
- Oral contraceptives (especially in women over thirty-five)
- Synthetic hormone replacement

Testing Techniques

The following tests help to assess your stroke risk:

Cardiovascular risk factors (cholesterol, homocysteine, fibrinogen, etc)—blood (see the Cardiovascular Disease section for more information)

Blood pressure

Hormone testing (thyroid, DHEA, cortisol, testosterone, IGF-1, estrogen, progesterone)—saliva, blood, or urine

Vitamin and mineral analysis (especially magnesium, E, potassium, CoQ10)—blood

Essential fatty acid balance—blood

Blood-sugar balance—blood

Toxic metals—hair or urine

TREATMENT

If you experience any of the symptoms listed previously, get medical help immediately. The following treatments will assist in the recovery from strokes or will prevent future strokes from occurring, but they cannot substitute for emergency care by doctors.

If you have arteriosclerosis, see the Cardiovascular Disease section for further suggestions. For high blood pressure, see Blood Pressure, High.

Diet

Recommended Food

Follow a diet consisting of whole, natural foods, including fresh fruits and vegetables, whole grains, beans, legumes, fish, nuts, and seeds. This eating plan, which is high in nutrients and fiber, will reduce your risk of forming blood clots. The antioxidants in these foods will also counteract free-radical damage, making you less likely to develop arteriosclerosis.

Fish are high in essential fatty acids and decrease your risk of stroke. They contain "good" fats that improve circulation and act as natural blood thinners. The Nurses' Health Study found a significant decrease in the risk of thrombotic stroke among women who ate fish at least two times per week, when compared with the risk in women who ate fish less than once per month. Although you should eat a wide variety of fruits and vegetables, try to have a couple of servings of those that are blue-red or purple in color at least twice a day. Purple grapes, berries, red cabbage, and eggplant are all high in anthocyanidins, a substance that lowers the risk of stroke and heart disease.

Potassium helps to reduce blood pressure and thereby decreases stroke risk. Good sources include leafy green vegetables, tomatoes, potatoes, and citrus fruits.

Consume green and white tea, which contains powerful antioxidants.

A review of studies in the *Journal of the American Medical Association* looked at the relationship between fruit and vegetable intake and the risk of ischemic stroke. This review included 75,596 women, ages 34 to 59 years, in the Nurses' Health Study and 38,683 men, ages 40 to 75 years, in the Health Professionals' Follow-Up Study. An increment of one serving per day of fruits or vegetables was associated with a 6 percent lower risk of ischemic stroke. Researchers found that cruciferous and green leafy vegetables, as well as citrus fruit and juice, were most helpful in decreasing ischemic stroke risk.

Food to Avoid

A diet that's high in saturated and trans-fatty acids is thought to be a leading cause of both arteriosclerosis and high blood pressure. Eliminate red meat, butter, fried and greasy food, and all junk food from your diet. You must also avoid margarine and shortening, as well as products made with these items. This includes many sweet baked goods. Vegetable oils should not be used for frying. The exception is canola oil.

Although we don't tend to think of sugar as a cause of heart disease, high amounts of it will increase the inflammation in artery walls. Decrease the amount of simple sugars in the diet, such as those from white breads, pastas, candy, and soda pop.

Sodium can send blood pressure levels soaring in many people. Don't use table salt, and avoid processed food, which is the leading source of sodium in the American diet.

Detoxification

If you've had a stroke, do not undergo any kind of fasting program until your doctor has told you that your condition is stable. Fresh vegetable juices are excellent for detoxification. Make them fresh or buy super green food powder drinks.

℞ Super Seven Prescriptions—Stroke

Super Prescription #1 High-potency multivitamin
Take as directed on the container. It contains a variety of antioxidants, as well as minerals that are associated with reducing the risk of stroke.

Super Prescription #2 Garlic (*Allium sativum*)
Take 300 to 500 mg of aged garlic twice daily. It reduces cholesterol levels and increases HDL cholesterol.

Super Prescription #3 Fish oil
Take a daily dosage of a fish oil product containing 1,000 mg of EPA and 500 mg of DHA. Fish oil reduces inflammation in the arteries and lowers cholesterol and triglyceride levels.

Super Prescription #4 Policosanol
Take 10 to 20 mg each evening. Numerous studies show that policosanol reduces total and LDL cholesterol and increases the good HDL cholesterol.

Super Prescription #5 Vitamin E
Take 400 IU daily of a mixed complex. It prevents cholesterol oxidation and is a natural blood thinner.

Super Prescription #6 Ginkgo biloba
Take 180 to 240 mg daily of a 24 percent flavone glycoside extract. Ginkgo has blood-thinning and antioxidant properties.

Super Prescription #7 Green tea (*Camellia sinensis*) **extract**
Take 500 to 1,500 mg of the capsule form. Look for a product standardized to between 80 and 90 percent polyphenols and between 35 and 55 percent epigallo-catechin gallate. Green tea contains a rich source of antioxidants and substances that assist detoxification.

General Recommendations

Pantetheine is a metabolite of vitamin B5 that has been shown in studies to reduce total and LDL cholesterol, as well to increase HDL. It can be particularly effective for people with diabetes. Take 600 to 900 mg daily.

Soy protein has been shown in studies to reduce total and LDL cholesterol and to increase HDL. Take 25 to 50 grams daily.

Reishi (*Ganoderma lucidum*) is a mushroom extract that reduces cholesterol. Take 800 mg two to three times daily.

Vitamin E prevents LDL oxidation. Take 400 to 800 IU of a mixed blend daily.

Vitamin C reduces total cholesterol and LDL levels and acts to prevent their oxidation.

Homeopathy

If you experience the symptoms of a stroke, you must get medical assistance at once. The following remedies may be helpful as part of a comprehensive stroke recovery protocol. Pick the remedy that best matches your symptoms in this section. Take a 6x, 12x, 6C, 12C, or 30C potency twice daily for two weeks to see if there are any positive results. After you notice improvement, stop taking the remedy, unless symptoms return. Consultation with a homeopathic practitioner is advised.

Aconitum Napellus will help calm someone who's panicked and afraid of dying while waiting for medical attention. Take a 30C potency or whatever potency is available.

Baryta Carbonica is a good remedy when there is mental weakness after a stroke and weakness on one side of the body. The person has childish characteristics as a result of the stroke.

Causticum is indicated for paralysis of the muscles of speech, paralysis of the bladder, and numbness of the hands and the feet. It is a specific remedy for right-sided paralysis.

Gelsemium Sempervirens is helpful for after effects of a stroke, characterized by muscle weakness and trembling, numbness of the face and the tongue, and the eyelids remaining half opened.

Lachesis Mutas is for left-sided paralysis after a stroke and for paralysis of the throat and the tongue.

Acupressure

- Gallbladder 20 and 21 stimulate circulation, especially to the head.
- Use Liver 3 to induce a sense of peacefulness and calm.

Bodywork

Massage
Have frequent circulatory massages to increase your energy and sense of well-being.

Reflexology
See pages 686–687 for information about reflexology areas and how to work them.

Work the spine to stimulate any damaged nerves and promote good circulation.

People who've suffered a stroke often have some numbness or paralysis on one side of their bodies. Reflexology can encourage the healing process. If your left side is damaged, work the big toe on the right foot. If the stroke has affected your right side, work the big toe on the left foot.

In addition, you should massage the regions that correspond to any affected body parts.

Other Bodywork Recommendations

Acupuncture can be very helpful in speeding recovery and as a complement to physical therapy. Acupuncture treatments should begin as soon as possible after one has suffered a stroke.

Aromatherapy

Mix a few drops of juniper with a carrier oil, and use in a massage to help break down toxins in the blood and carry them out of the body. You can also add juniper to a bath.

Black pepper, ginger, and rosemary all stimulate circulation. Again, you can use them in a massage or a bath.

If you feel fatigued, geranium, jasmine, neroli, bergamot, and rose can give a lift to your energy levels and your mood. These oils can also aid in stress reduction. Use them in any preparation you like.

Stress Reduction

General Stress-Reduction Therapies

Stress-reduction techniques, which include exercise, prayer, yoga, and positive mental imagery, should be incorporated as part of stroke recovery.

Bach Flower Remedies

Following are some suggestions, but you should consult the chart on pages 648–650 to determine the best remedy for your particular needs. Once you've chosen a remedy, place 10 drops of the liquid under your tongue. Hold the drops in place for thirty seconds and swallow. Use as often as needed.

If you feel defeated and believe that nothing will ever make you feel better, take Gorse.

Impatiens is for highly efficient people who cannot tolerate those who think or move slowly.

If you tend to be controlling and overprotective, especially around family members, use Chicory.

Perfectionists who find it hard to work or live with people who do not share their views should use Beech.

Crab Apple will help people who are debilitated by a stroke and are ashamed of their ailments.

Other Recommendations

- Hyperbaric oxygen therapy may help you to recover from a stroke, as it improves oxygen flow to the brain. Consult with a doctor who was trained in this therapy.
- As with other circulatory conditions, exercise is an important factor in both recovery from and prevention of stroke. You don't have to climb mountains—a daily walk or swim will suffice. Try to exercise in the early morning sunshine, which will lift your spirits.
- Stop smoking. This habit increases the risk of high blood and arteriosclerosis, the two most frequent causes of stroke.
- If you have diabetes, you're at risk for circulatory diseases like strokes and heart problems. You must eat well, exercise, manage stress, and work closely with an experienced doctor. For more information, see Diabetes.

- People who are overweight are more vulnerable to strokes than the rest of the population is. The diet and exercise guidelines here should help you lose weight, but if you want further suggestions, see Obesity.

REFERENCES

Joshipura, K. J., A. Ascherio, J. E. Manson, M. J. Stampfer, E. B. Rimm, F. E. Speizer, C. H. Hennekens, D. Spiegelman, and W. C. Willett. 1999. Fruit and vegetable intake in relation to risk of ischemic stroke. *Journal of the American Medical Association* 282(13):1233–39.

Skerrett, P. J., and C. H. Hennekens. 2003. Consumption of fish and fish oils and decreased risk of stroke. *Preventative Cardiology* 6(1):38–41.

Substance Abuse (Drug and Alcohol Addiction)

Substance abuse is a dependency—whether psychological, physical, or both—on drugs (including on prescription medications and alcohol). No one knows why some people develop such a dependency while others don't, but evidence indicates that genetics, environment, and individual psychology all have roles to play in the illness.

Drugs and alcohol can cause severe damage to almost every system in the body. Both of them have a toxic effect on the liver, an organ whose functioning is crucial to many bodily systems. Obviously, brain damage is always a concern. Aside from the very real possibility of a fatal overdose—the likelihood of which increases if drugs and alcohol are mixed—abusing drugs can create several life-threatening conditions.

The free radicals in these substances are carcinogenic, and addicts experience a high rate of breast, mouth, esophageal, and liver cancers. Cocaine and heroin can severely damage the heart. Shared needles can lead to AIDS and hepatitis transmission. Drugs can also cause mental disorders, such as anxiety, panic, and depression; kidney failure from excessive urine production (this is especially a problem for alcoholics); stroke and impotence, as a result of a depressed central nervous system; and a host of other disorders that result from a suppressed immune system. Substance abuse is the leading cause of traffic fatalities and plays a significant role in homicides, suicides, spousal and child abuse, and other violent acts.

Effective treatment begins when an addict makes the decision to give up drugs or alcohol. The process, however, rarely ends there. Many people suffer from withdrawal symptoms, which include heart problems, sweats, tremors, dehydration, seizures, and hallucinations. It is often a good idea to have medical supervision during this period. In addition, most serious users will need to address the psychological components of their addiction and may benefit from therapy or from a support group such as Narcotics Anonymous or Alcoholics Anonymous. Spiritual support is also strongly advised.

Biochemical imbalances can predispose one to drug dependency. For example, people who are prone to biochemical depression may use alcohol or drugs as a crutch. People with alcoholism often have a blood-sugar imbalance and candidiasis (see the Candidiasis section for more information), which increase their alcohol cravings. Other nutrient deficiencies may worsen their susceptibility to becoming addicted.

Complementary therapies for drug dependency and withdrawal focus on balancing the body's systems and address underlying emotional, mental, and spiritual disorders. Detoxification using natural therapies improves the person's vitality.

SYMPTOMS: HOW DO YOU KNOW IF IT'S A PROBLEM?

If you're trying to determine whether you or someone you know has a problem with drugs, it's important to realize that addiction can take many forms and that there is no one pattern of abuse. Usually, an addiction develops over time, as occasional social drinking or drug use progresses into heavy use and then to total dependency, but some people find themselves addicted from their first drink, puff, or hit. Some alcoholics drink only wine, beer, or certain kinds of hard liquor; others will drink anything that contains a trace of alcohol, including mouthwash and perfume. The frequency of use also varies. Some addicts will use small amounts of substances throughout the day (alcoholics may spike coffee, juice, tea, or other beverages with liquor), while others may stay sober for long periods in-between binges. The personalities of people who abuse substances also comprise a wide range, from the stereotypical violent, angry, sloppy addict to one who maintains a composed and polished front. Substance abuse can occur at any age and in either sex. (One general rule does seem to apply: If you require drugs or alcohol not just to release tension but to feel "normal," then you are in a late stage of addiction and need to seek help as soon as possible.)

ROOT CAUSES

It's unclear why some people are more prone to addiction than others are. Following are some of the leading possibilities.

- A genetic tendency toward addiction
- Psychological problems, including depression
- Environmental factors, such as the general availability of drugs and social pressure
- Nutritional deficiencies
- A blood-sugar imbalance (alcoholism)

Testing Techniques

The following tests help assess possible reasons for substance abuse tendencies:

Vitamin and mineral analysis (especially magnesium, B vitamins, chromium)—blood

Digestive function and microbe/parasite/candida testing—stool analysis

Food and environmental allergies/sensitivities—blood, electrodermal

Blood-sugar balance—blood

Amino acid balance—blood or urine

TREATMENT

Diet

Recommended Food

You need to rebuild your damaged body systems. Start by eating well-rounded meals of natural foods. A variety of fresh fruits and vegetables, whole grains, beans, nuts, seeds, and lean animal protein will help you feel balanced and energetic again.

If you haven't been eating much as a result of your addiction, you may find it difficult to sit down to three large meals a day. Instead, plan several smaller snacks. This strategy will also keep your blood-sugar levels even and help you avoid cravings.

Drink a glass of clean water every two waking hours. You'll be surprised at how much better you feel when you're properly hydrated, and you'll be less tempted to fill up on junk food. Water also helps flush the accumulated toxins out of your system.

You may experience some trouble sleeping without the aid of drugs or alcohol. If that's the case, try eating a snack of turkey or chicken on whole-grain crackers before you go to bed. These foods are all good sources of tryptophan, a chemical that activates the sleep-inducing neurotransmitter serotonin. For additional suggestions, see Insomnia.

Food to Avoid

As you're trying to kick the habit, you may instinctively reach for sugary treats or caffeinated beverages. Avoid this temptation, as caffeine and refined sugar will only increase your cravings for drugs.

Obviously, alcohol use is out of the question, even if you haven't formerly had a problem with alcohol.

Detoxification

Complete abstention from solid food is not recommended if you are going through withdrawal, as balanced nutrition will help curb your cravings. Once you've been sober for a while, however, you should go on supervised detoxification protocols to eliminate all the poisons you've consumed via drugs or alcohol. You can (and should) drink plenty of juices, herbal teas, and broths while detoxifying. It will take at least four months of good eating and monthly fasts to fully detoxify your body.

If you haven't been eating lots of fiber—and few substance abusers do—you may be severely constipated. Following the previously described eating plan will help, but it's also important to get the toxic matter out of your bowels. If you are having problems, see the Constipation section.

℞ Super Seven Prescriptions—Substance Abuse

Super Prescription #1   High-potency multivitamin
Take as directed on the container. It supplies a combination of vitamins and minerals that assists detoxification and improves your mood.

Super Prescription #2   Milk thistle (*Silybum marianum*)
Take 250 mg three times daily of a product standardized to 80 to 85 percent silymarin extract. Milk thistle supports liver detoxification and has been shown to reduce elevated liver enzymes.

Super Prescription #3   B-complex
Take 50 mg twice daily. Many of the B vitamins are required for detoxification, as well as for mood and energy support.

Super Prescription #4   Homeopathic Nux Vomica
Take a 30C potency twice daily for up to two weeks. It reduces withdrawal symptoms of irritability, nausea, constipation, and fatigue.

Super Prescription #5   Chromium
Take 200 mcg two to three times daily. It reduces sugar (and possibly alcohol) cravings.

Super Prescription #6   L-glutamine

Take 500 mg three times daily on an empty stomach. It improves mood and energy levels.

Super Prescription #7   5-hydroxytryptophan (5-HTP)

Take 100 mg three times daily on an empty stomach. It reduces the depression and the anxiety that come on during withdrawal symptoms. Taken before bedtime, it also promotes restful sleep. *Note:* Do not take this if you are on a pharmaceutical antidepressant or antianxiety medication.

General Recommendations

DL-phenylalanine helps fight depression and low energy. Take 500 mg three times daily on an empty stomach.

If you suffer from mild or moderate depression, take Saint-John's-wort (*Hypericum perforatum*). It will lift your mood and help you face your daily challenges. It will also bolster your weakened immune system. Use 300 mg three times daily of a 0.3 percent hypericin extract. *Do not take Saint-John's-wort if you are already on medication for depression or anxiety.*

Super green food supplements, such as spirulina, chlorella, or a blend of greens, promote healthful detoxification. Take as directed on the container.

If you need some help getting to sleep, drink a cup of valerian (*Valeriana officinalis*) tea before going to bed.

Many people who are trying to kick a drug or alcohol habit feel nervous and anxious. Passionflower (*Passiflora incarnata*) is a gentle yet effective herb to use. Take 3 ml of the tincture form or 500 mg of the capsule version three times daily. Hops (*Humulus lupulus*), kava (*Piper methysticum*), oatstraw (*Avena sativa*), and valerian (*Valeriana officinalis*) are other good herbal options. (See the Anxiety section.)

Reishi (*Ganoderma lucidum*) extract improves liver and immune system function. It also helps with concentration and focus. Take 800 mg twice daily.

Calcium and magnesium relax the nervous system; they are especially good if you experience twitches and cramps. Take 500 mg of calcium and 250 mg of magnesium twice daily.

People with alcoholism may benefit from supplementing niacin. Take 500 mg twice daily of the flush-free version.

N-acetylcysteine increases levels of glutathione, an important antioxidant. Take 300 mg three times daily.

Vitamin C is important for detoxification, and it increases glutathione levels. Take 1,000 mg three times daily.

Vitamin B1 (thiamine) is particularly important for people with alcoholism, to prevent cognitive dysfunction, memory impairment, and visual changes. Take up to 200 mg daily. For severe deficiencies, intravenous or injection forms given by a doctor are required.

Eleutherococcus/Siberian ginseng works to help the body adapt to mental and physical stress by improving adrenal gland function. Take 600 to 900 mg of a standardized product daily.

A study was completed that included 507 people with alcoholism, who were treated with 3 grams or more of niacin daily for five years. Results suggested that a majority benefited from supplementation, by experiencing symptom reduction and less relapses.

Homeopathy

Pick the remedy that best matches your symptoms in this section. Take a 6x, 12x, 6C, 12C, or 30C potency twice daily for two weeks to see if there are any positive results.

After you notice improvement, stop taking the remedy, unless symptoms return. Consultation with a homeopathic practitioner is advised.

Arsenicum Album is indicated when one feels tremendous restlessness, fatigue, and anxiety. There may be burning pains that feel better from warmth. Symptoms are worse between midnight and 2 A.M.

Ignatia Amara is for hysteria and emotional breakdown. The person has constantly changing mood and symptoms, cries but wants to be left alone, has a sensation of a lump in the throat, is anxious, and has twitches and spasms.

Lachesis is for people with addictions who get violent. They have intense feelings of jealousy, paranoia, and suspiciousness. They tend to be warm and feel worse from heat. There is an intolerance of anything touching the throat.

Lycopodium (*Lycopodium clavatum*) is indicated for people with an alcohol or drug addiction. They are irritable and have low self-esteem. They are chilly and feel better from warmth. They usually have a strong craving for sweets and often have digestive problems, such as gas and bloating.

Nux Vomica is good for emotional withdrawal symptoms that include irritability and anger, as well as physical symptoms of nausea, constipation, chilliness, and fatigue. There is great sensitivity to sound, light, odors, and touch.

Sulphur is a good remedy for people who crave alcohol and go on binges. They tend to feel warm and feel better from cool air and cold drinks. There is a craving for spicy foods. Skin rashes are common.

Acupressure

See pages 668–675 for information about pressure points and administering treatment.

- Stomach 36 improves your ability to absorb nutrients and gives you an overall sense of well-being.
- Spleen 10 will speed up the detoxification process.
- For anxiety or depression, work Lung 1.
- If you are fatigued, use Gallbladder 20.

Bodywork

Massage
A lymphatic massage will break down toxins that have been stored in fatty deposits.

Reflexology
See pages 686–687 for information about reflexology areas and how to work them. To encourage the release of toxins, give extra attention to the liver and the kidneys.

Hydrotherapy
Constitutional hydrotherapy supports detoxification. See pages 676–677 for directions.

Other Bodywork Recommendations
Acupuncture has a strong history of successfully treating addictions of all kinds. Consult a licensed practitioner who has experience in treating this problem.

Aromatherapy
Juniper breaks up poisons and speeds their exit from the body. Mix some with a carrier oil and use it in a lymphatic massage, or add a few drops to a hot bath.

Lavender, bergamot, and chamomile are antidepressants. Use them in any way you like to lift a case of the blues.

If you find that you're hungry all the time, inhale bergamot to suppress the appetite and reduce stress.

Stress-Reduction

General Stress-Reduction Therapies

Substance abuse is often an unproductive way of coping with stress or emotional pain. If you are to remain sober, then you must find another, more healthful way to manage stress. Read about various techniques in the Exercise and Stress Reduction chapter and experiment until you find one or two that you like enough to use regularly.

Bach Flower Remedies

Consult the chart on pages 648–650 to determine the best remedy for your particular needs. Once you've chosen a remedy, place 10 drops of the liquid under your tongue. Hold the drops in place for thirty seconds and swallow. Use as often as needed.

If you are plagued by vague fears that you can't name, take Aspen.

Cherry Plum will help if you have violent thoughts or impulses.

If you are ashamed of your illness, take Crab Apple.

People who hide their insecurity behind a mask of hostility will benefit from Holly.

Mustard is for people who suffer from severe depression that comes and goes without warning.

Star of Bethlehem will help people who need help coping with a shock or a crisis, even if the event occurred years ago.

Other Recommendations

- If you have problems with alcohol, be aware that some everyday products contain small amounts that may throw your good intentions off track. Avoid mouthwash, and read the labels on cold and flu medicines.
- Many people who abuse stimulants are actually trying to jump-start an underactive thyroid. For more information about testing yourself for this problem, see Hypothyroidism.
- If you've been abusing heroin, barbiturates, tranquilizers, or other depressants, you should be under medical supervision during your withdrawal period, which may last anywhere from a few weeks to a couple of months. It's too dangerous for you to quit cold turkey; instead, you should check yourself into a respected program that allows you to gradually and safely reduce your dependence on the drug.
- People who have been taking hallucinogens also need help as they pass through the acute stage of withdrawal. A health-care professional should be present to help them handle the uncontrollable, frightening, and sometimes violent thoughts that can occur during this time.

REFERENCES

Smith, R. F. 1974. A five-year trial of massive nicotinic acid therapy of alcoholics in Michigan. *Journal of Orthomolecular Psychiatry* 3:327–31.

Syndrome X

Syndrome X refers to a group of health problems that may include high blood pressure, overweight, and abnormal blood fats (cholesterol or triglycerides) and always includes a metabolic disorder known as insulin resistance. Insulin resistance is the resistance of one's cells to the blood sugar–transporting hormone insulin, which results in poor glucose metabolism. Excessive production of insulin leads to obesity, increased blood pressure, and high blood fats (triglycerides). Other terms that are sometimes used by doctors to describe syndrome X include metabolic syndrome, glucose intolerance, insulin resistance, and prediabetes.

The letter "X" in syndrome X, was so named because researchers in the past did not fully understand this syndrome, and X represents the unknown. Today syndrome X is a recognized condition and is well understood as a metabolic disorder. People who have untreated syndrome X are more prone to inflammatory disorders, such as cardiovascular disease, cancer, diabetes, and other chronic illnesses.

The modern American diet of refined carbohydrates and low fiber and a deficiency of essential fatty acids, combined with nutritional deficiencies and a lack of exercise, sets the stage for insulin resistance. Once insulin resistance has occurred, the cluster of symptoms known to accompany syndrome X, such as a weight problem or obesity, high blood pressure, high cholesterol, and high triglycerides, becomes evident. If you have two or more of these symptoms, many experts feel that you have syndrome X. People with syndrome X often have an "apple"-shaped body, as insulin promotes fat storage around the belly.

Syndrome X is best prevented and treated through nutrition, nutritional supplements, exercise, and other natural methods. As a matter of fact, we find that once a patient has been identified as having Syndrome X and follows our specific natural protocol, there is often a dramatic reduction in weight, blood lipids, and blood pressure, as well as an improved energy level.

SIGNS AND SYMPTOMS

- Insulin resistance and glucose intolerance (as diagnosed by blood testing)
- High blood pressure
- Abnormal blood lipids (high total cholesterol and triglycerides, and low HDL cholesterol)
- Excess fat around the belly or the chest

Testing Techniques

The following tests help assess possible reasons for syndrome X and insulin resistance:

Hormone testing (thyroid, DHEA, cortisol, testosterone, IGF-1, estrogen, progesterone)—saliva, blood, or urine

Intestinal permeability—urine

Vitamin and mineral analysis (especially magnesium, chromium, vanadium, zinc, B vitamins)—blood

Digestive function and microbe/parasite/candida testing—stool analysis

Food and environmental allergies/sensitivities—blood, electrodermal

---

ROOT CAUSES

- Heredity
- Unhealthful diet
- Chronic stress and the resulting stress hormone imbalance
- Nutritional deficiencies, especially of chromium, B vitamins, zinc, vanadium
- Obesity
- Lack of exercise

TREATMENT

Diet

The most important therapy for syndrome X and insulin resistance is a healthful diet. These dietary suggestions will help regulate your levels of sugar and also reduce your risk of complications, such as cardiovascular disease.

Recommended Food

Follow a diet that's high in fiber (vegetables, nuts, seeds, whole grains). Water-soluble fiber, as found in oat bran, beans, nuts, seeds, and apples, for example, helps to balance blood sugar. Ground flaxseeds should be consumed daily. Consume 1 teaspoon with each meal or ¼ cup daily. Make sure to drink plenty of water when you start taking flaxseeds (10 ounces per tablespoon). A daily total of 35 to 50 mg of fiber daily is a great goal.

Consume vegetable protein (legumes, nuts, seeds, peas) or lean animal protein (turkey, chicken, fish) with each meal and most snacks. Protein drinks that have low sugar levels can be consumed. Protein helps smooth out blood-sugar levels. Many people with diabetes find benefit by increasing the relative amount of protein in the diet.

Focus on quality fats. Fish such as salmon is excellent, as are nuts and seeds. Use olive and flaxseed oil with your salads.

Instead of eating three large meals, have several smaller meals throughout the day to keep your insulin and blood-sugar levels steady. Or have three main meals, with healthful snacks in-between. *Do not go longer than three hours without eating.*

A chromium deficiency contributes to blood-sugar problems, so eat plenty of brewer's yeast, wheat germ, whole grains, cheese, soy products, onions, and garlic. Onions and garlic will also help lower blood-sugar levels and protect against heart disease.

Enjoy plenty of berries, plums, and grapes, which contain phytochemicals that protect your vision.

Focus on foods with a low glycemic index and load value. See the Diabetes entry on pages 189–196 for more information.

Food to Avoid

Stay away from simple sugars. Obvious ones to avoid are candy, cookies, sodas, and other sweets.

White, refined bread also spikes blood-sugar levels. Whole-grain breads, cereals, and pastas are better choices, although you need to read the labels because they may contain an overabundance of carbohydrates. Brown rice, barley, oats, spelt, and kamut are complex carbohydrates that are good choices.

Eliminate alcohol and caffeine from your diet, as they can spike blood-sugar levels and thus insulin for some people.

Cut back on your consumption of saturated fat. Found in red meat and dairy products, it has been shown to increase the risk of diabetes and heart disease.

Avoid artificial sweeteners. Instead use diabetic-safe and more healthful natural sweeteners such as stevia, or xylitol.

Stay away from oils and foods that contain trans-fatty acids. Margarine, deep-fried foods, and most packaged foods, such as cookies, crackers, and pastries, contain hydrogenated oils. These land mines of trans-fatty acids promote insulin resistance.

Avoid high glycemic–load foods.

Detoxification

Consume detoxifying super green foods, such as chlorella, spirulina, wheatgrass, barley grass, or a mixture of super green foods. These foods also stabilize blood-sugar levels.

R̪ **Super Seven Prescriptions—Syndrome X**

Super Prescription #1   Chromium
Take a daily total of up to 1,000 mcg. Chromium improves glucose tolerance and balances blood-sugar levels.

Super Prescription #2   *Gymnema sylvestre*
Take 400 mg of a 25 percent gymneic acid extract daily. Gymnema lowers blood-sugar levels.

Super Prescription #3   Alpha lipoic acid
Take 300 to 1,200 mg daily. Alpha lipoic acid improves insulin sensitivity.

Super Prescription #4   Vanadyl sulfate
Take 100 to 300 mg daily. It improves glucose tolerance in people with insulin resistance. Higher dosages should be used under the supervision of a doctor.

Super Prescription #5   Biotin
Take 9 to 16 mg daily. Biotin is involved with proper glucose metabolism.

Super Prescription #6   High-potency multivitamin
It supplies many of the nutrients involved with blood sugar metabolism. Take as directed on the container.

Super Prescription #7   Essential fatty acids
Take a formulation that contains a mixture of omega-3, 6, and 9 fatty acids. Flaxseed or fish oil, combined with evening primrose oil, is common. Take as directed on the container. This supplement provides essential fatty acids that are needed for proper insulin function.

General Recommendations

An antioxidant formula supplies additional antioxidants, which are generally required in higher amounts in people with insulin resistance. Take as directed on the container.

B-complex vitamins are involved in blood-sugar metabolism. Take a 50 mg B-complex daily.

Zinc is required for proper insulin production and function. Take a daily total of 30 mg daily.

Vitamin C helps prevent oxidative damage, which is more common with this condition. Take 1,000 mg two to three times daily.

Magnesium is involved with insulin production and utilization. Take a daily total of 500 to 750 mg. Reduce the dosage if loose stools occur.

In a study of 180 men and women with type 2 diabetes, twice daily the participants were given a placebo, 100 mcg of chromium picolinate, or 500 mcg of chromium picolinate. Insulin values decreased significantly in both groups that received supplemental chromium after two and four months.

Vitamin E-complex improves glucose regulation and prevents cholesterol oxidation. Take 800 to 1,200 IU daily of a formula containing tocotrienols and tocopherols.

Milk thistle has been shown to improve blood-sugar levels. Take 600 mg of silymarin extract daily.

Banaba leaf has been shown in both animal and human studies to lower blood-sugar levels. Take 16 mg three times daily.

Adrenal extract supports adrenal gland function, which is also important for blood-sugar regulation. Take 500 mg twice daily on an empty stomach or as directed on the container.

DHEA is often low in people who have insulin resistance. If tests show that you have low levels, take 5 to 25 mg daily under a doctor's supervision.

Psyllium will reduce blood-sugar levels. It is a good source of fiber. Take up to 5 grams daily.

Asian ginseng (*Panax ginseng*) has been shown in a study to help improve blood-sugar levels. Take 200 mg daily.

Bitter melon (*Momordica charantia*) can help balance blood-sugar levels. Take 5 ml twice daily of the tincture or 200 mg three times daily of a standardized extract.

Garlic (*Allium sativum*) is an important herb for stabilizing blood sugar and helps reduce your risk of heart disease and other circulatory disorders by improving blood flow, lowering elevated blood pressure, and reducing levels of "bad" cholesterol. Take 300 to 450 mg twice daily.

Fenugreek (*Trigonella foenum-graecum*) is another herb that stabilizes blood sugar. Take a product with an equivalent dosage of 15 to 50 grams daily.

Policosanol is a good supplement to use for elevated cholesterol levels. Take 10 mg with the evening meal.

Homeopathy

Consultation with a homeopathic practitioner is advised to individualize homeopathic treatment.

Acupressure

- See an acupressurist for a specific treatment based on your symptoms.

Bodywork

Massage

Diabetics and people with unhealthy blood-sugar levels often suffer from poor circulation. A massage is a relaxing way to improve blood flow. Regular massaging of the feet may be especially beneficial to help ward off foot ulcers.

Reflexology

See pages 686–687 for information about reflexology areas and how to work them.

Work the points that correspond to the pancreas, the liver, and the thyroid, pituitary, and adrenal glands. You will probably have to massage these points every day for several months to see an effect.

Aromatherapy

Have fun trying the many different relaxing oils. Refer to page 658 for more information on aromatherapy oils; you may want to start with bergamot, jasmine, lavender, rose, sandalwood, or ylang ylang. Use them in a massage, a bath, lotions, or any of the other methods listed in the Aromatherapy chapter.

Stress Reduction

General Stress-Reduction Therapies

Insulin resistance puts additional stress on almost every part of your body and every area of your life. Keep up your emotional health by experimenting with the stress-reduction techniques discussed in the Exercise and Stress Reduction chapter. When you find one or two you like, practice them on a regular basis.

Other Recommendations

- Don't smoke or expose yourself to secondhand smoke. If you have insulin resistance, you are vulnerable to heart and kidney damage, both of which are linked to smoking. You may also have circulation problems, and smoking impairs blood flow.
- If you are overweight, it is imperative that you lose weight safely. Read the Obesity entry on pages 390–397.
- Exercise regularly to maintain optimal blood-sugar levels. Walking after meals is effective for some people.

REFERENCES

Anderson, R. A., N. Cheng, N. A. Bryden, M. M. Polansky, N. Cheng, J. Chi, and J. Feng. 1997. Elevated intakes of supplemental chromium improve glucose and insulin variables in individuals with type 2 diabetes. *Diabetes* 46(11):1786–91.

TMJ (Temporomandibular Joint) Syndrome

The temporomandibular joint connects the jawbone to the skull. When it is functioning properly, the bones of the joint allow the mouth to open smoothly and easily. Sometimes, however, there is a misalignment of the teeth or the jaw. In more serious cases, the cartilage that protects the joint wears down. Without cartilage to act as a cushion, the bones rub against each other.

TMJ can be caused by anything that places unusual pressure on the joint. A blow to the jawbone, habitual gum chewing, and poor orthodontic work are all possible factors. But by far the most frequent cause of TMJ is frequent grinding or clenching of the teeth. This seemingly benign habit is usually brought on by stress that causes muscles in the jaw to tighten. Another common underlying cause of TMJ is a structural misalignment of the jaw or the teeth (called *malocclusion* by doctors and dentists) or the cranial or facial bones can be involved. In addition, imbalanced musculature and spinal alignment in other areas of the body can be an underlying root cause of TMJ syndrome. Finally, deficiencies of nutrients such as magnesium can make this problem worse, because muscles tend to spasm and tighten more easily.

No matter what the cause, TMJ is at best uncomfortable and at worst almost unbearably painful. The first sign of a problem may be difficulty opening the mouth all the way or perhaps a popping or clicking sound when yawning or chewing. As the disorder progresses, the jaw muscles will begin to feel tender. This tenderness may develop into an ache or a sharp pain, which can spread to the neck, the ears, or the face.

A note of caution: Despite what some doctors or dentists may tell you, TMJ syndrome is real. But there have been many reports of unscrupulous professionals touting "miracle" cures for TMJ in the form of expensive and invasive treatments, including surgery. Before you undergo any aggressive measures, try the gentle home care and relaxation therapies suggested here. Chances are that they'll bring you substantial, if not total, relief. If you try these therapies and still have a great deal of pain, consult with a reputable, qualified specialist—and as always, ask for a full explanation of any procedure before you agree to it. Many naturopathic, osteopathic, or chiropractic physicians can help people with TMJ syndrome, using nonsurgical techniques. Acupuncture can also be quite helpful, as can stress-reduction techniques.

SYMPTOMS

- Clicking, popping, or grating noises when chewing or opening the mouth
- Difficulty opening the mouth all the way
- Stiffness, tenderness, or pain in the jaw
- Neck pain
- Earache
- Facial pain
- An asymmetrical appearance to the face
- Dizziness
- Ringing in the ears

ROOT CAUSES

- Tooth grinding or clenching (usually, the result of stress or a blood-sugar imbalance)
- Misalignment of the teeth or the jaw
- Poor orthodontia or dental work
- Injuries to the jaw
- Postural problems
- Frequent gum-chewing
- Prolonged thumb-sucking
- Muscle and spinal alignment imbalance
- Nutritional deficiencies (e.g., magnesium, calcium)

TREATMENT

Diet

Recommended Food

If your TMJ syndrome is acute, eat foods that require less chewing or that are not as hard to chew. Examples include soups, stews, steamed or cooked vegetables, and protein shakes.

Focus on foods that will stabilize your blood-sugar levels. Vegetables, beans, whole grains, nuts and seeds, soy products, and fish should be the mainstays of your diet. Instead of eating three large meals, plan on five or six smaller ones through the day. You'll keep your blood sugar in balance and won't be tempted to snack on sweet treats.

Food to Avoid

Avoid sugary foods like candy, chocolate, sodas, and most baked goods. They disturb blood-sugar levels and contribute to stress.

Testing Techniques

The following tests help assess possible reasons for TMJ syndrome:

Spinal and posture assessment—visual exam and x-ray

Vitamin and mineral analysis (especially magnesium, calcium)—blood

Food and environmental allergies/sensitivities—blood, electrodermal

Blood-sugar balance—blood

Stay away from caffeine, which causes muscles to tighten. Tea and coffee are obvious sources of caffeine, but chocolate, some pain-relievers, and over-the-counter cold medications have high amounts as well.

Alcohol has been linked to teeth-grinding. Although a drink or two may seem like a good way to relax, herbal teas are a much wiser choice for people with TMJ.

Don't chew anything that's hard on your jaw. Gum, caramels, bagels, animal meats, and hard or gooey candy are off-limits.

Detoxification

Go on a one- to three-day juice fast to cleanse your body of excess sugars. Support your fast with broths, herbal teas, and vegetable juices. If you must have some fruit juice, dilute it with water first.

℞ Super Seven Prescriptions—TMJ Syndrome

Super Prescription #1   Magnesium
Take 250 mg two to three times daily. This mineral relaxes the nervous system and the musculature around the jaw. *Note:* Reduce the dosage if loose stools occur.

Super Prescription #2   Calcium
Take 500 mg twice daily. It works synergistically with magnesium to relax tight muscles.

Super Prescription #3   Kava (*Piper methysticum*)
Take a standardized product containing 70 mg of kavalactones three times daily. Kava relaxes the nervous system and tight muscles. It is also very good for stress and anxiety. *Note:* Do not take with alcohol or any psychiatric medication.

Super Prescription #4   Methylsulfonylmethane (MSM)
Take 1,000 mg three times daily. MSM reduces muscle spasms and inflammation.

Super Prescription #5   Homeopathic Magnesia Phosphorica
Take 3 pellets of the 6x potency three times daily. This remedy relaxes tight muscles.

Super Prescription #6   B-complex
Take a 50 mg complex twice daily to reduce the effects of stress.

Super Prescription #7   *Valerian officinalis*
Take 3 ml or 300 mg three times daily to reduce the effects of stress and relax tight muscles.

General Recommendations

Glucosamine sulfate builds cartilage. Take 1,500 mg daily if you have cartilage deterioration in the TMJ.

Homeopathy

Pick the remedy that best matches your symptoms in this section. For acute TMJ pain, take a 30C potency four times daily. For chronic TMJ pain, take a 6x, 12x, 6C, 12C, or 30C twice daily for two weeks to see if there are any positive results. After you notice improvement, stop taking the remedy, unless symptoms return. Consultation with a homeopathic practitioner is advised.

Arnica (*Arnica montana*) is the classic homeopathic remedy for deep, bruising pain. It is especially helpful for TMJ pain that occurs immediately after an injury.

Hypericum Perforatum is indicated when there is a shooting, radiating nerve pain in the jaw area.

Ignatia (*Ignatia amara*) is for someone who is highly sensitive to stress that results in tight jaw muscles and TMJ pain. It is specific for TMJ syndrome that occurs after emotional grief or a trauma.

Kali Phosphoricum reduces the effects of stress and nerve pain.

Magnesia Phosphorica is a good general remedy for tight muscles that spasm and that feel better with warm applications.

Rhus Toxicodendron is for a stiff jaw that loosens up during the day and then stiffens up again in the evening. The jaw feels better with warm applications.

Acupressure

See pages 668–675 for information about pressure points and administering treatment.

- Large Intestine 4 is a point that will relieve pain and relax the muscles of the head and the jaw.
- Another point for pain located anywhere on the neck and head is Gallbladder 20.
- If you clench or grind your teeth at night, devote a few minutes before bedtime to working Lung 1. Breathe deeply, and try to clear your mind of obsessive thoughts.
- Pericardium 6 will ease panic or anxiety. Because it's located on the wrist, you can easily work this point whenever you feel your jaw tense up, even if you're in public.

Bodywork

Because it gently relaxes muscles *and* eases stress, bodywork offers some of the most effective treatments for TMJ. Experiment until you find the ones that work best for you.

Massage

A massage of the neck, the shoulders, the scalp, the jaw, and the muscles inside the mouth can do wonders. See a professional for an initial treatment, and then ask a loved one to practice home massage for daily maintenance.

A light facial massage can help you relax and develop a greater awareness of your jaw muscles.

Reflexology

See pages 686–687 for information about reflexology areas and how to work them.

Work the areas corresponding to the jaws, the neck, the ears, and the solar plexus.

Hydrotherapy

For immediate relief of pain, lie down with a warm compress held against your jaw. Add any of the essential oils suggested under Aromatherapy in this section for a stronger relaxing effect.

Other Bodywork Recommendations

A chiropractic adjustment can often relieve pain and bring the bones back into proper alignment. Consult a practitioner who has experience in working with TMJ patients. Naturopathic doctors and osteopathic doctors are also good choices.

Craniosacral therapy is a gentle way to align facial and cranial bones that contribute to TMJ.

Aromatherapy

Marjoram, black pepper, and rosemary have a warming and relaxing effect on clenched muscles. For best relief, add a few drops of oil to a warm compress.

Experiment with several of the relaxing oils until you find a few you like. Lavender, jasmine, rose, and bergamot are always good choices. Use them in any preparation you like, but don't rely on just one for a prolonged period of time, as you might become immune to its calming effects.

Stress Reduction

General Stress-Reduction Therapies

Many TMJ sufferers report good results from biofeedback, which teaches awareness of the bones and the muscles in the jaw.

If you suffer from a high degree of stress, you may want to supplement biofeedback with another technique, such as meditation or yoga.

Bach Flower Remedies

Consult the chart on pages 648–650 to find the remedy best suited for your own personality and tendencies. Following are some suggestions to get you started. Once you've chosen a remedy, place 10 drops of the liquid under your tongue. Hold the drops in place for thirty seconds and swallow. Use as often as needed.

For recurring thoughts that seem to go around in circles inside your head, especially at night, take White Chestnut.

If you can't stop worrying about loved ones, Red Chestnut will help.

Pine is for hardworking people who blame themselves when things go wrong, even if the fault is clearly belongs to someone else.

If you are a perfectionist and deny yourself even the simplest pleasures, Rock Water will help you create a more healthful balance in your life.

If you're a high-strung workaholic, try Nervain.

Other Recommendations

- Try to retrain your jaw posture. Every few minutes, stop to ask yourself whether your jaw is clenched; if it is, relax it. Proper jaw position is slightly relaxed, with your lips closed.

- Check your other postural habits. Do you tend to cradle the telephone between your jaw and shoulder? Do you slump forward at your desk? Try to sit up straight, as a general rule, and if you must speak on the phone for long periods, use a speaker phone or a headset.
- Clenching and grinding can be hard habits to break. If, despite your own attempts at relaxation and retraining, you still tense your jaw muscles, ask your dentist about a bite guard. He or she can fit one to your mouth, and you can wear it at night to prevent unconscious jaw damage.

Thrush. *See* Candidiasis

Underactive Thyroid. *See* Hypothyroidism

Ulcers

Peptic ulcers most frequently affect the stomach and the duodenum, which is the upper part of the small intestine. Both the stomach and the duodenum process high quantities of gastric juices. These juices have to be strong in order to break food down into digestible particles; in fact, they're composed largely of hydrochloric acid, a substance that can dissolve not just last night's dinner but body tissues as well. To protect the stomach and duodenum walls against damage from gastric acid, both organs are coated with a protective mucus layer. In addition, bicarbonate ions are secreted by the lining of the stomach and the duodenum. Under normal conditions, this mucus layer and the alkalinizing bicarbonate ions prevent the acid from eating away at the digestive tract lining. But when the lining is too weak and there is decreased bicarbonate secretion, some of the stomach tissues may be eroded. An eroded spot is called a peptic ulcer.

Most people know that stress increases the output of gastric acid. If you have an ulcer, reducing the levels of tension and anxiety in your life will go a long way toward healing the physical wound. But many other factors can cause or contribute to ulcers as well. Some drugs are notorious for increasing acid production—most notably, aspirin and the class of medications called nonsteroidal anti-inflammatory drugs (NSAIDs, for short). People who take aspirin or NSAIDs like ibuprofen on a regular basis are at a high risk for getting stomach ulcers. Smokers develop ulcers much more often than nonsmokers do. And as with every digestive disorder, a poor diet, especially one that includes spicy foods, citrus fruits, soda pop, caffeine, and alcohol, is frequently at the root of the problem. Food allergies or sensitivities can cause problems as well. One must also consider that low antioxidant status appears to predispose one to ulcers.

The bacteria *Helicobacter pylori* has been strongly linked to ulcer formation. Studies show that some people with ulcers have this bacterium in the affected organ, and elimination of *H. pylori* often helps with healing. Antibiotic therapy, as well as natural therapies, can be very effective for this infection. Make sure to supplement with probiotics to replace the helpful bacteria that antibiotics destroy. These good bacteria also play a role in preventing *H. pylori* infection.

Conventional therapy generally focuses on antacid medications. This group of medications suppresses stomach acid formation. For severe acute ulcer problems, such as a bleeding ulcer, these medications can be very effective and warranted. However, for many people these medications are prescribed on a long-term basis that does not treat the cause of the ulcer. In addition, long-term use can contribute to digestive problems in other areas of the digestive tract, as hydrochloric acid is required for protein digestion and the liquefaction of foods. Without proper stomach acid digestion, there is additional stress on the rest of the digestive organs. Also keep in mind that stomach acid is a natural barrier to bacteria such as *H. pylori,* as well as to other microbes. Suppression of this acid in the long term theoretically makes you more prone to an infection in the digestive tract. Finally, you require stomach acid to absorb minerals, so with long-term acid suppression you are prone to mineral deficiency.

Ulcers are a common complaint, but that doesn't mean they should be ignored. Without treatment, the pain and the burning will only get worse. In fact, the eroded area may grow larger and deeper until it begins to bleed. The ulcer may even perforate the stomach or intestinal wall. Bleeding or perforating ulcers should be treated as medical emergencies; if left unattended, they can be fatal.

SYMPTOMS

- Burning or gnawing pain in the upper abdomen that usually occurs when the stomach is empty or about an hour after eating. Pain may also come on at night.
- Loss of appetite
- Increased appetite (sometimes food actually soothes the ulcer)
- Nausea
- Vomiting

ROOT CAUSES

- Stress
- Medications, including aspirin and nonsteroidal anti-inflammatory drugs
- Dietary factors, including food allergies
- Smoking
- Alcohol use
- Infection with *H. pylori* (you are more susceptible if you have low stomach acid and not enough friendly flora)

Caution: If your stools or vomit are dark or bloody, or if you have intense abdominal pain that doesn't go away, you may have a bleeding or perforating ulcer. Consult a doctor immediately.

Testing Techniques

The following tests help assess possible reasons for ulcers:

H. pylori—blood, stool

Digestive function and microbe/parasite/candida testing—stool analysis

Antioxidant status—blood, urine

Food and environmental allergies/sensitivities—blood, electrodermal

---

Know Your NSAIDs

Nonsteroidal anti-inflammatory drugs—NSAIDs, for short—are some of the most commonly used medications in the world. Millions of people are dependent upon them for relief of back pain, headache, arthritis, and other conditions. Unfortunately, these drugs also increase the amount of gastric acid and can lead to peptic ulcers.

Following are some common and brand names for NSAIDs. If you've been using any NSAID for a prolonged amount of time, you may be at risk for peptic ulcers. Consider switching to an herbal preparation for effects that are just as potent but far gentler to your body.

If a doctor has prescribed an NSAID for you, consult with him or her before changing your regimen.

Popular NSAIDs include
- Advil
- Clinoril
- Feldene
- Ibuprofen
- Nalfon
- Nuprin
- Orudis
- Oruvail
- Relafen
- Tolectin
- Voltaren

TREATMENT

Diet

Recommended Food

Although you may not feel like eating, good nutrition is essential for healing ulcers. Eat several small meals a day to avoid placing a heavy burden on your digestive system.

Eat plenty of fiber. Although the smooth foods of the famous "bland diet" were once thought safest for ulcer patients, increased fiber intake has been shown to repair ulcers. Focus on sources of soluble fiber, such as oats.

Vitamin K has been shown to repair damage from gastric juices. Eat several servings of green leafy vegetables a day, and drink lots of green juices.

Studies have shown that cabbage juice has remarkable healing powers for ulcers. Drink a quart of cabbage juice daily. It may be diluted with water or carrot juice.

Cultured products will provide the friendly "bacteria" that fight *H. pylori*. Drink kefir milk or eat some live cultured yogurt every day.

Zinc is healing to the digestive tract. Good sources include pumpkin seeds and whole grains.

Consume garlic with your meals; test tube studies show it has anti-*Helicobacter pylori* properties.

Food to Avoid

Avoid sugar, spicy foods, citrus fruits and juices, coffee, black tea, and alcohol. They all contribute to high levels of gastric acid or are irritating to the stomach lining.

Consult the Food Allergies section, and use the elimination diet to determine whether a food allergy is causing or aggravating your ulcer. Although a reaction to any food can conceivably cause an ulcer, milk allergies are strongly linked to gastric problems.

In a single-blind study of 100 people with peptic ulcers, participants took DGL (760 mg three times daily) or the pharmaceutical Tagamet (cimetidine). Researchers found that both groups showed equal healing of ulcers after 6 and 12 weeks. Another study of 874 people found DGL as effective as antacids and the anti-ulcer medication Tagamet.

One double-blind trial compared 1 gram of mastic gum per day with a placebo in the treatment of thirty-eight people with duodenal ulcer. After only two weeks of treatment, symptoms improved significantly in 80 percent of those receiving mastic gum. Endoscopic (visual exam with a scope) examination verified healing in 70 percent of the mastic group but in only 22 percent of the placebo group.

Doctors once prescribed milk as a remedy for ulcers, but that practice has largely stopped. We now know that milk actually encourages stomach acid to form. In addition, many cases of ulcers are linked to a milk allergy.

Detoxification

Do a three-day juice fast to alkalinize your digestive tract. Stay away from acidic fruit juices during this time, and focus on green drinks and vegetable juices instead.

To keep your colon clean, take an enema on the first and last day of your fast and then once a month afterward.

℞ Super Seven Prescriptions—Ulcer

Super Prescription #1   Licorice root (DGL) (*Glycyrrhiza glabra*)
Chew 500 to 1,000 mg twenty minutes before meals or between meals, three times daily. DGL (deglycyrrhizinated licorice) stimulates the regeneration of the mucus layer and has anti-inflammatory effects. Preliminary research shows an inhibiting effect on the growth of *H. pylori.*

Super Prescription #2   Mastic gum (*Pistachia lentiscus*)
Take 500 mg three times daily. This supplement comes from the mastic tree and has been shown in test tube studies to destroy *H. pylori* and in human studies to be effective in healing ulcers.

Super Prescription #3   Aloe vera
Drink ¼ cup three times daily. Aloe promotes healing of the lining of the intestinal tract and has antimicrobial benefits.

Super Prescription #4   Homeopathic Nux Vomica
Take a 30C potency three times daily. This is the most common remedy for ulcers. See Homeopathy in this section for other helpful remedies.

Super Prescription #5   Probiotic
Take a product containing at least 4 billion active organisms twice daily, thirty minutes after meals. It supplies friendly bacteria, such as *Lactobacillus acidophilus* and *bifidus,* that prevent infection and aid digestion. It is particularly important to take if you are using antibiotics.

Super Prescription #6   Slippery elm (*Ulmus fulva*)
Take 3 ml or 500 mg of the capsule form or suck on a lozenge three times daily between meals. Slippery elm has a soothing and healing effect on the lining of the digestive tract.

Super Prescription #7   Chamomile (*Matricaria chamomilla*)
Drink a fresh cup of tea four times daily. Animal studies show that it has anti-ulcer activity, and it also relaxes the nervous system.

General Recommendations

Zinc promotes tissue healing. Take 30 mg daily, along with 2 mg of copper.

Vitamin A stimulates the healthy growth of intestinal cells and improves immune function. Take 25,000 IU daily, with a doctor's supervision. *Note:* Pregnant women or women planning for pregnancy should avoid doses above 5,000 IU.

Vitamin C acts as an antioxidant in the stomach lining and has been shown to retard *H. pylori* growth. Take 500 to 1,000 mg three times daily. Make sure to use a nonacidic vitamin C. Reduce your dosage if loose stools occur.

Essential fatty acids have been shown to help heal gastric and duodenal ulcers. Take 4,000 mg daily of fish oil or 1 tablespoon of flaxseed oil daily. Also, take 400 IU of vitamin E to prevent oxidation of these essential fatty acids.

L-glutamine promotes healthy intestinal cells. Take 1,000 mg three times daily on an empty stomach.

Homeopathy

Pick the remedy that best matches your symptoms in this section. For relief of acute ulcer pain, take a 30C potency every fifteen minutes, up to four doses. For chronic ulcer problems, take a 6x, 12x, 6C, 12C, or 30C twice daily for two weeks to see if there are any positive results. After you notice improvement, stop taking the remedy, unless symptoms return. Consultation with a homeopathic practitioner is advised.

Arsenicum Album is helpful for a burning sensation in the stomach that is alleviated by drinking milk or frequently sipping warm water and sitting up. The person feels anxious and restless.

Lycopodium (*Lycopodium clavatum*) is for gas and bloating, as well as for stomach pain. Symptoms are usually brought on by anxiety and a lack of confidence. The person feels worse when wearing tight clothes and better when sipping warm drinks. There may be a sour taste in the mouth. Symptoms are often worse in the late afternoon and the evening.

Nux Vomica is for people with heartburn and reflux that occur from stress, spicy foods, and alcohol. They are generally chilly, irritable, and oversensitive to stimuli (noise, light). Constipation is often a problem as well.

Pulsatilla (*Pulsatilla pratensis*) is helpful if your ulcer feels worse after you eat rich and fatty foods. Your symptoms feel worse in a warm room and better with fresh air. You also tend to feel tearful when ill, and you greatly desire comfort.

Phosphorous helps when you have a burning pain in the stomach that feels better from cold drinks. However, soon after drinking, you feel nauseous and may vomit.

Sulphur is for burning pain and belching, accompanied by diarrhea. You tend to be very warm and get relief from ice-cold drinks.

Acupressure

See pags 668–675 for information about pressure points and administering treatment.

- To strengthen your entire gastrointestinal tract, work Stomach 36.
- Another point that benefits the digestive system is Spleen 16. Work it on a daily basis to relieve the pain of ulcers and to restore your appetite for healthful food.

Bodywork

Massage
The primary benefit that massage offers the ulcer sufferer is stress relief.

Reflexology
See pages 686–687 for information about reflexology areas and how to work them.

Work the areas corresponding to the stomach, the duodenum, the diaphragm, and the solar plexus.

Side effects from the use of antibiotics are quite common. One study found that people supplementing probiotics while on antibiotic therapy (three antibiotics concurrently) had a significant reduction in diarrhea, nausea, and taste disturbance, as compared to those taking a placebo with their antibiotics.

Acupuncture
See a qualified practitioner for acupuncture and Chinese herbal therapy.

Hydrotherapy
Constitutional hydrotherapy is an excellent treatment that focuses blood flow back to the stomach to promote healing. See pages 676–677 for directions.

Aromatherapy
Lavender, ginger, and clary sage will calm gastric upset. Try them in a massage or add them to a bath or a warm compress.

Many oils have potent stress-relieving properties. Refer to page 658 for more information on aromatherapy oils; you may want to start with one or more of the following: lavender, rose, bergamot, and jasmine. Find a few that you like, and rotate them so that you don't become immune to their effects. You can use these oils in any preparation.

Stress Reduction

General Stress-Reduction Techniques
General stress-reduction techniques, such as deep breathing, prayer, yoga, and positive mental imagery, are helpful for recovery.

Bach Flower Remedies

If the following suggestions don't apply to you, consult the chart on pages 648–650. Once you've chosen a remedy, place 10 drops of the liquid under your tongue. Hold the drops in place for thirty seconds and swallow. Use as often as needed.

If you are strong-willed to the point of being inflexible, Vine will help you develop more tolerance.

Centaury will help quiet, kind people who take on too much work in order to please others.

Willow is for people who are bitter and resentful. Those who benefit from Willow often feel that life has been unfair to them.

Other Recommendations

- Tobacco smoke causes ulcers. Don't smoke or expose yourself to secondhand smoke.
- Do not take any NSAIDs or aspirin if you have a history of ulcers. If your doctor has prescribed these for you, check with him or her about a less-irritating alternative, or, better yet, work with a holistic doctor for a natural alternative.

REFERENCES

Al-Habbal, M. J., Z. Al-Habbal, and F. U. Huwez. 1984. A double-blind controlled clinical trial of mastic and placebo in the treatment of duodenal ulcer. *Clinical Experimental Pharmacology and Physiology* 11(5):541–44.

Armuzzi, A., F. Cremonini, F. Bartolozzi, F. Canducci, M. Candelli, V. Ojetti, G. Cammarota, M. Anti, A. De Lorenzo, P. Pola, G. Gasbarrini, and A. Gasbarrini. 2001. The effect of oral administration of *Lactobacillus GG* on antibiotic-associated gastrointestinal side-effects during *Helicobacter pylori* eradication therapy. *Alimentary Pharmacology and Therapeutics* 15(2):163–69.

Kassir, Z. A. 1985. Endoscopic controlled trial of four drug regimens in the treatment of chronic duodenal ulceration. *Irish Medical Journal* 78(6):153–56.

Morgan, A. C., et al. 1982. Comparison between cimetidine and Caved-S in the treatment of gastric ulceration, and subsequent maintenance therapy. *Gut* 23:545–51.

Uterine Fibroids. *See* Fibroids, Uterine

Vaginitis

Vaginitis is an inflammation of the mucous membrane that lines the vagina. The symptoms usually include burning or itching and may extend to abnormal vaginal discharge, painful urination, and pain during sexual intercourse. The vast majority of women will experience vaginitis at some point during their lives, and the unpleasant symptoms usually send women to their doctors for treatment.

Vaginitis is commonly caused by an overgrowth of yeast (*Candida albicans*). Common symptoms may include vaginal itch and/or soreness, burning, a cottage cheese–like discharge, and pain during intercourse. A physician can make a diagnosis, after a microscopic examination and a culture of the vaginal secretion. Other common conditions can mimic vaginal yeast infections. These include bacterial vaginosis (BV); the symptoms of this bacterial infection can include an abnormal grayish-white vaginal discharge and a foul-smelling vaginal odor. Another common cause is trichomonas vaginitis. This is a sexually transmitted disease caused by a one-celled microorganism called *Trichomonas vaginalis*. Symptoms include a foul-smelling, yellowish-green vaginal discharge and itching. Symptoms worsen during menstruation. This section focuses on yeast-related vaginitis. It is important to see your doctor to discover the cause of your vaginitis, because certain infections can be quite serious.

Women who experience chronic yeast infections often have a common history of being on repeated courses of antibiotics. While antibiotics may destroy harmful bacteria, they also have the potential to wipe out helpful normal flora in the vagina, as well as in the urinary and digestive tracts. Good bacteria, such as *Lactobacillus acidophilus,* play an important role as part of the local immune system in the vaginal area. They function to prevent the overgrowth of yeast and other opportunistic organisms that can cause infection. In addition, these good acidophilus species help to maintain an acidic pH in the vagina, which makes it less likely that an overgrowth of yeast will occur. These good bacteria also produce hydrogen peroxide, which is a natural antimicrobial agent that kills bacteria and fungus. Acidophilus supplements taken internally, as well as applied directly into the vagina (insert at night and cover with a pad), are an effective means to prevent and treat yeast infections. This remedy is best done under the supervision of a doctor. In addition, it's helpful to eat yogurt that is rich in friendly bacteria. A 1992 study found that women who consumed 8 ounces of yogurt daily had three times less incidence of vaginal yeast infections, as compared to women who did not eat the yogurt.

A key dietary factor that will help prevent reoccurring vaginal yeast infections is to reduce simple sugars in the diet. Yeast thrives on sugar, and too much of it has a suppressive effect on the immune system. Finally, be aware that food sensitivities can aggravate yeast infections for some women.

The immune system is constantly on the lookout for opportunistic organisms such as the yeast *Candida albicans*. When functioning optimally, it keeps unhealthful organisms in check. High stress, poor nutrition, and other factors can impair immune function, allowing for the overgrowth of candida. Many conventional doctors argue that only people with severe immune suppressive diseases, such as HIV/AIDS, have immune systems that are weak enough to allow for the overgrowth of yeast. This appears to be untrue, and a surprising number of seemingly healthy persons suffer from a weakened immune system, linked to systemic candidiasis.

Hormone balance is important in preventing vaginal yeast infections. These infections commonly occur one week prior to the beginning of a woman's menstrual flow. This is a sign that hormone balance plays a key role in the susceptibility to vaginal yeast infections. It is not unusual for women who experience PMS to also have problems with yeast overgrowth. Imbalanced estrogen and progesterone levels lead to an unfavorable vaginal pH. Typically, many of these cases are caused by what doctors call "estrogen dominance." The normal increase of progesterone does not occur during ovulation, and as a result, the relative balance of estrogen is too high. We have also found that many women resolve their chronic susceptibility to vaginal infections once they discontinue the use of the birth control pill. It is a well-known fact that this medication increases the incidence of yeast infections.

In summary, natural approaches are your best bet to resolve chronic cases of vaginal yeast infections. They can also be effective for relieving acute cases, when used under the supervision of a medical professional. If you are pregnant, do not start any therapy unless instructed to do so by your doctor.

SYMPTOMS

Vaginal:

- Itch
- Soreness
- Burning
- Cottage cheese–like discharge
- Pain during intercourse

ROOT CAUSES

- Antibiotics
- Poor diet (especially, too many simple sugars)
- Pregnancy
- Stress
- Birth control pills
- Sexually transmitted diseases
- Tight clothing
- Excessive douching
- Poor hygiene
- Food allergies or sensitivities
- Candidiasis (systemic)
- A suppressed immune system
- Diabetes
- HIV
- A hormone imbalance
- Flora imbalance

TREATMENT

Diet

Recommended Food

Fortify your immune system by eating a diet that's focused on natural, whole foods.

One of the best dietary strategies for restoring the natural balance of vaginal flora is to eat a cup of unsweetened live yogurt every day. Make sure the yogurt contains *L. acidophilus* and other friendly flora.

Garlic and onions can be consumed liberally for their antifungal properties. Flaxseeds also fight yeast infections. Take 1 to 2 tablespoons daily, along with 10 ounces of water.

Women with vaginitis often suffer from dehydration. Drink a glass of clean water every two waking hours.

Testing Techniques

The following tests help assess possible reasons for reoccurring vaginal yeast infections:

Immune system imbalance or disease—blood

Hormone testing (thyroid, DHEA, cortisol, testosterone, IGF-1, estrogen, progesterone)—saliva, blood, or urine

Digestive function and microbe/parasite/candida/flora testing—stool analysis

Food and environmental allergies/sensitivities—blood, electrodermal

Blood-sugar balance—blood

Diet

Food to Avoid

If you have vaginitis, you have two reasons to avoid sugar. For one, many of the organisms, such as *Candida albicans,* that cause vaginal infections feed on sugar. Second, sugar depresses the immune system, making it difficult to recover from your current infection and leaving you vulnerable to repeated cases of vaginitis. Do not eat any refined sugars, and restrict your intake of simple sugars from fruits, honey, molasses, and other natural sources.

Avoid foods that are high in yeast or mold, especially alcohol, aged cheese, dried fruit, nuts, and nut butters. You must also stay away from fermented foods, including vinegar, pickles, tempeh, and soy sauce.

Food allergies may be the cause of recurring vaginitis. Read the Food Allergies section and follow the elimination diet there. If your symptoms disappear when you stop eating a certain food, eliminate that product from your diet.

℞ Super Seven Prescriptions—Vaginitis

Super Prescription #1   *Lactobacillus acidophilus*
Insert 1 capsule intravaginally each evening, and cover with a pad overnight. Repeat for seven consecutive days for acute infections. Also, take a probiotic supplement (with friendly bacteria such as *Lactobacillus acidophilus*) orally that contains at least 4 billion organisms twice daily, thirty minutes after meals. These friendly bacteria fight yeast overgrowth.

Super Prescription #2   **Homeopathic Combination Vaginitis Formula**
Take as directed on the container. It contains the most common homeopathic remedies used for vaginal yeast infections.

A study of women who had recurrent vaginal yeast infections looked at the effects of daily ingestion of yogurt that contained *Lactobacillus acidophilus.* Women who consumed 8 ounces of yogurt daily for six months had a threefold decrease in infections and in vaginal candida colonization.

In a study, one hundred women with chronic vaginal yeast infections who were unresponsive to prolonged conventional therapy were treated with 600 mg of boric acid suppositories twice daily for two or four weeks. As a result, 98 percent of the women who were unresponsive to common antifungal treatments were cured.

Echinacea (*Echinacea purpurea*) has been shown to enhance immune function and have antifungal properties. A German study looked at the effect of oral echinacea supplementation on women who had a history of reoccurring vaginal yeast infections. Of the sixty women taking echinacea, only ten had recurrences of yeast infections.

Super Prescription #3   Boric acid

Insert a 600 mg capsule intravaginally each morning and evening for seven days for acute infections (cover with a pad). For a chronic infection, repeat for a total of two to four weeks. Vitamin E oil can be used on the external genitalia to prevent burning and discomfort. *Note:* Do not ingest boric acid orally.

Super Prescription #4   Echinacea (*Echinacea purpurea*)

Take 3 ml or 500 mg four times daily for immune support.

Super Prescription #5   Vitamin C

Take 1,000 mg two to three times daily for immune support.

Super Prescription #6   Oregon grape root (*Mahonia aquifolium*) or goldenseal (*Hydrastis canadensis*)

Take 3 ml or 500 mg four times daily for immune support.

Super Prescription #7   Oregano oil (*Origanum vulgare*)

Take 500 mg of the capsule form or 0.5 ml of the liquid twice daily or as directed on the container. Oregano oil has potent antifungal effects and is very important for women who have repeated vaginal yeast infections due to systemic candidiasis.

General Recommendations

Pau d'arco (*Tabebuia avellanedae*) has antifungal properties. Take 100 mg or 0.5 to 1.0 cc three times daily.

Garlic (*Allium sativum*) counteracts yeast infections and improves the immune system's defenses. Use several drops of garlic oil in a douche. For extra strength, you can also take garlic orally. Take 300 to 450 mg twice a day.

Vitex (chasteberry) is effective for women with hormone imbalance who experience repeated, cyclical vaginal yeast infections. Take 180 to 240 mg of a 0.6 percent standardized extract daily. *Note:* It should not be taken in conjunction with the birth control pill.

Homeopathy

Pick the remedy that best matches your symptoms in this section. For an acute vaginal yeast infection, take a 30C potency four times daily. For a chronic vaginal yeast infection, take a 6x, 12x, 6C, 12C, or 30C potency twice daily for two weeks to see if there are any positive results. After you notice improvement, stop taking the remedy, unless symptoms return. Consultation with a homeopathic practitioner is advised.

Borax is a remedy to use when you have a vaginal discharge that resembles egg whites or a white paste and have a feeling that warm water is flowing out. Vaginitis that responds to Borax often appears midway between the menstrual periods.

Calcarea Carbonica is a good choice when a woman experiences burning and vaginal itching before and/or after the menstrual period. Women who require this remedy are usually chilly, are overweight, and crave sweets, milk, and eggs. They become fatigued and overwhelmed easily.

Kali Bichromium is useful when the discharge is thick yellow and makes the external genitalia itch and burn.

Kreosotum is the most common remedy for acute vaginal yeast infections. There is a burning discharge with a putrid odor, along with great itching. The discharge is worse before menses or during pregnancy.

Natrum Muriaticum is used when the burning discharge resembles an egg white.

There is often vaginal dryness, along with the discharge. The woman craves salt and tends to be reserved. She feels worse in the sun and in warm rooms.

Pulsatilla (*Pulsatilla pratensis*) is indicated when there is a creamy-white or yellowish discharge. Symptoms often change throughout the day. The woman feels better in the open air. She has a strong craving for sweets and a desire for company.

Sepia is helpful when the vaginal discharge is yellow and itchy or white and offensive-smelling. A woman who requires this remedy often feels run down and irritable and wants to be left alone. She may feel a bearing-down sensation in the pelvic area.

Sulphur is used when the discharge is yellowish and offensive smelling, with great burning and itching. The woman's symptoms may worsen from warmth and bathing.

Acupressure

See pages 668–675 for information about pressure points and administering treatment.

- If you have a vaginal discharge, use Conception Vessel 4 and 6.
- Work Lung 1 to ease stress.

Bodywork

Reflexology

See pages 686–687 for information about reflexology areas and how to work them.

Work all the female reproductive areas to stimulate blood flow and encourage healing.

To stimulate the immune system, especially the production of antibodies, work the lymph and the spleen.

Hydrotherapy

Add several cups of organic apple cider vinegar to your bath, and soak for fifteen to thirty minutes. Allow the water to flow into your vagina.

Aromatherapy

Tea tree oil, a natural antiseptic, is a highly potent remedy for vaginitis. You can use the oil in a douche or in a compress two times a day, as needed, until the inflammation is under control. Tea tree oil is sometimes irritating, so start off by using just two or three drops of oil; if you don't have a reaction, you can try a few drops more.

To relieve tension, use lavender, rose, geranium, bergamot, or jasmine in a bath, a diffuser, or whatever preparation suits you best.

Stress Reduction

General Stress-Reduction Techniques

Some women who have a history of sexual abuse experience chronic vaginitis. Besides the recommendations in this section, seek counseling and spiritual support.

Bach Flower Remedies

Following are some suggestions, but you should consult the chart on pages 648–650 to determine the best remedy for your particular needs. Once you've chosen a remedy, place 10 drops of the liquid under your tongue. Hold the drops in place for thirty seconds and swallow. Use as often as needed.

If vaginitis makes you feel unclean, take Crab Apple.

Women who find it difficult to turn down others' requests should take Centaury to develop a clear sense of their own desires and to build their inner strength.

Elm is for women who take on too much responsibility and wind up exhausted or depressed, "overwhelmed."

After an extended period of stress that results in deep fatigue and exhaustion, Olive will help.

Other Recommendations

- Avoid sexual intercourse during the course of treatment to avoid irritation and reinfection. For some chronic cases of yeast-related vaginitis, the male partner needs to be on an antifungal protocol (see the Candidiasis section).
- Wear loose cotton clothing that allows your genitals to breathe. Avoid tight jeans and pantyhose with nylon crotches.
- If you go swimming, change out of your wet bathing suit quickly. Otherwise, you'll create a breeding ground for bacteria.

REFERENCES

Coeugniet, E., and R. Kuhnast. 1986. Recurrent candidiasis: Adjuvant immunotherapy with different formulations of Echinacin®. *Therapiewoche* 36:3352–58.

Hilton, E., H. D. Isenberg, P. Alperstein, et al. 1992. Ingestion of yogurt containing *Lactobacillus acidophilus* as prophylaxis for candidal vaginitis. *Annals of Internal Medicine* 116:353–57.

Jovanovic, R., et al. 1991. Antifungal agents vs. boric acid for treating chronic mycotic vulvovaginitis. *Journal of Reproductive Medicine* 36(8):593–97.

Varicose Veins

Two primary kinds of blood vessels exist in the circulatory system. Arteries are one kind; they deliver blood away from the heart to the rest of the body. Veins are the second type of blood vessel, and their function is to conduct blood back to the heart. Of the two kinds of vessels, veins have the more difficult task. Unlike the arteries, they cannot rely upon the heart's direct pumping motion to propel the blood to its destination. Instead, the pumping action comes from the contracting and relaxing effect of muscles surrounding the veins. Luckily, however, the veins are equipped with a series of valves that help keep the blood flowing in one direction only: toward the heart.

When one of these valves malfunctions, or when a vein wall is somehow weakened, the blood cannot continue to flow properly. Instead, it pools and accumulates within the veins, which are burdened by the excess blood. They grow weaker, and they begin to stretch and bulge. These enlarged, raised blood vessels are called varicose veins. They usually appear on the legs—especially on the thigh or the back of the calf—where the veins have to fight strong gravitational pressure as they push blood back up to the heart. Varicose veins can also appear in other parts of the body, including the anus, where they are called hemorrhoids. (For more information about anal varicose veins, see Hemorrhoids.)

Varicose veins may be tender and painful and may cause the legs to feel tight and swollen, but in general, they do not pose a health risk. They are also quite common:

about 50 percent of middle-aged Americans have some varicose veins. In many people, the condition is brought on by a genetic weakness in a vein wall or valve, but it can also be caused by anything that puts excess pressure on the veins. A diet that's high in fat and low in fiber can stress the veins (because this contributes to constipation), as can inactivity, obesity, and long periods of sitting or standing. Many women develop varicose veins during pregnancy, when the legs are burdened with a great deal of extra pressure. We often see women with hormone imbalances who have problems with varicose veins, particularly women taking a synthetic hormone replacement.

Although no one has a cure for varicose veins, home treatment is quite effective at reducing the pain and the swelling. Home therapies can also strengthen the vein walls and prevent the condition from growing worse. Of particular importance is a group of herbs known as venotonics. This class of herbs improves the tone of the venous wall. Horse chestnut (*Aesculus hippocastanum*) and butcher's broom (*Ruscus aculeatus*) are two prime examples and are discussed in this section. We find that the natural therapies in this section often prevent a further progression of varicose veins, and in some cases, there is a mild improvement. In most cases, patients find that their circulation improves. Sometimes, however, professional care is in order. In rare cases, varicose veins deep in the leg can lead to a more serious circulatory disorder, such as phlebitis or a blood clot that can travel to the lungs, resulting in a life-threatening pulmonary embolism. If you have an intense pain deep in your legs, or if you experience persistent swelling in one or both your legs, consult your doctor.

SYMPTOMS

- Swollen, raised veins that may be tender and painful
- Heavy, tight, swollen, or fatigued legs
- Bruising in the affected area
- Itchy skin near the varicose veins
- Ulceration over the varicose veins

ROOT CAUSES

- A genetic weakness in the vein or a vein's valve
- A diet that's low in fiber and high in fatty and refined food
- Obesity
- Inactivity
- Long periods of sitting or standing
- Liver disease
- A hormone imbalance
- Nutritional deficiencies

Testing Techniques

The following tests help assess possible reasons for varicose veins:

Blood pressure

Hormone testing (thyroid, DHEA, cortisol, testosterone, IGF-1, estrogen, progesterone)—saliva, blood, or urine

Vitamin and mineral analysis (especially vitamin C, E)—blood

Digestive function and microbe/parasite/candida testing—stool analysis

Food and environmental allergies/sensitivities—blood, electrodermal

TREATMENT

Diet

The low-fiber Western diet leads to constipation. Straining during bowel movements puts intense pressure on the veins of the lower body; over time, it can cause veins to weaken and enlarge. Therapies that encourage regular elimination are an important part of the treatment for varicose veins.

Recommended Food

A high-fiber diet is your best weapon against varicose veins. Reduce your risk of constipation by eating plenty of fresh vegetables and fruits, whole grains, and nuts and seeds.

Consume 1 to 2 tablespoons of ground flaxseeds, along with 10 ounces of water, daily to obtain healthful fiber.

Certain kinds of flavonoids will strengthen the walls of the veins and improve their elasticity. Berries that have a bluish-red color—cherries, blueberries, and blackberries, for example—are rich in the flavonoids you need, so enjoy them often as snacks or dessert. Buckwheat, as a food and in tea form, is a good source of a flavonoid called rutin, which increases the strength of capillaries. Use it in whole-grain pancakes or breads.

To improve circulation, flavor your meals with garlic, onions, ginger, or cayenne pepper.

Vitamin E is good for the circulation and also helps prevent blood clots. Wheat germ is an excellent source, as are soybeans and leafy greens.

Food to Avoid

Saturated fats, along with hydrogenated or partially hydrogenated oils, slow down your circulation and worsen the inflammation of the blood vessels. Avoid them.

Sugar and other refined carbohydrates can lead to weight gain and constipation. Dramatically reduce your intake of sweets and refined foods.

Caffeine and alcohol are dehydrating, and they worsen varicose veins.

Detoxification

If you are chronically constipated, a three-day juice fast will help clear out your bowels and give you a fresh start. During your cleanse, drink a wide variety of juices; aloe, carrot, apple, and green drinks will help to speed waste through your system.

℞ Super Seven Prescriptions—Varicose Veins

Super Prescription #1   Horse chestnut (*Aesculus hippocastanum*)
Take a standardized extract that contains 100 mg of aescin daily. This herb strengthens vein walls and valves and also improves circulation and reduces swelling.

Super Prescription #2   Butcher's broom (*Ruscus aculeatus*)
Take a standardized extract that gives you 200 to 300 mg of ruscogenins daily. Ruscogenins are constituents within this herb that are believed to reduce inflammation of veins.

Super Prescription #3   Grape seed extract or **maritime pine bark extract**
Take 200 to 300 mg daily. These supplements contain proanthocyandins, constituents that improve circulation and strengthen the integrity of the vein wall.

In one study of 240 people, horse chestnut extract was found to be as effective as conventional methods that used specialized compression stockings and diuretic therapy. Preliminary studies have shown that horse chestnut extract reduces the formation of enzymes that contribute to varicose veins.

Super Prescription #4   Bioflavonoid complex

Take 1,000 mg two to three times daily. Various flavonoids, such as rutin and hesperidin, have been shown to be effective as accessory nutrients in treating varicose veins.

Super Prescription #5   Bilberry (*Vaccinium myrtillus*)

Take a standardized extract containing 25 percent anthocyanosides at 160 mg twice daily. Bilberry improves the circulation and strengthens capillary walls.

Super Prescription #6   Vitamin E

Take 400 IU of a mixed complex twice daily. Vitamin E acts as a natural blood thinner, to promote blood flow and reduce inflammation of the veins.

Super Prescription #7   Witch hazel (*Hammamelis virginiana*)

Apply as a gel or a cream to external hemorrhoids, or add 1 ounce to a sitz bath daily. Witch hazel has an astringent effect on external varicose veins.

General Recommendations

Gotu kola (*Centella asiatica*) is an herb that improves blood flow and strengthens the integrity of the vein walls. Take a product that provides 60 mg of triterpenic acids daily.

A high-potency multivitamin provides a base of nutrients for healthy veins. Take as directed on the container.

Vitamin C is important for healthy vein walls. Take 500 mg two to three times daily.

Bromelain reduces inflammation of the veins and may help prevent blood clots. Take 500 mg three times daily, between meals. Look for products standardized to 2,000 M.C.U. (milk-clotting units) per 1,000 mg or 1,200 G.D.U. (gelatin-dissolving units) per 1,000 mg. Protease enzyme products also have this benefit.

Essential fatty acids are important for reducing the inflammation of blood vessels. Take 400 mg of fish oil or 1 tablespoon of flaxseed oil daily, along with 1,000 mg of evening primrose oil (*Oenothera biennis*).

A greens drink that contains a blend of super green foods, such as chlorella, spirulina, and so on, provides fiber and improves liver function. Take as directed on the container.

Ginkgo biloba is a popular treatment for all circulatory disorders. Find an extract standardized to 24 percent flavone glycosides and take 60 to 120 mg twice daily.

Vitamin C strengthens the rectal tissue. Take 500 mg two to three times daily.

Dandelion root (*Taraxacum officinale*) promotes bile flow and improved regularity. Take 300 mg or 2 ml of tincture three times daily.

Psyllium is a good fiber supplement and has been shown to reduce the pain and the bleeding associated with hemorrhoids. Take 5 to 7 grams daily, along with 10 ounces of water.

Homeopathy

Pick the remedy that best matches your symptoms in this section. Take a 6x, 12x, 6C, 12C, or 30C potency twice daily for two weeks to see if there are any positive results. After you notice improvement, stop taking the remedy, unless symptoms return. Consultation with a homeopathic practitioner is advised.

Aesculus Hippocastanum is for distended, purple veins that cause hot, sticking pains. Symptoms are worse when walking and in the cold.

Arnica (*Arnica montana*) is for veins that look and feel bruised. The veins are swollen and painful to touch.

Bellis Perennis is for varicosities that occur during pregnancy and make it difficult to walk. There is a deep bruising pain.

Carbo Vegetabilis is a good remedy when one experiences mottled skin with distended veins. One's legs feel heavy, weak, and chilly, yet have burning pains. The symptoms are worse from warmth and lying down and feel better from elevating the feet.

Hamamelis is for varicose veins of the thighs and the legs, in which there is a feeling of heaviness and bruising, with signs of swelling. The veins can become itchy. Symptoms are worse from touch, jarring, and pressure and feel better from motion.

Lachesis is for a blue-red swelling of varicose veins. The veins may bleed easily. The person tends to be hot and intolerant to heat. Symptoms often come on with menopause or pregnancy.

Pulsatilla (*Pulsatilla pratensis*) is for swollen veins in the legs that are bluish and have stinging pain. The symptoms are worse in the heat and feel better in the fresh air. Pulsatilla is a common remedy for varicose veins that occur during pregnancy.

Sepia is for purplish, congested veins that have lost their elasticity. The problem comes on with pregnancy or during menopause. The woman is prone to constipation and being chilly. She has a craving for sour, salty, and chocolate foods. The symptoms are better from exercise and warmth.

Acupressure

See pages 668–675 for information about pressure points and administering treatment.

- To encourage bowel movements, work Conception Vessel 6 and Large Intestine 4.
- Large Intestine 11 strengthens the colon. If you tend to be constipated, work this point on a daily basis.
- To improve circulation to your legs, work Gallbladder 34.

Bodywork

Reflexology

See pages 686–687 for information about reflexology areas and how to work them.
Work the areas corresponding to the colon, the liver, and the endocrine glands.

Hydrotherapy

Hot and cold hydrotherapy is a gentle but highly effective way to stimulate circulation and reduce inflammation in the legs. You can alternate hot and cold baths, if you like, or use a shower nozzle to spray your legs directly.

A wet compress is another gentle treatment for varicose veins. Apply it directly to the affected area. For added benefit, you can make the compress with any of the essential oils listed under Aromatherapy in this section or with witch hazel, which has a toning effect.

Other Bodywork Recommendations

Try to find ten minutes a day to lie down with your feet elevated. You'll encourage the blood to flow in its proper direction, and you'll reduce the pressure and the swelling.

Aromatherapy

To stimulate circulation and tone the legs, use rosemary, geranium, black pepper, or ginger. Don't massage the oil into the weakened veins; instead, add the oils to a bath or a wet compress.

Other Recommendations

- Exercise is one of the best ways to improve varicose veins. Bicycling is highly recommended, as it works the legs without putting a great deal of pressure on them.
- Avoid long periods of standing and sitting, if you can. Take frequent breaks to walk around or to put your feet up.
- Elevate the foot of your mattress so that it's five to eight inches higher than the head. When you sleep, your blood will flow to your heart more easily, instead of pooling in your veins.
- Support hose will take pressure off your veins and improve circulation. To get the maximum results, lie down with your legs raised before putting on the hose, so that you aren't trapping blood in the lower half of your body.
- If you're obese, you can significantly reduce varicose veins by losing weight. The dietary suggestions in this section will give you a start; if you'd like further help, see Obesity.
- Don't wear tight clothes that restrict your circulation. Tight pants, garters, and poorly fitting pantyhose will just make the condition worse.

REFERENCES

Diehm, C., et al. 1996. Comparison of leg compression stocking and oral horse chestnut seed extract therapy in patients with chronic venous insufficiency. *Lancet* 347:292–94.

Kreysel, H. W., H. P. Nissen, and E. Enghofer. 1983. A possible role of lysosomal enzymes in the pathogenesis of varicosis and the reduction in their serum activity by Venostasin. *Vasa* 12:377–82.

Warts

These bumpy small mounds of overgrown skin usually appear on fingers, hands, knees, elbows, or toes. Warts are usually brown or fleshy colored and have rough, dry surfaces.

Although anyone at any age can develop warts, they seem to strike more often during childhood and adolescence. They tend to recur and spread.

Warts are caused by a host of viruses and can be spread to other parts of the body or other people through direct contact. Experts have identified at least seventy different types of the human papilloma virus (HPV) that are known to infect the skin and leave warts.

Warts are usually identified by their location. A few of the more dominant ones are

- Common warts: This type tends to surface on the skin of the hands and the fingers. These warts usually don't hurt and are caused by HPV types 2 and 4.
- Plantar warts: This type usually appears on the soles of the feet and tends to grow down into the skin, instead of creating mounds. Caused by HPV type 1, plantar warts are painful and attack blood vessels that are embedded deeply in the skin.
- Plane warts: These are small, flat, and flesh-colored warts that grow in clusters.

- Venereal warts: This type (known medically as condyloma acuminata or genital warts) affects the genital and anus areas. These moist, fleshy mounds of skin feature surfaces that resemble cauliflower. At least four different types of HPV cause this type of wart, which is spread through sexual contact.

Children's and many adult cases of warts often disappear over time without treatment.

The conventional treatment for warts is a topically applied acid (salicylic acid) to slowly peel away the skin. Also, cryosurgery involves freezing the wart with liquid nitrogen, which destroys the wart cells. The last resort is to surgically remove a wart. This may be done for stubborn plantar warts that cause foot pain while one is walking or standing.

Natural therapy generally focuses on enhancing immune function to eradicate or suppress the virus that causes wart development.

Note: Venereal warts need to be treated by a doctor.

Testing Techniques

The following tests help assess possible reasons for warts:

Immune system imbalance or disease—blood

Intestinal permeability—urine

Detoxification profile—urine

Vitamin and mineral analysis—blood

Food and environmental allergies/sensitivities—blood, electrodermal

---

TREATMENT

Diet

Recommended Food

Eat a variety of whole, nutritious foods for optimal immune health.

Food to Avoid

Avoid simple sugars, which can reduce the effectiveness of the immune system against the virus that causes the warts.

R̲x̲ Super Seven Prescriptions—Wart

Super Prescription #1   Homeopathy
Pick the remedy that matches your warts in the Homeopathy section. We find that homeopathy is the most effective treatment, but it requires an individualized remedy to be effective.

Super Prescription #2   Thuja (*Thuja occidentalis*)
Apply one drop of Thuja oil to the wart(s) twice daily for four weeks. Thuja has a caustic effect on the wart and also has antiviral properties.

Super Prescription #3   Olive leaf extract (*Olea europa*)
Take 500 mg twice daily. Olive leaf has antiviral properties.

Super Prescription #4   Garlic (*Allium sativum*) **oil**
Apply one drop of garlic oil to the wart(s) twice daily for 4 weeks. Garlic oil has antiviral properties.

Super Prescription #5   Echinacea (*Echinacea purpurea*)
Take 2 ml or 300 mg twice daily. Echinacea enhances immune function and has antiviral properties.

Super Prescription #6   Selenium
Take 200 mcg daily. A selenium deficiency makes it easier for viruses to replicate.

Super Prescription #7   Vitamin E
Take 400 IU daily. Vitamin E is important for immune function and to combat viral infections.

General Recommendations

Take a high-potency multivitamin for general immune support. Take as directed on the container.

Homeopathy

Pick the remedy that best matches your symptoms in this section. Take a 6x, 12x, 6C, 12C, or 30C potency twice daily for two weeks to see if there are any positive results. After you notice improvement, stop taking the remedy, unless symptoms return. Consultation with a homeopathic practitioner is advised.

Antimonium Crudum is specific for hard, flat warts that are often located on the tips of the fingers or the toes (plantar warts) and under or around the nails.

Causticum should be used for large, fleshy, and soft warts that bleed easily. They are often located on the hands, the arms, and the face.

Dulcamara is indicated for large, smooth warts found on the back of the hand or on the palm.

Nitric Acid is a good choice for cauliflower-looking warts that bleed easily and are painful. They are often found on or near the genital area, the mouth, and the anus.

Thuja (*Thuja occidentalis*) is used for extensive crops of warts (usually large) that tend to come back after being burned off or surgically removed. It is also used for warts that have formed after one has a vaccination.

Bodywork

Aromatherapy
Place 1 drop of lemon and 1 drop of tea tree (*Melaleuca alternifolia*) oil on a Q-tip and dab onto the wart(s). Cover with a band-aid. Repeat daily for two to three weeks.

Other Bodywork Recommendations
Tape a new piece of banana peel to the wart with adhesive tape every day (plantar's wart) for two to four weeks. It contains a substance that kills warts.

Visualization and Hypnosis
Visualize your warts falling off. Some studies have shown this technique to be effective.

One six-week controlled trial found that hypnosis sessions twice weekly resulted in greater wart disappearance than did medication, placebo, or no treatment.

Hypnosis is another alternative treatment that is successful for some people with warts. The emerging field of psychoneuroimmunology demonstrates the powerful connection between the mind, the nervous system, and the immune system. The immune system can eradicate the virus that causes warts when it is working properly.

REFERENCES

Spanes, N. P., V. Williams, and M. I. Gwynn. 1990. Effects of hypnotic, placebo, and salicylic acid treatments on wart progression. *Psychosomatic Medicine* 52:109–14.

Yeast Infection. *See* Candidiasis

PART TWO

The Essentials of Natural Medicine

Diet and Nutrition

A nutritious diet is essential to having good health and vitality. Few "health experts" would disagree with this statement, since history and medical science have proven it to be true. The concept is so simple that many people forget that food provides the fuel and the building blocks that allow the body to function. This section of the book will guide you on what foods you should eat and why they are healthful. In addition, we will help you learn about the foods that contribute to disease so that you don't let them inhibit your vitality.

Modern Poisons

A century ago, our meals were prepared from fresh, whole foods. Generally, food crops were grown on local land that was considered a valuable commodity. People took time to prepare their food and enjoy the intrinsic flavors and aromas. Today, the combination of technology and globalization has turned much of our food supply into semisynthetic, genetically engineered, nutrient-lacking packaged goods. Take a look at your local supermarket. Most of the food you see is stuffed into boxes or other packages. It contains preservatives that ensure a long shelf life. Many North Americans tend to be overfed, yet simultaneously malnourished. What a paradox!

Tips for Adopting a Healthful Diet

- Learn as much as you can about nutrition. This book and many others are loaded with sound, effective advice on optimal nutrition.

- Influence your children positively by being a role model for how to eat nutritiously. Kids learn more by watching than from listening to us preach to them. Follow the same recommendations yourself that you instruct your children to follow. You will find that this is a powerful way to develop healthful eating habits in your children.

- Be enthusiastic about eating healthfully.

Enthusiasm begins with the belief that you really can make a difference in the quality of your health and vitality.

- Be patient. In a society where junk food is the norm, it takes time to adapt to a healthful diet.

- Take action. You can immediately affect how your children feel by controlling what goes in their mouths. Also, you can play a major role in preventing diet-related illnesses, such as obesity, diabetes, cancer, fatigue, anemia, and most other chronic diseases.

Back to Eden

Nature produces a variety of foods designed by our Creator that are perfectly compatible with the human body. History shows that the further we get away from these naturally occurring foods, the worse our health becomes. Some of the most interesting research in this regard was done by Dr. Weston Price, a dentist with a passion for anthropology and health. He traveled the world to study primitive cultures and their dietary habits. He found that people who consumed a traditional diet, consisting of plant foods they could collect and animals they could catch (especially fish), had superior health and longevity. More than ever, health-conscious people in America are choosing to eat fresh, organic whole foods. This great trend, we predict, will gain momentum as nutritional research continues to demonstrate the multitude of health benefits that accrue from eating natural foods.

Avoiding the SAD Diet

The rates of obesity, diabetes, cancer, heart disease, and many other chronic diseases continue to skyrocket, due in large part to the standard American diet (SAD). The obvious solution is not to eat what most Americans are consuming, if you want to be healthy.

The standard American diet is high in refined carbohydrates (a technical term for, basically, sugar), saturated and trans-fatty acids (the types of fats that are linked to disease), and animal protein. Most commercial foods are loaded with artificial sweeteners, dyes, and preservatives. Meals commonly consist of fast food or frozen foods, or they are skipped altogether. Meals do not usually include plant foods, such as fruits, vegetables, legumes, whole grains, nuts, and seeds. Instead of water, people drink coffee, alcohol, soda, or sweetened fruit juice. Pesticides, herbicides, and other toxic chemicals are present in the food supply (even in the leading brands of baby food). From childhood through the adult years, people have abandoned their basic instincts to eat nutritious food and have succumbed to television commercials that promote fake foods. For example, the *Journal of the American Dietetic Association* reported on a study of preschool children, in which researchers found that the most commonly eaten foods were fruit drinks, carbonated beverages, 2% milk, and French fries. Vegetables dominated the lists of children's least favorite foods.

The Pyramid Scam

In 1992, the United States Department of Agriculture published the *Food Guide Pyramid.* In our opinion, and in the opinion of most nutrition-oriented physicians, this recommended pyramid is a representation of why so many Americans are confused about what they should eat. Furthermore, we find that people who follow this type of nutritional program are more likely to be obese and to develop other chronic illnesses.

It is sad to say, but the USDA may not have your best health interests at heart. This department has what many would call a "conflict of interest." It represents the food industry and is in charge of developing policy for and educating consumers about nutrition. Look at the emphasis on the number of servings of bread, rice, cereal, and pasta. These are exactly the types of foods that, for the most part, are eaten in excess and that contribute to weight problems, heart disease, and many other insulin-associated conditions. Another problem is that the USDA sparingly recommends fats and oils. Any nutrition expert will tell you that essential fatty acids are crucial for good health, and most of the population is not consuming these fats.

USDA FOOD GUIDE PYRAMID

KEY
☐ Fat (naturally occurring and added)
▼ Sugars (added)

Fats, Oils, & Sweets
USE SPARINGLY

Milk, Yogurt, & Cheese Group
2–3 SERVINGS

Meat, Poultry, Fish, Dry Beans, Eggs, & Nuts Group
2–3 SERVINGS

Vegetable Group
3–5 SERVINGS

Fruit Group
2–4 SERVINGS

Bread, Cereal, Rice, & Pasta Group
6–11 SERVINGS

Source: United States Department of Agriculture (USDA) and the Department of Health and Human Services (HHS)

Balch and Stengler Food Guide Pyramid

Following is the type of pyramid we recommend to our patients. It is in line with modern nutrition research and promotes optimal health.

Dairy products —optional

Quality protein (fish, lean poultry, eggs) 2–4 servings

Whole grains (low glycemic) 3–5 servings/Legumes 2–3 servings

Healthful oils (Oils: olive, canola, flax, hemp) Nuts and seeds 3–4 servings

Vegetables 5–7 servings/ Fruit 2–3 servings

Water 6–8 glasses (48–64 ounces)

Macronutrients: The Essentials of Good Health

Macronutrients make up the basis of our foods and provide us with energy. These include carbohydrates, proteins, and fats.

CARBOHYDRATES

A *carbohydrate* is a compound that contains carbon and water molecules. Actually, individual sugar molecules joined together make up carbohydrates. The simplest of sugar molecules are glucose, fructose (fruit sugar), and galactose (a milk sugar). These are known as monosaccharides, as they each contain one sugar molecule. Within the category of carbohydrates are simple and complex carbohydrates. Examples of simple carbohydrates include table sugar, honey, and fruit sugars.

As you read in the description of the standard American diet, most people consume far too many simple carbohydrates. Although the body ultimately breaks carbohydrates down into glucose (the simplest of sugars), most simple carbohydrates, such as candy, potato chips, soda, and refined flours (white breads, crackers, chips, cookies, muffins), have little to no fiber, vitamins, minerals, or phytonutrients. These carbohydrates are often called empty calories. When consumed in excess, especially on an empty stomach, they lead to immune system suppression, mood swings, attention problems, and weight gain (fat deposition). Many of these effects are due in large part to the spike in blood sugar that results after they are eaten. As a result, the hormone insulin is released to help transport blood sugar to the cells. As a by-product of this, the pancreas (which produces insulin) is overtaxed, immune cells are weakened, and the body stores fat. Too high a percentage of simple carbohydrates in the diet predisposes people to develop obesity, diabetes, cavities, and heart disease. The question then arises: What about fruits, because most of them contain simple carbohydrates? Research has shown that many types of fruits are good to eat, when consumed in moderation. As it turns out, fruits contain a great deal of fructose. This simple sugar does not cause a rapid rise in glucose and insulin levels because fructose must first be converted into glucose by the liver, to be available for the body to use. Fructose has a much more stable effect on blood-sugar levels than do other common sugars, such as sucrose, maltose (found in rice syrup and malt), dextrose, and honey. Certain fruits, such as apples, contain fiber that helps to normalize blood-sugar levels.

Glycemic Index

Glycemic index (GI) has become a popular term; it is more meaningful than the label *simple carbohydrate*. GI refers to the rise in your blood sugar after you ingest a specific food. This numerical value is compared to the GI of glucose at a value of 100. It is recommended that people with obesity, diabetes, and insulin resistance eat foods that have lower glycemic values. For example, a Coca-Cola soft drink has a glycemic index of 63, whereas as a serving of kidney beans has a value of 23.

A GI of 70 or more is considered high.

A GI of 56 to 69 is considered medium.

A GI of less than 55 is considered low.

Glycemic Load

Recently, doctors and researchers have placed more value on the glycemic load (GL) value of foods. The glycemic load takes into account the amount of carbohydrates in one serving of a particular food. The glycemic index tells us how quickly a carbohydrate turns into blood sugar, but it neglects to take into account the amount of carbohydrates in a serving, which is important. The higher the glycemic load value, the higher the blood-sugar level and the resulting stress on insulin levels. This value is derived by multiplying the amount of carbohydrates contained in a specified serving size of the food by the glycemic index value of that food, and then dividing by 100. For example, an apple has a GI of 40, compared to that of glucose, which is the baseline at 100, but the amount of carbohydrates available in a typical apple is 16 grams. The GL is calculated by multiplying the 16 grams of available carbohydrates times 40 and then divided by 100, to arrive at a decimal number of approximately 6. Compare this to a serving of Rice Krispies, which has a glycemic index of 82 and 26 available carbohydrates and has a glycemic load of 21. And a serving of macaroni and cheese has a glycemic load of 32.

A GL of 20 or more is considered high.

A GL of 11 to 19 is considered medium.

A GL of 10 or less is considered low.

Complex carbohydrates should be the dominant type of carbohydrates in the diet. They provide a longer-lasting energy source, help us to feel fuller, maintain our blood-sugar balance, contain fiber that helps us with elimination, and contain more vitamins, minerals, and phytonutrients than simple carbohydrates do. Examples of complex carbohydrates include whole grains (such as whole wheat pasta, whole grain breads and cereals, and oatmeal), beans, brown rice, peas, and most root vegetables.

Consuming carbohydrates along with protein, fiber, and fat (good fats) helps to smooth out their effect on blood-sugar levels. This is another reason why a balance of all the nutrients is so important.

One study found a 50 percent reduction in people's white blood cell activity (good immune cells) for two hours after they ingested a sugar solution. Studies have found that this negative effect can last for five hours or more.

PROTEINS

Protein is found in both plant and animal foods. The body uses protein as a fuel source and to form or repair tissues, organs, and muscles. Protein consists of enzymes and hormones and is found in every cell of the body. Amino acids are the individual building blocks of protein. There are approximately twenty different amino acids. Ten of the amino acids are known as "essential amino acids," which means that our bodies cannot manufacture them, so it is essential that we consume them in our diets. The remaining ten nonessential amino acids can be manufactured in the body.

Debate continues among nutritionists about whether humans should consume animal protein, as compared to plant protein. We must remember that humans are omnivores, and that our digestive tracts (including our teeth) were designed to handle both animal and plant foods.

Animal protein contains complete proteins, which means that it contains all of the essential amino acids. It has a higher biological value, meaning that animal proteins are more digestible and easily utilized by the body. However, certain types of animal meat, especially the red meats, tend to be much higher in saturated fats. Another concern is that contaminants, such as hormones, antibiotics, and microbes (parasites, bacteria, virus), may be found in animal products. This is it is so important to buy organic meat products and cook them properly. Also, our fish supply has become increasingly contaminated with toxins, including heavy metals such as mercury.

Plants also contain protein that is vital to our health. One advantage of eating plants, aside from their protein content, is their fiber content. In addition, they are a valuable source of phytonutrients, from which researchers continue to discover a host of health benefits. Keep in mind that most plants are an incomplete protein source. However, this is not a problem, because a variety of combined plant foods provides all the essential amino acids. It is important to consume organic fruits and vegetables to limit the amount of pesticides and herbicides your body is exposed to. People with insulin resistance or diabetes may fare better by not having a completely vegetarian diet and often benefit from eating animal foods. Also, people who have celiac disease or a gluten intolerance must avoid most types of grains.

Quality protein sources include soy, eggs, poultry, legumes, fish, nuts, and occasional amounts of red meat. For infants, breast milk is the best source of protein.

FATS

Most people fear fat, because they associate it with obesity. However, to be healthy, humans require fat in the diet. The key is to eat the right kind of fats and to reduce or avoid harmful fats. Fat is required to produce energy; for healthy brain development and function; for normal growth and development; to absorb fat-soluble vitamins; for healthy skin, nails, and hair; for a healthy immune system; and for many other vital functions. All fats are composed of carbon, hydrogen, and oxygen molecules. The differences between fats come down to the number of carbon atoms in each type of fat and the way they are arranged. There are three main categories of fats:

Monounsaturated fat refers to fatty acids that have one double bond. The double bond affects the function of the fatty acids and makes the fat useful for certain cell functions. Monounsaturated fatty acids are healthful and are found in foods such as avocados and olive oil.

Polyunsaturated fats comprise all of the essential fatty acids. Essential fatty acids must be obtained through the diet, as the body cannot manufacture them. Polyunsaturated fatty acids contain more than one double bond. Good sources are fish such as salmon and mackerel, as well as flaxseeds and flaxseed oil, walnuts, soybeans, and certain other plant foods. See the next section for more information on essential fatty acids.

The term *saturated fats* means that all the carbon molecules are filled (saturated) with hydrogen molecules. This makes the fats solid to semisolid at room temperature. Examples of foods that are high in saturated fats include red meat, pork, and dairy products. Lard is another one. Some oils, such as palm and coconut oil, contain high amounts of saturated fats. There is a role for saturated fats in the body. For example, they are one component of brain cells. However, most people tend to go overboard with foods that contain saturated fats; the consumption of these fats is associated with an increased susceptibility to cancer, heart disease, and inflammatory conditions. Saturated fat is also known to be a storehouse for many different types of toxins.

Fats to Avoid

Read ingredient labels closely to determine which foods contain hydrogenated or partially hydrogenated fats. These "synthetic fats" cause oxidation and cell damage. Common food sources include margarine, cookies, crackers, salad dressings, and many commercial baked items. Alternative foods that do not contain these harmful fatty acids are available.

Essential Fatty Acids

It is important that you not only consume foods with essential fatty acids but also maintain a proper balance of these good fats. As mentioned earlier, the body cannot manufacture essential fatty acids. They are so vital to life, humans cannot live without them. Two types of fatty acids are considered essential. They are alpha linolenic acid (ALA), of the omega-3 family, and linoleic acid (LA), from the omega-6 family.

Three Families of Fatty Acids

Most of the research in regard to fatty acids has been done with omega-3 and omega-6 fatty acids. A third type, known as omega-9 fatty acids, is also important, but not much is yet known about all of its roles. The numbering of fatty acids (e.g., omega-3) is in reference to the first double bond location. Following is a summary of the omega families:

Omega-3 Fatty Acids

Alpha linolenic acid (ALA)

Eicosapentaenoic acid (EPA)

Docosahexaenoic acid (DHA)

Omega-6 Fatty Acids

Linoleic acid (LA)

Gamma-linolenic acid (GLA)

Arachidonic acid (AA)

Omega-9 Fatty Acids

Oleic acid

The Two Essential Fatty Acids

All the fatty acids are important. The body requires about twenty fatty acids to function properly. However, unlike the other fatty acids, alpha linolenic acid and linoleic acid cannot be manufactured by the body and must be obtained from the diet.

Alpha linolenic acid.   ALA is a member of the omega-3 fatty acid family. You have probably heard of it in regard to the health benefits of eating fish and flaxseeds. Other examples of foods that contain ALA include walnuts, green leafy vegetables, and canola oil.

Linoleic acid.   LA is a member of the omega-6 family. This fatty acid is found in foods such as sunflower, safflower, corn, and sesame, borage, and evening primrose oils.

What Are Essential Fatty Acids Used For?

Essential fatty acids are part of the cell membranes. They are needed for cells to carry out their normal functions. Here is a sample of the roles that essential fatty acids play:

Brain and retina development	Proper circulation
Balanced mood	Kidney function
Hormone synthesis	Nerve transmission
Regulation of pain and inflammation	Energy production
Immune Function	Skin, nail, and hair health

Physical signs of essential fatty acid deficiency or imbalance include

Dry skin, cracked skin	Dry eyes
Dandruff	Poor wound healing
Irritability	Frequent urination
Soft nails, nails that break easily	"Chicken skin" on the back of the arms
Dry, listless hair	
Excessive thirst	

Conditions associated with fatty acid deficiency or imbalance include

Arthritis	Diabetes
Asthma	Eczema
Attention deficit disorder	Fatigue
Cardiovascular disease (heart attack, stroke)	Hair loss
	Hypertension
Cancer	Lupus
Depression	Memory problems
Dry skin	Schizophrenia

The Importance of Fatty Acid Balance

Think of a scale, with the omega-3 fatty acids on one side and the omega-6 fatty acids on the other. To maintain a balance, each side must be equal. The problem with most children's diets in our modern society is that this scale is tipped in favor of the omega-6 fatty acids. This imbalance can lead to a whole host of problems, including behavioral changes, decreased immunity, cardiovascular problems, joint problems, skin problems, and a variety of other medical conditions. Researchers have stated that the Western diet contains anywhere from fourteen to twenty times more omega-6 fatty acids than omega-3s.

Dr. Ronald Rudin, an expert in essential fatty acids, estimates that over the last seventy-five years, our omega-3 fatty acid consumption has decreased by 80 percent. Following are some major reasons why this imbalance has occurred:

- Decreased consumption of foods that are rich in omega-3 fatty acid (fish, flaxseeds, whole grains)
- Refining of grains
- Increased sugar intake (interferes with fatty acid metabolism)
- Increased intake of trans-fatty acids (fast foods and margarine)
- Increased hydrogenation of oils
- Nutritional deficiencies (certain minerals, such as B6, are needed for fatty acid metabolism)
- Increased use of pharmaceutical medications (these may deplete nutrients and fatty acids)
- Infant formulas are not balanced with essential fatty acids
- Digestive problems

Harmful Fats

Saturated fats, described earlier, make up one category of unhealthful fats (see page 534). Hydrogenated fats and trans-fatty acids refer to the unsaturated fatty acid molecules from vegetable oils that have had hydrogen molecules added. This results in unnatural fats that are now semisolid or solid. Trans-fatty acids are found in margarine, salad dressings, commercial breads, cookies, and crackers. They should be avoided, due to their harmful effects on the body. They have no known beneficial function. As a spread or for baking, butter is a better option than margarine is. Oils such as canola and olive oil should be used for frying.

Fatty Acids Worthy of Description

DHA (docosahexaenoic acid) is an omega-3 long-chained fatty acid that's found in high concentrations in breast milk and fish. Humans have the ability to make DHA from the essential fatty acid ALA, but the efficiency of this process varies, depending on the individual. DHA plays a pivotal role in the development of a baby's brain and retinas. It also plays an important role in joint health and cognitive function. Sources of DHA include fish, especially cold-water fish, such as salmon, mackerel, herring, and tuna. Other good sources include eggs and some types of algae.

EPA (eicosapentaenoic acid) is an omega-3 fatty acid that helps to regulate inflammation, the immune system, blood clotting, and circulation (including to the brain). It is also found in DHA-rich fish.

GLA (gamma linoleic acid) is a member of the omega-6 family. It has a powerful effect on the functions of the brain, on joint health, and on hormone balance. Sources include borage oil, evening primrose oil, and black current seed oil.

AA (arachidonic acid) is first found in the mother's breast milk, where it helps with her infant's brain development. At approximately one year of age, an infant can make its own AA. Many animal products, such as beef and turkey, contain AA, so a deficiency is rare in our society. Too much AA can act as a precursor to inflammatory conditions in the body. Linoleic acid can also be converted into AA. Sources include animal fat, peanuts, and some algae.

Gotta Get Your Fiber

One key to a healthful diet is making sure that you get enough fiber on a daily basis. Plant foods are the only source of fiber. There are two types of fiber. Soluble fiber means that the fiber dissolves in water. An example would be oat bran or dried beans and peas. This type of fiber helps to slow the absorption of glucose from the intestines into the bloodstream and thus improves the blood sugar balance. It also helps to lower cholesterol. Insoluble fiber does not dissolve in water, and it helps to bind water and bulk up the stools to allow for efficient bowel movements. It also helps to bind excess fats and toxins in the digestive tract, to be excreted out with the stools. Populations that consume a lot of fiber have less risk of developing colon and other cancers. Fiber also provides a sense of fullness, without containing empty calories. It is recommended you get at least 25 grams of total fiber a day.

Constipation, straining at a bowel movement, abdominal pain, or hard stools can all be signs that you are not getting enough fiber. People with sensitive digestive systems (who are prone to bloating, gas, cramps, etc.) often do better by starting with steamed or cooked vegetables, such as broccoli, carrots, and cauliflower. Over time, they can convert to larger quantities of raw vegetables. Also, enzyme supplements are helpful for people who have trouble digesting raw vegetables. By including five or more servings of fruits and vegetables a day in your diet, you will obtain enough fiber. Essentially, try to get in a good source(s) of fiber with every meal.

FIBER CHART

	Serving Size	Soluble Fiber (grams)	Insoluble Fiber (grams)	Total Fiber (grams)
Fruits				
Apples	1 apple	0.4	2.6	3.0
Banana	1 banana	0.5	1.3	1.8
Blueberries	½ cup	0.2	1.9	2.1
Blackberries	½ cup	0.4	4.5	4.9
Grapes	10 grapes	trace	0.5	0.5
Grapefruit	½ grapefruit	0.1	0.3	0.4
Honeydew, Melon	½ cup	0.1	0.4	0.5
Peach	1 peach	0.6	1.1	1.7
Raisins	¼ cup	0.2	1.4	1.6
Vegetables				
Artichoke (fresh, cooked)	1 medium	3.5	2.9	6.4
Beans (black, dry, cooked)	½ cup	0.1	2.7	2.8
Broccoli	½ cup	1.6	1.0	2.6
Brussels sprouts (frozen, cooked)	½ cup	0.4	2.8	3.2
Lettuce	½ cup	0.2	0.3	0.5
Spinach (canned, cooked, or raw)	½ cup cooked or canned			
	2 cups raw	0.3	2.0	2.3
Vegetable soup (canned)	1 cup	0.6	1.6	2.1
Grains				
Bread (white or Italian)	1 slice	0.2	0.6	0.8
Bread, rye	1 slice	0.2	0.5	0.7
Bread, whole wheat	1 slice	0.3	2.2	2.5
Cereal, Total cornflakes	1 cup	trace	0.8	0.9
Cereal, Rice Krispies	1 cup	0.1	0.4	0.5
Cereal, Special K	1 cup	0.1	0.7	0.8
Cookies, oatmeal	1 large	0.3	0.6	0.9
Cookies, plain sugar	1 cookie	0.1	0.1	0.2
Crackers, Ritz	4 crackers	0.1	0.2	0.3

	Serving Size	Soluble Fiber (grams)	Insoluble Fiber (grams)	Total Fiber (grams)
Muffin, blueberry	1 small	0.2	0.6	0.8
Oats, whole	½ cup	0.5	1.1	1.6
Pancake	2 pancakes	0.2	0.7	0.9
Rice, medium grain	½ cup	trace	0.3	0.4
Nuts				
Almonds, roasted	(22 whole)	0.1	2.4	2.5
Peanuts	(30 to 40 whole)	0.1	1.9	2.0
Walnuts	14 halves	trace	1.0	1.1
Legumes				
Beans, black, dry, cooked	½ cup	0.1	2.7	2.8
Lentils, dry, cooked	½ cup	0.1	2.8	2.9
Peas (green, canned, or frozen)	½ cup	0.3	2.8	3.1

Water

An adequate water intake is very important for both children and adults. Most of our body consists of water, making it a crucial substance that enables all the cells, the organs, and the tissues of the body to work properly. This includes the brain. Mild dehydration can interfere with concentration and cause headaches. Most people do not consume enough water on a daily basis. Infants should consume 1.5 ounces of water per pound of body weight daily. Infants who are breastfed do not need to drink water, as they get plenty in the breast milk. Children should drink an average of 40 ounces a day. Adults should drink 48 to 60 ounces a day. A warm climate, exercise, soft drinks, and high-sodium foods lead to dehydration. Also, a person may need more water to help recover from an illness.

The other consideration in regard to water is quality. Tap water in North American homes is laced with chemicals. Chlorine is a good disinfectant but should not be consumed, as it destroys the good bacteria in the digestive tract and is linked to bladder and rectal cancer. It can be removed with a filtration system and with a charcoal filter in the showerhead. Fluoride is contained in the municipal water supply, depending on which area of the country you live in. Fluoridation of the water supply is a controversial topic; fluoridation may be a serious health hazard. Pesticides, heavy metals (e.g., lead) and other contaminants are found in the water supply. Parasites and bacteria are in higher-than-acceptable concentrations in some areas of this country's water.

The optimal solution is to install a reverse-osmosis system in your home or drink distilled water. Have your drinking water tested by a certified water-testing company in your area. You can also contact the

Drink before You Think

Do not wait until you have the sensation of feeling thirsty to start drinking water. By the time you feel thirsty, you are likely to be mildly dehydrated. Regular water intake throughout the day is encouraged.

Environmental Protection Agency Safe Drinking Water Hotline (1-800-426-4791 or www.epa.gov) to get more information about water safety standards and testing.

Whole Foods Diet

Your diet should focus on whole foods that are unprocessed and as fresh as possible. Although it's difficult to have a diet that is 100 percent whole foods, shoot for this as a goal when you prepare meals. A whole foods diet will be much richer in nutrients and enzymes than packaged, processed foods are.

Examples of whole foods include whole grain breads and cereals; fruits; vegetables; fresh fish, poultry, and meats; and nuts and seeds. Essentially, foods that have not been processed are whole foods—just the way nature intended them to be.

Variety in the Diet

A healthful diet includes a wide a variety of foods. Every food has a different nutritional profile. By eating as many different healthful foods as possible, you expand the amount and the types of nutrients you take in. In addition, your taste and desire for a wide variety of foods will increase after you experience so many different flavors, textures, and so on. Furthermore, a varied diet prevents food sensitivities from developing, thus you will avoid present and future problems (see the Food Sensitivities section for more information). Try to eat fruits and vegetables in every color of the rainbow: green, yellow, red, and so on. They all contain different phytonutrients, which are so valuable for preventing serious illnesses.

Why Organic Foods Are Best

Over 1 billion pounds of pesticides and herbicides are sprayed on U.S. crops each year. Yes, it is realistic to assume that you are ingesting these potential toxins.

The long-term effects of pesticide and herbicide exposure are unclear, but a scary picture is beginning to emerge. Population studies on adults suggest a link with certain types of cancers and neurological diseases. As parents and doctors, we do not want to wait until "absolute" scientific evidence links these chemicals to various diseases. Pesticides that had been considered safe and were used for decades are now being banned. For example, methyl parathion, a type of organophosphate, was recently banned from being sprayed on apples.

GO ORGANIC

Foods are one of the few environmental substances that we can specifically control in regard to our health. It's hard to control the air we breathe outdoors unless we move to a different area. But we can control the safety of our food, to a certain extent, and it starts when we buy organic.

Organic means foods that have not been sprayed with synthetic chemicals and have

According to the Environmental Protection Agency, "Adverse effects of pesticide exposure range from mild symptoms of dizziness and nausea to serious, long-term neurological, developmental and reproductive disorders. Americans use more than a billion pounds of pesticides each year to combat pests on farm crops, in homes, places of business, schools, parks, hospitals, and other public places. For the first time, the EPA is calling for hundreds of additional studies on pesticides to better understand their effects on children specifically (developmental neurotoxicity, acute and subchronic neurotoxicity). In addition, the EPA has developed new tests and risk assessment methods to target the factors unique to infants and children."

been grown in safe soil. Look for foods that are labeled "certified organically grown." Organic foods may not be totally pesticide-free, due to cross contamination from other crops and circumstances beyond anyone's control. A 1997 *Consumer Reports* study of one hundred pounds of organic and nonorganic food (randomly selected from grocery stores around the country) found that 25 percent of the organic samples had traces of pesticides, while 77 percent of the nonorganic food did. Yes, organic foods cost more, but your health is worth it. Be wary of the following fruits and vegetables, as they contain some of the highest amounts of toxic pesticides:

Peaches	Grapes
Apples	Strawberries
Pears	Raspberries
Winter squash	Spinach
Green beans	Potatoes

Baby food is contaminated with pesticides and chemicals as well. Fortunately, well-known baby food brands are now selling organic. The next best thing to buying certified organic food is to buy fruits and vegetables at local farmer markets. Get to know local farmers who do not use pesticides on their crops. You can also purchase poultry and meat products made from chickens, sheep, and cattle that consumed nonpesticide feed and are free of hormones and antibiotics. Organic milk is now available as well.

Organic Is More Nutritious Than Other Food

One study compared the amounts of healthful and toxic minerals in organically and conventionally grown foods. Following are the results, which highly favor organically grown foods.

Healthful Minerals

Boron—70% higher in organically grown

Calcium—63% higher in organically grown

Chromium—78% higher in organically grown

Cobalt—same in both groups

Copper—48% higher in organically grown

Iodine—73% higher in organically grown

Iron—59% higher in organically grown

Lithium—118% higher in organically grown

Magnesium—138% higher in organically grown

Molybdenum—68% higher in organically grown

Nickel—66% higher in organically grown

Phosphorous—91% higher in organically grown

Potassium—125% higher in organically grown

Rubidium—28% higher in conventionally grown (not a desirable mineral)

Selenium—390% higher in organically grown

Silicon—86% higher in organically grown

Sodium—159% higher in organically grown

Strontium—133% higher in organically grown

Sulfur—20% higher in organically grown

Vanadium—8% higher in organically grown

Zinc—60% higher in organically grown

Toxic Minerals

Aluminum—40% higher in conventionally grown

Cadmium—5% higher in organically grown

Lead—29% higher in conventionally grown

Mercury—25% higher in conventionally grown

Clean Your Fruits and Vegetables

All foods, whether organic or not, should be washed and cleaned thoroughly to rinse off bacteria, as well as pesticides. The problem with soft foods, such as pears, is that pesticides saturate into the core of the fruit. We recommend washing your fruits and vegetables with dish detergent or special soaps that dissolve pesticides.

Fish

As we mentioned, fish are an excellent source of protein and essential fatty acids. Unfortunately, certain species of fish are known to contain dangerous levels of mercury and other toxins. The following boxed text lists fish that are deemed to be safe from mercury and those that are considered borderline or unsafe. The quality and the safety of fish depend on the area where you live. You can check the status of the contamination of fish in your area at the government Web site, www.epa.gov, or contact your local state department.

Don't Skip Meals

It is important that you eat regular meals. This will help you to maintain regular blood sugar levels. Regular meals improve concentration, mood, and energy levels. Snacks between meals are important for people who are very active or are prone to blood sugar problems, such as hypoglycemia, insulin resistance, diabetes, and obesity.

Mercury and Fish

Fish That Are Generally Low in Mercury	*Fish That Are Generally High in Mercury*
Anchovy	Chilean seabass
Catfish	Cod, Atlantic
Clams	Groupers
Cod, Pacific	Flatfish, Atlantic
Crab	Halibut
Flatfish, Pacific	Lobster
Herring	Mackerel
Mahimahi	Ocean perch
Oysters	Orange roughy
Pollock, Pacific	Oreo dory
Salmon, wild Alaskan	Pollock, Atlantic
Sardines	Rockfish, Pacific
Scallops, farmed	Shark
Tilapia, farmed	Snappers
	Striped bass
	Swordfish
	Tuna

Bring Your Lunch to School and Work

Well-known fast-food chains infiltrate many schools. Although fast foods pose no problem if you have them only on occasion (once a week), your child should not eat them for lunch on a regular basis. They are loaded with harmful trans-fatty and saturated acids, artificial preservatives and sweeteners, and sugars. Many adults eat out at lunchtime. It is more economical and healthful to bring your own lunch. When you do eat out, choose reputable, more healthful restaurants.

Tips for Eating Out

You can enjoy eating out and still get a relatively healthful meal. Following are some tips:

- Tell the waiter that you do not want a dessert menu or sample at the end of the meal.
- Choose fruit juice, milk, or water over soda.
- Choose fruit instead of french fries as a side dish.

- Avoid fried foods.
- Order a salad with the dressing on the side (so that you can use a small amount instead of the heaping that usually drenches the salad).
- Give your children menu options that do not include fried foods.

Acid/Alkaline Levels

Our bodily fluids' pH registers on a scale of 0.0 to 14.0. Seven is neither acid nor alkaline. The higher the number over 7, the more alkaline it is. Anything 0 to 7.0 is increasingly acidic, and it increases at an exponential rate, with 9 on the scale being 10 times higher than 8, and so on—as the number drops. Alkalis offset acids, and acids neutralize alkalis.

While our bodies routinely produce and expel acids and alkalis, most of the foods we choose to eat produce an acidic effect in the blood. Most of the acid in our bodies is eliminated by breathing, but acid that is introduced to our bodies via our diets is expelled through our kidneys, taking many minerals with it. These minerals are needed to neutralize acids as they leave our bodies. Without a large-enough reserve of minerals, these acidic toxins can accumulate to a critically dangerous point.

The problem is that sugar, meat, dairy products, and most refined grains all have acidifying effects on our blood and tissues. Because our diets rely so strongly on these acid-producing foods, we use more and more of our minerals to flush them out. The scales keep dipping further and further out of balance. This is one reason many health experts believe that most people have suboptimal health. An acidic blood condition adversely affects enzymatic reactions in the body, contributing to a host of problems.

Fruits and especially vegetables contain the kind of organic minerals needed to keep your body's pH level in balance. There is, of course, organic acid in fruits. But these substances easily disintegrate and blow away with respiration, your body's exhaust system. Green vegetables, such as green lettuces, broccoli, and zucchini, and super green foods, such as spirulina, chlorella, and wheatgrass, as well as sea vegetables like dulse, nori, wakame, and hijiki, apparently can neutralize acidic tissues due to their alkalinizing effect. Eat multiple servings of these alkalinizing foods each day.

Phytonutrients

A major area of interest in nutritional science concerns the therapeutic benefits of phytonutrients, also known as phytochemicals. These naturally occurring substances give plants their characteristic flavor, color, aroma, and resistance to disease. When consumed, they also help people resist disease. Thousands of phytonutrients have been identified in fruits, vegetables, grains, seeds, algae, and nuts. They have tremendous benefits for people by helping to prevent illnesses such as cancer and cardiovascular disease. For example, two phytochemicals found in cruciferous vegetables (such as broccoli and cauliflower), known as indole-3 carbinol and sulforaphane, help the body to metabolize toxins and are associated with preventing certain types of cancers. Flavonoids, found in citrus fruits, protect us against heart disease, stroke, and cancer. Many phytochemicals are powerful antioxidants that protect against cell damage and environmental pollutants. Others also help cells to detoxify more efficiently. For example, green vegetables are high in chlorophyll, a potent detoxifying phytochemical. We need all the support that nature has to offer in our modern but toxic world.

Bottom line: You are what you eat. People who grow up eating whole food diets, including abundant amounts of plant foods, stand a better chance of avoiding cancer, heart disease, and other maladies. Many health benefits of phytochemicals are yet to be discovered.

Phytochemical	Source	Properties	Conditions
Allylic Sulfides	garlic, onions	detoxification support	cancer
Bioflavonoids	fruits and vegetables	antioxidant, cancer prevention	arthritis, cancer, circulatory diseases
Catechins	berries, tea (especially green tea)	antioxidant, detoxification	high cholesterol, cancer and heart disease prevention
Chlorophyll	green plants and other colored vegetables	antioxidant, contains vitamin K	anemia, detoxification, burns and wounds, cancer prevention
Curcumin	turmeric	anti-inflammatory, antioxidant	arthritis, inflammatory bowel disease, cancer
Ellagic Acid	berries, grapes, apples, tea	detoxifying	cancer prevention
Flavoglycosides	ginkgo, black tea	antioxidant, improved blood flow	heart disease, kidney disease, varicose veins, depression, poor memory
Fructooligosaccharides (FOS)	Jerusalem artichoke, chicory root, garlic, bananas	detoxification, increase beneficial bacteria	digestive conditions such as irritable bowel syndrome, Crohn's disease, ulcerative colitis, yeast overgrowth, cancer, vaginitis

Phytochemical	Source	Properties	Conditions
Gallic Acid	green tea, red wine	antioxidant, immune enhancing	infections, heart disease
Glucosinolates	cruciferous vegetables (broccoli, cauliflower, kale, brussels sprouts)	detoxifying, hormone balance	cancer prevention, general detoxification
Indoles	cruciferous vegetables (broccoli, cauliflower, kale, brussels sprouts)	detoxifying, hormone balancing	cancer prevention (especially hormone-dependent, such as breast and prostate)
Isoflavones	soy	hormone balancing	PMS, menopause, cancer prevention
Isothiocyanates	broccoli, cabbage, cauliflower, horseradish	detoxification	cancer prevention
Lignans	flaxseeds, walnuts	immune enhancement, hormone balance	cancer and cardiovascular disease prevention
Limonoids	citrus fruits and peels	detoxification	cancer and cardiovascular disease prevention
Lycopene	tomatoes, red grapefruit	antioxidant	cancer prevention and treatment
Organosulfur compounds	garlic, onions, chives	antioxidant, immune enhancing, detoxification	cancer and cardiovascular disease prevention, immune enhancement, general detoxification
Phenolic Acids	broccoli, berries, tomatoes, cabbage, whole grains	antioxidant	cancer prevention
Sulforaphane	cruciferous vegetables (broccoli, cauliflower, kale, brussels sprouts)	detoxification, hormone balance	cancer prevention
Terpenes	citrus fruit	anticancer	cancer prevention, hormone balance

References

Bernstein, J., S. Alpert, K. Nauss, and R. Suskind. 1977. Depression of lymphocyte transformation following glucose ingestion. *American Journal of Clinical Nutrition* 30:613.

EPA Web site. 2000.

Marlett, J., and T. Cheung. 1997. Database and quick methods of assessing typical dietary fiber intakes using data for 228 commonly consumed foods. *Journal of the American Dietetic Association* 97:1139–47.

Ringsdorf, W., E. Cheraksin, and R. Ramsay. 1976. Sucrose, neutrophilic phagocytosis, and resistance to disease. *Dental Survey* 52:46–48.

Rudin, D. O., and C. Felix. 1987. *The Omega 3 Phenomenon.* New York: Rawlinson Associates.

Skinner, J. D., B. R. Carruth, K. S. Houck, W. Bounds, M. Morris, D. R. Cox, J. Moran, 3rd, and F. Coletta. 1999. Longitudinal study of nutrient and food intakes of white preschool children aged 24 to 60 months. *Journal of the American Dietetic Association* 99(12):1514–21.

Smith, B. 1993. Organic foods versus supermarket foods. Element levels. *Journal of Applied Nutrition* 45:35–39.

Fasting

Fasting has been used for thousands of years as a medical therapy to help the body detoxify and rejuvenate from all kinds of health problems. It is defined as voluntarily not eating food for various lengths of time. Many of the world's oldest systems of health relied upon fasting for healing and as a way to prevent disease. The father of Western medicine, Hippocrates, found that fasting helped the body to heal itself, and he extolled its tremendous healing potential in his writings. Most world religions have used fasting as a way to improve physical and spiritual clarity. The Bible makes frequent references to the benefits of fasting, combined with prayer. Currently, fasting is becoming a more accepted method of detoxification for health practitioners throughout North America.

How Does Fasting Work?

The primary way in which fasting is beneficial is by simply giving the body time to rest. Specifically, the digestive organs are given a break from digesting food. A tremendous amount of energy is required for digestion, and the body can use this "saved" energy for healing and regeneration. In addition, a time of fasting prevents more toxic substances from entering the body and simultaneously allows for the expulsion of toxins. This is particularly true for the liver, which has to break down and metabolize all the toxic substances that enter the body. In addition, the immune system is also given a break from dealing with toxins from our food and water supply, as well as from our environment.

During the first day of a fast, the body burns stored sugar, known as glycogen. After this, the body begins to burn fat for fuel. There is one exception, though, and this occurs with the brain, which requires blood sugar. During the second day of a fast, some muscle tissue may be broken down into amino acids, which are converted by the liver into glucose to feed the brain. During the second to third day of fasting, the body goes into what is called ketosis. During this state, the liver converts stored fat into chemicals called ketones, which can be used by the brain, the heart, and the muscles for energy. Generally, during this period of time, people lose their hunger pains and have increased energy and a heightened sense of awareness, which often includes clarity of the mind and the spirit. People may lose up to two pounds a day during this stage. As fat is increasingly burned for fuel, stored toxins (such as pesticides and other chemicals) are released into the bloodstream, to be metabolized by the liver and the kidneys. (Bear in mind, however, we do not advocate fasting as a weight loss protocol.)

Length of a Fast

The length of a fast really depends on a person's health. The healthier one is, the longer one can fast. Many practitioners recommend two- to three-day fasts with each change of the season. More commonly, a spring fast is recommended to cleanse the body of toxins that accumulated during the dormant winter season. Some people enjoy preventative fasts of one day per week.

The most basic fast is the water fast, in which you consume only water for a specified amount of time. This is the most aggressive type of fast and is best used by people in good health or those who are experienced in fasting. If you are trying it for the first time, it is recommended that you start with just one day. You should consume at least 80 ounces of purified water daily. People who are more experienced at fasting may drink only water for up to five days.

Juice fasts are also very popular. They are not as intense as a water fast because the naturally occurring sugars from vegetable and fruit juices prevent ketosis from occurring. Common juices include carrot, lemon, apple, beet, celery, and various greens, such as wheatgrass, spirulina, barley grass, and other super green foods. You should consume approximately 64 ounces of fresh juices daily. This type of fasting is indicated for people who are fasting for the first time or for those who cannot take time out of their schedules for a more intense fast.

Getting Started

It is important to start and stop a fast properly. The best way to start is to gradually lighten the amount of food consumed three days before the fast. Also, you should avoid heavier foods, such as dairy products and meats. The day before the fast, your diet should consist of easily digested foods, such as light salads, fresh soups, fruits, and herbal teas.

A Good Ending

The end of the fast should be similar to the days before you began the fast. You should transition to light foods for a few days and then gradually incorporate heavier foods. Remember to keep drinking plenty of water, because detoxification will still be occurring.

Safety

A fast lasting longer than three days should be supervised by a medical doctor or a naturopathic physician. People with blood-sugar problems, such as hypoglycemia or diabetes, should consult with a doctor before starting any fast. This is also true of any other systemic disease you may have.

It is not uncommon for people to experience symptoms of detoxification during a fast. These can include fatigue, headache, bad breath, nausea, skin rash, or feeling as if they have the flu or a cold. These symptoms should clear up as the fast progresses beyond the second or third day.

It is important to get plenty of rest during a fast. Exercise should be very light, as should mental activities. In all, you should choose a fast that is most suitable to your particular needs and health. Fasting truly is nature's way of cleansing and regenerating the body.

Nutritional Supplements

Nutritional supplements have become regular items in the households of most Americans. For decades, people have intuitively known that deficiencies of nutrients contribute to poor vitality and disease. Holistic doctors such as ourselves have seen the difference that nutritional supplements can make in the prevention and the treatment of most health conditions.

To the detriment of the public, most conventional doctors in the past have had little support for the use of these nontoxic nutrients. Fortunately, times are changing. Two decades ago, the prestigious *Journal of the American Medical Association (JAMA)* advised that there was no evidence that healthy people would benefit from taking multivitamins. In June 2002, *JAMA* published an article that was a complete turnaround on the use of nutritional supplements. The authors of the study concluded that vitamin deficiency was an apparent cause of chronic diseases. Considering that only 20 percent of the population consumes the recommended minimum servings of fruits and vegetables each day, nutritional deficiencies are undoubtedly a widespread problem. Added to this is the fact that pharmaceutical medications, pollution, high stress levels, nutrient-depleted soils, and refined and packaged foods all contribute to nutritional deficiencies.

This chapter and the protocols in this book go well beyond general recommendations for nutritional supplements. We have provided not only the minimal doses people should strive for (such as the RDA) but also the optimal dosages to prevent diseases and deficiencies. In the conditions sections, we give the therapeutic amounts for each nutritional supplement, as well as the exact type to use to optimize your results.

Vitamins and Minerals

WHAT ARE VITAMINS?

A vitamin is an organic substance that is essential (i.e., vital) for life. Most vitamins cannot be synthesized in the body and so must be obtained from the diet or supplements. Vitamins fall into two main groups. Fat-soluble vitamins require a certain amount of fat to be absorbed. They are also stored longer in the body. Common examples of fat-soluble vitamins include vitamins A, D, K, and E. The second major group of vitamins is termed *water-soluble*. Vitamins in this group do not need fat to be absorbed and are excreted out of the body much more readily than fat-soluble vitamins are. Vitamins C and B are water-soluble.

WHAT ARE MINERALS?

Minerals are inorganic substances that are important components of tissues and fluids. They are necessary for the proper functioning of vitamins, enzymes, hormones, and other metabolic activities in the body. Minerals compose 4 percent of the body's weight. Most minerals, such as calcium, phosphorous, and magnesium, are found in the bones. Some minerals are required in minute amounts; these are called *trace minerals*. Chromium is an example of a trace mineral, because it is required in micrograms (1/100th of a milligram), as opposed to minerals like calcium, which are required in milligrams.

DOSAGE RECOMMENDATIONS

More people are becoming aware of the new Dietary Reference Intakes (DRI) that have been released by the Food and Nutrition Board of the National Academy of Science. The Dietary Reference Intakes refer to four nutrient reference values that can be used to assess diet, as well as for other purposes. The DRIs are a replacement for the well-known RDAs (Recommended Dietary Allowances) of the United States, which have been published since 1941 by the National Academy of Sciences, and the RNIs (Recommended Nutrient Intakes) of Canada . These new values are the collaborative work of the Standing Committee on the Scientific Evaluation of Dietary Reference Intakes of the Food and Nutrition Board, the Institute of Medicine, the National Academy of Sciences, and Health Canada. Unlike the RDAs, which establish the minimal amounts of nutrients required to protect against possible deficiencies, the new DRIs are designed to reflect a more modern understanding of nutrient requirements, to optimize health in people and groups of people.

The DRIs are comprised of four reference values. These include the RDA and three other values:

Recommended Daily Allowance (RDA): The average daily dietary intake level that is sufficient to meet the nutrient requirement of nearly all (97 to 98 percent) healthy individuals in a group. In other words, the RDA is the amount of vitamins and minerals that a healthy person requires to stay healthy. These amounts will prevent obvious vitamin deficiencies, such as scurvy and rickets. However, these values are really quite conservative, and most nutritionally trained doctors like ourselves feel that they are generally too low for optimal health.

Adequate Intake (AI): A value based on observed or experimentally determined approximations of nutrient intake by a group (or groups) of healthy people. Used when an RDA cannot be determined.

Tolerable Upper Intake Level (UL): The highest level of daily nutrient intake that is likely to pose no risk of adverse health effects to almost all individuals in the general population. As intake increases above UL, the risk of adverse effects increases.

Estimated Average Requirement (EAR): A nutrient intake value that is estimated to meet the requirement of half the healthy individuals in a group.

Note: In our discussion of each vitamin and mineral we have included our own adult Optimal Intake reference ranges. The Optimal Intake references are our estimates of the dosages of vitamins and minerals that provide the best chance of bringing about optimal health and not just the prevention of disease.

RDA SUMMARY TABLE

Compound	Adult Males (31–50 yrs)	Adult Females (31–50 yrs)	Children (4–8 yrs)	Infants (7–12 mths)	Pregnant and Lactating Women*
Vitamin A (daily RE[†])	1,000	800	700	375	1,300
Vitamin D (daily IU)	200[†]	200[†]	200[†]	200[†]	200[†]
Vitamin E (daily mg alphaTE[†])	10	8	7	4	12
Vitamin K (daily mcg)	80	65	30	10	65
Vitamin C (daily mg)	60	60	45	35	95
Folate (daily mcg)	400[‡]	400[‡]	200[‡]	80[†]	500–600[‡]
Thiamin (B1) (daily mg)	1.2[‡]	1.1[‡]	0.6[‡]	0.3[‡]	1.4[‡]
Riboflavin (B2) (daily mg)	1.3	1.1	0.6	0.4	1.4–1.6
Niacin (daily mg)	16	14	8	4	17–18
Pyridoxine (B6) (daily mg)	1.3	1.3	0.6	0.3	1.9–2.0
Cyanocobalamine (B12) (daily mcg)	2.4	2.4	1.2	0.5	2.6–2.8
Biotin (daily mcg)	30	30	12	6	30–35
Pantothenic Acid (daily mg)	5	5	3	1.8	6–7
Choline (daily mg)	550	425	250	150	450–550
Calcium (Ca) (daily mg)	1,000*	1,000	800	270[†]	1,000[†]
Phosphorus (P) (daily mg)	700[‡]	700[‡]	500[‡]	275[†]	700[‡]
Iodine (I) (daily mcg)	150	150	120	50	200
Iron (Fe) (daily mg)	10	15	10	10	30
Magnesium (Mg) (daily mg)	420	320	130	75[†]	320–360
Copper (Cu) (daily mg)	1.5–3	1.5–3	1–2	0.6–0.7	1.5–3
Zinc (Zn) (daily mg)	15	12	10	5	19
Selenium (Se) (daily mcg)	70	55	30	15	75
Chromium (Cr) (daily mcg)	50–200	50–200	50–200	10–60	50–200
Molybdenum (Mo) (daily mcg)	75–250	75–250	50–150	15–40	75–250
Manganese (Mn) (daily mg)	2–5	2–5	2–3	0.3–1.0	2–5
Fluoride (F) (daily mg)	4.0[†]	3.0[†]	1.0[†]	0.50[†]	3.0[†]
Sodium (Na) (daily mg)	500	500	400	120–200	500
Chloride (Cl) (daily mg)	750	750	600	180–300	750
Potassium (K) (daily mg)	2,000	2,000	1,600	500–700	2,000

Note:

g = grams

mg = milligrams (0.001 g)

mcg = micrograms (0.000001 g)

IU = International Units

RE = Retinol Equivalent (1 RE = 3.33 IU vit A or 6 mcg beta carotene)

Alpha TE = Alpha Tocopherol Equivalent

*Generally the higher number was reported.

[†]AI (Adequate Intake) from the new Dietary Reference Intakes, 1997: Calcium, Phosphorus, Magnesium, Vitamin D, and Fluoride. Dietary Reference Intakes, 1998: Thiamin, Riboflavin, Niacin, B6, Folate, B12, Pantothenic Acid, Biotin, and Choline. Values have changed from previous RDA.

[‡]RDA (Recommended Dietary Allowance) from the new Dietary Reference Intakes, 1997: Calcium, Phosphorus, Magnesium, Vitamin D, and Fluoride. Dietary Reference Intakes, 1998: Thiamin, Riboflavin, Niacin, B6, Folate, B12, Pantothenic Acid, Biotin, and Choline. Values have changed from previous RDA.

VITAMINS IN DETAIL

Vitamin A (Retinol, Retinal)

Function: Vision; growth and development; strengthens immune system—especially respiratory tract and mucous membranes; antioxidant

Sources: Liver, chili peppers, carrots, vitamin A–fortified milk, butter, sweet potatoes, parsley, kale, spinach, mangoes, broccoli, squash

RDA: Infants under 1 year: 1,875 IU (375 RE)

      1–3 years: 2,000 IU (400 RE)

      4–6 years: 2,500 IU (500 RE)

      7–10 years: 3,500 IU (700 RE)

      11 years to adult:

      Men 5,000 IU (1,000 RE)

      Women 4,000 IU (800 RE)

Note: One RE (retinol equivalent) = 3.33 IU (International Units)

Optimal Intake: Adult men: 5,000 IU (1,000 RE)

               Adult women: 2,500 IU (500 RE)

Deficiency Signs: Night blindness, infectious disease susceptibility, follicular hyperkeratosis (bumps on the skin—mainly, the back of the upper arm, the shoulders, the neck, the buttocks, and the lower abdomen), faulty tooth and bone formation, impaired growth

Toxicity: Overdoses of vitamin A can produce symptoms of vomiting, joint pain, abdominal pain, bone abnormalities, cracking, dry skin, headache, irritability, and fatigue. Symptoms disappear after supplementation has been discontinued. Pregnant women or those with liver disease should avoid vitamin A supplementation dosages above 2,500 IU (500 RE).

Carotenoids (Carotenes)

Examples of carotenoids include beta carotene, alpha carotene, gamma carotene, beta zeacarotene, cryptoxanthin, lycopene, zeaxanthin, lutein, canthaxanthin, crocetin, capsanthin).

Function: There are over 600 identified carotenoids. Approximately 50 act as precursors to vitamin A. Carotenoids are potent antioxidants, help with immune function, and are involved with the growth and the repair of tissues.

Sources: Yellow vegetables (carrots, pumpkins, squash, sweet potatoes); green vegetables (broccoli, peas, collard greens, endive, kale, lettuce, peppers, spinach, turnip greens); fruits (apricots, cantaloupe, papaya, peaches, watermelon, cherries, tomatoes)

RDA: None established

Optimal Intake: 5,000 to 25,000 IU of mixed carotenoids

Deficiency Signs: Increased susceptibility to developing certain cancers and cardiovascular disease

Toxicity: Relatively nontoxic. Too high of an intake can lead to carotenemia (yellowing of skin), which disappears after reduction of carotenoid intake.

Vitamin D (Vitamin D2-Ergocalciferol, Vitamin D3-Cholecaciferol)

D2—derived from plant sources

D3—derived from animal sources

Function: It promotes calcium and phosphorous absorption from intestines, increases calcium deposition into bones, mobilizes calcium and phosphorous from bones. It prevents certain cancers and is required for proper thyroid function.

Sources: Cod liver oil, cold-water fish (salmon, herring, sardines, mackerel), milk (fortified with vitamin D), egg yolk, small amounts in dark-green leafy vegetables and mushrooms. Sunlight is converted into vitamin D.

Optimal Intake: 400 to 800 IU

Deficiency Signs: Rickets—softening of the skull bones, bowing of the legs, spinal curvature, a contracted pelvis, abnormal enlargement of the head, and an increased joint space; delayed tooth eruption; osteoporosis

Toxicity: Nausea, anorexia, weakness, headache, digestive disturbance, kidney damage, calcification of soft tissues, and hypercalcemia

Vitamin K (Phylloquinone, Menaquinone)

Phylloquinone = K1, derived from plants

Menaquinone = K2, derived from gut bacteria

Menadione = K3, derived synthetically

Function: Blood clotting, bone formation, antioxidant

Sources: Dark-green leafy vegetables, parsley, broccoli, cabbage, spinach, soy, egg yolks, liver, legumes, and synthesized by intestinal bacteria

Optimal Intake: 50 to 100 mcg

Deficiency Signs: Blood-clotting problems, osteoporosis, menstrual cramps

Toxicity: Hemolytic anemia

Vitamin E-Complex (Tocopherol, Tocotrienols)

Includes alpha, beta, and gamma tocopherol, as well as tocotrienols. Most supplements refer to alpha tocopherol.

Function: Antioxidant, immunity, wound healing, red blood cell formation, estrogen metabolism, nerve health

Sources: Vegetable oils, seeds, nuts, brown rice, and whole grains

Optimal Intake: 400 IU

Deficiency Signs: Severe deficiency is rare. Dry skin, hemolytic anemia of newborns, muscle and neurological disorders.

Vitamin B1 (Thiamin)

Function: Energy metabolism (carbohydrate metabolism), neurological activity, brain and heart function

Sources: Pork, beef, liver, brewer's yeast, whole grains, brown rice, legumes

Optimal Intake: 5 to 10 mg

Deficiency Signs: Beriberi, a condition characterized by fatigue, anorexia, weight loss, gastrointestinal disorders, fluid retention, weakness, heart abnormalities, stunted growth, cyanosis, convulsions, poor memory

Toxicity: None reported

Natural vitamin E has been shown to have significantly greater bioavailability than synthetic vitamin E. Make sure to look for natural forms of vitamin E, listed as d-alpha-tocopherol, as opposed to synthetic, which is listed as dl-alpha-tocopherol.

Vitamin B2 (Riboflavin)

Function: Energy production, fatty acid and amino acid synthesis

Sources: Organ meats such as liver, milk products, whole grains, green leafy vegetables, eggs, mushrooms, broccoli, asparagus, fish

RDA:

0–0.5 year	0.4 mg
0.5–1 year	0.5 mg
1–3 years	0.8 mg
4–6 years	1.0 mg
7–10 years	1.2 mg

Optimal Intake: 10–15 mg

Deficiency Signs: Cracking at the corners of the mouth, inflamed tongue, reddening of the eyes, vision problems, dermatitis, nerve damage, decreased neurotransmitter production, malformations and retarded growth in children and infants

Toxicity: None reported

Vitamin B3 (Niacin)

Function: Energy production, formation of steroid compounds, red blood cell formation, cognitive function and mood

Sources: Organ meats, peanuts, fish, yeast, poultry, legumes, milk, eggs, whole grains, orange juice

Optimal Intake: 50–100 mg

Deficiency Signs: Pellagra, a condition characterized by dermatitis, diarrhea, dementia; depression, schizophrenia, weakness, lassitude, anorexia

Toxicity: Large doses can cause dilation of the blood vessels and flushing of the skin. Use a nonflushing form (inositol hexaniacinate) if you are sensitive to regular niacin. Time-released niacin products may result in liver damage.

Vitamin B5 (Pantothenic Acid)

Function: Metabolism of carbohydrates, proteins, and fats for energy production; production of adrenal hormones and red blood cells

Sources: Organ meats, fish, chicken, eggs, cheese, whole grains, avocados, cauliflower, sweet potatoes, oranges, strawberries, yeast, legumes

Optimal Intake: 50–100 mg

Deficiency Signs: Numbness and shooting pains in the feet; fatigue

Toxicity: None reported

Vitamin B6 (Pyridoxine)

Function: Formation of body proteins, neurotransmitters, red blood cells; immunity

Sources: Meats, poultry, egg yolk, soy, peanuts, bananas, potatoes, whole grains, cauliflower

Optimal Intake: 10–25 mg

Deficiency Signs: Mood abnormalities, sleep problems, anemia, impairment of nerve function, eczema, cracking of the lips and the tongue, premenstrual syndrome, depression

Toxicity: Very high dosages can cause nerve symptoms—numbness and tingling.

The risk of bearing a child with a common birth defect known as a neural tube defect is reduced by 60 percent if a 400 mcg folic acid supplement is taken daily by the mother one month prior to conception and through the first trimester. It also decreases the risk of limb and urinary defects.

Folic Acid (Folacin, Folate)

Function: Prevents neural tube defects (must be taken by the mother in early pregnancy). Methyl donor that is required for many processes in the body (reduces homocysteine levels). Cardiovascular health. Red blood cell production. Skin and nail health.

Sources: Dark green vegetables—spinach, kale, broccoli, asparagus—as well as organ meats, kidney beans, beets, yeast, orange juice, whole grains

Optimal Intake: 400 to 800 micrograms (mcg)

Deficiency Signs: Macrocytic anemia, fatigue, irritability, weakness, weight loss, anorexia, dyspnea, sore tongue, palpitations, forgetfulness, digestive upset, diarrhea

Interesting Fact: Even though folic acid is added to many foods, folic acid deficiency is the most common vitamin deficiency in the world.

Toxicity: None

Vitamin B12 (Cobalamin)

Function: Synthesis of DNA, red blood cells; nerve development

Sources: Gut bacteria synthesis, organ meats, clams, oysters, soy, milk products, cheese, chlorella, spirulina

Optimal Intake: 50–200 micrograms (mcg)

Deficiency Signs: Macrocytic anemia; glossitis; spinal cord degeneration; digestive upset; fatigue; mental abnormalities, including irritability, depression

Toxicity: None reported

Biotin

Function: Metabolism of fats, proteins, and carbohydrates; nail and hair growth

Sources: Gut bacterial synthesis, organ meats, cheese, soybeans, eggs, mushrooms, whole wheat, peanuts

Optimal Intake: 300 micrograms (mcg)

Deficiency Signs: Seborrheic dermatitis (cradle cap) and hair loss in infants; brittle nails and hair

Toxicity: None reported

Vitamin C (Ascorbic Acid)

Function: Antioxidant, immunity, collagen formation, bone development, cancer prevention and treatment, gum health, hormone and amino acid synthesis, adrenal gland hormones, wound healing

Sources: Citrus fruits, tomatoes, green peppers, dark-green leafy vegetables, broccoli, cantaloupe, strawberries, brussels sprouts, potatoes, asparagus

Optimal Intake: 500–1,500 mg

Deficiency Signs: Scurvy (rare in North America), signs of which include bleeding gums, poor wound healing, joint tenderness and swelling, recurrent infections, and profuse bruising

Toxicity: The first symptom of too much vitamin C is generally diarrhea, which disappears when the dosage is reduced.

MINERALS IN DETAIL

Calcium

Function: Bone and tooth formation, muscle contraction, heartbeat, blood clotting, and nerve impulse

Sources: Kelp, cheese, collards, kale, turnip greens, almonds, yogurt, milk, broccoli, and soy

Optimal Intake: 1,000 to 1,500 mg

Deficiency Signs: Bone deformity (rickets), growth retardation, insomnia, muscle and leg cramps

Toxicity: Normally, there are no toxic effects with large doses. Some researchers feel that people with a tendency to develop kidney stones should avoid high doses of calcium, although this has not been proven.

> An 8-ounce glass of milk contains 300 mg of calcium. The absorption of calcium from milk is 25 to 30 percent. Therefore, about 75 mg of calcium are actually absorbed.

Magnesium

Function: Bone and teeth formation, energy production, glucose metabolism, muscle and nerve impulses

Sources: Whole grains, nuts, legumes, soy, green leafy vegetables

Therapeutic Dosage: 400–600 mg

Deficiency Signs: Weakness, confusion, mood changes, muscle spasms/tremors, nausea, poor coordination, heart disturbances, insomnia, susceptibility to kidney stones

Toxicity: People with kidney disease or on heart medications should not supplement magnesium unless instructed to do so by their doctor. Diarrhea is usually the first symptom of too much magnesium.

Phosphorous

Function: Growth, bone production, energy production, kidney function

Sources: Meats, fish, eggs, poultry, milk products

Optimal Intake: 800–1,200 mg

Deficiency Signs: Deficiency is very rare. Symptoms may include muscle cramps, bone abnormalities, and dizziness.

Toxicity: Too much phosphorous in the form of phosphoric acid leads to urinary calcium excretion.

Potassium

Function: Nerve transmission, water balance, acid-base balance, heart function, kidney function, adrenal function

Sources: Fruits and vegetables, especially apples, bananas, carrots, oranges, potatoes, tomatoes, cantaloupe, peaches, plums, strawberries, meat, milk, fish

Optimal Intake: 2,000–3,000 mg

Deficiency Signs: Muscle wasting, weakness, and spasm; fatigue, mood changes, heart disturbances, nerve problems

Toxicity: Impaired heart and kidney function; people with heart or kidney conditions or on blood pressure medication should not take potassium unless instructed to do so by a physician.

Sodium

Function: Acid-base balance, muscle contraction, nerve impulse, amino acid absorption

Sources: Naturally occurring in meats, milk products, water, eggs, poultry, and fish; abundant in canned foods and other commercially processed foods

Optimum Intake: 2,000 mg

Deficiency Signs: Deficiency is very uncommon, except in the case of dehydration through profuse sweating or diarrhea. Symptoms can include muscle weakness and cramping, low blood pressure, muscle twitching, mental confusion, anorexia, and fainting.

Toxicity: High blood pressure, especially when potassium intake is low

Manganese

Function: Required for enzyme systems involved with energy production, blood-sugar control, fatty acid synthesis, thyroid hormone function, connective tissue and bone formation, sprains and strains

Sources: Liver, kidney, whole grains, nuts, spinach, green leafy vegetables

Optimal Intake: 5–10 mg

Deficiency Signs: No symptoms have been observed in humans. Animal studies show growth problems.

Toxicity: Too much manganese can interfere with iron absorption and can cause iron deficiency.

Chromium

Function: Blood sugar control

Sources: Whole grains, meats, potatoes, liver, brewer's yeast

Optimal Intake: 200 micrograms

Deficiency Signs: Elevated blood-sugar levels

Toxicity: Chromium appears to be safe, with no major toxic side effects reported.

Copper

Function: Collagen formation, red blood cell formation, bone formation, energy production, mental function, many other enzyme systems

Sources: Whole grains, shellfish, nuts, eggs, poultry, organ meats, peas, dark-green leafy vegetables, legumes

Deficiency Signs: Rare but could include low immune function, poor collagen and connective tissue strength, bone and joint abnormalities, anemia

Optimal Intake: 2–3 mg

Toxicity: Nausea, vomiting, and dizziness

Iron

Function: Hemoglobin production to supply oxygen to cells, collagen synthesis, normal immune function

Sources: Liver and organ meats, beef, legumes, dark-green leafy vegetables, kelp, blackstrap molasses

Chromium is an essential nutrient that is required for sugar and fat metabolism. Normal dietary intake of Cr for humans is suboptimal. Insufficient dietary intake of Cr leads to signs and symptoms that are similar to those observed for diabetes and cardiovascular diseases. Supplemental Cr given to people with impaired glucose tolerance or diabetes leads to improved blood glucose, insulin, and lipid variables.

Deficiency Signs: Iron deficiency is characterized by fatigue, paleness, poor memory and concentration, developmental delays and behavioral disturbances, chronic colds, and weakened immunity, as well as a craving for indigestible materials (e.g., pencils, dirt, ice).

Optimal Intake: Men—10 mg

Women with a normal cycle or no cycle—10 mg

Women with a heavy cycle—20 mg

Toxicity: Too much iron is associated with an increased risk for developing heart disease and cancer. Acute iron poisoning in children can result in damage to the intestinal tract, liver failure, nausea and vomiting, shock, and death.

> Iron sulfate, the most widely prescribed form of supplemental iron, can be constipating and irritating to the digestive tract. We recommend other forms, such as iron citrate, iron glycinate, and other types of chelated iron.

Selenium

Function: Antioxidant, cancer prevention, immunity, thyroid function, development of the fetus during pregnancy

Sources: Liver, kidney, meats, seafood. Grains and vegetables are good sources, but selenium content depends on the level in the soil where they are grown.

Deficiency Signs: Selenium deficiency is associated with an increased risk for heart disease, cancer, and poor immune function.

Therapeutic Dosage: 200 mcg

Toxicity: Teeth abnormalities, depression, nausea and vomiting

Iodine

Function: Required to manufacture the thyroid hormone

Sources: Iodized salt and water; seafood; seaweeds, such as kelp

RDA:
0–0.5 yrs.	40 mcg
0.5–1 yrs.	50 mcg
1–3 yrs.	70 mcg
4–6 yrs.	90 mcg
7–10 yrs.	120 mcg

Deficiency Signs: Goiter (enlargement of thyroid gland), fatigue, depression

Optimal Intake: 250 mcg

Toxicity: Too much iodine can interfere with thyroid activity (hypothyroid) and may cause acne eruptions.

Molybdenum

Function: Active in enzyme systems involved with the metabolism of alcohol, uric acid, and sulfur

Sources: Meats, whole-grain breads, legumes, leafy vegetables, organ meats, and brewer's yeast

Deficiency Signs: None known, but the inability to detoxify sulfites (preservatives in foods) is reported.

Optimal Intake: 200 mcg

Toxicity: None reported

Silicon

Function: Bone, cartilage, and ligament formation; skin elasticity

Sources: Unrefined grains, cereals, and root vegetables

RDA: There is no RDA and little information exists about dosages for silicon.

Optimal Intake: 50 mg

Deficiency Signs: None known, but brittle hair and nails are suspected.

Toxicity: Miners who were exposed to large dosages of silicon over a prolonged period of time have developed silicosis—a fibrotic formation of the lungs. The amounts found in foods and multivitamins appear to be very safe.

Vanadium

Function: Blood-sugar balance, bone and teeth development

Sources: Shellfish, mushrooms, black pepper, and buckwheat

Optimal Intake: 50 mg (as vanadyl sulfate form)

Deficiency Signs: None known, but blood-sugar imbalances are suspected.

Toxicity: Little is known, but very high amounts may lead to cramps and diarrhea.

Zinc

Function: Involved in over 200 enzymatic reactions; required to manufacture many hormones; immunity; skin healing; growth; vision; blood-sugar metabolism; antioxidant support; reproductive development and fertility

Sources: Oysters, herring, shellfish, red meat, whole grains, legumes, and nuts

Optimal Intake: 15–30 mg

Deficiency Signs: Hair loss, poor wound healing, poor immune function, diarrhea, skin conditions (acne), mental disturbance, white spots on the nails

Toxicity: Rare. Very high dosage (above 150 mg) can lead to immune system suppression, digestive upset, or anemia.

Alpha Lipoic Acid

Function: Antioxidant; energy production; potentiates the effects of vitamins C and E

Sources: Liver, yeast, potatoes, spinach, red meat

RDA: None given

Optimal Intake: 50–100 mg

Deficiency Signs: No specific symptoms given, but people with diabetes and diabetic neuropathy tend to benefit from supplementation.

Toxicity: None known

Choline

Function: Required to manufacture the neurotransmitter acetylcholine; metabolism of fats

Sources: Grains, legumes, egg yolks, whole grains, and soy

Optimal Intake: 500 mg

Deficiency Signs: Potential liver and kidney dysfunction

Toxicity: Rare, but symptoms of fishy breath, sweating, salivation, low blood pressure, and liver toxicity

Inositol

Function: Component of cell membranes; used for depression and to prevent complications of diabetes

Sources: Citrus fruit, whole grains, nuts, seeds, and legumes

Optimal Intake: 250 mg

Deficiency Signs: None known

Toxicity: None known

Coenzyme Q10

Function: Antioxidant, heart activity, energy production

Sources: Meat, seafood

Optimal Intake: 30 to 100 mg

Deficiency Signs: Gum disease, heart failure, fatigue, hypertension, atherosclerosis

Toxicity: None known

L-Carnitine

Function: Energy production, heart function, triglyceride metabolism

Sources: Meat, dairy products

Optimal Intake: 250 to 500 mg

Deficiency Signs: Loss of muscle tone, recurrent infections, brain swelling, heart irregularities, high triglycerides, fatigue, and failure to thrive

Toxicity: None

Selecting Vitamins and Minerals

Make sure to purchase vitamins and minerals that are free of artificial sweeteners and preservatives or fillers. Work with a knowledgeable nutritional professional to select the highest-quality supplements. Most nutrients are available in tablet, capsule, powder, and liquid forms. Multivitamins should be taken with a meal for optimal absorption and to prevent digestive upset. If you are taking pharmaceutical medications, check with a holistic doctor to see which nutrients are known to be depleted by the drug(s) you are taking. Also, check to see if there are any possible adverse reaction problems known with your medications and supplements.

Nutritional Supplement Guide

The following section contains common nutritional supplements you will find on the shelves of most health food, pharmacy, and grocery store shelves. We have included a brief description of each supplement, conditions that it is indicated for, precautions, and dosage recommendations. For information on vitamin, herbal, and homeopathic supplements, please see their corresponding sections.

Acetylcarnitine

Description: Acetylcarnitine is a modified form of the amino acid–like substance L-carnitine. The acetyl group allows this nutrient to be readily absorbed across the blood-brain barrier and is used to make the brain neurotransmitter acetylcholine. L-carnitine is used to transport fatty acids into the cell mitochondria for energy production. Acetylcarnitine allows for energy production within brain cells. This supplement is mainly used to enhance cognitive function. Studies have found that it delays the progression of early-stage Alzheimer's disease.

Indications: Age-related cognitive decline

Alzheimer's disease

Amenorrhea

Depression

Down's syndrome

Infertility (male)

Peripheral neuropathy

Precautions: Side effects are uncommon, although skin rash, body odor, and digestive upset have been reported.

Dosage: Take 1,500 to 3,000 mg daily.

Acidophilus

Description: Lactobacillus acidophilus is known as a probiotic. It is a beneficial bacteria that inhabits several areas of the body, including the mouth, the throat, the lungs, the digestive tract, the urinary tract, and the vagina. Acidophilus produces substances called bacteriocins, which act as a natural antibiotic to destroy or keep harmful microorganisms in check. It also helps break down undigested fiber from fruits, vegetables, and milk sugar (lactose). This good type of bacteria is also involved in the manufacturing of vitamins and amino acids. Finally, acidophilus helps with the proper detoxification of hormones and other substances. Many supplements combine it with *Bifidobacterium bifidusm.*

Indications: Cancer prevention

Candidiasis

Canker sores

Constipation

Eczema

Food allergies

Immune support

Inflammatory bowel disease

Irritable bowel disease

Lactose intolerance

Leaky gut syndrome

Traveler's diarrhea

Vaginitis

Precautions: People with candida overgrowth may notice die-off symptoms, including nausea, diarrhea, bloating, and so on, when they first begin acidophilus supplementation. If you use antibiotics, take acidophilus at least two hours away from the antibiotics dose.

Dosage: Adults should take a product containing at least 4 billion active organisms twice a day, thirty minutes after a meal.

Activated Charcoal

Description: Activated charcoal is used to reduce digestive flatulence and also to absorb harmful toxins, including infectious agents that cause diarrhea.

Indications: Diarrhea

Flatulence

Toxin absorption

Precautions: Take it with a large glass of water, two hours away from other medications and supplements.

Dosage: Take 500 to 1,000 mg three times daily for up to three days.

Adrenal Extract

Description: Adrenal extracts are supplements derived from bovine adrenal glands or the adrenal cortex. They may contain minute amounts of naturally occurring corticosteroids. Many researchers believe that the nutritional profile, including RNA and polypeptides, supports human adrenal gland function. In the human body, the adrenal glands are located on top of each kidney. The adrenal glands are responsible for producing stress hormones such as cortisol, to control the effects of stress and inflammation. Fatigue is the most common reason to take adrenal extract supplements.

Indications: Allergies

Arthritis

Autoimmune conditions

Fatigue

Lower back pain

Precautions: Sensitive individuals may experience anxiety, irritability, headache, or insomnia.

Dosage: Take 1 to 2 capsules or tablets two to three times daily on an empty stomach.

Alanine

Description: Alanine is a nonessential amino acid that helps to build protein. It is used as a nutritional supplement to reduce the symptoms of prostate enlargement.

Indications: Prostate enlargement

Precautions: People with liver or kidney disease should not supplement amino acids unless under the direction of a health-care professional.

Dosage: Men with prostate enlargement can supplement 390 to 780 mg per day, along with the amino acids glycine and glutamic acid at the same dosages.

Amino Acids

Description: Amino acids are the individual building blocks of protein. There are approximately twenty different amino acids. Ten of the amino acids are known as "essential amino acids," which means that our body cannot manufacture them, so it is essential that we consume them in our diets. The remaining ten nonessential amino acids can be manufactured in the body.

Indications: Amino acid supplements are used for a variety of conditions, as mentioned throughout this book. Individual amino acids will be described in this section.

Precautions: People with liver or kidney disease should not supplement amino acids unless under the direction of a health-care professional.

Dosage: Generally, take 250 to 500 mg three times daily, between meals.

Androstenedione

Description: Androstenedione is a hormone that occurs naturally in the body. It is currently available as a supplement and is popular among bodybuilders and athletes. Studies have shown this hormone to increase testosterone levels in women. Studies with men have been mixed, with one showing an increase in estrogen and testosterone, and others showing an increase in estrogen only. Bodybuilders and other athletes also use similar hormones, known as androstenediol and norandrostenedione, but they have not been well studied.

Indications: Menopausal or postmenopausal women with low estrogen or testosterone levels

Precautions: Androstenedione and related supplements should be used only with a doctor's guidance. The National Football League has banned androstenedione and related substances.

Dosage: Take 100 to 300 mg daily.

Arginine

Description: Arginine is one of the better-studied amino acids that has been shown to be helpful for several conditions.

Indications: Angina
>Congestive heart failure
>High blood pressure
>HIV
>Impotence
>Infertility
>Interstitial cystitis
>Surgical recovery
>Wound healing

Precautions: People with liver or kidney disease should not supplement amino acids unless under the direction of a health-care professional. Arginine should not be used by people with oral or genital herpes.

Dosage: Dosage recommendations vary, depending on the condition. Most conditions require anywhere from 3 to 20 grams daily.

Bee Pollen

Description: Bee pollen is the pollen produced by flowering plants, which clings to bees as they gather nectar. Bee pollen contains many vitamin and minerals, as well as flavonoids such as rutin and quercitin. It is thought that the minute amounts of pollens desensitize a person for the same pollen allergies.

Indications: Allergies (mainly, hay fever)
>Arthritis

Fatigue

Immune support

Precautions: People who are allergic to bee stings should avoid bee pollen. To make sure you are not allergic to a bee pollen product, try a minute amount first on the skin or the tip of the tongue before beginning a regular dosage.

Dosage: Take 500 to 1,000 mg daily.

Bentonite

Description: Bentonite is a type of clay that is used internally and externally to absorb toxic substances. It is often a component of "colon cleansing" protocols.

Indications: Colon cleansing

Ingestion of toxic substances

Precautions: Take it three hours away from any medication or supplement. It is best used short term, and you must drink 8 to 16 ounces of water with each teaspoonful to prevent constipation or bowel obstruction.

Dosage: Take 1 teaspoonful daily or as directed by a health-care practitioner.

Beta Glucan

Description: Beta glucan refers to a type of polysaccharide that is extracted from the cell walls of medicinal mushrooms, oats, barley, and baker's yeast. The structure and the activity of various beta glucans differ, depending on the source.

Indications: Blood sugar balance

High cholesterol

Immune support

Precautions: Immune-enhancing beta glucan products should be avoided by people who are on immunosuppressant medications.

Dosage: Dosage recommendations vary greatly, depending on the product. Follow the label recommendations.

Beta-Sitosterol

Description: Beta-sitosterol is a plant sterol that is used as a supplement to lower cholesterol and reduce the symptoms of prostate enlargement.

Indications: High cholesterol

Prostate enlargement

Precautions: This supplement appears to be very safe, with no known precautions.

Dosage: Doses of up to 10 grams are used for high cholesterol, and up to 130 mg daily are used for prostate enlargement.

Betaine Hydrochloride

Description: This hydrochloric acid (HCL) supplement is derived from sugar beets. It is used to increase stomach acid levels for people who have an HCL deficiency.

Indications: Acne

Anemia

Arthritis

Asthma

Candidiasis

> Fatigue
>
> Food sensitivities
>
> Gallstones
>
> Inflammatory bowel disease
>
> Irritable bowel syndrome
>
> Skin rashes
>
> Vitiligo

Precautions: People with a history of heartburn, gastritis, or reflux should use caution.

Dosage: Take 1 or more capsules with each meal. Reduce the dosage if you feel a warming or burning sensation in your stomach.

Boric Acid

Description: Boric acid is a substance that's mainly used for the treatment of vaginal yeast infections. It is available in suppository or powder form. It has also been shown to shorten the duration of cold sores, when applied topically.

Indications: Cold sores

> Vaginal yeast infections

Precautions: Boric acid should never be ingested internally, especially by children. It should also never be applied topically to the skin of infants and children. Do not use boric acid on open wounds.

Dosage: Boric acid suppositories are used intravaginally by inserting 1 to 2 capsules (300–500 mg each) nightly, for up to two weeks.

Bovine Cartilage

Description: This is cartilage extracted from cow trachea. This connective tissue contains collagen, mucopolysaccharides, calcium, sulfur, and proteins. It is mainly used for arthritis, although some doctors prescribe it for cancer, as it is thought to inhibit tumor growth. More research is needed to confirm any benefit for these uses.

Indications: Arthritis

> Cancer

Precautions: There are no good data on precautions or concerns with supplementing bovine cartilage.

Dosage: A typical dosage is 1,000 to 3,000 mg three times daily.

Branched-Chain Amino Acids

Description: The three branched-chain amino acids include L-isoleucine, L-leucine, and L-valine. They are referred to as branched-chain because of their chemical structure. They are essential amino acids, meaning that the body cannot manufacture them, so they must be present in the diet. They play a key role in maintaining and building muscle tissue.

Indications: Athletic training and performance

> Liver cirrhosis
>
> Phenylketonuria
>
> Tardive dyskinesia

Precautions: People with Lou Gehrig's disease, amylotrophic lateral sclerosis (ALS), should avoid supplementation unless instructed to do so by a health-care professional. People with liver or kidney disease should not supplement amino acids unless under the direction of a health-care professional.

Dosage: The typical daily dosage is 50 mg per 2.2 pounds of body weight.

Brewer's Yeast

Description: Brewer's yeast is made from the dried, pulverized cells of a type of fungus known as *Saccharomyces cerevisiae.* It is rich in B vitamins, chromium, amino acids, and selenium. Real brewer's yeast has a bitter taste.

Indications: Diabetes
Diarrhea
Fatigue
High cholesterol

Precautions: Brewer's yeast is a safe supplement to use, although occasional reports of allergic reaction occur. Caution should be used for people on diabetic drugs, as the chromium in brewer's yeast may lower the requirements for these medications.

Dosage: Take 1 to 2 tablespoons daily.

Carnitine

Description: L-carnitine is an amino acid–like substance that is responsible for transporting fatty acids into the mitochondria (energy factories) of cells to produce energy. L-carnitine is manufactured from the amino acids in the body. The richest food source is red meat. It has also been shown to have several benefits for cardiovascular system problems, such as congestive heart failure and high triglycerides.

Indications: Angina
Anorexia
Arrhythmias
Athletic performance
Cardiomyopathy
Chronic fatigue syndrome
Congestive heart failure
Diabetes
Down's syndrome
Heart attack recovery
High cholesterol
HIV
Intermittent claudication
Kidney disease
Liver disease
Male infertility
Premature infants

Precautions: There is no toxicity with L-carnitine, but it should not be taken along with the drug pentylenetetrazol.

Dosage: Take 1,000 to 3,000 mg daily.

Carnosine

Description: This antioxidant substance is composed of the amino acids histidine and alanine. It occurs naturally in the body, especially in muscle, the brain, and the heart, as well as in food. Nerves and muscle cells contain high levels of carnosine. A zinc-carnosine complex has been shown to be effective against *Helicobacter pylori* infection.

Indications: Antioxidant support

  Diabetes

  Hepatitis C (zinc L-carnosine form)

  Peptic ulcer (zinc L-carnosine form)

  Wound healing

Precautions: No side effects have been reported.

Dosage: A dosage of 150 mg (zinc carnosine complex) twice daily is recommended for the treatment of *Helicobacter pylori* infection. Otherwise, up to 1,500 mg of carnosine can be used daily as an antioxidant.

Cetyl Myristoleate (CMO)

Description: CMO is a fatty acid substance that occurs in certain animals and is used as an anti-inflammatory supplement for arthritis.

Indications: Rheumatoid arthritis and osteoarthritis

Precautions: Too high of a dosage may cause diarrhea. The safety of CMO has not been established for pregnant women and nursing mothers.

Dosage: Take 500 mg daily.

Chlorella

Description: Chlorella is a blue-green algae whole food supplement. It contains more than twenty different vitamins and minerals and is a rich source of amino acids, iron, and chlorophyll. It is commonly used as a daily detoxification supplement.

Indications: Athlete's support

  Bad breath

  Constipation

  Detoxification

  Fatigue

  Heavy metal toxicity

  Skin conditions (rashes, etc.)

Precautions: No side effects are known.

Dosage: Take 1,000 to 3,000 mg daily.

Chlorophyll

Description: Chlorophyll is the pigment that gives plants their green color. It is regarded as a phytonutrient that has antioxidant, detoxifying, blood building, and anti-inflammatory properties.

Indications: Anemia

  Bad breath

  Constipation

Precautions: No side effects are known.

Dosage: Take 100 to 300 mg daily.

Chondroitin Sulfate

Description: Chondroitin sulfate is a nutritional supplement extract made from cow's cartilage. It consists of glycosaminoglycans, substances that form cartilage. This supplement is mainly used for osteoarthritis.

Indications: Osteoarthritis

Sprains/strains

Precautions: Very high dosages may cause nausea.

Dosage: The dosage used to treat osteoarthritis is 1,200 mg daily.

Colloidal Silver

Description: Colloidal silver refers to silver particles that are suspended in a water solution. Historically, silver was used topically to treat infections and is still used today to prevent eye infections in newborns. This trace mineral supplement appears to have potent antibacterial effects.

Indications: Bacterial infections

Burns

Conjunctivitis

Precautions: Colloidal silver products appear to vary greatly in quality and potency. They are best taken on a short-term basis, unless used under the guidance of a doctor. Long-term use of high dosages has been reported to result in a condition known as argyria. This permanent condition is characterized by gray or bluish-gray skin.

Dosage: Take 1 teaspoon daily for up to two weeks. Concentrations vary from 1 part per million to 100 parts per million.

Colostrum

Description: Colostrum is the component of breast milk that is formed during the first forty-eight hours after birth. Supplemental colostrum is generally derived from bovine (cow) colostrum. It is rich in antibodies (immunoglobulins) and various growth factors.

Indications: Immune support

Precautions: No side effects are known.

Dosage: Take 1,000 to 5,000 mg daily.

Conjugated Linoleic Acid (CLA)

Description: CLA is a varied form of the essential fatty acid linoleic acid. It is found in the red meat of cattle that are fed natural grasses. It is also found in eggs, poultry, and safflower and corn oil. CLA is mainly used as a supplement to reduce body fat. Animal and test tube studies have demonstrated its anticancer properties, but these results have yet to be proven in human studies.

Indications: Cancer prevention

Weight loss

Precautions: There are occasional reports of digestive upset.

Dosage: Take 1,000 mg two to three times daily.

Creatine

Description: Creatine is a naturally occurring substance in the body and in foods, which is made up of three amino acids—arginine, glycine, and methionine. Creatine is used by the body's muscle cells to create energy and maintain muscle mass.

Indications: Athletic support

Congestive heart failure

Maintaining muscle mass in seniors

Precautions: Diarrhea and muscle cramping are the most common side effects. People with liver or kidney disease should check with their doctors before using creatine.

Dosage: Take 2 to 5 grams daily.

Cysteine

Description: Cysteine is a nonessential amino acid that contains the mineral sulfur. It is a component of the antioxidant glutathione and is required for the synthesis of the amino acid taurine. It plays an important role in detoxification and healthy immune system function.

Indications: Antioxidant support

HIV

Precautions: Do not use it if you are prone to developing cysteine-related kidney stones. People with liver or kidney disease should not supplement amino acids unless under the direction of a health-care professional.

Dosage: Take 500 to 1,500 mg daily.

D-Glucarate

Description: D-glucarate is the supplemental form of glucaric acid, a phytonutrient found in fruits and vegetables. D-glucarate is used by the liver to detoxify hormones, as well as carcinogenic agents. This phytonutrient inhibits an enzyme known as beta glucuronidase, which increases toxic hormones that may be reabsorbed into circulation.

Indications: Cancer prevention

Detoxification

Fibrocystic breast syndrome

PMS

Precautions: There are no known side effects.

Dosage: Take 400 mg daily.

DHEA (Dehydroepiandrosterone)

Description: DHEA is currently a hormone that is available over the counter. It is the most abundant hormone produced by the adrenal glands. It has several functions, including but not limited to supporting the body's reaction to stress; controlling inflammation; and enhancing the libido, cognitive function, immune modulation, and metabolism. DHEA is a precursor hormone to testosterone and androstenedione.

Indications: Alzheimer's disease

Arthritis

> Chronic fatigue syndrome
>
> Depression
>
> Diabetes
>
> Erectile dysfunction
>
> Heart disease prevention
>
> Immune support
>
> Inflammatory bowel disease
>
> Lupus
>
> Menopause
>
> Osteoporosis
>
> Prednisone withdrawal

Precautions: Too high of a dosage may cause facial hair growth and acne breakout. Pregnant women and breastfeeding mothers should avoid using DHEA. People with an existing cancer should also avoid it.

Dosage: A starting dose of 5 to 15 mg is recommended and is increased depending on the clinical situation and laboratory testing.

DMAE (2-Dimethylaminoethanol)

Description: DMAE is a substance that has a chemical composition similar to that of choline. DMAE is used to improve mental alertness and reduce age-related cognitive decline. It has also become popular as a topical agent for skin wrinkles.

Indications: Age-related cognitive decline

> Alzheimer's disease
>
> Wrinkles

Precautions: DMAE is believed to be nontoxic.

Dosage: Take 100 to 400 mg daily.

Enzymes

Description: Enzymes are protein molecules that are found in every cell. They are required for the life-sustaining enzymatic reactions that occur in the body. Digestive enzymes help to break down food, while metabolic enzymes are involved in energy production, detoxification, immunity, and several other activities. Raw and lightly cooked foods provide enzymes, but there is debate as to whether they really increase the body's endogenous supply. Supplemental enzymes can be taken for a variety of health benefits. There are three main types of supplemental enzymes. Plant enzymes are derived from plants. The most common examples are bromelain from pineapple stems and papain from unripe papayas. Both help you to digest proteins, and bromelain has anti-inflammatory effects when taken on an empty stomach.

Microbial or fungal enzymes (also sometimes labeled as plant enzymes) are derived from the fermentation of fungus. The enzymes are then purified and available for therapeutic use. These types of enzymes can be used as digestive aids. Protease enzymes break down protein, lipase enzymes are for fats, amylase is for carbohydrates, and many others are available to break down other food components. Similar to bromelain, microbial-derived protease enzymes have blood-thinning and anti-inflammatory effects when taken between meals. These types of enzymes tend to have the best stability out of the three categories of enzymes.

The third category is animal enzymes. These enzymes are typically derived from animal organs. For example, pancreatic enzymes are usually derived from a sheep or pig pancreas.

Indications: Arthritis (protease enzymes taken between meals)

> Autoimmune conditions
>
> Cancer
>
> Candidiasis
>
> Celiac disease
>
> Colic
>
> Digestive disorders (most kinds)
>
> Food sensitivities
>
> Infections
>
> Sport injuries

Precautions: Side effects are uncommon. Protease enzymes are known to aggravate some users who have an active ulcer or gastritis. People taking blood-thinning medications should check with their doctors first before using enzymes. People with chronic candidiasis may experience yeast die-off symptoms, such as nausea, diarrhea, bloating, and so on, when they first begin enzyme supplementation.

Dosage: For digestive support, you would usually take 1 to 2 digestive enzyme complexes with each meal. Individual enzymes may be taken between meals for therapeutic effects. Take as directed by a health-care professional.

Evening Primrose Oil (EPO)

Description: Evening primrose oil is rich in an omega-6 fatty acid known as GLA (gamma linolenic acid). GLA has been shown to have anti-inflammatory effects and is required for proper brain function.

Indications: Arthritis

> Attention deficit disorder
>
> Fibrocystic breast syndrome
>
> Diabetes
>
> Dry skin
>
> Eczema
>
> Multiple sclerosis
>
> Peripheral neuropathy
>
> PMS

Precautions: Digestive upset and headaches are rare side effects. People with epilepsy should use EPO only under the guidance of a doctor. Evening primrose oil is best taken in conjunction with omega-3 fatty acids, such as fish, flaxseed, or perilla oil.

Fish Oil

Description: Fish oil is the richest source of the omega-3 fatty acids DHA (docosahexanoic acid) and EPA (eicosapentaenoic acid). Both DHA and EPA have anti-inflammatory effects. DHA plays an important role in brain function and joint health. EPA regulates inflammation, the immune system, blood clotting, and circulation.

Indications: Arthritis

Asthma

Attention deficit disorder

Bipolar disorder

Cancer

Cardiovascular disease

Chronic obstructive pulmonary disease

Depression

Diabetes

High blood pressure

High cholesterol and triglycerides

Inflammatory bowel disease

Lupus

Osteoporosis

Preeclampsia

Pregnancy

Schizophrenia

Precautions: Digestive upset (especially reflux and burping) may occur if the fish oil product is not enteric coated. Fish oil has a mild blood-thinning effect, so consult with your doctor before supplementation if you are on a blood-thinning medication. Some people may have a rise in LDL cholesterol. This can be prevented with garlic supplementation.

Dosage: Take 3 to 5 grams total of EPA and DHA together for therapeutic purposes. Otherwise, take 1 to 2 grams total EPA and DHA together for preventative purposes.

Flaxseed Oil

Description: Flaxseed oil is a rich source of alpha linolenic acid, an omega-3 fatty acid. Alpha linolenic acid is converted into DHA (docosahexanoic acid) and EPA (eicosapentaenoic acid). It is used to reduce inflammation; promote healthy circulation and healthy skin, hair, and nails; as well as to improve constipation. However, it has not been as well studied as fish oil has.

Indications: Arthritis

Asthma

Attention deficit disorder

Bipolar disorder

Cancer

Cardiovascular disease

Chronic obstructive pulmonary disease

Constipation

Depression

Diabetes

High blood pressure

High cholesterol and triglycerides

Inflammatory bowel disease

Lupus

Osteoporosis

Preeclampsia

Pregnancy

Schizophrenia

Precautions: Too much flaxseed oil can cause diarrhea. Men with prostate cancer should avoid supplementation with flaxseed oil and use ground seeds instead. Flaxseed oil has a mild blood-thinning effect, so consult with your doctor before supplementation if you are on blood-thinning medication.

Dosage: Take 1 to 2 tablespoons or 8 to 12 capsules daily.

FOS (Fructooligosaccharides)

Description: FOS refers to short chains of fructose molecules that are incompletely digested by humans. They serve as food or as a probiotic for healthy bacteria such as *Lactobacillus acidophilus* and *Bifidobacterium bifidusm.*

Indications: Diabetes

Digestive disorders

High cholesterol

Immunity

Precautions: High doses may cause diarrhea. Initial use may increase gas and flatulence, due to alterations in gut flora.

Dosage: Take 2,000 to 3,000 mg daily.

GABA (Gamma-Amino Butyric Acid)

Description: GABA is an amino acid–like substance that has a calming effect on the nervous system. It is naturally produced in the brain from the amino acid glutamate. Nutrition-oriented doctors use it as a calming agent for epilepsy and anxiety.

Indications: ADHD

Anxiety

Epilepsy

Muscle tightness

Precautions: GABA should not be combined with pharmaceutical psychiatric or anticonvulsant medications. It is best used under the guidance of a nutrition-oriented doctor.

Dosage: Take 250 to 500 mg three times daily.

Glandulars

Description: Glandulars refer to nutritional supplements made from animal tissue or animal tissue extracts. Research has found that amino acids, enzymes, and other nutrients from glandular supplements are absorbed into the bloodstream. In addition, minute quantities of hormones are likely present in many glandular products. It is thought that glandular supplements work by supplying minute amounts of hormones and specific nutrition to improve the functioning of the targeted gland. Preparations are available for most glands, such as thyroid, pancreas, adrenals, thymus, and many others. Most products are derived from cow or sheep organs.

Indications: Support for any underfunctioning or imbalanced gland

Precautions: A small percentage of users experience digestive upset. Look for organic products, to minimize the likelihood of using a contaminated product.

Dosage: The typical adult dosage is 1 to 2 capsules or tablets two to three times daily between meals. Take as directed on the label, as product potencies vary.

Glucosamine

Description: Glucosamine occurs naturally in the body and is involved in the manufacturing of cartilage. Supplemental glucosamine is mainly derived from the chitin (shell) of shellfish, such as crabs, shrimps, and lobsters. Glucosamine has been shown to support cartilage formation and reduce arthritic pain. The two forms of supplemental glucosamine are glucosamine sulfate and glucosamine hydrochloride. Most of the research to date has been done with the sulfate form.

Indications: Osteoarthritis

Sprains/strains

Precautions: Digestive upset, including diarrhea. Persons who are allergic to shellfish don't normally have a problem, as this reaction is usually to the protein found in the meat of shrimps and in crabmeat. People who are allergic to sulfa drugs do not need to be concerned, as the source of the drugs is different from the mineral sulfur that is part of glucosamine sulfate.

Dosage: Take 1,500 mg daily.

Glutamic Acid

Description: Glutamic acid is an amino acid that is suited to build protein and has been studied for the symptoms of prostate enlargement.

Indications: Prostate enlargement

Precautions: People with liver or kidney disease should not supplement amino acids unless under the direction of a health-care professional.

Dosage: Men with prostate enlargement can supplement 390 to 780 mg per day, along with the amino acids glycine and alanine at the same dosages.

Glutamine

Description: Glutamine is the most abundant and metabolically active amino acid in the body. It also serves as an energy source, because it can be converted to glucose, especially for the cells of the intestinal tract.

Indications: Alcohol withdrawal

Athletic performance

Gastritis

HIV

Surgical recovery

Ulcers

Precautions: People with liver or kidney disease should not supplement amino acids unless under the direction of a health-care professional.

Dosage: Take 1,500 to 3,000 mg daily.

Glycine

Description: Glycine is an amino acid that is used to build proteins, reduce prostate enlargement symptoms, improve cognitive function, and aid in liver detoxification.

Indications: Detoxification

Prostate enlargement

Schizophrenia

Precautions: People with liver or kidney disease should not supplement amino acids unless under the direction of a health-care professional.

Dosage: Men with prostate enlargement can supplement 390 to 780 mg per day, along with the amino acids glutamic acid and alanine at the same dosages.

Grapefruit Seed Extract

Description: Grapefruit seed extract is, as the name implies, the extract of grapefruit seeds. This supplement is mainly used for the treatment of infections, particularly fungal and bacterial infections. It is also available as a nasal spray to treat sinusitis.

Indications: Infections

Irritable bowel syndrome (related to candida overgrowth)

Sinusitis

Precautions: The internal use of this supplement should be avoided by pregnant women and breastfeeding mothers.

Dosage: Take 10 to 20 drops or 200 mg three times daily.

Grape Seed Extract

Description: Grape seed extract is, as the name implies, the extract of grape seeds. This supplement contains a class of flavonoids known as proanthocyanidins. Grape seed is mainly used as an antioxidant and to improve the stability of collagen and elastin, two substances that are important for healthy skin, joints, ligaments, tendons, and blood vessels. It is also used to improve microcirculation throughout the body.

Indications: Antioxidant support

Bruising

Macular degeneration

Retinopathy

Varicose veins

Precautions: No side effects have been reported.

Dosage: Take 50 to 300 mg daily.

Green Tea

Description: This tea or supplemental extract is derived from the leaves of *Camella sinensis,* the same plant that is used to make white and black tea. The leaves are lightly steamed and less processed than those of black tea, which accounts for its high antioxidant properties. It has been found to contain very potent antioxidant activity, and it improves detoxification. Green tea is commonly available in liquid, tablet, and capsule form.

Indications: Cancer

Cardiovascular disease

Detoxification

Digestive health

Gingivitis

High cholesterol

Tooth decay

Weight management

Precautions: Green tea that has not had the caffeine removed may cause irritability, insomnia, nervousness, and a fast heartbeat. However, these side effects are less common with green tea than with black tea, since it contains an amino acid known as L-theanine, which has a calming effect on the nervous system.

Dosage: Drink up to 10 cups of green tea daily, although 2 to 3 cups daily will provide good antioxidant protection. The supplement form should be standardized to 80 to 90 percent polyphenols and 35 to 55 percent epigallocatechin gallate, the potent antioxidant in green tea.

Glutathione

Description: Glutathione is a protein made up of the amino acids glycine, cysteine, and glutamic acid. It is one of the most important antioxidants and plays a key role in detoxification. There is concern whether oral glutathione supplements actually are effectively absorbed and utilized in the body. Nutrition-oriented doctors report good results with the intravenous form of glutathione. It is known that vitamin C, alpha lipoic acid, whey protein, and other nutrients increase the blood levels of glutathione.

Indications: Antioxidant

Cancer

Chronic fatigue syndrome

Emphysema (use the aerosol form)

Infertility (male)

Parkinson's disease

Precautions: No side effects have been reported.

Dosage: Take 500 to 1,500 mg daily.

Histidine

Description: Histidine is an amino acid that is considered nonessential in humans but may be essential in some children.

Indications: Rheumatoid arthritis

Precautions: People with liver or kidney disease should not supplement amino acids unless under the direction of a health-care professional.

Dosage: Take 250 to 500 mg three times daily between meals.

Huperzine A

Description: Huperzine A is a substance that is extracted from club moss (*Lycopodium serratum*). It has been shown to have some benefit for people with Alzheimer's disease and age-related cognitive decline. Huperzine A prevents the breakdown of the neurotransmitter acetylcholine.

Indications: Age-related cognitive decline

Alzheimer's disease

Precautions: Do not use it if you are currently taking a pharmaceutical medication for Alzheimer's disease.

Dosage: Take 100 to 200 mcg two to three times daily.

Hydroxycitric Acid (HCA)

Description: Hydroxycitric acid is a compound found in the fruit known as *Garcinia cambogia*. Animal but not human studies have found that HCA suppresses appetite and causes weight loss.

Indications: Weight loss

Precautions: No side effects are known.

Dosage: Take 500 to 1,000 mg three times daily before meals.

5-Hydroxytryptophan (5-HTP)

Description: The supplement 5-HTP is an amino acid–like substance used as a precursor to make the neurotransmitter serotonin. Serotonin is important for balanced mood, sleep, pain control, and other important functions of the body. This supplement is extracted from the seeds of the African plant *Griffonia simplicifolia*.

Indications: Anxiety

> Depression
>
> Fibromyalgia
>
> Food cravings (carbohydrates)
>
> Insomnia
>
> Migraine headaches
>
> Seasonal affective disorder
>
> Weight loss

Precautions: Large amounts may cause digestive upset, headaches, or sleepiness. It should not be taken in conjunction with pharmaceutical antidepressant, antianxiety, or other psychiatric medications.

Dosage: Take 50 to 100 mg three times daily on an empty stomach.

Indole-3 Carbinol

Description: Indole-3 carbinol is a phytonutrient found in cruciferous vegetables, such as broccoli, cauliflower, brussels sprouts, cabbage, and kale. Preliminary research has demonstrated anticancer properties. It also supports healthy estrogen metabolism. Studies have shown that it stopped or reduced the formation of precancerous lesions of the respiratory tract and the cervix of the uterus.

Indications: Cancer prevention

> Cervical dysplasia
>
> Estrogen metabolism

Precautions: There are no known side effects.

Dosage: Take 400 mg daily.

Ipriflavone

Description: Ipriflavone is a synthetic copy of a soy flavonoid known as daidzein. It is used as a supplement for the maintenance and the enhancement of bone density. Animal and human studies have shown that when combined with calcium and other minerals, it stimulates bone building by increasing the cells that form bone (osteoblasts) and reducing the activity of cells that break down bone (osteoclasts).

Indications: Hyperparathyroidism

Kidney failure (to maintain bone density)

Osteoporosis

Otosclerosis

Paget's disease

Precautions: Digestive upset is the most common side effect, which can be ameliorated by taking ipriflavone with food. One study found that lymphocyte count decreased in 29 out of 132 women who were supplementing ipriflavone. This reduction was not regarded as clinically significant, but it is recommended to have your doctor monitor these white blood cells.

Dosage: Take 600 mg daily.

Kelp

Description: Kelp is a type of sea vegetable that's rich in iron and several minerals. It is used as a supplement to support thyroid function.

Indications: Goiter

Hypothyroid

Precautions: People with any type of thyroid disease should check with their doctors before supplementing kelp.

Dosage: Take 2 to 4 capsules daily, or take as directed on the label or as advised by a health-care professional.

Lutein

Description: Lutein is a member of the carotenoid family. It has antioxidant activity and is known to be a key component of the macula, an area of the retina that is responsible for vision. It is mainly used as a supplement to prevent and treat macular degeneration.

Indications: Cataracts

Macular degeneration

Precautions: No side effects have been reported.

Dosage: Take 15 mg daily if you have macular degeneration and up to 5 mg daily as a preventative dosage.

Lycopene

Description: Lycopene is a member of the carotenoid family. It has received much attention because studies have shown that it has a protective effect against prostate and other cancers. Studies have also shown that lycopene enhances immune function and protects against heart disease. Tomatoes, watermelon, and pink grapefruit are all good food sources of lycopene.

Indications: Asthma

Atherosclerosis prevention

Cancer prevention

Immune support

Macular degeneration

Prostate cancer

Precautions: No side effects have been reported.

Dosage: Take 5 to 10 mg daily, as a good preventative dosage against cancer. Men with prostate cancer should supplement 30 mg daily.

L-Theanine

Description: L-theanine is an amino acid found in green tea. It has a calming and relaxing effect on the body.

Indications: Anxiety

          Insomnia

Precautions: No side effects have been reported. If you are taking pharmaceutical antianxiety medications, talk with your doctor first before using this supplement.

Dosage: Take 200 to 400 mg daily.

Lysine

Description: Lysine is an essential amino acid that must be obtained in one's diet, as the body cannot manufacture enough of it (gut bacteria synthesize small amounts of lysine). It is found in chicken, cottage cheese, avocados, and wheat germ. It is involved in the growth of children and in bone formation. It is most commonly used as a supplement to prevent and treat herpes outbreaks.

Indications: Cold sores

          Genital herpes

          Osteoporosis

          Shingles

Precautions: High dosages may cause digestive upset.

Dosage: Take 1,500 to 3,000 mg for the treatment of acute herpes outbreaks and 500 to 1,000 mg to prevent herpes outbreaks.

Malic Acid

Description: Malic acid is a naturally occurring substance that is found in fruits and vegetables, especially in apples. It helps with the production of ATP within cells for energy production. Some holistic doctors use it as a therapy, along with magnesium, for fibromyalgia and aluminum detoxification.

Indications: Aluminum detoxification

          Fibromyalgia

Precautions: There are no known side effects.

Dosage: Take 1,200 to 2,400 mg daily.

Medium-Chain Triglycerides (MCTs)

Description: Medium-chain triglycerides are fatty acids that are found in coconut and palm oil, as well as in butter. They are used by athletes for training and may have mild weight-loss properties. Some nutritionists claim that they support thyroid function. MCTs have been shown to have a mild blood glucose–lowering effect.

Indications: Athletic training

          Diabetes

          Hypothyroidism

Precautions: Digestive upset is known to occur for some users. They should be used under a doctor's care if you have diabetes or liver disease.

Dosage: The typical dosage is 15 to 30 grams, although athletes often use 50 grams or more.

Melatonin

Description: Melatonin is a natural hormone produced in the brain's pineal gland that regulates the body's biological clock and sleep cycles. Melatonin is produced in response to darkness. This hormone has been shown to be helpful for insomnia, seasonal affective disorder, and other mood disturbances. It has potent antioxidant properties and also protects against radiation damage.

Indications: Aging

Cancer (breast and prostate)

Cluster headaches

Insomnia

Jet lag

Radiation exposure

Seasonal affective disorder

Tardive dyskinesia

Precautions: Pregnant women or nursing mothers should avoid supplementing melatonin unless instructed to do so by their physicians. People with cancer should also consult with their doctors first before supplementing melatonin. Children should not supplement melatonin unless instructed to do so by their doctors. People on steroid medications should avoid taking melatonin unless their doctors feel it is appropriate.

Dosage: Take 0.3 to 0.5 mg as a starting dosage for insomnia and jet lag.

Methionine

Description: This essential amino acid is necessary for growth, detoxification, and normal metabolism.

Indications: Detoxification support

HIV

Pancreatitis

Parkinson's disease

Precautions: B vitamins, especially B6, folic acid, and B12, should be supplemented along with methionine to prevent the build-up of homocysteine, a risk factor for cardiovascular disease. People with liver or kidney disease should not supplement amino acids unless under the direction of a health-care professional.

Dosage: Take 500 mg one to two times daily.

MSM (Methylsulfonylmethane)

Description: MSM is a naturally occurring component in the body and is found in many foods, especially green vegetables. It is a good source of the mineral sulfur. MSM is used as a supplement primarily to reduce pain and inflammation.

Indications: Allergies

Arthritis

Asthma

Autoimmune diseases

Fibromyalgia

Hair and nail health

Headaches

Heartburn

Muscle spasms

Sports injuries

Precautions: Rare reports of digestive upset, such as diarrhea, cramping, and stomach upset, occur with too high a dosage. Otherwise, MSM is nontoxic. People on blood-thinning medications should check with their doctors first before using MSM, as it has mild blood-thinning effects.

Dosage: Take 500 to 2,000 mg for preventative purposes and up to 10,000 mg daily for severe pain and inflammatory disorders.

N-Acetylcysteine

Description: This is a varied form of the amino acid acetylcysteine. It is commonly used to increase the levels of glutathione in the body, for detoxification, and as a mucus thinner.

Indications: Angina

Antioxidant support (via glutathione production)

Bronchitis

Chronic obstructive pulmonary disease

Cystic fibrosis

Gastritis

HIV

Pneumonia

Postnasal drip

Precautions: Long-term use may deplete zinc and copper levels. Nausea, vomiting, headache, dizziness, and abdominal pain have been reported with supplementation. People with liver or kidney disease should not supplement amino acids unless under the direction of a health-care professional.

Dosage: Take 500 to 1,500 mg daily.

NADH (Nicotinamide Adenine Dinucleotide)

Description: NADH is the coenzyme form of vitamin B3 (niacin), which plays a role in cellular energy production. Preliminary research has shown NADH to be helpful for chronic fatigue syndrome and depression. It may also hold promise in reducing the symptoms of Alzheimer's disease and Parkinson's disease, although these uses have not been proven.

Indications: Alzheimer's disease

Chronic fatigue syndrome

Depression

Parkinson's disease

Fibromyalgia

Precautions: NADH appears to be nontoxic.

Dosage: Take 5 to 10 mg daily on an empty stomach.

Ornithine

Description: This amino acid is used in the body for tissue regeneration.

Indications: Athletic training
Liver cirrhosis
Wound healing

Precautions: High doses, above 10 grams, may cause digestive upset. People with liver or kidney disease should not supplement amino acids unless under the direction of a health-care professional.

Dosage: Take 5 to 20 grams daily.

Pectin

Description: Pectin is a soluble fiber derived from apples, grapefruit, or other citrus fruits.

Indications: Diabetes
High cholesterol

Precautions: Pectin supplements may cause digestive upset.

Dosage: Dosages of up to 15 grams a day are used.

Perilla Oil

Description: Perilla oil is an extract of the Asian beefsteak plant. It is a rich source of alpha linolenic acid. As with other essential fatty acid supplements like flaxseed oil, perilla oil helps to reduce inflammation, improve circulation, and enhance brain function and has several other uses.

Indications: Allergies
Arthritis
Cancer prevention
Cardiovascular disease prevention
Inflammatory bowel disease
Memory and concentration
Neurological health

Precautions: Perilla has mild blood-thinning effects. Consult with your doctor before supplementing if you are taking a blood-thinning medication.

Dosage: Take 6,000 mg daily.

Phenylalanine

Description: This amino acid serves to build protein and acts as a precursor to L-tyrosine, L-dopa, norepinephrine, and epinephrine. L-phenylalanine occurs naturally in foods. The supplemental form, D-phenylalanine (DPA), is not naturally occurring in the body but can be converted into phenylethylamine to elevate mood and decrease pain. Also, a common supplement form that combines L-phenylalanine (LPA) and D-phenylalanine (DPA) is known as DLPA (DL-phenylalanine).

Indications for DPA: Depression
Lower back pain
Osteoarthritis
Parkinson's disease

Rheumatoid arthritis

Pain

Indications for DLPA: Alcohol withdrawal

Depression

Precautions: People with phenylketonuria and tardive dyskinesia must not supplement phenylalanine. Rare instances of heartburn, nausea, and headaches have been reported. People with liver or kidney disease should not supplement amino acids unless under the direction of a health-care professional.

Dosage: DLPA is usually taken at a dosage of 500 mg, two to three times daily between meals. LPA is used in dosages of up to 3,500 mg daily.

Phosphatidylcholine (PC)

Description: Phosphatidylcholine is an extract from lecithin that supplies a form of choline that is used as a building block for cell walls and the neurotransmitter acetylcholine. Lecithin contains anywhere from 10 to 20 percent phosphatidylcholine. PC is important for proper brain and neurological function and supports healthy liver detoxification.

Indications: Alzheimer's disease

Bipolar disorder

Hepatitis

High cholesterol

Liver cirrhosis and detoxification

Precautions: Digestive upset, such as diarrhea or nausea, may occur with high dosages.

Dosage: Take 1,500 to 9,000 mg daily.

Phosphatidylserine (PS)

Description: PS is a type of phospholipid extracted from soy that is used to build and maintain healthy cell membranes. It is used as a supplement to improve memory and depression, as well as to balance stress hormones. It is one of the few substances known to slow down early-stage Alzheimer's disease.

Indications: Age-associated memory impairment

Alzheimer's disease

Attention deficit hyperactivity disorder

Brain injury

Dementia

Depression

Stress hormone imbalance

Precautions: There are no known side effects.

Dosage: Take 100 to 500 mg daily, although most studies used 300 mg.

Policosanol

Description: Policosanol is a naturally occurring compound extracted from sugarcane wax, beeswax, or rice bran wax. Nearly all of the published studies have been done on the sugarcane extract form. It is composed of a combination of fatty alcohol groups that includes octacosanol. Comparison studies have shown policosanol to be equally effective as pharmaceutical cholesterol-lowering medications. Policosanol appears to do a better job of increasing the good HDL cholesterol.

Indications: Angina

High cholesterol, including total and LDL cholesterol, and lipoprotein(a)

Intermittent claudication

Stroke prevention

Precautions: Pregnant women or breastfeeding mothers should not use policosanol.

Dosage: Take 10 to 20 mg with the evening meal.

Pregnenolone

Description: Pregnenolone is a steroidal hormone produced in large part by the adrenal glands. It is a precursor hormone that the body uses to manufacture DHEA and progesterone. It is commonly used by holistic doctors for arthritis and autoimmune conditions such as lupus.

Indications: Arthritis (especially rheumatoid form)

Depression

Lupus erythematosus

Poor memory

Psoriasis

Precautions: Pregnenolone should be avoided by people who have seizure disorders or a history of hormone-related cancers.

Dosage: Take 10 to 50 mg daily.

Progesterone

Description: Progesterone is a hormone that's found in both men and women. For women, it is involved in regulating the menstrual cycle and reproductive function. Progesterone is mainly produced and secreted by the ovaries during ovulation. It is also manufactured by the adrenal glands, the brain, and the placenta in pregnant women. Natural progesterone cream is a popular supplement for the treatment of PMS, menopausal symptoms, endometriosis, and several other conditions.

Indications: Autoimmune conditions

Endometriosis

Fibrocystic breasts

Infertility (female)

Irregular menses

Menopausal symptoms

Osteoporosis

Ovarian cysts

PMS

Uterine fibroids

Precautions: Natural progesterone cream has a good safety record. Women with a history of cancer should consult with a doctor before using it. Women using the birth control pill or synthetic progestin should avoid it.

Dosage: The dosage depends on the condition being treated. Menopausal women generally apply a quarter teaspoon (20 mg) to the skin one to two times daily.

Propolis

Description: Propolis is "bee glue," the resinous substance that is formed when bees gather propolis from the buds and the bark of trees. The worker bees, with their salivary secretions and wax flakes, seal the chambers and the entrance of the beehive. Propolis has antimicrobial, antioxidant, and anti-inflammatory properties.

Indications: Gingivitis

Herpes

Infections

Mouth ulcers

Parasites

Peptic ulcers

Periodontal disease

Ulcerative colitis

Wound healing

Precautions: There are rare reports of allergic reactions, such as skin itching and redness.

Dosage: Take 500 to 1,000 mg of the capsule form or 1 to 3 ml of the tincture form, or use it topically as a cream or a spray.

Psyllium

Description: Psyllium is a fiber supplement. Psyllium seed husks are popular for the treatment of constipation. Psyllium has also been shown to lower cholesterol levels.

Indications: Constipation

Diabetes

Diarrhea

Diverticulitis

Hemorrhoids

High cholesterol

Irritable bowel syndrome

Precautions: Psyllium should be taken two to three hours away from any medications or supplements, as it may hinder absorption.

Dosage: Take 5 grams three times daily, with at least 8 ounces of water.

Pyruvate

Description: Pyruvate is a by-product of carbohydrate and protein metabolism in the body. It is available as a supplement and is mainly used for weight loss. It has also been shown to have antioxidant effects and may improve one's exercise endurance.

Indications: Antioxidant support

Athletic support

Weight loss

Precautions: High dosages may cause digestive upset.

Dosage: Take 5 to 30 grams daily for weight loss.

Red Yeast Rice

Description: Red yeast rice, the fermented product of rice on which red yeast (*Monascus purpureus*) is grown, is a supplement that's used to lower cholesterol. Historically, red yeast rice was described in ancient Chinese texts as an aid to improve circulation. Human studies have shown it to effectively reduce cholesterol levels.

Indications: High cholesterol

Precautions: Mild digestive upset may occur. It should be avoided by pregnant women and breastfeeding mothers, people with liver disease, and those on pharmaceutical cholesterol-lowering medications. It is recommended that coenzyme Q10 (10–200 mg daily) be supplemented while you take red yeast rice extract, as some researchers theorize that it may cause a deficiency of this nutrient.

Dosage: The dosage used in studies was 1.2 to 2.4 grams of red yeast rice standardized to 10 to 13.5 mg of monacolins. However, FDA regulations do not allow supplement manufacturers to list the concentration of monacolins in their products.

Resveratrol

Description: Resveratrol is a compound found in red wine that has potent antioxidant activity. Preliminary research has demonstrated cardiovascular benefit and possible anticancer properties.

Indications: Antioxidant
Cancer prevention
Cardiovascular disease prevention

Precautions: There have been no reported side effects.

Dosage: Take 500 mcg to 50 mg daily.

Royal Jelly

Description: Royal jelly is the substance that worker bees secrete to feed the queen bee. It contains B vitamins and other nutrients. Holistic doctors use it for energy support. It has been shown in studies to lower cholesterol.

Indications: Fatigue
High cholesterol
Stress

Precautions: People who are allergic to bee pollen or honey should not use royal jelly.

Dosage: The typical adult dosage is 50 to 100 mg daily.

Rye Pollen

Description: Rye pollen is a supplement used for the treatment of chronic prostatitis and benign prostatic hyperplasia.

Indications: Benign prostatic hyperplasia
Chronic prostatitis

Precautions: There are no reported side effects.

Dosage: Take 3 tablets twice daily.

SAMe (S-Adenosylmethionine)

Description: SAMe is a naturally occurring substance in the body that is made from combining the amino acid methionine with ATP. It is regarded as a methyl (CH_3)

that enables a variety of biochemical reactions to occur properly. SAMe is mainly used for the treatment of osteoarthritis, depression, and fibromyalgia.

Indications: Depression

Detoxification

Fibromyalgia

Hepatitis

Liver cirrhosis

Osteoarthritis

Precautions: SAMe is very safe. However, it is not recommended for people with bipolar disorder. It can be used in conjunction with pharmaceutical antidepressants as long as you are being monitored by a physician.

Dosage: Take 400 to 1,200 mg daily.

Shark Cartilage

Description: Shark cartilage is used as a supplement for the treatment of cancer and arthritis. It has been reported that shark cartilage prevents the growth of new blood vessels that feed tumors. The health benefits of shark cartilage lack scientific validity. However, some practitioners report obvious clinical improvement in patients.

Indications: Arthritis

Cancer

Precautions: Pregnant women and breastfeeding mothers should avoid the supplementation of shark cartilage.

Dosage: Take 50 to 100 mg daily.

Soy Isoflavones

Description: Phytoestrogen compounds that are extracted from soy, such as daidzein, genistein, and glycitein, are known as soy isoflavones. They are commonly used to reduce menopausal, PMS, and other female hormone–related conditions. They have been shown to help improve bone density, protect against bone loss, and reduce cholesterol levels. Interestingly, men with prostate problems are also helped.

Indications: High cholesterol

Menopause

PMS

Prostate enlargement

Vaginitis

Precautions: Women with a history of breast or uterine cancer should avoid isolated soy isoflavone supplementation until further research shows benefit.

Dosage: Take 100 to 300 mg daily.

Spirulina

Description: Spirulina is a type of blue-green algae that has been consumed as a food by Mexicans for many centuries. It is a rich source of amino acids, chlorophyll, B vitamins, GLA, carotenoids, and other nutrients. Spirulina has been shown to have immune-enhancing effects, it detoxifies heavy metals, and it protects against radiation sickness. A phytonutrient in spirulina known as phycocyanin has been shown to stimulate the production of blood cells.

Indications: Anemia

        Cancer

        Detoxification

        High cholesterol

        Immune support

        Radiation poisoning

        Vitamin A deficiency

Precautions: No side effects are known.

Dosage: Take 2,000 to 3,000 mg daily.

Sulforaphane

Description: Sulforaphane is a phytonutrient found in broccoli sprouts and other cruciferous vegetables. It has potent antioxidant effects, supports healthy detoxification, and improves estrogen balance.

Indications: Cancer prevention

        Detoxification

Precautions: There are no known side effects.

Dosage: Take 400 mg daily.

Taurine

Description: Taurine is an amino acid–like substance that is an important part of bile for fat absorption. It is also essential for the development of the nervous system and for heart function.

Indications: Cardiomyopathy

        Congestive heart failure

        Cystic fibrosis

        Diabetes

        Epilepsy

        High blood pressure

        Surgical recovery

Precautions: People with liver or kidney disease should not supplement amino acids unless under the direction of a health-care professional.

Dosage: Take 1,500 to 5,000 mg daily.

TMG (Trimethylglycine)

Description: TMG, also called betaine, is a supplement that's used to lower homocysteine levels and improve liver detoxification.

Indications: Hepatitis

        High homocysteine levels

        Liver detoxification support

Precautions: No side effects are known.

Dosage: Take 500 to 3,000 mg daily.

Tyrosine

Description: This amino acid is derived from another amino acid known as phenylalanine. L-tyrosine is a precursor for the formation of the neurotransmitters L-dopa dopamine, norepinephrine, and epinephrine. The skin also converts tyrosine into melanin, the pigment that protects the skin against harmful UV radiation. In addition, this amino acid is required for the synthesis of thyroid hormone.

Indications: Depression

　　　　　　　Hypothyroidism

　　　　　　　Parkinson's disease

　　　　　　　Phenylketonuria

Precautions: People with liver or kidney disease should not supplement amino acids unless under the direction of a health-care professional.

Dosage: Take 250 to 500 mg twice daily between meals.

Vinpocetine

Description: Vinpocetine is an extract from the leaf of the periwinkle plant. It has been shown in studies to dilate blood vessels, enhance circulation in the brain, improve oxygen utilization, make red blood cells more pliable, and inhibit aggregation of platelets. Studies have shown it to benefit cognitive function for people with dementia.

Indications: Dementia

　　　　　　　Hearing loss

　　　　　　　Memory problems

　　　　　　　Tinnitus

Precautions: Pregnant women or breastfeeding mothers should not take vinpocetine. Use caution if you are currently taking blood pressure medications.

Dosage: Take 10 to 20 mg daily.

Whey Protein

Description: Whey is a component of cow's milk and is a good source of branched-chain amino acids, which are required for the maintenance and the building of muscle mass. Whey protein has also been shown to increase the body's levels of glutathione, a very important antioxidant.

Indications: Athlete's support

　　　　　　　Meal replacement

Precautions: People with kidney or liver disease should check with their physicians before supplementing whey protein.

Dosage: Take 25 grams daily.

Antioxidants

What are antioxidants?

The use of antioxidant supplements has become very popular with consumers and health professionals. Researchers are continuing to find that many diseases are prevented or improved with the help of antioxidants, either from a healthful diet or from supplementation. The role of antioxidants is to prevent or control oxidation—hence the prefix *anti* (meaning "against"). Oxidation refers to the burning of oxygen as fuel in cells and the subsequent creation of substances known as free radicals. Free radicals are unstable molecules that are very reactive and can damage cell DNA and various tissues. Researchers estimate that our cell DNA receives anywhere from 75,000 to 100,000 hits from free radicals every day. A free radical is missing an electron (a charged particle) and seeks out another molecule to pair up with, to gain an electron. This process actually creates more free radicals.

THE PROCESS OF OXIDATION

A good example of the oxidation process is an apple that has been sliced open. Within a small period of time, the flesh of the apple will turn a brownish color. This occurs because of oxygen interacting with the exposed apple. If you were to slice an apple and immediately squirt lemon juice on it, you would find that the brownish discoloration (oxidation) occurs over a much longer period of time. This protective effect occurs from the antioxidants vitamin C and bioflavonoids that exist in lemon juice. Within our bodies, similar reactions are occurring all the time. For example, antioxidants protect cholesterol from becoming oxidized. Researchers have found that cholesterol really becomes a villain only when it becomes oxidized and makes the process of atherosclerosis more likely. For people who consume a diet that's high in fruits and vegetables, our richest source of antioxidants, the risk of cardiovascular disease is reduced. The same is true for a variety of cancers and other chronic diseases.

SOURCES OF FREE RADICALS

Besides free radicals that are produced in the life-giving process of energy production within our cells, we are also exposed to a variety of other factors that increase our free radical exposure. Ionizing radiation from the sun, X-rays, and other sources is common. Too much exposure may result in skin cancer, wrinkles, and cataracts. Also, industrial pollution contributes to the burden with toxic metals (arsenic, mercury, and others), smoke, and many other toxins. We then have to consider that many pharmaceutical medications create free radicals in users. In addition, people with chronic diseases such as diabetes generate more free radicals than a healthy individual does. Athletes produce a higher amount of free radicals as a by-product of exercise. Smoking, alcohol, fried foods, and high-fat diets all are notorious sources of toxic free radicals.

ANTIOXIDANT ENZYME SYSTEM

Our bodies have a built-in antioxidant system. This includes key enzymes such as catalase, superoxide dismutase (SOD), and glutathione peroxidase. Minerals such as selenium, manganese, zinc, and copper are required to keep these enzyme systems working efficiently.

COMMON ANTIOXIDANTS

Since the typical North American diet is deficient in antioxidant-rich plant foods, it is important for people to supplement additional antioxidant nutrients. Well-known antioxidants include vitamins A, C, and E, as well as selenium, glutathione, CoQ10, and beta-carotene. Additional ones include lutein, lycopene, and other carotenoids. Grape seed extract, N-acetylcysteine, alpha lipoic acid, and tocotrienols are also great antioxidants. Phytonutrients, as found in herbs such as green tea, turmeric, ginkgo biloba, and milk thistle, have some of the most potent antioxidant activity ever discovered. Each of the antioxidants plays a key role in neutralizing free radicals and optimizing immune system function. These are just a few examples of the antioxidants that are available in foods and supplements.

TESTING ANTIOXIDANT STATUS

There are several different ways you can test your antioxidant status. One is to have a blood test that measures the levels of key antioxidants found in your blood. Another is to have a blood or urine test that measures the level of oxidative stress in your body. This gives an assessment of your body's oxidative stress status and antioxidant reserves. And, finally, a newer technology uses a computer-guided low-energy, blue light laser to scan the palms of your hands and measure the carotenoid antioxidant level.

References: Nutritional Supplements

Anderson, R. A. 1997. Chromium as an essential nutrient for humans. *Regulatory Toxicology and Pharmacology* 26(1 Pt 2):S35–41.

Bower, C., F. Stanley, and D. Nicol. 1993. Maternal folate status and risk for neural tube defects. *Annals of the New York Academy of Sciences* 678:146–55.

Fairfield, K. M., and R. H. Fletcher. 2002. Vitamins for chronic disease prevention in adults: Scientific review. *Journal of the American Medical Association* 287: 3116–29.

Ferslew, K. E., R. V. Acuff, E. A. Daigneault, T. W. Woolley, and P. E. Stanton, Jr. 1993. Pharmacokinetics and bioavailability of the RRR and all racemic stereoisomers of alpha-tocopherol in humans after single oral administration. *Journal of Clinical Pharmacology* 33(1):84–88.

Recker, R. R., A. Bammi, J. Barger-Lux, and R. P. Heaney. 1988. Calcium absorbability from milk products, an imitation milk, and calcium carbonate. *American Journal of Clinical Nutrition* 47:93–95.

Werler, M., S. Shapiro, and A. Mitchell. 1993. Preconceptual folic acid exposure and risk of occurent neural tube defects. *Journal of the American Medical Association* 269:1257–61.

Herbal Medicine

History

Herbal medicine is the oldest therapy in world history, predating by tens of thousands of years the rich herbal remedies of ancient China, India, and Egypt. Herbs have been found in archaeological explorations in the most ancient of civilizations.

Much later on, around 400 B.C., the Greeks began to systematize and codify medical principles. Hippocrates, whom we recognize as the father of Western medicine, and the doctors who followed him, believed that there were four basic types of body fluids and that health was maintained by keeping each of these types in its proper balance. They relied upon herbs such as rosemary, fennel, and saffron, in conjunction with exercise, massage, and other gentle therapies, not just to treat the symptoms of an illness, but to stimulate a person's inner healing powers and to bring the unbalanced fluid back to its appropriate level.

Roman physicians took their cues from the Greeks. Before Roman soldiers went into battle, doctors painted the soles of the soldiers' feet with garlic oil as a way of stimulating the immune system in case of injury and promoting quick healing. One doctor, Dioscorides, detailed four hundred herbal remedies in his work *De Materia Medica*. Another doctor, Galen, expanded upon the body-fluid theories of the Greeks and further encouraged the idea of health as a matter of balance.

As the Romans conquered most of the Middle East and Europe (thanks to the garlic, no doubt), they brought their doctors, their medical treatises, and their remedies with them. By the time the Roman Empire fell, an herbal healing system had been firmly established throughout the continent. Garlic was recognized as an effective guard against colds and fever, and peppermint was widely known to encourage good digestion. Europeans knew that basil eased their cramps and that parsley acted as a diuretic. More important than the use of any one herb was the idea that plants in general were agents that, with the proper application, could be used to stimulate the body's natural healing response.

But by the medieval era, European medical practice had grown much more aggressive and invasive. Doctors began to rely upon emetics and purgatives for treating most illnesses—strategies that probably killed more patients than healed them. Worse, these doctors began to attack the local healers who used herbs. It's now thought that the witch hunts of early modern Europe were really ways for the medical establishment to remove the women who had knowledge of herbs and healing from their positions of power within the villages.

One fifteenth-century physician, Paracelsus, was so disgusted by the state of medical practice that he devoted his career to gentle, natural herbal therapies. He not only studied European sources, but also took care to include the considerable work of Middle Eastern herbalists. He learned which herbs could cure disease, and he taught other physicians that foods and herbs contained energy that could be absorbed and utilized by the body. Paracelsus didn't have everything right—he believed that a plant's shape was indicative of the part of the body it could cure—but he was a strong, credible voice that brought serious attention back to herbal treatment.

Since the time of Paracelsus, European medicine has been a battle between the holistic philosophy of herbalism and an increasingly mechanized view of the body. And as Europeans began to explore and colonize, this battleground spread to North America, where Native Americans had been using herbal remedies for centuries, if not millennia. Nevertheless, herbalism remained an important and respected tradition in Europe, as well as in America, up through the early 1900s.

By the middle of the twentieth century, however, herbal remedies were almost completely eclipsed by the development of synthetic "wonder drugs." Scientists learned how to isolate the active ingredients in herbs and patent them as medications like morphine and aspirin. Pharmaceutical companies made huge profits from the sales of their products and used the money in part to fund medical schools that shunned teaching herbalism. Soon herbs—the very source of many of the "legitimate" pharmaceuticals—were ridiculed as ineffective and untested.

It's not hard to understand the deep distrust that exists between pharmaceutical companies and many natural health-care doctors and practitioners. Pharmaceutical companies can't put a patent on a natural remedy like herbs, and, therefore, they can't control profits in the same way they can with synthetic drugs.

But it's deeper than mere greed. We've grown only too familiar with Western medicine's approach to disease, which views the body as a machine with parts to be either fixed or replaced. Symptoms of disease—fatigue, cough, constipation, and so on—are treated with drugs or procedures, while the cause, which is often improper living, goes ignored. In the United States, health is too often considered the absence of any obvious disease. Get rid of the symptoms, you have gotten rid of the disease. Right? Not really!

Since the days of Hippocrates, Western herbalism has taken a radically different approach. Although we no longer believe in Hippocrates' theory of body fluids, we continue his emphasize on balance, on building and protecting our natural constitutions. With a strong constitution, the regular waves of viral diseases, like the flu epidemics that hammer so many of us over and over again, can be successfully resisted. And while disease may afflict us from time to time, many herbs in nature's pharmacy can treat the root cause of the ailment—an essential part of preventing its reoccurrence. With herbs, we not only cure periodic illness, but also prevent fresh onslaughts from weakening our constitutions and unnecessarily shortening our lives.

Keep in mind that 80 percent of the world's population relies on herbs as a primary form of medicine. Many cultures use herbal therapies as a first line of treatment for illness. For example, hospitals in China train doctors to specialize in herbal medicine for all the different categories of disease (cardiology, dermatology, etc.). Most medical doctors in Germany utilize herbal therapies in their practices. As herbal therapy enters mainstream medicine, more doctors are becoming educated and willing to recommend these treatments to their patients. By following the guidelines in this chapter, you can strengthen the various organ systems of your body and feel a difference in your health. If you are new to herbal medicine, start with common herbs, such as peppermint for an upset stomach or echinacea for the common cold. Your confidence will grow with each successful use of these wondrous herbs.

Mixing Herbs and Pharmaceuticals

As herbals became America's fastest-growing branch of alternative medicine, the Western medical community was the last to find out. Herbs are ignored in medical school and have only recently begun to make occasional appearances in medical journals. When doctors are oblivious to the benefits of herbal remedies, patients are often reluctant to reveal that they are taking herbals because of embarrassment at the prospect of a stern lecture on the subject.

Sometimes, the only time a doctor finds out about an herbal-pharmaceutical mix is when a patient suddenly exhibits strange symptoms not seen with the pharmaceutical alone. At times, that mix can be deadly. Add a commercial stimulant to ginseng, and we now know that we are increasing the likelihood of a potential bad reaction. Cardiac glycosides, herbal ingredients that act on the heart, can cause arrythmia—an irregular heartbeat—when taken with a prescription diuretic. The side effects of certain selective serotonin reuptake inhibitors (SSRIs) that are used to treat cases of major depression—marketed under names such as Prozac, Paxil, or Celexa—may be magnified by Saint-John's-wort, a popular herb intended for mild to moderate cases of depression.

But most often, herbs can be an effective complement to conventional therapies. Ginger, for example, has been shown in clinical trials to limit nausea from chemotherapy. Reports from Europe—where herbs have been used longer and studied much more intensely than in the United States—indicate that pharmaceutical-herbal interactions are unusual. The symptoms of an adverse reaction are likely to be muted, if you consider the generally mild nature of herbs. When there is a reaction, it's first likely to surface as an upset stomach or a feeling of discomfort. Your first response should be to stop the remedies and get in touch with a health-care professional.

The use of standardized extracts, which are made up of specified quantities of herbal ingredients in commercially prepared remedies, is a good thing, but is likely to further complicate the use of pharmaceuticals combined with herbals. As herbal remedies are better prepared and quantified, they become more effective—and more dangerous when unknowingly mixed with pharmaceuticals.

Pharmaceutical companies have been quick to pick up on the popularity of herbs and have been careful to note which herbs and which pharmaceuticals may provoke harmful side effects. On the positive side, that has helped educate the public on the dangers of mixing. On the negative side, I've noticed that pharmaceutical companies are also quick to take the knee-jerk position of warning against all mixing—no doubt, at least in part to avoid any potential litigation, as well as a result of the age-old grudge match at work between pharmaceutical giants, which are a virtual global cartel now, and the herbal companies.

Even as doctors are being advised in a growing flood of special alerts about herbs to watch for, don't rely on your physician to make the connection. Too often, doctors are still struggling to understand the basics of herbal remedies. Medical schools typically avoid the subject of herbs in medicine. Pharmacists may understand little or nothing about herbalism, even if they can make the connection between herbs and the active ingredients in many prescription medications.

That means you have to make the connection yourself. Before mixing any herbs with any prescription medication, err on the side of caution. Aggressively go after the facts for yourself, and then go in prepared to ask your doctor questions.

Don't take "no" for an answer. If your doctor flatly rules out an herbal remedy, ask why. If you're not satisfied with your doctor's response, why not track down another physician? Wait until you find a qualified physician who has taken the time to learn how herbs work. Even if he or she may be suspicious of herbs' long-term health effects, you need to see a doctor or a qualified herbalist who can review the potential interactions and help weed out beneficial herbal remedies from the questionable ones.

Always keep in mind that there may be several different herbal and pharmaceutical remedies to choose from, and seeing how each will interact can offer you some healthful substitutes while enabling you to avoid any toxic reactions. In some cases, you may decide to take a mix of herbs, supplements, and vitamins instead of a drug. Instead of an SSRI tranquilizer, for example, you may decide on a mix of DHA, which is included in the omega-3 fatty acids derived from seafood, and vitamin-B complex (containing B12, B6, and B5) along with Saint-John's-wort.

In this New World of digital information, millions of people are turning to the World Wide Web to gain an unprecedented education in medicine. Use it to its full advantage, and bring a skeptical attitude to help find the most authoritative answers to your health questions. Health is the number one category for searches on the Internet, and this curiosity on the part of the public will force doctors to spend more time on continuing education or risk falling behind many of their patients on the latest advances in their field.

Safe Use

The proper use of herbal preparations should pose no health dangers to you. There are herbs that are toxic and should not be used by the public. Most toxic herbs are not available in your typical health food store, drugstore, or supermarket supplement section. If you are unfamiliar with an herb or a combination of herbs and cannot find any valid literature, then simply do not use it. Please pay particular attention to how you should calculate a specific dosage for your child, which is discussed later in this section. This is important, to help you achieve a therapeutic effect with the herbs.

When purchasing quality herbal products:

- Make sure the label provides easy directions and recommended dosages.
- The label should list all ingredients in order of potency.
- Look to see if the specific parts of the plants used are identified. For example, some herbs work better when their leaves are used; other herbs house their medicinal ingredients in the roots, not the leaves.
- Purchase products that are wrapped in safety seals to prevent tampering and preserve freshness.
- Make sure the label lists an expiration date and a lot number.
- Buy products that are certified to be organic. This ensures that no pesticides or herbicides were used in harvesting and preparing.
- Cautions should be listed on the container.
- The company should be known for high standards in quality control.

Herbal Preparations

TINCTURE

A tincture, or liquid extract, is the preservation of herbs in water and alcohol. This is one of the most common forms of herbal medicines, along with capsules and teas. Since it is in a liquid form, tinctures are easy to absorb and assimilate. Some herbs require an alcohol extraction process so that certain medicinal constituents are pulled out of the plant and made available to the user. Some people do not like the taste, due to the alcohol. The taste can be improved by adding the herbs to a small cup of hot water and letting it sit for a few minutes, allowing some of the alcohol to evaporate, and then adding it to juice. Glycerine-based tinctures have had the alcohol removed and are more palatable for children and people averse to a product that contains alcohol.

CAPSULES

Capsules contain the dry powder of the herb. They are popular because of their convenience—they're easy to take, because no taste is involved, and easy to store in containers. The downside is that they can be used only by older children or adults who can swallow capsules. If the herb(s) you purchase are available only in capsule form and your child cannot swallow capsules, you can open the capsules up and mix the contents in water, juice, or food.

TABLETS

Tablets contain powdered herbs that have been compressed with binders and substances that make the tablet smooth and easy to swallow. The advantage is that more material can be compressed into a tablet. The downside is that many children and some adults cannot swallow tablets.

LOZENGES

Herbs can be made into a dissolvable lozenge. A common example is echinacea/zinc lozenges.

COMPRESSES

A compress involves the application of a hot or cold herbal extract to the skin. The herb can be put directly on the skin, or it can be applied to the skin using a cloth that has been saturated with the herb.

TEAS (DECOCTION/INFUSION)

A tea consists of an herb or an herbal combination soaked in water. There are two main methods of doing this.

A decoction is used for harder plant parts, such as the bark, the root, and the seeds. These require more time and heat, in order to extract the medicinal ingredients. First, you heat the herb (1 tablespoon of the dry herb or 3 tablespoons of the fresh herb) in water until it boils, then let it simmer (covered with a lid) for 15 to 25 minutes. Next, let it sit for 10 minutes, strain, and serve. An example of a tea that would involve making a decoction is one made from raw ginger root.

The more common preparation for a tea is an infusion. This uses the softer parts of herbs, such as leaves and flowers. It is effective for herbs like peppermint leaf; the tea can be drunk more quickly to capture the volatile oils. Commercial preparations of tea bags are available, or you can use dry or fresh herbs. If using a tea bag, add 1 bag to a cup of boiling water and let it sit for 10 to 15 minutes. For dry or fresh herbs, bring 1 cup of water to a boil in a kettle and add 1 tablespoon of the dry herb or 3 tablespoons of the fresh herb to the water. Cover it with a lid, and let it sit for 10 to 15 minutes. Strain and serve.

FOMENTATION

With this method, a cloth is soaked in a prepared infusion or a decoction. The wet cloth is then applied to the affected area. This preparation is good for skin rashes or local inflammation.

GLYCERITE

This is an herbal extract in a glycerin base. Glycerin is made from soaps and oils. It preserves herbs and is great for kids. It has no toxicity and can be sweetened easily for a taste kids love.

ESSENTIAL OIL

Medicinal herbs are preformulated to be highly concentrated and the volatile oils are extracted. They can be applied topically or smelled for a therapeutic effect.

CREAM

The desired herb is blended with an emulsion of water in oil. This allows the oily mixture to blend with skin secretions and penetrate the skin for healing purposes.

SALVE

This is a mixture of herbal oils or extracts with beeswax.

LINIMENT

This is a topical herbal preparation in oil.

POULTICE

A poultice consists of plant material applied to the skin, by first mixing the herb into a paste and applying it to the affected area between two thin pieces of cloth.

STEAM

Herbs or herbal (essential) oils are added to steaming hot water. This therapy is useful for ailments of the upper respiratory tract.

SUPPOSITORIES

Herbs are inserted into the rectum (e.g., for hemorrhoids) or the vaginal opening for a local treatment. Suppositories also provide a good way to get the herb into the bloodstream.

SYRUP

Syrups can be added to sweeten decoctions and infusions.

BATHS

Herbs can also be delivered through the skin. Adding herbal preparations to a warm bath can be effective. An example is an oatmeal bath for itchy skin breakouts or rashes.

STANDARDIZED EXTRACT

This is an herbal extract that has been standardized to certain levels of active compounds. It can be important to duplicate the level of active compounds that were used in positive studies. At this time, many herbs have unknown active constituents.

Herbal Terms

The following terms are used to describe the properties and the actions of herbs. We have avoided most of these terms in this book and have instead used common terms. However, this list can be helpful when you consult other works on herbal medicine.

abortifacient   A plant that causes miscarriage or expulsion of the fetus. It is important that a pregnant woman avoid this type of plant. An example is the herb pennyroyal.

adaptogen   Helps the body adapt to stress, whether it be physical, mental, or emotional. It is often referred to as a "tonic." It supports energy levels. Many adaptogen herbs work in part by supporting adrenal gland function. Ginseng is a classic example.

alterative   An herb that helps improve general health by balancing and tonifying body functions. Alteratives boost nutritional status through improved digestion and elimination. They are sometimes referred to as "blood purifiers." Alteratives generally have a low potential for toxicity and can be used on a long-term basis. A good example is burdock root.

analgesic   Pain reliever. Also termed an anodyne (e.g., white willow).

anticatarrhal   Decreases mucus production (e.g., goldenseal, mullein).

antidepressant   Relieves feelings of depression (e.g., Saint-John's-wort).

antidote   Counteracts the effect of a poison.

anti-emetic   Prevents vomiting (e.g., ginger).

antifungal   Destroys or prevents fungal infections.

antigalactic   Reduces or stops breast milk secretion (e.g., sage).

antihelmintic   An herb that destroys parasites (e.g., garlic, wormwood, black walnut).

anti-inflammatory   Reduces inflammation in the body (e.g., licorice root, bromelain, boswellia, white willow, black cohosh).

antimicrobial   Prevents or destroys microbe (virus, bacteria, fungus, etc.) growth.

antioxidant   Prevents the damage of cells by free radicals (e.g., ginkgo, astragalus, hawthorne berry, milk thistle, thyme, wild oregano).

antiparasitic   Prevents the growth of or destroys parasites (e.g., black walnut, clove, garlic, wormwood).

antipyretic   Reduces fever (e.g., yarrow).

antiseptic   Prevents the growth of microbes on the skin (e.g., calendula, propolis).

antispasmodic   Prevents or reduces muscle spasms (e.g., black cohosh, chamomile, kava, valerian, wild yam).

antitussive   Relieves or suppresses coughing (e.g., horehound, wild cherry bark).

antitumor   Fights or suppresses tumor growth (e.g., astragalus, echinacea).

astringent   An herb that causes contraction of the tissues. It's useful in conditions such as bleeding or diarrhea (e.g., geranium, sage, witch hazel, yarrow).

bitters   Bitter-tasting herbs that stimulate the digestive organ secretions and actions—stomach, liver, gallbladder, pancreas. They can also help increase an abnormally low appetite (e.g., gentian root, burdock, goldenseal, dandelion root).

bronchodilator   An herb that causes relaxation and dilation of the bronchial tubes (respiratory passageway). They're often used in coughs, bronchitis, and asthma (e.g., peppermint, ma huang, yerba santa).

calmative   An herb that gently calms the nerves (e.g., chamomile, hops, kava, passionflower, valerian).

carminative   Prevents or reduces gas (e.g., ginger root, fennel, anise, peppermint).

cathartic   An herb that stimulates bowel evacuation (laxative) (e.g., cascara sagrada, senna, rhubarb).

cholagogue   Stimulates bile flow from the gallbladder (e.g., dandelion root).

choleretic   Stimulates bile production in the liver (e.g., milk thistle, burdock, dandelion root).

demulcent   An herb that has a soothing and healing effect on the mucous membranes of the body (e.g., slippery elm is a demulcent for the digestive tract).

diaphoretic   An herb that causes perspiration. This can be useful with a cold, to help the immune system expel the virus (e.g., yarrow, boneset).

diuretic   Promotes urination (e.g., dandelion leaf, parsley).

emetic   An herb that causes vomiting (e.g., ipecac).

expectorant   An herb that promotes the expulsion of mucus from the respiratory tract (e.g., horehound, lungwort, yerba santa).

febrifuge   An herb that reduces fever (e.g., white willow).

galactagogue   Stimulates milk flow (e.g., blessed thistle, fennel, fenugreek).

hemostatic   An herb that stops bleeding (e.g., cinnamon, yarrow).

hepatic   An herb that acts on the liver to stimulate bile flow (e.g., burdock, milk thistle, licorice, dandelion root, yellow dock, artichoke).

hypnotic   An herb that induces sleep (e.g., valerian).

hypotensive   An herb that lowers blood pressure (e.g., hawthorne berry, garlic).

immunomodulator   An herb that supports the action of the immune system (e.g., astragalus, echinacea, garlic, lomatium, Oregon grape, osha).

laxative   An herb that promotes fecal expulsion (e.g., cascara sagrada, senna, aloe, rehmania).

lymphagogue   Stimulates activity of the lymphatic system (e.g., burdock, ceanothus, pokeroot).

mucolytic   An herb that thins mucus secretions.

nervine   An herb that relaxes and calms the nerves (e.g., chamomile, passionflower, valerian, skullcap, lavender).

nutritive   An herb that is nourishing to the body (e.g., nettles).

palliative   Relieves symptoms but does not cure the disease (e.g., a child sleeps well when taking passionflower before bedtime, but cannot sleep unless he or she uses passionflower).

prophylactic   Herbs used to prevent a disease or a condition.

rubefacient   Herbs that are irritating to the skin and the mucous membranes. They're used to increase blood flow to the affected area (e.g., horseradish opens up the sinuses).

sedative   A calming herb (e.g., valerian, passionflower, chamomile).

stimulant   Increases energy or has an exciting action (e.g., ginseng).

synergist   An herb that acts to increase the effectiveness of another herb or herbs in a formula so that the sum of the herbs is greater than its parts (e.g., licorice root).

tonic   Nourishes and restores normal function (e.g., Siberian ginseng).

vermifuge   Promotes the expulsion of intestinal worms (e.g., wormwood).

vulnerary   Promotes tissue healing (e.g., calendula applied topically on cuts and scrapes or aloe for burned skin).

Storing Herbs

Most of the herbs used today come in commercial packaging. Therefore, it is easy to store them. General guidelines to remember:

- Tinctures—Store in the cupboard so that they are not exposed to light.
- Capsules and tablets—Make sure the lid is closed at all times, and do not store them in an area with high humidity.
- Teas—Bagged teas should be kept in an area that is dry and out of the light.
- Herbs bought in bulk should be stored in airtight glass containers. The temperature should be between 55 and 65 degrees F. Make sure to keep bulk teas out of the light as well.

Safety note: As with pharmaceutical medications, make sure to store herbal products out of the reach of children.

Helping Your Child with Herbs

The following information offers creative ways to administer herbs to children. Medicine doesn't have to taste bad to be good. In fact, many herbal medicines not only work better than conventional medicines but also taste better!

For example, if a tincture that has an alcohol base is used, put the desired amount of herb in a quarter cup of hot water for five minutes to let the alcohol evaporate, let it cool, and then add the tincture to water or juice. One of our favorites is to mix herbal teas with juice! Other strategies include

1. Mixing herbal capsules in foods, such as oatmeal, apple sauce, and jam.
2. Using a dropper to put the desired amount of tincture in the child's juice (dilute juice with 50 percent water). Concord grape juice hides bad-tasting herbs well.
3. For children who are stubborn, who refuse to eat or drink anything with herbs, or who will not take any medicine, there is one aggressive solution left. Use a dropper and squirt the desired amount in the side of the child's mouth. This way, the child can't spit it out. Be careful that the child does not bite the glass dropper while you use this technique.

PRECAUTIONS

As with any substance, whether it is a food, a drug, or a pollen, allergic reactions can occur with herbs. Although it is rare, you could be allergic to a single herb or an herbal formula. When using an herb or an herbal formula for the first time, take a small amount—such as 3 drops or a dab of the powder form, and see whether an adverse reaction happens in the next two hours. Chances are, there won't be a problem. If a severe allergic reaction does occur, such as wheezing, difficult breathing, or hives, seek medical attention immediately and discontinue any further use of the herb. If more mild reactions occur, such as itching or a mild rash, choose another herb that has a similar action.

Quality Herbs

We feel that it is important to use only high-quality herbs. Organically grown herbs are recommended. Consult with a naturopathic doctor or a reputable herbalist, a nutritionist, or a holistic doctor to find out which brands are of the highest quality. Many health food store and pharmacy employees will be able to help you as well.

Frequency of Use

This book provides detailed information on how to take the recommended herbs and supplements for each condition. Following are general guidelines on how frequently you should take herbal supplements.

Acute conditions: Take the recommended dosage every two to three waking hours to relieve symptoms and support the body's response. For infectious conditions, continue the herbal treatment for two days after the symptoms have resolved to prevent a relapse.

Chronic conditions: Take the recommended dosage two to three times daily.

Note: Herbs can be taken with or between meals. If you are prone to digestive upset, take the herbs with meals. If the herbs are being used to strengthen digestion, we recommend that they be taken close to mealtime.

HANDY CHART: CALCULATING DOSAGE FOR CHILDREN

Dr. Stengler's Quick Dosage Guide for Children

Here is a simplified calculation that parents can use to calculate the dosage for their children:

5 to 30 pounds: ⅕ the adult dosage

30 to 60 pounds: ¼ the adult dosage

60 to 90 pounds: ⅓ the adult dosage

90 to 120 pounds: ½ the adult dosage

120 to 150 pounds: ¾ the adult dosage

HERB CHART

Note: Common medicinal uses for children are listed. More uses may be indicated for adults.

Alfalfa (Medicago sativa)

Medicinal Use: Arthritis, indigestion, menopause, high cholesterol, ulcers, anemia, skin disorders

Parts Used: Mainly the leaves, but the seeds are used also.

Form Used: Capsules, tablets, bulk herb

Potential Side Effects: Caution for people with systemic lupus erythematosus. High doses should not be taken by people on blood-thinning medications.

Comments: It's used for detoxification, hormone balancing, and alkalinizing properties.

Aloe Vera (Aloe vera)

Medicinal Use: Externally for burns, scrapes, canker sores and general wound healing. Take internally for inflammatory bowel disease, ulcers, candida, intestinal infections, constipation, and other disorders of the digestive tract; psoriasis; diabetes; HIV

Parts Used: Leaves

Form Used: Gel, cream, salve, and aloe juice preparation taken internally

Potential Side Effects: Aloe latex form (not commonly available) should not be taken by people with inflammatory bowel disease, pregnant or nursing mothers, or children.

Comments: One of nature's top healing herbs for the skin and the digestive tract. Use food-grade juice when taking internally.

Anise (Pimpinella anisum)

Medicinal Use: Intestinal gas, colic, parasites, bronchitis, and coughs

Parts Used: Seeds

Form Used: Tea or tincture

Potential Side Effects: None known

Comments: It has a sweet taste that children like; often blended with bad-tasting herbs.

Artichoke (Cynara scolymus)

Medicinal Use: High cholesterol and triglycerides, indigestion, poor fat digestion, constipation, poor liver function

Parts Used: Leaves

Form Used: Capsule, tincture

Potential Side Effects: Too high of a dose may cause loose stools.

Comments: Avoid it if you have an obstructed bile duct.

Ashwagandha (Withania somniferum)

Medicinal Use: Stress, immune support, memory enhancement, osteoarthritis, aging, anemia, fatigue

Parts Used: Root

Form Used: Tincture, capsules

Potential Side Effects: None known

Comments: It's an excellent stress hormone balancer.

Astragalus (Astragalus membranaceus)

Medicinal Use: Supports immune system (common cold, sore throat, preventative purposes), adaptogen, fatigue, hepatitis, heart function, chronic diarrhea, chemotherapy and radiation support

Parts Used: Root

Form Used: Tincture, capsule, tea

Potential Side Effects: Do not use if you have a fever.

Comments: It can be used on a long-term basis for immune support.

Barberry (Berberis vulgaris)

Medicinal Use: Candida, intestinal infections, parasites, diarrhea, immune support, skin ailments (psoriasis, eczema)

Parts Used: Root and stem bark

Form Used: Tincture, capsule, ointment

Potential Side Effects: Avoid during pregnancy and when breastfeeding. Not to be used by infants.

Comments: It has very similar properties to goldenseal.

Basil (Ocimum basilicum)

Medicinal Use: Constipation, indigestion, diabetes, hypothyroid

Parts Used: Seeds and leaves

Form Used: Tablet, capsule, tincture

Potential Side Effects: Avoid during pregnancy and when breastfeeding. Do not supplement if you have kidney or liver disease.

Comments: It has potent antioxidant properties.

Bilberry (Vaccinium myrtillus)

Medicinal Use: Diabetes, retinopathy, macular degeneration, cataracts, diarrhea, eyestrain, glaucoma, hemorrhoids, night vision, varicose veins

Parts Used: Berries

Form Used: Tincture, capsule, tablet, tea

Potential Side Effects: None known

Comments: It's one of the best herbs for the eyes.

Bitter Melon (Momordica charantia)

Medicinal Use: Diabetes, indigestion

Parts Used: Fruit

Form Used: Tea, capsule, tablet, tincture

Potential Side Effects: Excessive amounts may cause abdominal pain and diarrhea.

Comments: It's a great herb for people with diabetes.

Black Cohosh (Cimicifuga racemosa)

Medicinal Use: Arthritis, fibromyalgia, depression, menopausal symptoms, menstrual cramps, PMS

Parts Used: Root and rhizome

Form Used: Tincture, capsule, tablet

Potential Side Effects: Do not use during pregnancy or when breastfeeding.

Comments: It's one of the best herbs for menopausal symptoms.

Bladderwrack (Fucus vesiculosus)

Medicinal Use: Hypothyroidism, constipation

Parts Used: Algae stem

Form Used: Tincture, capsule, tablet, tea

Potential Side Effects: None known, but choose a product screened for toxins and contaminants.

Comments: It supports thyroid function.

Black Walnut (Juglans nigra)

Medicinal Use: Prevent or treat infections from parasites, worms, and yeast

Parts Used: Husk

Form Used: Tincture, capsule

Potential Side Effects: Large doses can be sedating to the circulatory system; not to be used during pregnancy.

Comments: Use under the guidance of a health professional for the treatment of worms, parasites; short-term use only.

Blessed Thistle (Cnicus benedictus)

Medicinal Use: Constipation, indigestion, insufficient milk supply of breastfeeding mother

Parts Used: Tincture, capsule, tea

Form Used: Leaves, stems, flowers

Potential Side Effects: None known, but use with caution during pregnancy.

Comments: It's an excellent herb to promote milk production for breastfeeding mothers.

Blue Cohosh (Caulophyllum thalictroides)

Medicinal Use: Amenorrhea, dysmenorrhea, labor pains

Parts Used: Root and flower

Form Used: Tincture, capsule

Potential Side Effects: Too high of amounts may cause headaches, nausea, high blood pressure. Only use during pregnancy under the guidance of a doctor.

Comments: It's a hormone balancer that is best used under the care of a knowledge-able practitioner.

Boswellia (Boswellia serrata)

Medicinal Use: Arthritis, sports injuries, ulcerative colitis, asthma, bursitis

Parts Used: Resin of the tree branch

Form Used: Capsule, tablet

Potential Side Effects: Very safe

Comments: It's a tremendous natural anti-inflammatory.

Bromelain

Medicinal Use: Arthritis, burns, cancer, cardiovascular disease, protein digestion, injuries, respiratory mucus, surgery recovery, thrombophlebitis, varicose veins, sinusitis, and prostatitis

Parts Used: Stem of pineapple

Form Used: Capsules, tablet

Potential Side Effects: Avoid combining with pharmaceutical blood thinners.

Comments: It's a natural anti-inflammatory when taken between meals and aids protein digestion when taken with meals.

Bugleweed (Lycopus virginicus)

Medicinal Use: Hyperthyroidism

Parts Used: Leaves and flowers

Form Used: Tincture, capsule

Potential Side Effects: Avoid if you have hypothyroidism. Do not use if you are pregnant or nursing.

Comments: It's one of the most effective supplements for cases of hyperthyroidism.

Burdock (Arctium lappa)

Medicinal Use: Skin conditions such as rashes and acne, to improve liver function, detoxification, antimicrobial

Parts Used: Root

Form Used: Tincture, capsule

Potential Side Effects: None known

Comments: It's a good general detoxifier, especially for skin conditions.

Butcher's Broom (Ruscus aculeatus)

Medicinal Use: Hemorrhoids, varicose veins

Parts Used: Roots and stems

Form Used: Tincture, tablet, capsule

Potential Side Effects: Nausea in rare cases

Comments: It's excellent for hemorrhoids and varicose veins.

Calendula (Calendula officinalis)

Medicinal Use: Cuts, scrapes, rashes, burns, antiseptic

Parts Used: Flowers

Form Used: Tincture (applied topically), creams, salves

Potential Side Effects: None

Comments: It's an excellent herb to promote healing and prevent infection of the skin.

Cascara (Rhamnus purshiana)

Medicinal Use: Laxative

Parts Used: Bark

Form Used: Tincture, capsule

Potential Side Effects: For short-term use only; long-term use can lead to electrolyte loss.

Comments: It's best used under the guidance of a health-care professional, if taken long term.

Catnip (Nepeta cataria)

Medicinal Use: Colic, fevers, restlessness, and digestive aid

Parts Used: Leaves and flowers

Form Used: Tea, tincture

Potential Side Effects: None

Comments: Only a few drops are needed for colic and restlessness for infants and children.

Cayenne (Capsicum frutescens)

Medicinal Use: Improves circulation, antiseptic, stimulates sweating in the first stages of colds, heals sore throats, and relieves pain

Parts Used: Fruit

Form Used: Tincture, capsule, and topical ointment

Potential Side Effects: Digestive upset

Comments: The topical ointment is used as a pain reliever. It's a powerful cardio-vascular tonic.

Chamomile (Matricaria recutita)

Medicinal Use: Indigestion, nervousness, colic, eczema, gingivitis, diarrhea, insomnia, anxiety, ulcers, and inflammatory bowel disease

Parts Used: Flowers

Form Used: Tea, tincture, capsule

Potential Side Effects: Rare allergic reaction

Comments: It's helpful for a wide variety of digestive ailments.

Cinnamon (Cinnamomum zeylanicum)

Medicinal Use: Colds, diarrhea, digestive upset, bleeding, heavy menstruation

Parts Used: Inner bark

Form Used: Tincture, tea, as a food

Potential Side Effects: None in normal dosages

Comments: It's a warming herb that improves circulation.

Clove (Syzgium aromaticum)

Medicinal Use: Topical anesthetic for teething

Parts Used: Flower buds

Form Used: Essential oil

Potential Side Effects: Too high a dosage can be irritating to the mucosa

Comments: Apply 1 to 2 drops of clove essential oil to gums during teething to reduce pain.

Comfrey (Symphytum officinalis)

Medicinal Use: Externally for sprains, burns, wounds, fractures

Parts Used: Root

Form Used: Poultice

Potential Side Effects: Not to be taken internally, due to toxic alkaloids

Comments: It speeds healing of wounds and skin conditions.

Cornsilk (Zea mays)

Medicinal Use: Bedwetting, urinary tract infections

Parts Used: Golden silk of corn

Form Used: Tea or tincture

Potential Side Effects: None

Comments: It's used as a tonic for the urinary tract.

Corydalis (Corydalis turtschaninovii, Corydalis yanhusuo)

Medicinal Use: Pain, insomnia, dysmenorrhea

Parts Used: Rhizome

Form Used: Tincture, capsule

Potential Side Effects: Vertigo, nausea, and fatigue; should be avoided by pregnant and nursing women

Comments: It's an excellent natural pain reliever.

Cranberry (Vaccinium macrocarpon)

Medicinal Use: Prevention and treatment of urinary tract infections

Parts Used: Ripe fruit

Form Used: Unsweetened juice or capsule

Potential Side Effects: None

Comments: It has potent antioxidant properties.

Damiana (Turnera diffusa)

Medicinal Use: Low libido, erectile dysfunction, depression

Parts Used: Leaves

Form Used: Tea, tincture, capsule, tablet

Potential Side Effects: Higher amounts may cause loose stools. Avoid during pregnancy.

Comments: Historically, it was used as an aphrodisiac for both men and women.

Dandelion (Taraxacum officinale)

Medicinal Use: Stimulates gallbladder and liver function; stimulates general digestion; leaf has a diuretic effect for edema; constipation; chronic skin problems.

Parts Used: Root and leaf

Form Used: Tea, tincture, capsule, tablet

Potential Side Effects: Diarrhea; do not use if gallstones are present.

Comments: It's an excellent liver tonic.

Devil's Claw (Harpagophytum procumbens)

Medicinal Use: Arthritis, lower back pain, indigestion

Parts Used: Root

Form Used: Tincture, tablet, capsule

Potential Side Effects: Avoid if you have an ulcer or gallstones.

Comments: It's an effective natural anti-inflammatory.

Dong Quai (Angelica sinensis)

Medicinal Use: Anemia, dysmenorrhea, irregular menses, PMS, menopause

Parts Used: Root

Form Used: Tincture, capsule tablet, tea

Potential Side Effects: Sun sensitivity. Avoid if you are pregnant or nursing.

Comments: It's used for many female conditions.

Echinacea (Echinacea purpurea or angustifolia)

Medicinal Use: Immune system enhancement, antiviral, antibacterial, antifungal

Parts Used: Roots and flowers

Form Used: Tincture, tea, capsule, tablet

Potential Side Effects: Caution for people who are allergic to the daisy family. Do not use on a long-term basis if you have an autoimmune condition.

Comments: It's effective for colds, flu's, sore throats, and respiratory tract infections; Nature's antibiotic.

Elderberry or Elder Flowers (Sambucus nigra)

Medicinal Use: Colds, flu's, coughs, and sinusitis

A study conducted by the Hospital for Sick Children in Toronto, in conjunction with the Canadian College of Naturopathic Medicine, looked at the safety of echinacea during pregnancy. In the study, 206 women who used echinacea during pregnancy for upper respiratory tract infections were analyzed, along with a control group of 198 pregnant women who had upper respiratory tract infections but never used echinacea. The researchers found no association between the use of echinacea and birth defects. There were also no differences in the rates of live births or spontaneous abortions between the two groups.

Another concern parents have is whether echinacea will affect fertility. This question is asked because of a 1999 press release about the topic. A study suggested that common herbal supplements, such as Saint-John's-wort, ginkgo, and echinacea, might adversely affect fertility. Researchers took hamster eggs, removed the outer coating, and exposed the eggs to the herbs. They then mixed in human sperm, which will usually penetrate the egg. At higher dosages, the herbs either impaired or prevented the sperms' ability to penetrate the eggs. High concentrations of *Echinacea purpurea* interfered with sperm enzymes.

Based on this, some researchers have prematurely concluded that echinacea may interfere with fertility. Is this a valid conclusion? No. There are several problems. In the body, any herb is first broken down by the digestive system. In this study, the researchers used the whole herb in relatively high concentrations, which would never contact sperm in real life. Also, the experiment was done in a laboratory petri dish. To be valid, human studies would have to be done. We have no problem recommending echinacea for short-term use in pregnancy or as needed for infections in people trying to conceive.

Parts Used: Berries, flowers

Form Used: Tincture, tea

Potential Side Effects: None

Comments: It's one of the best herbal medicines for the flu.

Elecampagne (Inula helenium)

Medicinal Use: Respiratory tract infections, digestive support

Parts Used: Root

Form Used: Tea, tincture

Potential Side Effects: None in normal doses; high doses can cause vomiting and digestive upset.

Comments: Use it as a lung tonic.

Ephedra or Ma Huang (Ephedra sinica)

Medicinal Use: Cough, asthma, hay fever, sinusitis

Parts Used: Stem

Form Used: Capsule, tea, tablet

Potential Side Effects: Hypertension, insomnia, heart arrhythmias or palpitations, dry mouth

Comments: Avoid during pregnancy or when breastfeeding. Best used under the guidance of a holistic doctor and never for long periods. Not available over the counter since 2004.

Eyebright (Euphrasia officinalis)

Medicinal Use: Conjunctivitis, pink eye, allergies affecting the eyes, sinus and nasal congestion, cough

Parts Used: Whole herb

Form Used: Tincture, capsule

Potential Side Effects: None

Comments: It can be used as an eyewash or taken internally.

Fennel (Foeniculum vulgare)

Medicinal Use: Reduces intestinal gas, colic, respiratory tract infections; increases nursing mother's breast milk supply

Parts Used: Seed

Form Used: Tincture, tea, capsule

Potential Side Effects: None in normal doses

Comments: It's an excellent digestive tonic; sweet tasting.

Fenugreek (Trigonella foenumgraecum)

Medicinal Use: Digestive tract inflammation, colic, blood sugar imbalances, high cholesterol, constipation

Parts Used: Seed

Form Used: Tincture, tea

Potential Side Effects: None

Comments: It's one of the better herbs for diabetes.

Feverfew (Tanacetum parthenium)

Medicinal Use: Migraine headaches, arthritis

Parts Used: Leaves

Form Used: Capsule, tincture

Potential Side Effects: Not recommended for children under two years of age or for pregnant and nursing women.

Comments: It's an excellent remedy for the prevention of migraine headaches.

Flaxseeds (Linum usitatissimum)

Medicinal Use: Inflammatory skin conditions, dry skin, constipation, arthritis

Parts Used: Seeds

Form Used: Ground-up seeds (powder) or oil

Potential Side Effects: Too much can cause diarrhea.

Comments: Excellent for chronic skin conditions, as it supplies essential fatty acids.

Garlic (Allium sativa)

Medicinal Use: Immune system support—antiviral, antibacterial, antifungal; ear infections; high cholesterol

Parts Used: Cloves

Form Used: Fresh cloves, tincture, capsule, tablet

Potential Side Effects: Digestive upset

Comments: It's commonly used as eardrops for ear infections; excellent for elevated cholesterol levels; anticancer.

Gentian (Gentian lutea)

Medicinal Use: Digestive stimulation, poor appetite

Parts Used: Root

Form Used: Tincture, capsule

Potential Side Effects: Can aggravate preexisting heartburn, gastritis, or ulcers.

Comments: It's useful for malabsorption and low appetite after an illness.

Ginger (Zingiber officinalis)

Medicinal Use: Reduces intestinal gas; sore throats; colds; anti-inflammatory; stimulates digestion

Parts Used: Root

Form Used: Tea, tincture, capsule

Potential Side Effects: None in normal doses

Comments: It's one of the best herbs for intestinal gas; a warming herb.

Ginkgo (Ginkgo biloba)

Medicinal Use: Poor memory, attention deficit disorder, improves circulation (Raynaud's disease), intermittent claudication, depression, high blood pressure, impotence, PMS, radiation toxicity, tinnitus, stroke recovery/prevention, macular degeneration, cataracts, retinopathy, vertigo, Ménière's disease, migraine headaches

Parts Used: Leaf

Form Used: Tincture, capsule

Potential Side Effects: Headache, digestive upset, blood thinning

Comments: It's one of the best herbs to improve circulation.

Ginseng: American ginseng (Panax quinquefolius), ***Siberian Ginseng*** (Eleutherococcus senticosus), ***and Chinese ginseng*** (Panax ginseng)

Medicinal Use: Counteract stress—physical, mental, and emotional; immune system support; fatigue. American ginseng is used for asthma.

Parts Used: Root

Form Used: Tincture, capsule, tea

Potential Side Effects: Chinese ginseng can cause overstimulation.

Comments: American ginseng is cooling, Siberian ginseng is cooling, and Chinese ginseng is warming.

Goldenseal (Hydrastis canadensis)

Medicinal Use: Colds, sore throats, flu, ear infections, digestive tract infections, fungal infections, sinusitis, diarrhea, urinary tract infections, parasites, vaginitis

Parts Used: Root

Form Used: Tincture, capsule

Potential Side Effects: Digestive upset. Avoid if you are pregnant or nursing. Not to be used on a long-term basis.

Comments: It's very bitter; one of the best herbs to use for infections of the mucous membranes.

Gotu Kola (Centella asiatica)

Medicinal Use: Poor memory, connective tissue healing, varicose veins, burns, sarcoidosis

Parts Used: Roots and leaves

Form Used: Tincture, capsule

Potential Side Effects: None known

Comments: It decreases scar tissue formation after an injury.

Green Tea (Camellia sinensis)

Medicinal Use: Cancer prevention, cardiovascular disease prevention, detoxification, digestive health, tooth decay prevention, weight loss

Parts Used: Leaves

Form Used: Tea, capsule, tablet, tincture

Potential Side Effects: Insomnia, anxiety

Comments: It contains some of the most potent antioxidants known.

Guggul (Commiphora mukul)

Medicinal Use: Atherosclerosis, elevated triglycerides and cholesterol, hypothyroidism

Parts Used: Resin from plant stem

Form Used: Capsule, tablet

Potential Side Effects: Digestive upset; pregnant or breastfeeding women should not use it.

Comments: It's an effective and popular natural remedy for high cholesterol levels.

Gymnema (Gymnema sylvestre)

Medicinal Use: Diabetes, insulin resistance

Parts Used: Leaves

Form Used: Tincture, tablet, capsule

Potential Side Effects: None known, but should be avoided during pregnancy or breastfeeding.

Comments: It's an excellent natural remedy for both types of diabetes.

Hawthorne (Crataegus oxycantha)

Medicinal Use: Heart conditions (congestive heart failure, angina, cardiomyopathy, arrhythmia), hypertension

Parts Used: Berry

Form Used: Tincture, capsule, tea

Potential Side Effects: Seek medical consultation when combining it with heart medications.

Comments: It's an excellent heart tonic.

Hops (Humulus lupulus)

Medicinal Use: Stomach ache due to anxiety, restlessness, insomnia, colic, insomnia

Parts Used: Fruiting bodies (strobile)

Form Used: Tincture, tea, capsule

Potential Side Effects: None known

Comments: It gently calms the nerves.

Horehound (Marrubium vulgaris)

Medicinal Use: Bronchitis, asthma, coughs

Parts Used: Flowering herb

Form Used: Tincture

Potential Side Effects: None known

Comments: It helps discharge mucus from the respiratory tract.

Horse Chestnut (Aesculus hippocastanum)

Medicinal Use: Back pain, hemorrhoids, varicose veins

Parts Used: Seeds

Form Used: Capsule, tablet, tincture

Potential Side Effects: Rare cases of digestive upset, headaches, and skin itching.

Comments: It's an excellent remedy for varicose veins and hemorrhoids.

Horsetail (Equisetum arvense)

Medicinal Use: Urinary tract infections

Parts Used: Stems

Form Used: Tincture, tea, capsule

Potential Side Effects: None

Comments: Good source of silica.

Huperzia (Qian ceng ta, Huperzine A)

Medicinal Use: Memory (Alzheimer's disease, age-related cognitive decline)

Parts Used: Moss

Form Used: Capsule, tablet, tincture

Potential Side Effects: No known side effects. Use under a doctor's guidance if you are taking a medication that affects acetylcholine metabolism.

Comments: It's a specific herbal remedy for poor memory.

Kava (Piper methysticum)

Medicinal Use: Anxiety, insomnia, hyperactivity, muscle spasms

Parts Used: Root

Form Used: Tincture, capsule, tea

Potential Side Effects: Skin rash rarely occurs. Avoid if you have liver disease or when consuming alcohol. Do not use while nursing or breastfeeding. Do not use if you are taking antianxiety or antidepressant pharmaceutical medications.

Comments: It's an excellent remedy for anxiety.

Lavender (Lavendula angustifolia)

Medicinal Use: Stress, anxiety, headache, muscle spasms, insomnia, indigestion

Parts Used: Flowers

Form Used: Tea, tincture, essential oil

Potential Side Effects: Best used externally

Comments: It's calming to the nervous system and the mind.

Lemon Balm (Melissa officinalis)

Medicinal Use: Respiratory tract infections, fevers, depression, antiviral, cold sores, genital herpes, hyperthyroidism (Graves' disease)

Parts Used: Whole herb

Form Used: Tincture, salve

Potential Side Effects: Not to be used if you have hypothyroidism or glaucoma.

Comments: It's a gentle calming herb.

Licorice (Glycyrrhiza glabra)

Medicinal Use: Immune system support, antiviral, coughs, sore throats, digestive tract inflammation, heartburn, adrenal gland support, liver support, antispasmodic, anti-inflammatory, asthma, chronic fatigue syndrome, ulcers, reflux, hepatitis, shingles

Parts Used: Root

Form Used: Tincture, tea, capsule, cream

Potential Side Effects: Large amounts can lead to water retention and thus increase blood pressure, so avoid if you have high blood pressure. Avoid during pregnancy.

Comments: It's sweet tasting. It reduces toxicity and increases the effectiveness of other herbs. Use as a topical gel for cold sores.

Lomatium (Lomatium dissectum)

Medicinal Use: Immune system support, antiviral, antibacterial, colds, urinary tract infections

Parts Used: Root

Form Used: Tincture, capsule

Potential Side Effects: Skin rash in a small percentage of users. Do not use during pregnancy.

Comments: It's an excellent antiviral herb for colds and flu's.

Maitake (Grifola frondosa)

Medicinal Use: General immune support, antiviral, antitumor, HIV, diabetes, high cholesterol, cancer, hepatitis

Parts Used: Fruiting body

Form Used: Tincture, capsule

Potential Side Effects: None known

Comments: It provides long-term immune support.

Marshmallow (Althea officinalis)

Medicinal Use: Urinary tract infections, respiratory infections, diarrhea, asthma, cough, ulcer, and inflammatory bowel disease

Parts Used: Root

Form Used: Tincture, capsule, tablet, tea

Potential Side Effects: None

Comments: It's a soothing herb for the mucous membranes of the body.

Milk Thistle (Silybum marianum)

Medicinal Use: Liver congestion and cirrhosis, hepatitis, gallstones, alcohol and drug addiction recovery, constipation, PMS, indigestion, skin conditions (acne, eczema)

Parts Used: Seed

Form Used: Tincture, capsule, tablet

Potential Side Effects: None known

Comments: It's the best-studied herb for hepatitis; protects and regenerates liver cells.

Motherwort (Leonurus cardiaca)

Medicinal Use: Amenorrhea, menopause, heart palpitations, anxiety

Parts Used: Leaves and flowers

Form Used: Tincture, capsule, tablet, tea

Potential Side Effects: Avoid during pregnancy.

Comments: It's used during menopause to reduce heart palpitations and anxiety.

Mullein (Verbascum thapsus)

Medicinal Use: Coughs and bronchitis, upper respiratory tract infections, externally for ear infections, asthma, chronic obstructive pulmonary disease

Parts Used: Flowers, leaves

Form Used: Tincture, capsule, oil for ear infections (topical), tea

Potential Side Effects: None known

Comments: It's a soothing herb for the respiratory tract.

Myrrh (Commiphora myrrha)

Medicinal Use: Sore throats, urinary tract infections, gingivitis, mouth sores, parasites

---

Interesting herbal facts:

- The Latin name for goldenseal, *Hydrastis canadensis,* means "a Canadian plant that accomplishes water." This refers to goldenseal's beneficial effect on the flow of mucus.

- Passionflower—The name "passionflower" is believed to come from its beautiful flowers, which are thought to represent the Passion of Christ, the story of the Crucifixion. The flowers look like a cross.

- An old-time remedy for sleeplessness in children is to stuff the pillow with hops before bedtime.

- Studies have shown that ginger is one of the most effective treatments for nausea and vomiting after surgery.

- Ginkgo biloba is the world's oldest living tree species. Fossil records date back more than 200 million years. The tree can live as long as 1,000 years. Medicinal use of ginkgo dates back to its use in Chinese herbal medicine 3,500 years ago.

- Garlic not only reduces "bad cholesterol" while increasing "good cholesterol," but regular use is also associated with a lower risk of stomach and colon cancer.

- Cranberry prevents bladder infections by stopping *E. coli* (the most common bacteria involved in bladder infections) from adhering to the bladder wall.

- Chamomile is a very popular medicine in Germany. In 1987, it was named "plant of the year." They, of course, use German chamomile, not Roman chamomile.

- According to Rudolph Weiss, M.D., the bitter taste of gentian root persists even in a dilution of 1:20,000! Gentian can help increase the appetite in people who are weak and have lost their desire for food. It does not increase food cravings in people with a normal healthy appetite.

- Horehound has been used as an herbal cough expectorant for over 2,000 years.

- Hawthorn berry improves the contractions of the heart muscle and improves blood flow through the coronary arteries.

- Milk thistle has been shown to help protect and regenerate liver cells.

Parts Used: Resin from the stems of the plant

Form Used: Tincture

Potential Side Effects: Large doses taken internally may cause kidney irritation and diarrhea.

Comments: It's commonly used for infections of the throat and the mouth.

Nettles (Urtica dioica)

Medicinal Use: Anemia, detoxification, rashes, arthritis, prostate enlargement, hay fever, brittle hair, edema

Parts Used: Leaves and root

Form Used: Tincture, capsule, salves, tea

Potential Side Effects: None known

Comments: Very nutritive, very high in minerals. The root is used for the prostate and the leaves used for all other conditions.

Oatstraw (Avena sativa)

Medicinal Use: Stress, depression, restlessness, fatigue, itchy skin

Parts Used: Seeds

Form Used: Tincture, capsule, seeds

Potential Side Effects: None

Comments: An oatmeal bath is used for itchy skin.

Oregano (Origanum vulgare)

Medicinal Use: Candidiasis, most infections

Parts Used: Leaves and dried herb

Form Used: Tincture, capsule

Potential Side Effects: Do not use during pregnancy.

Comments: It's a powerful antifungal herb.

Oregon Grape (Mahonia aquefolium)

Medicinal Use: Respiratory tract and urinary tract infections, diarrhea, psoriasis, parasites

Parts Used: Root and stem bark

Form Used: Tincture, capsule

Potential Side Effects: Avoid during pregnancy.

Comments: It's often used as an alternative to goldenseal for infections of mucous membranes.

Passionflower (Passiflora incarnata)

Medicinal Use: Insomnia, anxiety and restlessness, heart palpitations

Parts Used: Flower

Form Used: Tincture, capsule, tea

Potential Side Effects: None known

Comments: It's a gentle nerve relaxer.

Pau D'Arco (Tabebuia aellanedae, Tabebuia impestiginosa)

Medicinal Use: Candida, infections, parasites, prostatitis, cancer

Parts Used: Bark

Form Used: Tea, capsule

Potential Side Effects: Large amounts may cause nausea, bleeding, and digestive upset. Avoid during pregnancy and breastfeeding.

Comments: It's commonly used for candida overgrowth; anticancer.

Peppermint (Mentha piperita)

Medicinal Use: Colic, indigestion, nausea, fevers, irritable bowel syndrome, headaches, gallstones

Parts Used: Leaf

Form Used: Tea, tincture, oil

Potential Side Effects: Heartburn in some individuals

Comments: It provides acute relief from digestive complaints.

Plantain (Plantain spp.)

Medicinal Use: Antiseptic, anti-inflammatory, urinary and respiratory tract infections, topically for wounds and bites

Parts Used: Leaf

Form Used: Tea, tincture

Potential Side Effects: None known

Comments: It works well topically for insect bites.

Pygeum (Pygeum africanum)

Medicinal Use: Prostate enlargement, prostatitis

Parts Used: Bark

Form Used: Capsule, tablet, tincture

Potential Side Effects: Mild digestive upset

Comments: It's a specific herb for prostate enlargement; works well combined with saw palmetto.

Red Raspberry (Rubus idaeus)

Medicinal Use: Diarrhea, nausea, vomiting, sore throat, pregnancy support

Parts Used: Leaf and berry

Form Used: Tincture, tea, food

Potential Side Effects: None known

Comments: Historically, it has been used by herbalists and naturopathic doctors as a uterine tonic before or during pregnancy.

Reishi (Ganoderma lucidum)

Medicinal Use: Allergies, bronchitis, tumors, HIV, viral infections, immune support during chemotherapy and radiation treatments, hypertension, poor memory, liver detoxification, hepatitis

Parts Used: Fruiting body

Form Used: Tincture or as a food

Potential Side Effects: None that are common; use caution during pregnancy

Comments: It's used for long-term immune support.

Rosemary (Rosemary officinalis)

Medicinal Use: Soothes nervous system, antioxidant, memory, lice, candida, hypothyroidism

Parts Used: Leaf

Form Used: Tea, tincture

Potential Side Effects: Avoid during pregnancy.

Comments: It's generally used in a condition-specific combination herbal formula.

Sage (Salvia officinalis)

Medicinal Use: Antimicrobial, reduces secretions, intestinal gas, hot flashes, sore throats, gingivitis, dries up breast milk

Parts Used: Leaves

Form Used: Tea, tincture

Potential Side Effects: Very high amounts may cause neurological symptoms. Best used short term (less than 2 weeks).

Comments: This herb has a drying quality.

Sarsaparilla (Smilax spp.)

Medicinal Use: Eczema, acne, psoriasis

Parts Used: Root

Form Used: Tincture, capsule

Potential Side Effects: Stomach upset. Do not take during pregnancy or breastfeeding.

Comments: It's used to clear up skin conditions.

Saw Palmetto (Serenoa repens, Sabal serrulata)

Medicinal Use: Acne, baldness, prostate enlargement, bladder infection prevention (men), polycystic ovarian syndrome, prostatitis

Parts Used: Berries

Form Used: Tincture, capsule, tablet

Potential Side Effects: Rare digestive upset

Comments: It's the most well-researched herb for the prostate.

Senna (Cassia senna)

Medicinal Use: Constipation

Parts Used: Leaves and pods

Form Used: Tincture, capsule, tea, tablet

Potential Side Effects: Chronic use may cause bowel sluggishness; diarrhea.

Comments: It's best used short term.

Shitake (Lentinus edodes)

Medicinal Use: General immune system support, HIV, hepatitis, cancer, bronchitis

Parts Used: Fruiting body

Form Used: Tincture or food

Potential Side Effects: Rare digestive upset

Comments: It provides long-term immune support.

Skullcap (Scutellaria lateriflora)

Medicinal Use: Nervousness, insomnia, anxiety, hyperactivity, poor digestion

Parts Used: Aerial part (above ground)

Form Used: Tincture, capsule, tea

Potential Side Effects: None

Comments: It's one of the best herbs to use for insomnia.

Slippery Elm (Ulmus fulva)

Medicinal Use: Soothes mucous membranes of respiratory tract, digestive tract, and urinary tract; bronchitis; colitis; ulcers; heartburn; gastritis; sore throats; and urinary tract infections

Parts Used: Inner bark

Form Used: Tincture, capsule, tea, and lozenge

Potential Side Effects: None known

Comments: It's a soothing herb for the mucous membranes.

Soy (Glycine max)

Medicinal Use: Cancer prevention, high cholesterol, menopausal symptoms, osteoporosis, PMS

Parts Used: Bean

Form Used: Capsule, tablet, powder

Potential Side Effects: Digestive upset. Do not use isoflavone extracts if you have cancer, unless instructed to do so by your doctor. Use with caution if you have hypothyroidism.

Comments: It's a great estrogen balancer.

Spirulina (Spirulina)

Medicinal Use: Anemia, cancer, high cholesterol, detoxification, immune support, radiation poisoning

Parts Used: Algae

Form Used: Capsule, tablet, powder

Potential Side Effects: None known

Comments: It's an excellent detoxifier and full of minerals.

Saint-John's-wort (Hypericum perforatum)

Medicinal Use: Anxiety; depression; viral infections; topically for burns, scrapes, nerve pain, bruises; seasonal affective disorder

Parts Used: Flowers, whole herb

Form Used: Tincture, capsule, oil

Potential Side Effects: Small percentage of users develops sensitivity to light. Should not be combined with pharmaceutical antidepressants.

Comments: It's a great herb for mild to moderate depression.

Stevia (Stevia rebaudiana)

Medicinal Use: Natural sweetener

Parts Used: Leaf

Form Used: Tincture, powder, crystals

Potential Side Effects: None known

Comments: It's a safe natural sweetener.

Tea tree (Melaleuca alternifolia)

Medicinal Use: Topically for skin fungus, burns, and acne, cold sores, mouth and gum infections, skin infections, vaginitis, warts

Parts Used: Leaves

Form Used: Tincture, oil

Potential Side Effects: Too high of a concentration to the skin can be irritating. Use cautiously on the face. Do not ingest internally (except for mouthwashes), unless under the guidance of a doctor.

Comments: It's excellent for athlete's foot.

Thuja (Thuja occidentalis)

Medicinal Use: Externally for warts

Parts Used: Branches, leaves, bark

Form Used: Oil, tincture

Potential Side Effects: Not to be taken internally by children

Comments: It's an excellent topical treatment for warts.

Thyme (Thyme vulgaris)

Medicinal Use: Respiratory tract infections (bronchitis) and urinary tract infections, topically for skin fungus, bad breath

Parts Used: Leaves and flowers

Form Used: Tincture, capsule, tea

Potential Side Effects: Too much of the essential oil can cause abdominal pain.

Comments: It's mainly used in respiratory tract infection formulas.

Turmeric (Curcuma longa)

Medicinal Use: Anti-inflammatory, antitumor, arthritis, indigestion

Parts Used: Rhizome (the part of the plant that's above ground)

Form Used: Tincture, capsule

Potential Side Effects: Do not take high amounts during pregnancy. Use with caution if you have gallstones.

Comments: It's one of the best anti-inflammatory herbs.

Usnea (Usnea barbata)

Medicinal Use: Cough, cold, infection

Parts Used: Entire lichen

Form Used: Tincture, capsule

Potential Side Effects: Use with caution during pregnancy and breastfeeding.

Comments: It helps clear up respiratory tract infections.

Uva ursi (Arctostaphylos uva ursi)

Medicinal Use: Urinary tract infections

Parts Used: Leaves

Form Used: Tincture, capsule

Potential Side Effects: None in normal doses, but higher doses may cause cramping, nausea, or vomiting.

Comments: It's one of the best herbs for urinary tract infections.

Valerian (Valeriana officinalis)

Medicinal Use: Insomnia, restlessness, spasms, pain

Parts Used: Root

Form Used: Tincture, capsule

Potential Side Effects: A small percentage of users feel drowsy in the morning if it's used as a sleep aid.

Comments: It's one of the stronger nerve-relaxing herbs.

Vitex (Vitex agnus-castus)

Medicinal Use: Acne, amenorrhea, fibrocystic breast syndrome, infertility, irregular menses, dysmenorrhea, improved lactation, hot flashes, ovarian cysts, PMS, uterine fibroids

Parts Used: Dried fruit

Form Used: Tincture, capsule, tea, tablet

Potential Side Effects: Occasional digestive upset, headaches, skin rash. Do not use if you are taking the birth control pill. Avoid during pregnancy unless specifically prescribed by a practitioner.

Comments: It's the most versatile female hormone–balancing herb.

Wild Cherry (Prunus serotina)

Medicinal Use: Cough, bronchitis

Parts Used: Bark

Form Used: Tincture

Potential Side Effects: None known

Comments: Not to be used in large amounts or for prolonged periods of time.

Willow (Salix alba and spp.)

Medicinal Use: Headaches, pain, fever, arthritis

Parts Used: Bark

Form Used: Tincture, capsule, tea

Potential Side Effects: Do not use if you are on blood-thinning medications or have hemophilia, as it thins the blood. Not to be used during viral infections.

Comments: It's a natural alternative to aspirin.

Witch Hazel (Hammamelis virginiana)

Medicinal Use: Gingivitis, eczema (topically), inflamed veins, cold sores, eczema, wound healing

Parts Used: Bark

Form Used: Tincture

Potential Side Effects: Internal use may cause stomach cramping.

Comments: It's excellent when used topically for hemorrhoids and varicose veins.

Wormwood (Artemisia absinthium)

Medicinal Use: Parasites, indigestion

Parts Used: Leaves, flowers, oil

Form Used: Tincture, capsule, tea

Potential Side Effects: High amounts used over long periods of time may cause digestive upset, diarrhea, and tremors. Do not use during pregnancy or when breastfeeding.

Comments: It's excellent for parasites and digestive tract infections.

Yarrow (Achillea millefolium)

Medicinal Use: Fevers, toothaches, digestive upset, improves circulation, cold, inflammatory bowel disease

Parts Used: Flowers, leaves

Form Used: Tincture, tea

Potential Side Effects: External application may result in a rash. Do not use during pregnancy or breastfeeding.

Comments: It's mainly used for feverish conditions.

Yellow Dock (Rumex crispus)

Medicinal Use: Sore throat, iron deficiency anemia, liver tonic, poor digestion

Parts Used: Root

Form Used: Tincture, capsule

Potential Side Effects: None

Comments: It's great for iron-deficiency anemia; contains small amount of iron and enhances the absorption of iron.

Yerba Santa (Eriodictyon californicum)

Medicinal Use: Bronchitis, laryngitis

Parts Used: Leaves

Form Used: Tincture, tea

Potential Side Effects: None

Comments: It helps to expel respiratory mucus.

References: Herbal Medicine

Gallo, M., et al. 1999. Pregnancy outcome following gestational exposure to echinacea, a prospective controlled study. The Motherisk Program, Division of Clinical Pharmacology, Hospital for Sick Children and the University of Toronto, Canadian College of Naturopathic Medicine.

Ondrizek, R. R., et al. 1999. Inhibition of human sperm motility by specific herbs used in alternative medicine. *Journal of Assisted Reproduction and Genetics* 16(2): 87–91.

Homeopathy

What Is Homeopathy?

Homeopathy is one of the fastest-growing alternative forms of medicine in North America. This form of medicine uses ultra-diluted amounts of plant, mineral, and animal substances to stimulate the healing systems of the body. Homeopathy is effective for a wide range of conditions and is available in health food stores, pharmacies, and shopping centers. Homeopathy can be used to strengthen the defense systems of the body and to stimulate healing of mental or emotional imbalances. Homeopathic remedies are an excellent therapy to stimulate or help repair a damaged immune system. Since homeopathic medicines are ultra-diluted, they are extremely safe for children. (No side effects or toxicity!)

Homeopathic researchers are finding that each homeopathic remedy has its own "fingerprint" on the electromagnetic spectrum. It appears that homeopathic remedies work on a vibrational/energetic level. Unlike most pharmaceutical or natural medicines, homeopathic remedies appear to work directly at the electromagnetic level. In some ways, each remedy has a different electromagnetic frequency and thus action, similar to the various actions of different acupuncture points.

History of Homeopathy

"Like cures like."

—SAMUEL HAHNEMANN

Few therapies owe as much to one man as does homeopathy. While many people have gone on to study and practice homeopathy, virtually everyone in the field bows to an influential eighteenth-century physician named Samuel Hahnemann.

Born in Germany and raised to practice medicine, Hahnemann was an enigmatic, easily angered man—and an entirely original thinker. At a time when bloodletting was still a commonly exercised and often fatal "cure," Hahnemann railed against the medieval quality of Western medicine, which often hurt or killed patients instead of healing them.

Disgusted by the harmful effects of the practice, Hahnemann quit medicine. But later, he hit upon a unique—and now widely practiced—therapy. His healing methods grew out of a heated public dispute with a Scottish herbalist over the medicinal powers of Peruvian bark, known as cinchona, which we now know contains quinine.

Today homeopathy is widely practiced in Europe and the United Kingdom and is rapidly gaining popularity in North America.

Spanish conquerors had brought cinchona back to Europe after discovering that it could be used to cure malaria, which was then ravaging much of the continent. According to an oft-told story, the Scottish professor William Cullen attributed cinchona bark's powers to its bitter taste. Cullen theorized that the bitterness acted as a tonic to the body and reduced malaria's often-fatal fever—a key symptom. Cullen's ideas fit neatly into medical thought at that time, when researchers looked for ways to eliminate the symptoms of a disease as a method for treating the illness itself.

Hahnemann decided to test the theory, using his own body as a guinea pig. While completely healthy, he started taking doses of cinchona, carefully keeping notes as his body began to experience many of the same symptoms as a malaria patient.

"My feet, finger ends, etc., at first became cold; I grew languid and drowsy; then my heart began to palpitate, and my pulse grew hard and small; intolerable anxiety, trembling, prostration throughout all my limbs; then pulsation, in the head, redness of my cheeks, thirst, and, in short, all these symptoms which are ordinarily characteristic of intermittent fever."

When he stopped taking cinchona, the symptoms stopped, only to be triggered again by a fresh dose.

Out of this one experience grew the entire field of homeopathy, now one of the most widely practiced forms of complementary medicine in the world. Hahnemann believed that the bark's curative power was reflected by its ability to create the same set of symptoms as the disease itself. From this, he established the "law of similars," maintaining that "like cures like." It's important to understand the concept, as it lies at the heart of homeopathic cures.

First, Hahnemann was an early believer that the human body typically comes fully equipped with the ability to fight off disease. It's the role of medicine, he felt, to facilitate that great internal healer with fresh cures that would make our bodies even better disease fighters.

Symptoms weren't the problem, Hahnemann wrote, but were signs that the body's powerful immune system was fighting a disease. When his fellow doctors were busy attacking the symptoms, he felt that they were using treatments that acted only to eliminate the symptom and thereby suppress the disease. Hahnemann believed that doctors, rather than helping a patient recover, were in fact damaging the body's natural ability to fend off disease, leaving the patient even less prepared to fight off an illness the next time it occurred.

When a body responded to a cold with a nasal discharge, Hahnemann saw it as a sign that the body's immune system had gone to work. He believed that the best course wasn't to devise drugs that would stop the nose from running, which wasn't the real problem to begin with, but to find new cures from substances that, in their crude form, recreate the same symptoms.

If these substances mimic the symptoms in a healthy body, he said, you'll find the source of new medicines that will help the immune system combat illness. It's important to understand that what causes symptoms in large doses can act as a remedy when administered in tiny amounts.

It wasn't the first time this thought had been expressed. The father of Western medicine, Hippocrates, wrote that "Through the like, disease is produced, and through the application of like it is cured." The word homeopathy is derived from the Greek—*homois* (similar) and *pathos* (suffering). This is exactly the same thinking that goes into the development of new vaccines and allergy medications. When we take small amounts of the virus that can cause disease and inject them into the body, we improve the immune system's ability to fight off that illness. Addressing immunity is one of the few areas of traditional Western medicine that homeopaths can completely agree with.

The Law of Proving

Using himself and his large family as his original test subjects, Hahnemann went on to test—or, as he called it, "prove," based on the German word for "test"—dozens of remedies drawn from minerals, herbs, and animal parts. "The Law of Proving," that you can determine a substance's medicinal effect by testing it on groups of people, is still practiced today much as it was in 1790.

In the beginning, Hahnemann and the early advocates of homeopathy would take small doses of different substances until these provoked a set of symptoms that they could record. At that time in history, animals were never used in proving, as the difference with human physiology would lead to a different set of symptoms. The only major difference between proving today and two hundred years ago is that now homeopaths will conduct a classic double-blind test, splitting a group in two and giving half the group a placebo and the other half the remedy under examination.

Hahnemann started by journeying into some dangerous areas. He experimented with belladonna, or deadly nightshade, and even arsenic, along with a whole range of toxic substances that could provoke a violent response in a patient when administered in their concentrated crude forms. During this proving process, the homeopath would carefully write down the symptoms that were caused by each substance. The most common symptoms were written in bold face, any symptoms experienced by a large group were written in italics, and infrequently experienced symptoms were written in plain text. The fact that homeopaths still find that people respond uniformly to many of these substances underlines the clinical accuracy that has characterized homeopathy from its beginning.

Once Hahnemann and his followers found a substance that would create the classic symptoms of a disease, they felt that they could use trace amounts of the material to fight the disease itself.

The Law of Potentization

The most meticulous of men, Hahnemann began to prepare various doses of his chosen substances, weakening and strengthening the remedies and carefully noting the symptoms produced with different concentrations. During this process, he found that he could improve the results by dissolving the substances in water or alcohol and vigorously shaking the mixture—a method he called "sucussion."

By successively diluting his remedies, a process he called "potentization"—the third law of homeopathy—Hahnemann showed in his home trials that the resulting remedy would grow in potency. Hahnemann found that patients started to recover from their illnesses, usually within forty-eight hours of beginning treatment. It was a slow and methodical process. Hahnemann would take 1 drop of his remedy and start by mixing it with 99 parts of a neutral liquid—alcohol, milk, or water—then he would shake it thirty times. That first dilution of the medication is ranked 1C. Then he would take the diluted substance and dilute it again into 99 parts of the neutral liquid, a routine he repeated as many as 30 times (30C) before he reached the desired amount of potentization.

Now here is an important point to remember, since the strengths of homeopathic medicines are still ranked by this same scale. In some cases, a homeopathic doctor will recommend a remedy diluted to 6C, at other times to 30C, and many other potencies are available. By the way, Hahnemann's home kitchen recipes have been entirely replaced by modern manufacturers' precise methods of sucussion and potentization.

Hahnemann's critics, and there were many, scoffed at the idea that such minute quantities of the original substance could have a therapeutic effect on a patient. But Hahnemann maintained, as his followers do today, that the process of sucussion released the vital energies inherent in the remedies. He theorized that those primary energies were most effective in bolstering the immune system.

Most often, if there is no improvement after two days with an acute illness, the homeopath is likely to switch to another remedy. Each person's body is unique (age, weight, hereditary predispositions, allergies, etc.), so remedies need to conform to each individual. Patients who continue to take the medication for a prolonged period run the risk of staging an accidental proving, where they begin to provoke more of the same symptoms. Homeopathy seeks a rapid recovery. No one is asked to take homeopathic medicines the way he or she might take daily doses of vitamins.

Homeopathic remedies are aimed at balancing your body's immune *system and all other healing systems of your body.*

The Hard Way

It was never an easy therapy to defend, though Hahnemann rarely seemed to do anything the easy way. Suffering in extreme poverty for much of his life, he remained a caustic critic of medicine as it was practiced in the nineteenth century.

In 1812, Hahnemann's theories were put to the extreme test when Napoleon allowed him to treat 180 people suffering from typhoid, a disease that was rampaging through France, killing thousands, and confounding most physicians. Only one of this group died, a remarkable result at that time, and homeopathy began to take hold in European medical practices as a well-regarded complementary practice.

In 1832, homeopaths were given credit for successfully combating a cholera epidemic. The epidemic helped to usher homeopathy into America, where it became one of the most popular therapies available in nineteenth-century American medicine.

Before he died in 1843, Hahnemann and his growing band of colleagues "proved" ninety-nine remedies. These medicines are now the core of more than five hundred medicines outlined in modern homeopathy's materia medica.

Homeopathy continued to thrive in Europe. It is one of the most common alternative therapies available in Germany. In Britain, homeopathy has even been adopted by the Royal Family to treat much of what ails them. And in America, the last decade has seen a definite increase in awareness of homeopathic remedies. These remedies are now taking their place at checkout counters in grocery and health food stores across the country.

If we look back to Hahnemann's time, it is easy to see in retrospect that any therapy that relied on the power of *the body's natural immune system* was often vastly superior to the toxic array of treatments then in vogue. In the eighteenth and early nineteenth centuries, people's chances of making a full recovery were often markedly higher if they trusted their bodies' natural recuperative powers, rather than any of the elixirs prescribed by physicians—a cause of considerable controversy then and now. Even in the present day, homeopaths often find themselves at loggerheads with conventional medicine, denouncing its reliance on suppressing drugs to wipe out symptoms without addressing the reasons why people get sick in the first place.

Most modern critics of homeopathy focus on its foundation stone: Toxic substances that can harm or kill a patient when taken in full strength will cure when weakened to the point that only trace elements remain. To the conventional physician who laughs at the healing powers of homeopathy, such a premise is illogical, even absurd.

But pharmacology has long recognized that while some poisons can kill, a reduced potion may only debilitate, and a tiny dose can stimulate a body and help fight disease. Recent research is showing that smaller doses of chemotherapy are more effective (and healthful) for people with certain cancers. Arsenic has emerged back on the scene, with small doses showing benefit against certain cases of cancer. In regard to the small doses of homeopathics, any doctor can tell you that epinephrine, which is often used for life-threatening allergic reactions, is quite effective at a dilution of 1:100,000. More recently, physicists have begun to explore the role of sucussion, speculating that the repeated shaking of the dose creates an internal electromagnetic pattern that can be duplicated ad infinitum in our bodies or that can influence our electromagnetic fields in positive and healthful ways.

Reasons for Using Homeopathy

There are five main reasons why homeopathy is gaining popularity among doctors and the public:

1. Homeopathy is highly effective for both chronic and acute diseases, including epidemics. It works to strengthen the immune and other healing systems of the body. It can be used to treat conditions for which conventional medicine has no effective treatment.
2. It is cost effective. Compared to pharmaceutical medications, homeopathic remedies are quite inexpensive.
3. It is a preventative medicine. One does not have to have a disease to be treated with homeopathy. It can be used to optimize health.
4. It can be used to treat the whole person. Homeopathy takes into account all the factors of a person's health, even a child's—the mental, the emotional, and the physical.
5. Side effects are not an issue, which is especially important when it comes to children and seniors, who are more prone to toxic side effects of medications.

Homeopathy, as with many of the natural therapies, works with the healing systems of the body. As we will see in the remedy chart located in this chapter, homeopathic medicines are prescribed not only for the disease itself (such as the flu or anxiety), but also for symptoms that are expressed by the person. This allows for an actual improvement in chronic health conditions, rather than just merely suppressing symptoms. Symptoms are used to differentiate the homeopathic remedy for the individual, thus allowing for the "whole" person to be treated.

Prescribing Homeopathy

There are two basic ways that people and practitioners can use homeopathy.

1. Combination remedies. This refers to homeopathic formulas that contain two or more homeopathic remedies. If the remedy a person needs is in the formula, then it will be helpful. If the homeopathic remedy one requires is not one of the ingredients, then usually nothing will happen or only minor improvements that do not last will occur. Combination remedies are available in most health food stores or pharmacies. They are prepared for certain conditions, including colds, flu, teething, colic, diarrhea, rashes, headaches, and others.

2. Single remedies. This is the system that's used by trained homeopathic practitioners. The one remedy that best matches the patient's symptoms is prescribed. In general, this system is more effective than combination remedies, but it requires a knowledgeable practitioner to pick the correct homeopathic. If the single remedy choice is obvious (as described in the remedy summary), then go ahead and use single remedies for yourself or a loved one.

Administering Homeopathics

Homeopathic remedies are generally available in a pellet, tablet, liquid, or cream form. They are best taken ten to twenty minutes before eating or drinking. For infants, pellets or tablets can be mixed in an ounce of purified water, and then a few drops are put in the child's mouth with a dropper or a teaspoon. Children like the sweet taste of the pellets and the tablets. The remedies are also best taken away from strong-smelling odors, such as eucalyptus or essential oils.

For acute conditions, homeopathic remedies are often taken every fifteen minutes or two hours, depending on the severity of the condition. For chronic conditions, homeopathics are usually taken one to two times daily, or less frequently, depending on the strength of the remedy prescribed.

Which Potency to Use

Potency refers to the strength of the remedy. The number behind the name of the homeopathic indicates the dilution and the strength of the medicine. The higher the number, the stronger the action of the remedy. For example, 30C is stronger than 12C, and 12x is stronger than 6x.

There are two common scales of homeopathy available in the marketplace. "X" means the lowest potencies used. X stands for a 1 in 9 dilution. So 1x is equal to 1 part of the original substance diluted in 9 parts solvent. Many stores carry the 6x and 12x potencies for the remedies.

In keeping with the third law of homeopathy, in which remedies become stronger the more they are diluted, "C" is more dilute and stronger than the X potencies. The first dilution—that is, 1C—is equal to 1 part of the original substance in 99 parts of solvent. Many stores carry the 12C and 30C potencies for the remedies.

HOMEOPATHIC REMEDIES FOR EVERYDAY AILMENTS

Remedies	Disorders	Physical Symptoms	Mental/Emotional Symptoms	Made Worse By
Aconite Aconitum Napellus	angina anxiety arrhythmia asthma common cold ear infections fevers flu insomnia sciatica	dry cough early stages of inflammation or fever first 24 hrs. of colds or fevers glassy-eyed great thirst for cold drinks headaches inflammations sensitive to noise	anxious fearful of future, death frantic fright panic attacks restless (physical & mental) shock tension	dry, cold winds hearing music in evenings (around midnight) smoke warm, airless rooms
Allium Cepa	allergies common cold ear infections flu hay fever sore throat	beginning of colds copious nasal discharge, as if peeling onions coughs runny nose teary eyes	fear of pain impatient moody	cold or damp evenings warm room
Antimonium Tartaricum	anorexia bronchitis constipation or diarrhea diarrhea eczema hair loss headaches indigestion nausea	cold sweat cold to touch drowsiness headaches (as if a tight band is around head) nausea pale face rattling cough vomiting	do not like to be touched irritable life is unbearable like to be left alone	at night damp cold lying down movement being touched warm rooms
Apis Mellifica	arthritis asthma backache benign prostate hyperplasia (BPH) common cold depression female disorders flu food allergies hives osteoarthritis shingles sore throat	burning sensation eye inflammation fever hot, burning, stinging pain red, glassy appearance red, swollen joints sore throat sweating	angry controlling deep sadness depression irritable jealous ongoing worry oversensitive workaholic	heat of bed late afternoon (3 P.M.) stuffy room touch warm room warmth
Arnica Montana (also in ointments and creams; first remedy after injury)	after stroke or heart attack arthritis backache carpal tunnel syndrome eczema fibromyalgia flu gastritis	aches and pains bruising physical trauma respiratory difficulties shock swelling	cannot concentrate deny anything is wrong impatient wants to be left alone tossing and turning in bed wary, on guard	after being touched damp environment exertion lying in one position too long using the injured area

(continued on next page)

Remedies	Disorders	Physical Symptoms	Mental/Emotional Symptoms	Made Worse By
Arnica Montana (*continued*)	headaches hemorrhoids injuries (bruises, burns, stings, and sprains) migraines pneumonia			
Arsenicum Album	rheumatoid arthritis sprains whooping cough			
	AIDS anxiety asthma bronchitis chronic fatigue syndrome chronic diarrhea common cold congestive heart failure depression digestive disorders dizziness eating disorders eczema environmental allergies flu food allergies hay fever headaches heart disease hemorrhoids insomnia irritable bowel syndrome psoriasis	burning sensation chills clear, watery mucus dry mouth exhaustion fever overall weakness pale sore throat stomach pain vomiting	afraid anxious controlling critical depressed fearful feels bruised hypochondriac insecure irritable obsessive/compulsive panicky	cold food cold drinks sight/smell of food touch worse at night
Belladonna	respiratory infections shingles ulcers			
	backache (lower back) common cold constipation dizziness ear infection fever flu gout headaches hemorrhoids high blood pressure insomnia menopause migraines	acute inflammation cold hands cold limbs colds with fever cough dizziness early onset of hemorrhoids fever flushed face glassy eyes headaches (intense, throbbing) reddened mucous membranes	excited fearful insomnia jumpy restless wild dreams	bending down exposure to heat and light at night head uncovered light lying down motion noise touching

Remedies	Disorders	Physical Symptoms	Mental/Emotional Symptoms	Made Worse By
Belladonna (*continued*)	osteoarthritis painful periods sinusitis stroke	redness sore throat swelling tenderness throbbing, pulsating abscesses violent onset		

Bryonia Alba	arthritis
	back pain
	  (lower)
	bronchitis
	carpal tunnel
	  syndrome
	common cold
	constipation
	diarrhea
	dizziness
	fibromyalgia
	flu
	gastritis
	gout
	headaches
	indigestion
	irritable bowel
	  syndrome
	migraines
	osteoarthritis
	rheumatoid
	  arthritis
	sciatica
	sprains
	ulcers
		bursting, splitting
		  pain
		does not want to
		  move
		dry, hacking cough
		fever
		painful breathing
		respiratory discom-
		  fort
		swollen, painful
		  joints
		very thirsty
			angry
			wants to be alone
			dull
			grumpy
			irritable
			tired
			worried
				bright lights
				dry winds/drafts
				excitement
				mornings
				noise
				slightest movement
				warm room causes
				  coughing, sneezing
				warmth

Calcarea Carbonica	acne
	anxiety
	arthritis
	asthma
	backache (lower)
	bronchitis
	carpal tunnel
	  syndrome
	cataracts
	chronic fatigue
	  syndrome
	common cold
	constipation
	depression
	eczema
	environmental
	  allergies
	fibromyalgia
	flu
	food allergies
	gout
	high blood
	  pressure
		catches colds easily
		cough
		cramps
		cravings for
		  indigestible
		  things (dirt,
		  chalk)
		exhaustion
		heartburn
		pale skin
		profuse sweating
		sore throat
		stiff in the mornings
		sweats easily
			anxious
			confused
			depressed
			fear of unknown
			fear of speaking
			  before others
			homesickness
			inflexibility
			insecurity
			need to control
			worry
				cold, damp wind
				diarrhea
				drafts
				exertion
				full moon
				winter

(*continued on next page*)

Remedies	Disorders	Physical Symptoms	Mental/Emotional Symptoms	Made Worse By
Calcarea Carbonica (*continued*)	irritable bowel syndrome menopause multiple sclerosis obesity osteoarthritis PMS psoriasis rheumatoid arthritis sciatica sinusitis sprains vaginitis			
Calcarea Phosphorica	anxiety arthritis backache carpal tunnel syndrome fibromyalgia insomnia osteoarthritis osteoporosis	indigestion muscle cramps painful bones and joints swollen neck glands	fidgety need for stimulation nervous restless worries	cold weather exertion grief/bad news in the morning tight clothing
Cantharis	baldness bladder infection bronchitis chemotherapy support cystitis dizziness	abdominal pains bloody stools burning pain inflammation need to urinate painful urination urgent thirst	extremely anxious insolent irritable violent	afternoon before, during, and after urination cold water movement touch
Carbo Vegetabilis	asthma bronchitis chronic fatigue syndrome dizziness environmental allergies headaches irritable bowel syndrome	cold sweat exhaustion faint feverish great fatigue indigestion poor circulation sluggishness weak	anxious confused fear of the dark lack of interest no vitality unreliable memory	fatty foods lying down warm, damp air worse at night
Chamomilla	asthma drug withdrawal diarrhea ear infection insomnia menopause pain periods PMS	coughs fever heavy periods hot hot flashes intense pains low threshold for pain night sweats one cheek red, the other pale overly sensitive to pain	abusive angry bad temper complains about pain impossible inner turmoil irritable rude spiteful violent	arguments at night does not want open wind in the ears does not want people nearby heat worse during menstruation

Remedies	Disorders	Physical Symptoms	Mental/Emotional Symptoms	Made Worse By
Cocculus Indicus	backache dizziness insomnia motion sickness painful periods	back pains exhaustion sore limbs and arms	emptiness nervous exhaustion profound sadness slowness in thinking	after eating after emotional disturbances cold air jolts loss of sleep menstrual periods noise touch
Coffea Cruda	depression headaches insomnia	sensitive to pain	depression despair extreme sensitivity mind chatter sleeplessness	at night in cold noise open air strong odors

Colocynthis	arthritis
	bladder infection
	cystitis
	diarrhea
	dizziness
	gout
	headaches
	irritable bowel
	  syndrome
		cramps
		extreme abdominal
		  pain
		nausea
		painful stools
		vomiting
			angry
			indignant
			irritable
				after eating and
				  drinking, especially
				  fruit
				cold
				dampness

Euphrasia	allergies common cold constipation eye problems hay fever headaches prostate disorders	cessation of periods inflammation from injuries painful periods watery mucus	[none in particular]	bright lights coughing evenings indoors warmth

Ferrum Phosphoricum	anemia
	arthritis
	backache
	beginning stages of
	  colds
	bronchitis
	diarrhea
	dizziness
	ear infection
	flu
	hay fever
	fibromyalgia
	miscarriage
	stroke
		abdominal pains
		early inflammation
		exhaustion
		no appetite
		pale skin
		paralysis
		vomiting
			nervous
			sensitive
				after eating
				at night/and
				  4–6 A.M.
				jarring
				rapid movements
				sun exposure
				too hot
				touch

Gelsemium	allergies
	anxiety
	arthritis
	chemotherapy
	  support
	childbirth
	chronic fatigue
	  syndrome
		chills
		exhaustion
		extremely fatigued
		fevers
		heavy eyelids
		heavy lidded/drowsy
		pulsating headaches
		  (back of head)
			anxiety
			apathy about illness
			depression
			dullness
			fears
			mind chatter
			nervousness
			phobias
				bad news
				damp weather/fog
				excitement
				mental exertion
				movement of
				  head
				open air
				sun and heat

(continued on next page)

Remedies	Disorders	Physical Symptoms	Mental/Emotional Symptoms	Made Worse By
Gelsemium (*continued*)	depression diarrhea dizziness fibromyalgia flu hay fever headaches (tension) migraines stroke	trembling visual disturbances due to headaches weak, heavy	sense of inadequacy terrified to be left alone	taking stimulants (coffee, alcohol, drugs)
Hepar Sulphuris	acne allergies anxiety arthritis bronchitis common colds diarrhea ear infections eczema sinusitis ulcers	cannot expectorate mucus chills fever foul, smelly discharges hoarse, dry cough joint pain laryngitis sore throat swollen glands	anxiety easily offended impulsiveness irritable very sensitive	being uncovered cold drafts/air cold drinks or food disturbances of any kind noise touch
Hypericum Perforatum	backaches contusions depression diarrhea headaches hemorrhoids impotence injured fingers/toes injury to nerves puncture wounds sprains tailbone and spinal injuries	indigestion nausea nerve pain neuralgia puncture wounds shooting pains	depression "drift away" forget what going to say shock sleepy	being touched cold, damp, foggy weather stuffy, warm rooms when uncovered
Ignatia Amara	anxiety asthma backaches (lower) bronchitis chronic fatigue syndrome common cold constipation depression eating disorders female disorders flu headaches (chronic) hemorrhoids insomnia migraines obesity	drowsiness dry, hacking cough frequent yawning fever/chills sore throat stabbing headaches	cries easily deep grief depression jealousy sentimental severe emotional shock sighs frequently very sensitive weepy	coffee, tobacco, alcohol cold air consolation rain smoky rooms strong smells or emotions winter worse in morning
Ipecacuanha	asthma back pain chemotherapy support	bleeding from any body part blood in expectorant	anxiety argumentative contemptuous	lying down movement warmth

Remedies	Disorders	Physical Symptoms	Mental/Emotional Symptoms	Made Worse By
Ipecacuanha (*continued*)	hemorrhaging migraines morning sickness motion sickness nausea in pregnancy	fever indigestion loose cough nausea red face swollen skin swollen eyes vomiting with coughing weak	fear of death irritable morose	winter
Kali Bichromicum	bronchitis colds with thick, heavy mucus earaches, ear infec- tions headaches (one small spot) migraines osteoarthritis rheumatoid arthritis sinusitis vaginitis	coughs with discharge hypersensitive to pain joint pain postnasal drip thick, stringy, sticky discharge	anxiety irritable	cold weather in the morning noise touch
Kali Carbonicum	common cold dizziness headaches PMS respiratory infections	dizziness headaches before periods headaches stiff stuffy nose yellowish phlegm	irritable nervousness overwhelmed scared unhappy worried about future	changes in weather coffee cold surroundings hot drinks touch
Lachesis	asthma chronic fatigue syndrome depression headaches heavy, painful periods hemorrhoids high blood pressure menopause migraines PMS	fatigue fevers hot flashes palpations sore throat (begins on left side) weak heart	depressed excitable irritable jealous restless sensitive suspicious talkative	after drinking alcohol bright light clothing around neck heat spring sun tight clothing touch waking in the morning
Ledum	alcoholism bladder infections bronchitis common cold flu gout headaches infections kidney infections osteoarthritis puncture wounds (immunizations, surgery, insect bites)	abscesses bleeds easily bruises easily chilly cold all the time headaches joint aches and pains puncture wounds sprains stings/bites throbbing pain	anxiety extreme anger impatient morose timid wants to be left alone	aggravated by heat lying down movement touch under warm covers warmth worse at night

(*continued on next page*)

Remedies	Disorders	Physical Symptoms	Mental/Emotional Symptoms	Made Worse By
Ledum (*continued*)	rheumatoid arthritis sprains			

Lycopodium	acne
	anxiety
	asthma
	baldness
	benign prostate
	  hyperplasia
	bladder infection
	bronchitis
	chronic fatigue
	  syndrome
	colitis
	common cold
	constipation
	Crohn's disease
	cystitis
	diabetes
	digestive/eating
	  disorders
	eczema
	flu
	food allergies
	heartburn
	impotence
	insomnia
	irritable bowel
	  syndrome
	kidney stones
	macular
	  degeneration
	migraines
	PMS
	prostate enlargement
	psoriasis
	rosacea
	seborrhea
	sinusitis
	urinary problems
		chronic mucus
		  formation
		coughs
		fever
		headaches
		indigestion
		prostate problems
		puncture wounds
		skin ailments
			anxious
			fear of failure
			hypochondriac
			impatient
			inferiority/superiority
			insecure
			lack of self-
			  confidence
			lack of self-control
			mental fatigue
			nervousness
			secretive
				chilled
				coughing
				covered up
				not eating regularly
				overeating
				stuffy rooms
				tight clothing
				worse at night

Magnesia Phosphorica	dizziness ear infection headaches leg cramps menstrual pains/cramps morning sickness sciatica (backache)	aches and pains cramps/spasms nausea	cannot think clearly complains moans and groans tired/exhausted	at night being touched cold, chilly weather drafts touch
Mercurius Solubilis	backaches common cold colitis ear infection fibromyalgia sinusitis ulcers	dry throat eye inflammation fever neuralgia sore throat thirst	anxiety dull irritable lack of will power nervous poor concentration and memory	at night being warm in bed dampness light temperature changes

Remedies	Disorders	Physical Symptoms	Mental/Emotional Symptoms	Made Worse By
Mercurius Solubilis (*continued*)	vaginitis		suspicious timid	

Natrum Muriaticum	anemia
	anxiety
	arrhythmia
	asthma
	backache (lower)
	chronic diarrhea
	chronic fatigue
	  syndrome
	common cold
	constipation
	depression
	digestive
	  disorders
	dizziness
	eczema
	environmental
	  allergies
	flu
	hay fever
	hemorrhoids
	high blood pressure
	irritable bowel
	  syndrome
	menopause
	migraines
	motion sickness
	obesity
	PMS
	psoriasis
	sciatica
	ulcers
	vaginitis
		cravings
		fever
		headaches
		irregular periods
		nausea/vomiting
		runny nose (clear
		  mucus)
		sore throat
		very thirsty
		weakness
		whooping cough
			brooding
			cannot express
			  feelings
			cries in deep sobs
			depression
			feels abandoned
			grief
			impatience
			loner
			low spirits
			moody
			sense of doom
			sentimental
			very irritable
				consolation
				crying in front of
				  others
				drafts
				extreme cold
				hot sun
				in morning
				jarring
				music
				noise
				warm room

Nux Vomica	alcoholism and drug
	  addiction
	asthma
	backache
	bladder infection
	chemotherapy
	  support
	chronic constipation
	chronic fatigue
	  syndrome
	colitis
	common cold
	Crohn's disease
	cystitis
	diarrhea
	dizziness
	endometriosis
	environmental
	  allergies
	fibroids
	flu
		chills/fever
		coughs
		flatulence
		heartburn
		indigestion
		labor pains
		nausea
		phlegm
			aggressive behavior
			angry
			anxiety
			competitor
			dislike touch
			fearful
			impatient
			indignant
			intimidates
			irritable
			jealous
			self-centered
			sensitive to criticism
			spiteful
			stressed out
			stubborn
				alcohol/hangovers
				cold wind
				dryness
				eating
				light
				noise
				smells
				spices
				touch
				upon waking
				warm rooms

(*continued on next page*)

Remedies	Disorders	Physical Symptoms	Mental/Emotional Symptoms	Made Worse By
Nux Vomica (*continued*)	gout hay fever headaches heart disease heavy, painful periods hemorrhoids high blood pressure insomnia irritable bowel syndrome kidney stones morning sickness motion sickness multiple sclerosis PMS stress			
Phosphorus	Alzheimer's disease anemia anxiety arthritis asthma bronchitis cataracts chronic fatigue syndrome common cold congestive heart failure constipation depression diabetes dizziness eczema fibromyalgia food and environmental allergies flu gastritis glaucoma hay fever hearing loss heart disease hemorrhaging hemorrhoids high blood pressure insomnia irritable bowel syndrome migraines morning sickness obesity psoriasis respiratory infections rheumatoid arthritis stomach ulcers	burning pains chills chronic phlegm cough deafness fevers headaches indigestion joint and muscle pain laryngitis sore throat swelling around the eyes very thirsty for cold, icy drinks vomiting	anxious bottles things up fear of being alone fears insanity indifference nervous tension seeks approval and love suicidal	cold drafts evenings mental and physical exertion noise strong odors touch warm food and drinks weather changes

Remedies	Disorders	Physical Symptoms	Mental/Emotional Symptoms	Made Worse By

Podophyllum	diarrhea
	headaches
	irritable bowel
	  syndrome
		abdominal pain
		bowel movements
		  containing mucus
		cramps, stomach
		growling stomach
		stiff joints and
		  muscles
		sudden urgency to
		  release stools
		thirst for cold drinks
		weak and faint
			depressed
			excitable
			moans in sleep
			talkative
				hot weather
				in the morning

Pulsatilla	acne
	allergies
	asthma
	backache
	benign prostate
	  hyperplasia
	bronchitis
	cataracts
	chronic fatigue
	  syndrome
	common cold
	cystitis
	depression
	diarrhea
	digestive
	  problems
	dizziness
	ear infection
	fibromyalgia
	flu
	hay fever
	headaches
	hemorrhoids
	irritable bowel
	  syndrome
	labor pains
	menopause
	morning sickness
	osteoarthritis
	painful periods
	PMS
	postnatal depression
	rheumatoid arthritis
	sciatica
	sinusitis
	ulcers
	vaginitis
		burning vaginal
		  discharge
		eye inflammation
		female problems
		hacking cough
		heartburn
		nausea
		pains move from
		  joint to joint
		swelling around the
		  eyes
		thick yellow or
		  greenish discharge
		thirstless
		upset stomach
			avoids confrontation
			depression
			desires sympathy
			fear
			longs for attention
			moody
			sensitive
			slow, gentle, quiet
			  mind
			weepy/clingy
				in evening
				lying down at night
				rapid movements
				rich, fatty foods
				sun/heat
				temperature changes
				warm room or bed

Rhus Toxicodendron	acne
	backache (lower)
	carpal tunnel
	  syndrome
	common cold
	depression
	dizziness
		acute arthritis pain
		dizziness
		fever blisters
		fevers
		great pain on initial
		  movement
		itchy sensation
			cries easily
			depressed
			irritable
			lonely
			nervous
			restless
				cold drinks
				damp, cold weather
				drafts
				intensifies at night in
				  bed
				rest
				wet weather
				(continued on next page)

Remedies	Disorders	Physical Symptoms	Mental/Emotional Symptoms	Made Worse By
Rhus Toxicodendron (*continued*)	eczema fibromyalgia flu gout headaches hives osteoarthritis psoriasis rheumatoid arthritis rosacea sciatica shingles sprains TMJ	joint and muscle pain rashes sore throat sprains/strains thirsty for cold beverages		
Ruta Graveolens	allergies arthritis asthma backache (lower) carpal tunnel syndrome common cold constipation fibromyalgia gout headaches (eye strain) osteoarthritis sciatica sprains	acute aches and pains coughs headaches hip problems sprains stiffness	anxiety contradictory depressed despair dissatisfied with self and others feels bruised noncaring nonemotional quarrelsome weakness	bending down cold, damp weather lying down overexertion sitting worse at night
Sepia	anemia backache (lower) bladder infection bronchitis chemotherapy support chronic fatigue syndrome constipation cystitis depression digestive disorders dizziness endometriosis headaches with nausea hormonal imbalance irritable bowel syndrome menopause migraines miscarriage morning sickness painful periods peptic ulcer PMS	chronic phlegm coughs exhaustion fatigue fevers menstrual pain nausea in pregnancy stiffness stomach upset	anxious aggressive bitter critical depressed feelings of disappointment forgetful independent indifference irritable nagging/bossy jumpy rude weepy	cold, damp, stormy weather exertion in heat jarring mental fatigue noise stuffy rooms walking

Remedies	Disorders	Physical Symptoms	Mental/Emotional Symptoms	Made Worse By
Sepia (*continued*)	sciatica seborrhea uterine pain vaginitis varicose veins women's health issues			

Silica	acne
	anemia
	bronchitis
	carpal tunnel
	  syndrome
	cataracts
	chronic fatigue
	  syndrome
	constipation
	diabetes
	diarrhea
	digestive disorders
	dizziness
	ear infections
	environmental
	  allergies
	food allergies
	infections
	insomnia
	migraine (right side)
	recurrent colds
	rheumatoid arthritis
	TMJ
		chills
		chronic phlegm
		fever
		pimples
		poor stamina
		sweat with sour smell
		tiredness
			anxiety
			faint-hearted
			fear of failure
			frustrated
			homesickness
			obstinate
			overwhelmed
			self-doubt
			spiteful
			yielding
				bathing
				damp drafts
				hot food
				in morning
				stuffy rooms
				uncovered
				wet, cold weather

Spongia Tosta	asthma chronic fatigue syndrome common cold flu	dry, barking cough exhaustion hoarseness sore throat wheezing cough	anxiety apprehension fear of dying tearfulness	cold drinks midnight moving about sweating touch
Staphysagria	benign prostate hyperplasia (BPH) bladder infection cystitis depression eczema headaches menopause PMS psoriasis	depression injuries nausea urinary problems	abuser blame self internal turmoil irritable "lash out" low self-esteem sensitive suppress emotions touchy violent outbursts	cold cold drinks dehydration during menstruation lack of sleep smoke touching
Sulphur	acne acute infections alcoholism anxiety arthritis asthma back pain bladder infection	coughs diarrhea exhaustion fever indigestion itching, burning skin muscle cramps	anxiety careless attitude center of attention constant excitement fear boredom mania selfish "7-year itch"	alcohol bathing blowing the nose coughing heat immobility open air standing

(continued on next page)

Remedies	Disorders	Physical Symptoms	Mental/Emotional Symptoms	Made Worse By
Sulphur (*continued*)	bronchitis chronic fatigue syndrome constipation diabetes diarrhea dizziness ear infections eczema fibromyalgia food allergies flu hay fever headaches hemorrhoids hypoglycemia indigestion insomnia irritable bowel syndrome menopause menstrual problems migraines multiple sclerosis pregnancy psoriasis rheumatoid arthritis ulcers vaginitis	red patch from one cheek over the nose to the other cheek sore throat stiff joints "sulphur mask"		sun swallowing talking 11 A.M. slump
Tabacum	anxiety dizziness morning sickness motion sickness	chills with cold sweat cold, clammy, pale skin nausea pale skin stomach upsets vomiting	anxious giddy	extremes of cold/heat and stuffy rooms movement, jarring physical effort
Urtica Urens	cystitis fibromyalgia gout hives insect bites kidney stones puncture wounds rheumatic arthritis shingles skin allergy reaction vaginitis	blotchy skin fevers itching, burning sensation joint aches and pains sore throat want to lie down	[none in particular]	bathing heat lying on right side overtax muscles and joints physical exercise snowy, damp, cold

Constitutional Homeopathic Remedies

One fascinating area of homeopathy consists of constitutional remedies, which are linked to physical, mental, and emotional characteristics. Based on a person's symptom profile, a homeopathic practitioner can accurately choose a constitutional homeopathic remedy to treat or prevent an imbalance by strengthening the person's overall healing and defense systems. This section describes common constitutional remedies. They are prescribed by homeopathic practitioners to improve a person's overall health and to treat chronic illness. If a remedy matches up closely to your constitution, then you can try taking a 30x, 12C, or 30C potency twice daily for a week and see if there are any changes. Once improvement has begun, stop the remedy unless progress halts, in which case take it again as needed. Otherwise, it is best to follow the advice of a qualified homeopathic practitioner.

Note: Some acute remedies, such as Sulphur, are also useful as constitutional remedies.

Common Constitutional Remedies

CALCAREA CARBONICA

Physical symptoms: People who fit this constitutional type tend to be plump or obese, tire easily, and be susceptible to infections, especially ear or upper respiratory infections. In general, they are chilly. For children, there can be a delay in development, such as a slow onset of walking or talking. People's nails may break or be brittle. They tend to sweat profusely on the back of the head when sleeping. They often crave eggs, sweets, and dairy products. The remedy is also indicated for people with chronic constipation.

Mental and emotional symptoms: They are easily overwhelmed; work oriented and organized; worriers; independent, stubborn, and curious.

LYCOPODIUM

Physical symptoms: People who fit the Lycopodium remedy picture have problems with the digestive system—bloating, gas, and burping—that get worse between 4 and 8 P.M. They often have large appetites and crave sweets. They are also prone to respiratory problems and tend to get problems on the right-side of their bodies.

Mental and emotional symptoms: They like having authority, are domineering but have low self-esteem.

NATRUM MURIATICUM

Physical symptoms: People who require this remedy often complain of headaches, some of which can be severe. Symptoms are usually worse between 10 A.M. and 3 P.M. They have a strong craving for salty foods. Their cold sores break out from sun exposure. Their skin and eyes are extremely sensitive to the sun.

Mental and emotional symptoms: They tend to be depressed and prefer to be alone. They often have a history of emotional grief, such as the death of a loved one or a divorce. They do not like to cry in front of others. It is important to them to be very neat and tidy in appearance.

PHOSPHOROUS

Physical symptoms: People who fit this constitutional type often have reoccurring nosebleeds for no apparent reason. Their colds have a tendency to turn into respiratory tract infections. Many people with asthma benefit from this remedy. Digestive upset, such as "tummy aches," can be common. They have a great thirst for cold drinks and crave sweets and ice cream.

Mental and emotional symptoms: The personality type is outgoing and very sociable. They like attention. They have sympathy for others and do not like to be alone, especially in the dark.

PULSATILLA

Physical symptoms: Their bodies get warm easily, and they desire to be outside in the fresh air. Children and adults are prone to getting ear and respiratory infections and sinusitis, which often has a greenish-yellow discharge. They crave sweets, especially pastries, and have little thirst.

Mental and emotional symptoms: They are generally shy, yet they crave attention. Their feelings are easily hurt.

SILICA

Physical symptoms: This remedy is for people with a very low resistance to infections, such as ear infections, colds, sinusitis, sore throats, and bronchitis. They are always coming down with an infection and have poor stamina. People who require Silica are often very thin and underweight and may have brittle skin, nails, and hair. They are chilly and cannot stand drafts of cold air.

Mental and emotional symptoms: They are usually stubborn and irritable, yet very shy and sensitive to criticism.

SULPHUR

Physical symptoms: People who require this remedy are prone to getting skin rashes and have bad body odor. They have a great thirst (cold drinks) and appetite, with strong cravings for sweets and spicy foods. They get overheated and sweat easily.

Mental and emotional symptoms: They tend to be very curious (always asking why and how something works) and are very sociable. They like to be the leaders in groups of people. They also tend to be messy and unorganized.

A Guide to the Twelve Cell Salts

WHAT ARE CELL SALTS?

Cell salts are simplified forms of homeopathic remedies that quickly and simply alleviate many childhood health problems. Dr. Schussler, of Germany, discovered that twelve inorganic minerals were key constituents of cells. His theory was that a deficiency or an imbalance of these cell salts led to disease. By supplementing these naturally occurring biochemical cell salts, one can stimulate the cells to assimilate nutrients more efficiently. Replenishing and balancing these minerals restores the proper structure and the function of each cell, tissue, and organ. Ferrum Phosphoricum cell salt, for example, is a homeopathic dilution of iron, making it an excellent treatment for anemia because it bolsters iron assimilation in the cells, increasing the oxygen-carrying capacity of red blood cells.

HOW TO USE CELL SALTS

Cell salts are used similarly to other homeopathics. Just like other homeopathics, they are available in pellet, tablet, or liquid form. The most common potencies available are the 6x. They are best taken ten to twenty minutes between eating or drinking. For infants, cell salt tablets can be crushed and mixed in an ounce of purified water; then a few drops are put in the child's mouth with a dropper or a teaspoon. They are best taken away from strong-smelling odors, such as eucalyptus or essential oils.

For acute conditions, take cell salts every fifteen minutes or two hours, depending on the severity of the condition. For chronic conditions, cell salts are usually taken one to three times daily. Since they are of a low potency, cell salts are often used on a long-term basis.

CELL SALTS

Name	General Theme	Indications
Calcarea Fluorica	connective tissue	ligament and tendon sprains/weakness, brittle teeth and gums, abnormal spine curvature
Calcarea Phosphorica	bone health	fractures, teething, growing pains, osteoporosis
Calcarea Sulphurica	wound healer	abscess, boils, acne
Ferrum Phosphoricum	iron metabolism, bleeding	anemia, stops bleeding, fever
Kali Muriaticum	mucus	fluid in ears, sore throat
Kali Phosphoricum	nerves	nerve injury, brain tonic, concentration, anxiety
Kali Sulphuricum	skin	discharges
Magnesia Phosphoricum	muscles and nerves	muscle spasms, cramps, stomach cramps, relaxes nervous system, seizures, hyperactivity
Natrum Muriaticum	water balance	skin dryness, hay fever, grief, cold sores
Natrum Phosphoricum	acid-base balancer	heartburn, vaginitis
Natrum Sulphuricum	detoxifier	jaundice of newborn, hepatitis, head injury, colitis
Silica	tissue cleanser	acne, boils (with pus discharge), sinusitis, weak immunity

Bach Flower Remedies

In the early 1900s, Dr. Edward Bach developed the Bach Flower Remedies from flower and plant extracts. He believed that physical problems were a result of emotional imbalances. By relieving emotional blockages with the flower remedies, he theorized that physical ailments would improve. This is another simple system of homeopathy that one can use. Bach's thirty-eight flower remedies focused on emotional problems, greatly addressing the stresses that people face. One of the beauties of this system is the lack of harmful side effects because of the microdilutions of the medicines. Bach Flower Remedies are gaining popularity in the health food arena because they are simple and easy to use. They are available in most health food stores and pharmacies.

How to Use Bach Flower Remedies

Pick the Bach Flower Remedy or Remedies that match your emotional theme. It is common to mix two or more remedies together to fit your emotional makeup or imbalance, or one remedy can be used by itself. Take the remedy three to four times daily for acute situations or one to two times daily for chronic imbalances. The correct Bach Flower Remedy or mixture will help move you in the direction of mental and emotional healing.

BACH FLOWER REMEDIES

Agrimony
apprehensive
covers up feelings
hide problems from self and others
suffers distress from arguing
may overindulge in food, alcohol, drugs
 to cope

Aspen
anxious
apprehensive
unknown vague fears

Beech
analytical
critical toward self and of others
judgmental
lacks tolerance

Centaury
cannot say "no" to requests of others
exploited by others
overly anxious to please and serve others

Cerato
always asking others for advice
doubts own judgment
indecisive
needs confirmation

Cherry Plum
fearful of doing horrible things
fearful of being out of control
irrational
verge of losing mind

Chestnut Bud
does not learn from experiences
makes same mistakes over and over and never
  learns from them

Chicory
manipulates others
overly protective
possessive
self-centered

Clematis
absent-minded
day dreams
lacks interest
loves to sleep a lot

Crab Apple
*** The Cleansing Remedy ***
(detoxifier physically)
feels dirty inside and out
self-disgust

Elm
feels overwhelmed with own problems or duties
periods of depression
undertakes too much

Gentain
"Dr. Doom"
depressed from known cause
despondent
everything is wrong
frustrated
just gives up
negative
pessimistic

Gorse
defeated
has given up hope
great despair
pessimistic

Heather
lonely
obsessed with personal problems
tells "all" to whomever will listen
overly talkative

Holly
harbors negative thoughts, such as envy,
  revenge, suspicion, hate
sharp-tongued, like the points of a holly leaf

Honey Suckle
dwells on past achievements or griefs
nostalgic

Hornbeam
feels fatigued
mental weariness
no energy
physical tiredness
procrastinates

Impatiens
frustrated by slow coworker
impatient
irritable
quick in thoughts and actions

Larch
expects failure
feels inferior to others
lacks confidence

Mimulus
fears everyday life
fears from a known cause
overly cautious
shy, timid
worrier

Mustard
"Doom and Gloom" that comes and goes
  for no apparent reason
dark cloud overhead
feels sorrowful
miserable for no reason

Oak
"workaholic"
great sense of duty
hurdles obstacles at own expense
never gives up
strong as an oak

Olive
drained
exhausted, both mentally and physically
has run out of steam; could be due to personal
  problems or illness

Pine
dissatisfied with self
feels guilty
lacks self-value
overly apologetic
perfectionist

Red Chestnut
anticipates misfortune
fears the worst will happen to friends, family, loved ones
gripped with fear for others
projects worry

Rock Rose
*** Remedy for Emergencies ***
("panic attacks")
fears losing control
feelings of terror and fright, due to illness or accidents

Rock Water
opinionated
puritanical
self-denying
strict with self, but not others
tries to be good example for others

Scleranthus
cannot make a choice between two things
does not ask others for their opinions
feels out of sorts
mood swings
PMS
vacillates

Star of Bethlehem
*** Comfort Remedy ***
(smoothes, calms, centers)
cannot be consoled
great distress
shock from serious illness or accident

Sweet Chestnut
feels dejection
mental torture from unbearable situation
pushed to the limits
unbearable anguish

Vervain
cannot see anything else
feels a need to fulfill
highly strung
overly enthusiastic
people who feel the need to convert others
will not be beaten by illness
workaholic

Vine
born leaders
"bossy"
capable people
confident
rigid
has to have his or her way!

Walnut
*** "Change" and "Transition" Remedy! ***
(for menopause, divorce, moving)
can be easily led astray on rare occasions
helps adapt to change

Water Violet
"loners"
calming to others
gentle, quiet individuals
independent
reserved

White Chestnut
inner turmoil
insomniac, due to racing thoughts
"mind chatter"
worrier

Wild Oats
indecision about current career, yet does not know where to go
"Life is passing me by!"
"not knowing what you want to do when you grow up"

Willow
blames others
feels weepy
has difficulty forgiving others
thinks life is unjust

***RESCUE REMEDY—This Bach remedy is widely utilized for emergency situations, such as taking exams, public speaking, a visit to the doctor, bad news, or any other stressful or fearful situation. Rescue remedy consists of the following five essences: Cherry Plum, Clematis, Impatiens, Rock Rose, and Star of Bethlehem. This remedy can be taken safely in conjunction with all other complementary healing programs. It also comes in a cream form, which can be used topically for burns, stings, or sprains.

Aromatherapy

Introduction

We've all experienced the rush of feeling that can accompany a familiar, long-forgotten smell. Whether it's the aroma of banana bread just like grandmother's or the scent of the cologne our first love wore, smells have the power to take us back in time. Suddenly, we remember the anticipation we felt that long-ago day in grandmother's kitchen or the heartache of saying good-bye to our lover. We feel the same way, all over again.

If its sole effectiveness lay in harnessing that power of remembrance, aromatherapy would doubtless be a useful tool. But the strength of aromatherapy goes even beyond this. The essential oils used in aromatherapy are extracted from plants and impart their healing powers to the body through the sense of smell, certainly, but also through their ability to permeate the bloodstream. They have antibiotic, antibacterial, and tonic qualities that can relieve pain and stress, help balance the body and the mind, and even prevent disease. Besides, aromatherapy is enjoyable, whether you visit an expert aromatherapist for a massage or soak at home in a bath scented with your favorite essential oils.

Specific essential oils have specific properties that can alleviate particular symptoms or conditions. For example, eucalyptus oil helps to clear congestion, while peppermint oil is good for relieving nausea. Familiarity with the characteristics of just a few essential oils and with the different ways they can be used gives us the power to self-treat many common ailments. Whether your trouble is physical, mental, or emotional, you may find relief in the use of aromatherapy.

History

Long before humans discovered the processes for extracting essential oils from plants, they found ways to use aromatic plants and other perfumes to enhance their lives. Picture an ancient Egyptian temple. Incense is burning, infusing the air with frankincense, myrrh, and sandalwood. A cadre of priests anoints the faithful with scented oils. Many of these pilgrims are already covered with various scents from their aromatic baths and perfumed cosmetics. And when they return to their homes, many of them will burn juniper or thyme to freshen the air and ward off evil spirits.

The Egyptians were among the first to indulge in aromatherapy. The same botanical knowledge that helped them embalm their dead was also used in daily life. But they were not the lone aromatherapists in the ancient world. While Egyptian priests and perfumers practiced their craft, to the east in India, Ayurvedic healers were recording the healing properties of such aromatic plants as coriander, ginger, and rose.

Farther east in China and Japan, aromatic woods and perfumes were used in religious rites and for personal beauty and hygiene. The ancient Greeks learned the secrets of aromatherapy from the Egyptians, and they became enthusiastic partakers of scent. They often used huge quantities of aromatic substances during religious rituals and adorned their bodies daily with perfume from head to toe, in hopes of gratifying the gods. But they also made the connection between scent and health. They believed that certain perfumes had therapeutic properties. Emotional or mental ailments could be healed with medicinal perfumes, and once the mind was healed, physical health would follow.

Hippocrates, the "father of medicine," prescribed perfumed therapies; Greek medical practice also yielded the label *iatralypte,* a physician who cured through the use of aromatic ointments. They passed their knowledge on to the Romans, who in turn spread the use of botanicals to each new land they conquered.

After the fall of Rome, aromatherapy in Europe dwindled. But the Arab world continued to add to the knowledge of perfumes' healing powers. By the tenth century, an Arabian physician, Avicenna, had discovered a way to distill the essential oils from rose petals. Soon, many other essential oils were available, and by the time trade resumed between Europe and the East, the use of essential oils was widespread. Oils such as juniper and pine were used to combat illness and keep it from spreading, and the use of perfumes for personal adornments and hygiene was commonplace.

Aromatherapy met an enemy with the Puritan movement, which lumped perfume and incense in with paganism and witchcraft. And with the advent of modern science, aromatherapy fell further from favor. The natural essential oils, so prized for generations, were replaced with synthetic scents in cosmetics, perfumes, and foods.

It wasn't until the 1920s that aromatherapy began a resurgence. The French chemist and perfumer Ren-Maurice Gattefoss actually coined the term *aromatherapy* after an accident in his laboratory left his hand badly burned. He immersed his hand in lavender oil and later noticed that the burn healed quite quickly and left no scar. This personal experience led him to delve further into the possibilities of healing with essential oils.

Dr. Jean Valnet, a French physician and a scientist, built upon the knowledge of Gattefoss by using essential oils as part of his medical practice to treat physical and psychiatric problems. Valnet later published a guide to the use of essential oils called *Aromatherapie.* One of his converts, Madame Marguerite Maury, established the first aromatherapy clinics in Paris, England, and Switzerland. There, she used essential oils in beauty therapies that were personalized for each subject. Her aromatherapy sought to rejuvenate clients with scents directed at their personalities and health problems. She published the fruits of her research in 1964 in *The Secret of Life and Youth.*

Today, their knowledge is passed on through aromatherapy courses, institutes, and seminars in North America and Europe. Many certified aromatherapists practice the same healing arts that Gattefoss and Valnet first used, and the availability of many books on the subject allows people to try it for themselves at home.

Aromatherapy Basics

The term *essential oil* is misleading. Essential oils are not oily or greasy; they evaporate readily, leaving no residue. As they evaporate, their aromatic molecules permeate the air. When we inhale the aroma, these molecules travel into the nose and to the olfactory receptors where our sense of smell originates. These receptors then transmit information about the odor to the limbic system in the brain.

The limbic portion of the brain not only processes smells, but also handles emotions, which may be one reason why smells can so easily trigger our feelings. In addition, the limbic portion of the brain influences the production of hormones, the immune system, and the nervous system. As such, aromatherapy can affect basic bodily functions and mental fitness.

The essential oil molecules do not stop in the nose, however. They travel on into the lungs and, from there, into the bloodstream, where they can improve health by acting on individual cells. They are also readily absorbed into the skin, but they are most often diluted in a carrier oil—such as almond oil—before application to prevent skin irritation.

Once the tiny essential oil molecules penetrate the skin, they can stimulate circulation and encourage cell regeneration. Some oils relieve muscle soreness, while others can help release tension and spasms. They can enter the bloodstream here, too, and go on to the internal organs and the lymphatic system.

Whether inhaled or absorbed through the skin, essential oils can fight bacteria, fungi, viruses, and other microbes inside the body and can stimulate the immune system to help renew health. Essential oils can also be taken internally, but this must be done only under the supervision of a qualified aromatherapy practitioner. Never ingest essential oils on your own, and make sure to keep your supply out of reach of children. Many essential oils are extracted from their plants in stills.

No, this isn't the kind of still used in the back woods to make moonshine. It's a specially constructed piece of equipment for distilling essential oils that uses pressurized steam. Fresh or dried plant material is placed in a special compartment, and steam is circulated through it. The heat forces open tiny pockets in the plants to release the essential oils, which evaporate and move into a condensation chamber. As the mixture cools, the steam condenses into water and the essential oil—which does not dissolve in water—floats on top. The oil is then skimmed off and packaged for sale.

Some plant materials don't lend themselves to steam distillation, so their essential oils are extracted by other means. Citrus oils, such as orange, lemon, and bergamot, are obtained by cold pressing.

Flowers with low concentrations of essential oils, such as jasmine, are put through a complex process called enfleurage. Their petals are placed in animal fat, which absorbs the essential oil; alcohol is then added to separate the essential oil from the fat. The alcohol evaporates, leaving the essential oil—more properly called an *absolute,* in this case—behind.

Alcohol is also used in solvent extraction, with tree sap that's too thick to use otherwise or with flowers when enfleurage is considered too inefficient.

A solvent such as hexane saturates the plant material and chemically extracts the essential oils; the resulting material is then dissolved in alcohol to remove the solvent. These essential oils often contain residue from the solvent. For this reason, we suggest that you avoid essential oils that were extracted with solvents other than alcohol.

How Oils Can Be Used

Remember when you were a child and your mother rubbed a menthol ointment on your chest to relieve chest congestion? She may also have put some of the ointment into a vaporizer to fill the room with a cloud of menthol-scented steam, to help you breathe more easily. This was a form of aromatherapy, and your mother was practicing it in different ways to maximize its healing powers. Likewise, aromatherapists not only match essential oils to particular symptoms, they also carefully choose the method of delivering aromatherapy.

There are several different ways for essential oils to be used, and different application methods are best suited to different ailments. Respiratory problems, such as sinusitis and bronchitis, respond well to steam inhalation and chest massage, while nervous complaints are best assuaged by a combination of massage, baths, and inhalation. Indigestion can be eased by directly inhaling the aroma of peppermint oil, while constipation responds to an abdominal massage with a blend of fennel and marjoram. In addition, different people respond to different oils in unique ways.

With a little practice and some common sense, you will soon learn how you can best treat yourself and your family with aromatherapy.

Massage

Aromatherapy massage combines two therapies into one very effective therapy for a multitude of complaints, whether physical, mental, emotional, or a combination of each. Besides, it's one of the most pleasurable experiences around. If you're given a prescription for a massage with sage and geranium for depression, or with eucalyptus and rosemary for a backache, you can rest assured that the treatment will be delightful all by itself—and its healing aftereffects will be an even greater bonus.

Massage alone stimulates circulation, releases toxins from the muscles, relaxes breathing and muscle tension, and soothes the nervous system.

With aromatherapy, massage becomes a multifaceted healer. It delivers aromatic molecules into the body through the skin and the nose to relax or stimulate the body as needed, while providing all the benefits of a full-body massage.

Although there's no substitute for a full-body massage from an experienced practitioner, the benefits of self-massage are well documented. A daily self-massage with a carrier oil that's infused with essential oils will not only moisturize the skin and boost circulation, it can also improve your overall well-being through aromatherapy.

And when you're experiencing a problem, massage can be used to help heal specific parts of the body. You can mix your own blend to use every day; use one-half to 1 teaspoon of essential oil per pint of unscented body lotion or botanical oil, such as sweet almond oil or sunflower oil. For specific ailments, use 1 ounce of a carrier oil to 10 to 20 drops of essential oil, follow a recipe recommended by a trusted expert, or follow the directions of your aromatherapist.

Here are some suggestions to get you started. A muscle sprain or strain can be massaged gently with lavender, juniper, or cypress oil, while varicose veins can be helped with a massage around the affected area with cypress or geranium oil.

Constipation can be treated with a gentle abdominal massage using black pepper, fennel, or marjoram; be sure to massage the area clockwise, from right to left, to follow the path that wastes take through the intestines.

A chest massage with eucalyptus, peppermint, or lavender oil can relieve chest infections, while a neck massage with one of these oils can calm a cough.

Massaging the face with eucalyptus or rosemary oil will clear the sinuses (make sure not to get close to the eyes).

Aromatherapy with massage can also focus on the face to improve circulation and reduce facial tension, bringing greater beauty to the skin. Using oils such as bergamot can help combat acne, while sandalwood is good for dry, dehydrated, or aging skin. Facial massage should be done gently and with upward motions only.

Bathing

Scented baths are a perfect way to enjoy the healing powers of essential oils.

You can take a page from Cleopatra's history and soak in a soothing, rose-infused tub, or get ready to face the day with an uplifting blend of black pepper and juniper. Add a total of 6 to 10 drops of oil to a bathtub full of warm water, and swish the water to mix in the oil.

If your skin is sensitive, or if you are preparing a bath for a child, dilute the essential oil in 1 ounce of carrier oil first, and then add up to 6 drops of the mixture to the tub.

Caution: Skin Irritants

Several of the essential oils are known to irritate the skin when used in baths or massages. People with sensitive skin should avoid these oils when bathing or receiving massages. Other people can use these oils if they are first diluted in a carrier oil before being added to the bath; use only 3 to 4 drops per bath. In massage, these oils should be used in concentrations of no more than 2 percent essential oil to carrier oil.

Irritants in Baths
Irritants in baths and massages include basil, cinnamon leaf, lemon, sweet fennel, lemon grass, Siberian fir needle, verbena, parley seed, melissa, pimenta leaf, peppermint, thyme, and tea tree.

A Simple Way to Use Aromatherapy

One of the easiest ways to use aromatherapy is to simply smell the essential oils, whether directly from the bottle, with steam, in your home with the help of a diffusor or an aromatherapy air freshener, or on your body with a personal perfume. In each case, the aroma is pleasant, and its healing properties are inhaled into the lungs and diffused throughout the body.

Grandma's smelling salts were aromatherapy of a kind; their strong smell of ammonia could rouse almost anyone from a faint. Luckily, using essential oils as inhalants is much more pleasant. Direct inhalation works particularly well for respiratory complaints, stress, emotional conditions, and nausea. You can use a suggested blend or simply select one or more of the oils recommended for treating your specific condition and mix them together in a small glass bottle. Make sure to choose oils with aromas you enjoy. You can either open the bottle and inhale the scent, or you can place 2 or 3 drops on a tissue to inhale periodically throughout the day. Sinus problems respond especially well to steam inhalations, although a mixture of steaming water and essential oils can also be used to treat other respiratory ailments, such as colds and the flu, sore throats, and nervous complaints, such as anxiety and stress.

To prepare a steam inhalation, use a large heat-proof bowl that's been placed securely on a tabletop. Fill it about halfway with steaming water and add between 3 and 6 drops of an essential oil or a blend. Lavender is a good one to start with, because it is effective for anxiety and depression, as well as respiratory problems. Sit comfortably, and place a towel over your head to trap the steam. Inhale deeply for five to ten minutes. Steam is also an effective way to use essential oils to cleanse the complexion.

For normal skin, use frankincense, geranium, jasmine, rose, vetiver, or a combination of several.

For dry skin, bergamot, fennel, geranium, myrrh, and sandalwood are recommended.

Oily skin can benefit from cedarwood, cypress, lemon, orange, peppermint, tea tree, and ylang ylang.

Sensitive skin responds best to chamomile, rose, and rosewood.

Air fresheners and diffusors allow you to perfume your home with healing essential oils.

For everyday use, choose an essential oil or a blend that the whole family enjoys.

In sickrooms, antiseptic, antibacterial, antiviral, and antifungal oils, such as tea tree, eucalyptus, bergamot, and geranium, can help purify and cleanse the air to help control germs.

In the office, you might want to select an antianxiety or antistress aroma, such as lavender, chamomile, or petitgrain.

For an aromatherapy air freshener, mix distilled water with 4 to 10 drops of essential oil per ounce of fluid and pour into a spray bottle. Spray the mixture into the room just as you would any air freshener. Make sure to shake well before each use. Diffusors distribute essential oil molecules into the air. Many of these devices work on electricity; you simply add your chosen oil or blend and plug it in. Others, such as aromatherapy lamps, use a candle to heat a mixture of water and essential oils to disperse the aroma.

To use a lamp, fill the bowl with water and add up to 20 drops of your oil or blend. Then light the candle and enjoy the scent wafting throughout the room.

Making your own personal perfume ensures that you can carry your favorite essential oils anywhere you go. You can choose a suggested blend or create your own by adding up to 20 drops of essential oils that you like to one-eighth of an ounce of jojoba oil. Dab the mixture on your pulse points and enjoy.

Compresses

Hot and cold compresses are often suggested for physical injuries, as well as for aches and pains due to chronic conditions, such as arthritis. By adding appropriate essential oils to these, you can increase their power to heal.

Compresses can relieve pain and reduce swelling and inflammation. Hot compresses are best for chronic conditions, particularly for backaches, arthritis, toothaches, and earaches. Cold compresses are an important first-aid measure for sprains; they also help to relieve headaches and, when used on large portions of the body, can help bring down a fever.

Often practitioners suggest alternating hot and cold compresses, once the initial injury care with cold compresses is complete. This helps sprains and strains to heal.

To make a hot compress, fill a bowl with water as hot as possible while still being bearable to the touch. Add 5 to 7 drops of an essential oil—try black pepper, chamomile, coriander, or a blend. Dip into the bowl a clean cloth folded several times to absorb more fluid, making sure to absorb the essential oils floating on top of the water. Wring the excess water from the cloth and apply it to the affected area. Replace with a fresh compress when the first one cools to room temperature.

For a cold compress, substitute ice water for the hot and prepare the same way. Change compresses when the one in use warms up to body temperature.

Mouthwashes and Gargles

Aromatherapy mouth treatments are helpful for a variety of problems, including mouth ulcers and gum disease. They can also be used on a daily basis for oral hygiene. Oils such as myrrh, rose, and tea tree are good for gingivitis, while cypress and tea tree oils can help heal and prevent bleeding gums. Myrrh, basil, bergamot, and tea tree oils are helpful for healing mouth ulcers.

The appropriate oils can be used either as a mouthwash/gargle or in oil for a gum massage.

To make a mouthwash, dissolve 3 to 5 drops of oil into a teaspoon of vodka, and then stir the mixture into a half-cup of warm distilled water. You may want to add a drop of peppermint oil to your recipe to improve the flavor. After brushing your teeth, or as needed, swish the mouthwash around in your mouth. To supplement the mouthwash, you may use a gum-massage oil. In a glass bottle with a dropper, mix one-fourth of an ounce of carrier oil with 20 to 25 drops of the desired essential oils, including 1 drop of peppermint or fennel for flavor. Before each use, turn the bottle upside down several times to mix, and then rub a few drops onto your gums.

Custom Hair and Skin Care

Women and men can easily include aromatherapy in their everyday cleansing routines by adding a few drops of essential oils to unscented shampoos, conditioners, lotions, and cleansers. The proper oils can help ease dryness or oiliness in your skin or scalp, assist in the regeneration of skin cells, improve the circulation of blood to your skin, and improve the condition of your hair. Make sure to choose high-quality base products, with no fragrance already added. Then add 8 to 10 drops of essential oil per ounce of product. Rose, jasmine, lavender, and neroli are good oils for normal or dry skin; dry skin can also benefit from fennel, benzoin, and cedarwood.

Oily skin is best treated with juniper, patchouli, peppermint, tea tree, and ylang ylang.

Aging skin responds well to myrrh and helichrysum; for sensitive skin, stick to chamomile, jasmine, rose, or rosewood.

For use on the hair, people with oily hair have the most choices; they can try bergamot, cypress, clary sage, juniper, pine, rosemary, tea tree, and lemon.

Dry hair responds well to chamomile, lavender, and rosemary; try a mix of the three. Normal hair can use lavender, chamomile, thyme, and ylang ylang.

To clear up dandruff, add tea tree, cedarwood, rosemary, and pine.

Besides using essential oils in prepared products, you can also add your chosen varieties to jojoba oil for a deep-conditioning treatment. Use 10 drops in 1 ounce of jojoba oil and leave on the hair overnight, if possible, or at least for half an hour. Then shampoo.

Using Essential Oils

To get started in aromatherapy, you, of course, need essential oils. But which to choose? High-quality oils can be expensive, and it's worthwhile to select oils that both meet your personal needs and are as versatile as possible.

For general use, focus on ten basic oils: rose, rosemary, peppermint, tea tree, lemon, eucalyptus, lavender, sandalwood, juniper, and rose geranium. These ten oils can be blended or used singly, as you desire. Of course, if you have a specific condition that calls for a special oil in treatment, add that one to the list. One caveat is worth mentioning here. Generally, if you do not like the scent of an essential oil, do not use it. Trust your nose to guide you to the essential oils that will be most beneficial to you.

And, as with any treatment, care is called for in aromatherapy. As previously mentioned, never ingest essential oils on your own initiative. Always dilute essential oils before applying them to the skin. And if you experience any discomfort, skin irritation, or sensitivity, stop using that particular oil.

Certain medical conditions require extra caution. If you are pregnant, consult your doctor before using aromatherapy. Likewise if you have cancer, asthma, high or low blood pressure, or epilepsy, or if you are taking any medications—prescription or over-the-counter. In addition, if you are using homeopathic remedies, aromatherapy can diminish their effects. Avoid using essential oils if you are under homeopathic care, or check with a homeopathic practitioner.

Whether you choose to use aromatherapy occasionally or every day, we think you'll find that it's a welcome addition. Sinking into a relaxing aromatherapy bath at the end of a long day's work or indulging in a weekly aromatherapy massage will not only help your body and mind, it will also soothe your spirit.

Of course, even frequent aromatherapy can't counteract the effects of a poor diet, a sedentary lifestyle, or a stressed-out approach to life. Whether you're trying to overcome a specific physical or mental problem or you're just seeking greater overall health, use aromatherapy to complement your good eating and exercise habits.

> Never apply essential oils before going out in the sun. Oils such as bergamot, cold-pressed lime, neroli, lemon, grapefruit, angelica root, cumin, ginger, lovage, and verbena can cause sun sensitivity.

Choosing and Storing Aromatherapy Supplies/Buying Oils

Because the key ingredient in aromatherapy is the essential oil, properly selecting your oils is paramount. Here are a few tips for buying wisely: Choose only pure essential oils. Though scientists have learned to create quite lifelike aromas in the laboratory, these substances are made from petroleum by-products, not plants. If that isn't enough to convince you of their uselessness in aromatherapy, consider this: In each essential oil are dozens of chemical compounds, many of which are present in only trace amounts. Synthetic scents may imitate the smell but can never replicate the exact molecular makeup of healing essential oils. And don't be fooled by "nature-identical" labels. If it doesn't say "pure essential oil," don't buy it.

Trust your nose. It sounds simplistic, but it's true: If you don't like the smell of an essential oil, it isn't likely to help you—even if it is recommended for your particular ailment.

God has been gracious in giving us alternatives. Simply choose another recommended oil that's more pleasing to you.

Consider the source. Buy only from reputable suppliers; well-established natural food stores are one good choice. If you're in doubt, consult a qualified aromatherapist for suggestions. Consider the price. Sadly, some manufacturers dilute essential oils with carrier oils or mix them with synthetics, without labeling them as such. A tip: A drop of pure essential oil placed on a tissue will evaporate completely without leaving any trace of oil. If a greasy spot is left behind, the oil has been adulterated.

But you may be able to tell the difference without even opening the bottle. The prices of true essential oils vary widely, according to the difficulty of extracting the pure plant oils from their host plants. Rose oil, for example, should be quite a bit more expensive than lavender oil because many pounds of rose petals are required to make just one ounce of rose oil. If a manufacturer sells all of its oils for the same price, or if its prices are substantially lower than those of other manufacturers, chances are the products are adulterated or otherwise inferior.

Essential Oil Care

Once you've bought your precious essential oils, be sure to store and use them properly to preserve their healing properties. Most oils will keep well for a year or more.

Keep your oils in a cool, dry place in dark glass bottles. Never allow your oils to stand in a damp environment or near light or heat.

Avoid touching the inside of the bottle cap, the rim of the bottle, or the dropper to your skin or to any other surface. This will help prevent contamination.

Uncap your oils only long enough to release the amount of oil you need. The oils are extremely volatile and will evaporate quickly.

Choosing Carrier Products

Second only to the quality of the essential oils in aromatherapy is the quality of the carrier oils, the lotions, and other products you use. As with essential oils, buy from a reputable supplier and read the labels carefully. Store all of your aromatherapy oils in the refrigerator, and allow them to come to room temperature before use.

Make sure to choose products that contain no additives.

Choose unscented, cold-pressed, organic vegetable oils.

Unrefined oils are preferred over refined oils.

Avoid mineral oil, which is a petroleum product, and coconut oil, which has molecules too large to be absorbed into the skin.

Be aware of the shelf life of the oils you purchase. Buy small quantities of oils that go rancid quickly and larger quantities only of those with a longer life. Different types of carrier oils are preferred for different uses.

Following is a selection of carrier oils and their properties:

Almond oil is often used in aromatherapy massage; it also relieves itching and inflammation. It spoils quickly, however.

Apricot kernel oil is a rich oil full of vitamin A, which is often used for dry, mature, sensitive, and dehydrated skin.

Avocado oil contains lots of vitamins A and E, so it is very helpful for skin problems. Its richness makes it especially valuable for mixing with other oils. It goes rancid quickly.

Canola oil is a light, penetrating oil that keeps well and works well in blends for massage and the skin.

Evening primrose oil is often used in beauty products because it promotes skin repair and health and helps prevent premature aging. It does spoil easily, however.

Flaxseed oil is full of vitamin E, making it valuable for skin healing and regeneration. It spoils quickly.

Grapeseed oil is a good choice for oily or acne-prone skin because it is light and slightly astringent.

Hazelnut oil helps skin maintain firmness and elasticity. It is expensive.

Jojoba oil, which is actually a wax ester, softens and moisturizes skin while helping to control acne and oily skin. Its antioxidant benefits extend to other oils with which it is mixed; it can extend the shelf life of your blends.

Olive oil has been used for centuries to beautify the skin and the hair, and its benefits are still recognized today. It mixes well with other carrier oils.

Sunflower oil is high in vitamin E and is good for sensitive skin.

Vitamin E oil is renowned for its skin-healing properties. It is best blended with other carrier oils; make sure to buy natural vitamin E, not synthetic.

Emergency Situations

Irritated Skin: To relieve skin irritated from essential oils, wash with soap and water or a mild detergent. If the rash does not clear up in a few days, seek medical attention. If there is blistering, seek medical attention right away.

Essential oil in the eyes: Place a small drop of plain carrier oil (e.g., olive oil) into the affected eye(s). The carrier oil helps to absorb the essential oil. Rinse with water and pat with a cloth. Seek medical attention immediately to have the eyes examined.

Sick and nauseated: If you become sick, nauseated, confused, or get a headache from the essential oils, then breathe some fresh air. Your symptoms should improve immediately and over the next couple of hours. If there is no improvement, seek medical attention.

If a child swallows an essential oil: Call 911 immediately. Do not try to induce vomiting.

Traditional Chinese Medicine: Acupuncture and Acupressure

Introduction

Traditional Chinese Medicine (TCM) is rooted deep in China's ancient past and has developed entwined with one of the world's oldest and most profound philosophies. At first glance by a Westerner, much of it may seem puzzling and alien, but a student of Chinese medicine can quickly gain an understanding of its basic tenets, as well as many practical remedies to ensure better health and prevent disease.

Few branches of alternative health care offer the wealth of experience associated with Chinese medicine. More than four thousand years ago, the healers in Chinese society began to experiment with various herbs to see which could cure physical and mental complaints. And not all their remedies came from plants. The medicines included a variety of minerals and animal extracts woven into a fantastic set of potions that were thought to have "magical powers."

Over the ensuing years, Chinese medicine grew up hand in hand with Chinese philosophy, following the Way, or the Tao, in search of simplicity and harmony in all things. For the Chinese physician, it was as important to understand the works of the philosopher Lao Tzu ("The Old Master," considered a contemporary of Confucius) as it was to study the collected masterworks of medicine. Central to this philosophy was the inevitability of change.

Meanwhile, in the laboratory of human experience, Chinese practitioners were able to test various remedies, losing much of the so-called magic as they improved their knowledge of medicine. But they made progress without using dissection, which was forbidden in Chinese society. As a result, TCM's anatomy is more figurative than literal and does not correspond to the body in ways that Westerners expect.

Through experimentation, they built a complex and rich tradition that extends to acupuncture, acupressure, Qigong, and Tai Chi. New methods of care were developed and systematically inscribed in their vast materia medica, the encyclopedic volumes listing TCM remedies.

From this combination of philosophy and trial and error, Chinese practitioners developed a holistic approach to treating patients that is all too often lacking in the West. By learning more about human nature and emphasizing harmony and balance as the source of good health, they were able not just to treat an illness, but to teach the patient about the importance of good nutrition, preventive remedies, and a balanced outlook on life that would help prevent disease from recurring.

Contemporary practitioners of Chinese medicine will begin much the same way Chinese physicians did thousands of years ago: watching, asking questions, observing the tongue and the skin, assessing personality traits, and listening carefully to the patient before making a diagnosis and devising a treatment.

Today we know that Traditional Chinese Medicine offers many practical *and long proven safe* remedies to some of our most common ailments. Over the last generation, we've seen a number of these practices gain widespread respect in the West for the benefits they offer everyone the world over. Chinese physicians' work on nutrition plays an important role in Chinese medicine, and we're seeing a growing number of independent clinical studies back up their claims. In addition, we're routinely discovering new uses for TCM that would surprise even an ancient practitioner.

The growing confidence in this field in the West has led to important attitudinal shifts in the uses of Chinese medicine. While Westerners were glad to begin using Chinese remedies for conditions like the flu, allergies, or menstrual cramps, only recently have we begun to see the possibilities in acute cases, such as heavy bleeding, appendicitis, and dangerously high fevers.

History

By the time Hippocrates began laying down the basic philosophy of Western medicine 2,500 years ago, Chinese medicine was already widely accepted and practiced. A coherent Chinese history, in both politics and medicine, reaches back to some 3,000 years B.C.

The oldest record of herbal remedies dates to the beginning of the Han Dynasty (206 B.C. to 220 A.D.). *Huang Di Nei Jing,* or *The Yellow Emperor's Inner Classic,* now almost two thousand years old, is one of the oldest medical texts still in use today. Scholars believe that it was compiled over a period of centuries. Written as a dialogue between the Yellow Emperor and Qi Bo, his leading minister, it is required reading for the serious student of Chinese medicine.

Like the *Huang Di Nei Jing,* the other weighty volumes that form the backbone of Chinese medical practice reflect many centuries of compilation and review. As leading healers tried new variations of herbal remedies, they carefully noted the effects and developed new forms of treatment.

Early on, Chinese medicine included many exotic remedies to cure people afflicted by demons. Magical potions mixed from herbs, minerals, and animal parts were concocted to influence the spirits. Remedies were often linked with alchemy and astrology. Many were based on astrological observations or relied on numerology to provide answers to a patient's health problems.

By the time of the Han Dynasty, such primitive magic had given way to a new system of medicine, based on careful observation. But TCM was not separated completely from its ancient past. Consider the number five. Han astronomers could identify five planets circling the earth. Five vital elements—fire, wood, earth, water and metal—constituted the primary building blocks of the planet. And five developed into one of the most important numbers in Chinese medicine, as physicians sought to understand the complex interaction of forces that influenced their patients' health.

They often would mix five different herbs to treat a disease, a practice that extends to the present day.

Near the end of the Han Dynasty, Zhang Zhong-Jing wrote *Discussion of Cold-Induced Disorders and Miscellaneous Diseases*. Many of the herbal remedies included in this classic of Chinese medicine are still in use today.

New volumes examining various remedies, herbal and otherwise, came along, and today those books are part of the classic TCM library. Chinese medicine grew to encompass not only herbal remedies for illnesses, but also forms of exercise and massage that could help heal the sick and prevent disease. Acupuncture developed into its own highly technical discipline.

After the Chinese Communists seized power fifty years ago, TCM experienced a brief period of decline, as its emphasis on the Tao and classic remedies came in confrontation with Western medicine. But within a decade, the Communists bowed to history and accepted TCM as an important practice.

In recent years, TCM has gained acceptance in the West as well. The areas of TCM that have translated best in the West include therapies that are widely respected for their clear health benefits.

Over the past two thousand years, Chinese herbalism has grown from a handful of notations in the *Inner Classic* to more than five thousand substances listed in the *Encyclopedia of Traditional Chinese Medicinal Substances*, gathered at the Jiangsu College of New Medicine.

Adherents of Tai Chi and Qigong, ancient methods of exercise aimed at restoring the natural balance in body and mind, are believed to have developed many of their key movements after observing them in the animal world. Practiced by millions around the globe, they are daily rituals for people seeking to restore physical and mental harmony.

Acupressure and acupuncture were subjected to the same system of trial and error, as Chinese physicians experimented to see which remedies carried lasting cures. Gradually, the sharpened bones used by the first acupuncturists were replaced by more carefully designed instruments.

Today, acupuncture and acupressure have gained widespread use in the West, even gaining the blessing of some insurance companies.

No other medical system in the world has the same wealth of historical experience to draw upon. And although many Western observers find the symbolic nature of TCM too fanciful, we are drawn back to Chinese medicine because of its repeatedly proven ability to heal the sick and keep the healthy well.

For many millennia, Chinese physicians relied on empirical research to back up their claims, cataloguing cures of chronic pain through acupuncture or the effect of Chinese herbal remedies on fever or fatigue. Of course, we're also learning through repeated clinical studies that many of TCM's herbal remedies, acupressure, and acupuncture have scientifically provable benefits. TCM has, in turn, had a profound effect on Western herbalism.

In TCM and Chinese philosophy, this balance is represented by yin and yang, complementary qualities that exist together in all things. Yin is cool or cold, fall and winter, wet and passive. Yang is its opposite: warm or hot, spring and summer, vibrant and dry. Yin is also bright and light; yang is dark. Yin is light; yang is heavy.

Just as the seasons change, cooling and heating the earth in turn, so do other elements. In each case, yin and yang are constantly transforming as the pendulum swings from one to the other. This concept is represented in the symbol for yin and yang, black and white that flow around and into each other.

The Yin/Yang Symbol

The curve dividing the circle indicates that yin and yang continuously flow together. They blend and transform into one another, creating peace and harmonic homeostasis. The small dots of opposite color indicate that nothing is strictly yin or yang, but rather there is a small element of the opposite in each entity, creating balance in life.

Meridians

TCM believes that qi (pronounced *chee* and also spelled "chi") energizes us as individuals, as well as the world around us; it is constantly in motion. Within our bodies, Chinese physicians have identified channels, or meridians, that circulate qi in much the same way that blood is circulated through veins.

But don't go looking for any physical evidence of meridians. These meridians are invisible, yet within TCM, they are the most important elements in a person's health. TCM views meridians, or *jing luo,* as crucial, because they are responsible for transmitting the essential life force, qi, throughout the body.

Over the centuries, Chinese physicians identified twelve main meridians and supporting channels that branch throughout the body. Each of the main meridians corresponds to a major organ and links organs, muscles, and all the body's many parts.

The Chinese physician relies on these meridians to treat the body. Herbal remedies are processed initially by the stomach, but their essential force is channeled through meridians to reach an affected organ. The energy created there goes on to improve the functions of related organs and to improve your health along the way.

Acupuncturists are trained to play the harmonic nature of the meridians with needles, seeking particular points that will in turn lead to a vital organ. In this way, they play your body much the same way you might use a bow to play the violin, and they seek to tune your system so that it plays the sweetest music. Or you may choose to treat yourself with acupressure, using fingers in place of needles to find the points that lead you to peace and rejuvenation.

Many Westerners have sought to tie the meridians to the body's nervous system, hoping to explain the clear benefits of acupuncture in clinical terms. Unfortunately for the literal minded, Chinese physicians are quick to point out that meridians are charted through areas where the nervous system could not be affected. Even without the link, though, Western acupuncturists have gained widespread acceptance for their treatment measures.

Just as we wouldn't be able to illuminate portions of our home without an electrical system, life itself would be impossible without meridians, according to Chinese philosophy, to channel qi throughout our systems.

Acupuncture

Acupuncture quickly assumed a vital role in Chinese medicine, offering a way to regulate the flow of qi in the meridians. Acupressure and acupuncture are very similar in the way that they stimulate the same points to encourage the flow of energy and relief from stress and pain.

But acupuncture picks up where the milder acupressure leaves off and can offer lasting relief for people with chronic pain.

In the early days, acupuncture needles were made from sharpened slivers of bone or bamboo, inserted into one of many acupuncture points linked along the meridians to the organs and identified because of their therapeutic properties in certain disorders. Today those needles are made from stainless steel or come with copper-coated tops. Some physicians prefer to use silver or gold needles. Most practitioners, in fact, have adopted the Western practice of using disposable needles. In the West, disposable needles are the preferred choice.

Today acupuncture is used to treat a whole range of modern maladies. The uses of acupuncture extend to backaches, colds, angina, headaches, tinnitus, glaucoma, tonsillitis, sunstroke, asthma, impotence, and psoriasis, to name only a few conditions. While it may not offer a cure-all for cancer or AIDS, acupuncture can help relieve many of the painful symptoms and the effects of the modern therapies used for those diseases. More and more of our colleagues are adding it to their list of useful therapies.

Acupuncture is most often used in the West to treat chronic conditions, but it is occasionally used to treat certain acute disorders. Within TCM, though, acupuncture is routinely used to help fine-tune the system and restore balance.

Think of an acupuncturist as a piano tuner, carefully checking each of the ivory and ebony keys and adjusting any sour note to conform to its harmonic whole. In our view, this is even more important today, as we deal with an ever-rising level of stress in our modern world. We need "new," yet tested, ways to dissolve the damaging array of stressors to which we are continually subjected.

Some sites on the body's map of meridians and acupuncture points, particularly at our extremities, are associated with treatments for specific disorders. The most commonly punctured points are between the elbows and the fingertips and between the toes and the knees.

Extremely fine needles are used for thin-skinned patients, while someone who is particularly fleshy may call for somewhat thicker needles. Needles also vary in length, from half an inch to three inches. In no case should the procedure cause pain. Most patients describe the feeling as a tingling sensation, though some people remark that a numbness may set in at the insertion point.

In all cases, a variety of points will be selected and needles inserted, often leaving the hand or some other extremity looking like a pincushion.

In order to help stimulate energy flow, a practitioner may occasionally stroke a needle, rotate it, or flick it with a finger. Some acupuncturists have elected to connect their needles to a small electric stimulator, which sends a slight electric charge through the needles into the tissue. The technique varies from one acupuncturist to the next, and for each patient.

There are now several Western theories to explain the undeniable benefits of acupuncture. Under the neurotransmitter theory, Western scientists postulate that these needles inhibit spinal cord nerve cells and release beta-endorphins and other substances that deaden pain and relieve patients.

Acupuncture, they theorize, also helps to stimulate anti-inflammatory cell activity, increase skin temperature, and stimulate the flow of blood.

Qualifications

When seeking an acupuncturist, look for someone who's thoroughly trained and certified. In China, acupuncturists are expected to complete a five-year course, which includes two years of herbal medicine. In the West, an acupuncturist should have completed at least a three-year course.

Other scientists have studied the interaction of copper and steel needles, suggesting that these metals create an electromagnetic field that can stimulate positive and negative ions. Acupuncturists refer to this as tonification and dispersal.

Treatment times will vary, according to the patient. A healthy adult may be left with needles inserted for up to twenty minutes. A child may be in and out in a matter of minutes.

In the East, some acute cases will be treated daily. Chronic conditions may call for visits once a week or every other week. Of course, periodic visits will allow the acupuncturist keep qi in harmony and prevent other disorders that lead to disease.

Acupressure

Never underestimate the healing power of human hands. The doctrine of the laying on of hands is based on sound principles.

Who among us hasn't massaged our temples to soothe a headache or asked a spouse to rub our back or feet to relieve tension and ease pain? Naturally, in the empirical system of Chinese medicine, this type of treatment would come in for a significant amount of study.

Thousands of years ago, Chinese doctors noticed that something beneficial was happening with massage. These traditional physicians wanted to define this benefit and harness its powers into an understandable therapy that could be taught to others. Over the years, this therapy became known as acupressure, which is closely related to acupuncture.

Understood properly, acupressure will help you treat many of the most common complaints of the modern age. We spend long hours at work, often sitting in uncomfortable chairs that encourage bad posture. We suffer from stress-related tension, bad diets, and virtually no exercise. It's no wonder, then, that the body responds with back and stomach aches and a whole gamut of additional pains, from head to toe.

Acupressure is one of the oldest, if not the oldest, self-practiced form of therapy in the world. And just as someone in China saw the benefits of acupressure more than four thousand years ago, you can also be helped by this ancient brand of TCM.

One of the most frequently diagnosed problems in Chinese medicine is stuck or stagnant qi, indicating a blockage in the healthy flow of vital energy through the network of meridians. This disharmony is manifested by all the aches and pains that I've just described.

Utilizing the same knowledge of meridians and diagnostic methods used in all branches of TCM, acupressure treats these symptoms by manipulating the acupressure points that will ease pain and release stagnant qi.

By manipulating these points with the hands and the fingers, applying pressure along crucial meridians, you can release endorphins and other natural substances in your body that block pain. By stimulating the flow of blood, you will also soothe sore muscles and relax the body, promoting the body's natural ability to heal itself.

One of the most frequently observed symptoms of stress is chest tension and difficulty breathing. An acupressurist knows which points need to be manipulated to relieve the tension and restore healthy breathing.

In the process, acupressure releases toxins that are built up in the body's tissues. It is always a good idea to flush these toxins with plenty of fluids after each session.

As the traditional Chinese physician always sought to treat the whole person and not just a particular disease, it was quickly noted that someone receiving acupressure not only found his or her body become relaxed but also felt day-to-day cares slip away as the mind was freed from immediate distractions and could resume its former acuity with peace.

The applications of acupressure are too numerous to list here, but let's consider a few. Sports medicine, for example, often incorporates acupressure to relieve the damage caused during a game or in practice. Many of these techniques date back to Chinese battlefields, when warriors noted that certain types of body contact would actually relieve some chronic pains.

Acupressure is an ancient form of beauty therapy as well. Certain facial massages can relax your features, easing old worry lines and preventing new ones from forming.

To begin, you may want to apply either firm pressure, a slow circular massage, or a hard rubbing motion to stimulate the point, depending on the desired physical response.

When you apply pressure, you can use your fingers, knuckles, palm, or thumbs.

As you gain more experience, you can try various methods to see which works best for you.

By applying pressure for about thirty seconds to one minute, you help ease pain, relieve stress, and calm your nervous system.

Slower circular motions are used on pressure points to sedate or stimulate them. By rhythmically squeezing and releasing these muscle groups (like kneading bread), you relieve stiffness and work on constipation and muscle spasms.

When you want to increase the flow of qi, use a harsh rubbing motion. It helps to heat the body and reduce swelling. Anyone who's been out in the cold too long and has come inside rubbing his or her frozen hands knows what we are talking about here.

Finally, you may find that tapping an acupressure point will stimulate the muscles in that area. You may want to use your fingers or a loosely balled fist, depending on how close the muscle groups are to the body's surface.

Over the years, Chinese physicians came to identify 365 acupressure points, the same ones used in acupuncture, which in turn lie along the body's meridians.

In the meticulous fashion of TCM, each point was named according to the benefit it offered.

Standard Meridian Abbreviations

Lu	Lung	K	Kidney
LI	Large Intestine	P	Pericardium
Sp	Spleen	B	Bladder
TW	Triple Warmer	GB	Gallbladder
St	Stomach	Lv	Liver
SI	Small Intestine	GV	Governing Vessel
H	Heart	EX	Extra Point
CV	Conception Vessel		

Basic Acupressure Techniques

- Locate the pressure point(s) from the illustrations that have been provided.
- Go to the designated areas and feel for the tender point.
- Use the corner of your thumb pad for rotating procedures or the entire pad to apply direct pressure. Also, fingers and knuckles can be used to apply direct pressure. You can tap on points using the index finger, instead of applying direct pressure, or you can knead muscle areas as if kneading dough.
- Use a slow, steady movement.

- Work the pressure points on both the right and the left corresponding positions, when applicable.
- Each pressure point treatment should last from ten to thirty seconds. Repeat the procedure five times.
- If the problem is acute (quick onset, short term), you can massage these points two to three times a day until symptoms subside.
- If it is a chronic problem, you can treat it once a day for a longer period of time for relief of pain or for respiratory or nervous disorders.

Common Acupressure Points

Take the Sea of Vitality Point (B23, B47). By seating yourself comfortably and manipulating its point at the lower left of your back, you may find it helpful to focus on your energy reserves filling back up again. In addition, Sea of Vitality can help alleviate acne or the ache of bruises elsewhere on your body.

Under each cheekbone, directly under the eyes, lies the Facial Beauty Point (ST3). Massaging this area can also relieve acne, stimulate your facial skin, and improve the tone of your skin.

On the top of your head between the cranial bones lies the One Hundred Meeting Point (GI20). You find it by tracing your fingers from the back of each ear to the top of the back of your head. Press at this point to help relieve stress and headache pain while restoring clear thinking and concentration.

Below the base of the skull lies the Gates of Consciousness Points (GB20), which can also improve concentration and memory and relieve pain.

Joining the Valley Point (LI4) offers some quick relief for frontal headaches and shoulder pain. It is also effective for labor pain, which is why you need to avoid it if you may be pregnant; it can stimulate premature contractions. In the angle that lies at the top of the hand between the thumb and the forefinger lies the Joining the Valley Point. Apply appropriate pressure to bear on this point, and you can feel your headache draining away.

In one of the simplest and most effective maneuvers in the books, you can take your forefinger and place it firmly between your eyebrows, pressing for several minutes. This *yintang* point will clear your head and relieve many headaches. Oftentimes, the affected pressure point is tender to touch. In this case, massage around this spot.

If you ever visit an acupressurist, you'll see that the physician doesn't just use the muscles in his hand to apply pressure. An experienced practitioner will lean into the massage point, using body weight to apply pressure. You'll find that this is just as effective when you work on your own points, as you are being asked to apply strong pressure for several minutes to each point.

You're not asked to deal with a lot of pain here. If you experience too much discomfort, ease up on the pressure or the rubbing.

Acupressure points of the head, front and side views

A session can last anywhere from a few minutes to a full hour, and you may want to experiment by practicing acupressure in a sitting or lying down position. Take long, deep breaths as you engage in acupressure. By balancing your breath, you help balance the body. Open yourself to the healing powers of acupressure, and clear your mind of daily clutter.

In order to give yourself the full benefits of acupressure, develop your own schedule for healing touch sessions. You can designate a spot in your office or at home. Make sure you follow through with a routine session at least once a day—more often, if it helps. Just exactly what kind of schedule you keep will be up to you and what you hope to achieve, whether it's reducing mild stress or dealing with chronic pain.

If you'd like to gain some help at acupressure, consider tracking down a specialist in acupressure massage. An acupressure masseur will start at the top of the back and gradually work downward, applying pressure with the thumb or the whole hand.

As with any professional massage, the subject experiences the exquisite pain of strong hands and is often left spent and rested.

As always, there are plenty of don'ts to be considered along with the do's.

- Don't get too strenuous while pregnant. You should check with a qualified acupressurist before using any points to see which exercises are helpful, though, as acupressure can relieve many of the aches and pains associated with pregnancy and childbirth. Make sure you moderate the finger pressure during pregnancy as well. Acupuncture at this time is not an option, as overstimulation of these points can trigger contractions.

- Certain sensitive areas, like portions of the throat or the groin, should be either avoided or only gently touched. Remember, you should never experience any excessive pain from this procedure.

- Burns, injuries, or any other physically damaged region should be allowed to heal before treating the area with acupressure. That is particularly true for fractured or broken bones, as well as for disk injuries and severe back pain. A physician should deal with injuries.

- Always remember that you're more vulnerable to cold after each session. You may need to put on an extra sweater or a sweatshirt to guard against the cold while staying comfortable.

Other than taking commonsense precautions, though, I think you'll find that acupressure can often be useful as an ongoing method of self-treatment. It's just as relevant today as it was to the ancient Chinese.

Many acupressure experts suggest that you keep a diary of your activities: by tracking your symptoms, you will be able to log your progress. Obviously, many conditions, like cancer or appendicitis, can only be peripherally treated by acupressure. But don't underestimate its long-term healing powers.

While Western pharmaceutical companies compete in the hunt for ever-more-expensive drugs, this is one class of treatment that is free for all.

Acupressure points of the upper body, front view

Acupressure points of the legs, front view

Acupressure points of the upper body, back view

B54

B54

B60

B60

Acupressure points of the legs, back view

LU1

LI11

TW5

LI4

LI3

Acupressure points of the upper body, side view

Acupressure points of the legs, side view

Hydrotherapy

Hydrotherapy is a type of bodywork that uses water as a healing agent. It can involve water in the form of a liquid, a solid, or a vapor. Water is used as a stimulus to improve energy levels and resistance to disease. The manipulation of your blood's circulation by using hydrotherapy can help many ailments, such as fevers, bronchitis, headaches, sinusitis, colds, insomnia, and various other conditions. Although a gentle treatment, hydrotherapy can have profound health benefits. In addition, hydrotherapy is an effective way to stimulate the immune system, optimize circulation, and promote detoxification.

History

The use of water as a healing tool has been recorded since ancient times. Records found from the Egyptians and the Babylonians are filled with descriptions about various forms of hydrotherapy. Ancient Greeks and Romans placed a high priority on baths for healing and disease prevention. Vincent Priessnitz, who lived from 1799 to 1852, was one of the most influential people in the hydrotherapy movement. As a boy, he observed how injured animals instinctively went to a nearby creek to let the cold, flowing water heal their injuries. Priessnitz experimented with various forms of hydrotherapy as a boy growing up on a farm in Europe. At age seventeen, he was run over by a wagon and pronounced untreatable by a local surgeon. Using hydrotherapy, he was able to recover from his broken ribs. From that point on, people came from around the country for his famed hydrotherapy treatments. Later in life, the Austrian emperor gave him a gold medal for civic merit. Father Sebastian Kneipp (1821–1897) was also a famous advocate of hydrotherapy, devising approximately 120 different uses of water for healing. His hydrotherapy treatments are still used by spas and clinics in Europe today.

Constitutional Hydrotherapy

The most powerful of the hydrotherapy treatments is constitutional hydrotherapy. It has been named constitutional since it has benefits to the entire constitution of a person.

1. Optimizes circulation
2. Detoxifies and purifies the blood

676

3. Enhances digestive function and elimination
4. Tonifies and balances the nervous system
5. Stimulates and enhances the immune system

It is particularly helpful for people suffering from digestive problems; respiratory problems, such as sore throats and bronchitis; or infections, such as a cold or the flu. *Note:* If a child has asthma, this procedure should be used only under the guidance of a physician.

FREQUENCY OF TREATMENT

Acute conditions: one to two times daily

Chronic conditions: five to seven times weekly

DIRECTIONS

Note: This treatment is best done with the help of an assistant.

1. The person lies in bed on his or her back.
2. An assistant covers the bared chest and the abdomen with two thicknesses of towels that had been placed in hot water and wrung out (wet towels can be heated in the microwave). Towels should be hot, yet tolerable, for children. Place a small section of the towel on the child first to make sure it is not too hot.
3. Cover the hot towels with a dry towel.
4. Cover the person with blankets to prevent the individual from getting chilled. Leave the towels on for five minutes.
5. After five minutes, remove the hot towels and replace with a single thickness of a thin towel that has been run under cold water and then wrung out (with some moisture left in the towel).
6. Place the cold towel on the bared chest and the abdomen. Cover with a dry towel and blankets. Leave on for ten minutes. The towel should be warm after ten minutes. If not, leave it on longer, or do not make the towel so cold or wet next time.
7. Take cold towel off, and have the person turn over and lie on the stomach. Repeat the same procedure on the back. Five minutes of hot towels, followed by ten minutes of a thin cold towel.

HOW IT WORKS

The alternation in hot and cold increases the immune system's white blood cells to help fight off infections. It also increases circulation to the digestive organs and other organs of elimination.

Foot Hydrotherapy

A more simple treatment than constitutional hydrotherapy, foot hydrotherapy helps to relieve respiratory congestion, headaches, and insomnia.

FREQUENCY OF TREATMENT

Acute conditions: one to two times daily

Chronic conditions: once daily

DIRECTIONS

1. Sit on a chair or a couch and place both feet in a bucket of warm water (make sure it is tolerable, if for a child) for five to ten minutes.
2. Remove your feet from the water and dry them.
3. Put on a pair of cotton socks that had been placed in cold water and wrung out.
4. Cover with a pair of wool socks (or cotton, if wool is not available).
5. Leave the socks on for a half hour or longer. You should be resting now and can even go to sleep with the socks on.

Comment: The foot hydrotherapy works by diverting blood flow to the feet and away from the upper body, thus reducing congestion.

Headache Treatment

You can alleviate a headache simply by putting your feet in warm water and placing an ice pack around your neck. This hot-cold water strategy causes blood to move away from the head toward the feet, relieving the head of congestion and pain.

Natural Hormones

Introduction

Hormones have been used as a form of medicine for centuries. Ancient Chinese texts describe how the elderly rejuvenated their sex lives with the use of natural hormones. Today, specific hormones are available as dietary supplements, and many holistic doctors recommend a variety of natural hormones in the prevention and the treatment of disease. Throughout this book, you will find specific conditions that can be prevented or improved with the help of natural hormone therapy. This section explains what natural hormones are and how to best use them.

The Study That Awakened the Establishment

Natural hormones have gained a lot of attention since July 2002. During this time, the *Journal of the American Medical Association* reported on a study known as the Women's Health Initiative. The study involved over 16,000 healthy women and was supposed to run until the year 2005. However, it was stopped prematurely, as investigators found significant increases in the women's risk of developing coronary heart disease, stroke, blood clots, and breast cancer. The only positive note was a reduction in the risk of colorectal cancer and fracture rates. However, researchers concluded that the harm from using the synthetic hormone replacement Premarin and Provera combination, known as Prempro, outweighed the benefit. After this information was released, many doctors and medical establishments recommended that women strongly consider discontinuing its use as a synthetic hormone replacement. This left many women in a quandary about what to do, because most of them were not offered any other options.

The Natural Choice

Holistic physicians have used natural hormones for several decades now. We define the term *natural hormone* as a hormone that is identical to what is produced and utilized in the human body. It is that simple. If a hormone does not have the identical structure to the one found in the human body, we classify it as "synthetic." The cells in our bodies were designed to be compatible with the hormones we naturally produce. On the other hand, synthetic hormones are recognized differently by our cell receptors and may initiate a different action, as compared to a natural version of the same hormone.

Perhaps the best example to illustrate this is to look at the widely prescribed estrogen hormone Premarin. This estrogen prescription is derived from the urine of horses—pregnant mares, to be exact. Now, one may think that the estrogen from a horse is natural, seeing as it is found in "Nature." However, many of the estrogens in Premarin are foreign to the human body. According to the *Physician's Desk Reference,* Premarin contains a group of estrogens known as equilins. This includes equilin, 17-dihydroequilin, equilenin, and 17-dihydroequilenin. These types of estrogens are not found in the human body. How the human body metabolizes and copes with these foreign estrogens is not exactly known. Yet in vitro studies have shown that Premarin metabolites damage the DNA of cells. This may be one reason why users of Premarin have an increased cancer risk.

Natural Hormones Available as Supplements

Currently, five natural hormones are available over the counter. This includes androstenedione, DHEA, melatonin, progesterone, and pregnenolone. All other hormones such as estrogen, testosterone, thyroid, and others, require a prescription from a doctor. Following is a summary of the hormones that are currently available as dietary supplements. Please note that we feel it is best to work with a knowledgeable doctor when using these hormones, instead of self-experimenting with them.

Androstenedione

Description: Androstenedione is a hormone that occurs naturally in the body. It is currently available as a supplement and is popular among bodybuilders and athletes. Studies have shown this hormone to increase testosterone levels in women. Studies with men have been mixed, with one showing an increase in estrogen and testosterone, and others showing an increase only in estrogen. Bodybuilders and other athletes also use similar hormones, known as androstenediol and norandrostenedione, but these have not been well studied.

Indications: It is indicated for menopausal or postmenopausal women with low estrogen or testosterone levels.

Precautions: Androstenedione and related supplements should be used only under a doctor's guidance. The National Football League has banned androstenedione and related substances.

Dosage: Take 100 to 300 mg daily.

DHEA (Dehydroepiandrosterone)

Description: DHEA is the most abundant hormone produced by the adrenal glands. It has several functions, including but not limited to supporting the body's reaction to stress, control of inflammation, libido, cognitive function, immune modulation, and metabolism. DHEA is a precursor hormone to testosterone and androstenedione.

Indications: Alzheimer's disease
Arthritis
Chronic fatigue syndrome

> Depression
> Diabetes
> Erectile dysfunction
> Heart disease prevention
> Immune support
> Inflammatory bowel disease
> Lupus
> Menopause
> Osteoporosis
> Prednisone withdrawal

Precautions: Too high a dosage may cause facial hair growth and acne breakout. Pregnant women and breastfeeding mothers should avoid using DHEA. People with existing cancers should also avoid it.

Dosage: A starting dose of 5 to 15 mg is recommended and is increased depending on the clinical situation and laboratory testing.

Melatonin

Description: Melatonin is a natural hormone produced in the pineal gland that regulates the body's biological clock and sleep cycles. Melatonin is produced in response to darkness. This hormone has been shown to be helpful for insomnia, seasonal affective disorder, and other mood disturbances. It has potent antioxidant properties and protects against radiation damage.

Indications: Aging
> Cancer (breast and prostate)
> Cluster headaches
> Insomnia
> Jet lag
> Radiation exposure
> Seasonal affective disorder
> Tardive dyskinesia

Precautions: Pregnant women or nursing mothers should avoid supplementing melatonin unless instructed to do so by their physician. People with cancer should also consult with their doctors first before supplementing melatonin. Children should not supplement melatonin unless instructed to do so by their doctors. People on steroid medications should avoid taking melatonin unless their doctors feel it is appropriate.

Dosage: Take 0.3 to 0.5 mg as the starting dosage for insomnia and jet lag.

Pregnenolone

Description: Pregnenolone is a steroidal hormone produced in large part by the adrenal glands. It is a precursor hormone that the body uses to manufacture DHEA and progesterone. Holistic doctors commonly recommend it for arthritis and autoimmune conditions such as lupus.

Indications: Arthritis (especially rheumatoid form)
> Depression
> Lupus erythematosus
> Poor memory
> Psoriasis

Precautions: Pregnenolone should be avoided by people who have seizure disorders or a history of hormone-related cancers.

Dosage: Take 10 to 50 mg daily.

Progesterone

Description: Progesterone is a hormone found in both men and women. For women, it is involved in regulating the menstrual cycle and reproductive function. Progesterone is mainly produced and secreted by the ovaries during ovulation. It is also manufactured by the adrenal glands, the brain, and the placenta in pregnant women. Natural progesterone cream is a popular supplement for the treatment of PMS, menopausal symptoms, endometriosis, and several other conditions.

Indications: Autoimmune conditions
Endometriosis
Fibrocystic breasts
Infertility (female)
Irregular menses
Menopausal symptoms
Osteoporosis
Ovarian cysts
PMS
Uterine fibroids

Precautions: Natural progesterone cream has a good safety record. Women with a history of cancer should consult a doctor before using it. Women using the birth control pill or synthetic progestin should avoid it.

Dosage: The dosage depends on the condition being treated (see the corresponding sections in this book, such as Premenstrual Syndrome or Menopause). Menopausal women generally apply a quarter teaspoon (20 mg) to their skin one to two times daily.

PRESCRIPTION NATURAL HORMONES

Most natural hormones, such as thyroid, testosterone, growth hormone, estrogen, and others, require a prescription. Holistic doctors generally prescribe these hormones with the help of a compounding pharmacy. Pharmacists at these specialized pharmacies are trained in formulating natural hormone prescriptions exactly to the requirement of each individual patient.

Testing Your Hormone Balance

Before using any of the natural hormones (or any hormones, for that matter), we recommend that you consult with a doctor to test your hormone levels. There are several ways that you can do this. They include blood tests, urine testing, and saliva testing. While all three methods have their strengths and weaknesses, we generally use saliva testing with our patients. Saliva testing offers an accurate, cost-effective, and convenient way to find out your hormone status.

References

1998. *Physician's Desk Reference,* 52nd Edition. Montvale, N.J.: Medical Economics Company, p. 311.

Pisha, E., et al. 2001. Evidence that a metabolite of equine estrogens, 5-hydroxy-equilenin, induces cellular transformation in vitro. *Chemical Research in Toxicology* 14(1): 82–90.

2002. Risks and benefits of estrogen plus progestin in healthy postmenopausal women: Principal results from the Women's Health Initiative Randomized Controlled Trial. *Journal of the American Medical Association* 288(3): 321–333

Bodywork

Since the dawn of humankind, bodywork has been used to heal people's injuries and illnesses and to promote relaxation. Bodywork refers to external therapies, applied to the outside of the body, that create relaxation and healing. The most common form of bodywork is massage. Almost everyone is familiar with massage, as it involves rubbing and pressing muscles and soft tissues. Yet many other forms of bodywork can help you prevent illness and recover from it. *Prescription for Natural Cures* includes specific recommendations in the areas of massage, acupressure, reflexology, craniosacral therapy, osteopathy, chiropractic, hydrotherapy, physiotherapy, magnet therapy, and others.

Healers have long realized that the external surface of the body can be used as a conduit or a reflex center to positively influence the internal organs. The body is a complex and intelligent network of muscles, soft tissues, and nerve structures that communicate with each other. A disruption or an imbalance in the soft tissues can lead to or contribute to an imbalance elsewhere in the body.

Everyone experiences injuries to the muscles, the bones, and the connective tissue many times in his or her life. In more serious cases, pharmaceutical medication may be required to treat severe pain and inflammation, but most cases require only stimulation of the body's healing mechanisms. Various forms of bodywork improve circulation and lymphatic flow, which allow the body's cells to detoxify and the tissues to recover from injury. Studies also show that bodywork enhances healthy immune cells that fight infection. An increasing number of people are turning to practitioners of bodywork to decrease the effects of stress on their bodies and minds.

The forms of bodywork described herein (and many others that are too numerous to mention) are very compatible with the dietary and nutritional supplements recommended in *Prescription for Natural Cures*. As a matter of fact, most people will do better with a synergistic combination of natural healing methods. Also, for people who need to use prescription drugs, bodywork is usually compatible with these and will speed the healing process. For a referral to various bodywork associations, please see the appendix—A Natural Health-Care Modalities and Resource Guide, on page 695.

Following are descriptions of the types of bodywork recommended in the conditions sections throughout the book.

Acupuncture/Acupressure

These therapies are based on the ancient Chinese medicine concept that the body contains twelve main channels of acupuncture/acupressure points. Through these channels runs the energy referred to as qi (pronounced *chee,* also written as "chi"). Disease arises when one or more of these channels (meridians) are blocked. Using needles (acupuncture) or pressing on specific points (acupressure) will reestablish energy flow and balance in the body. There are hundreds of acupuncture/acupressure points. Each point has one or more indications. Practitioners of Oriental medicine use acupuncture and acupressure in their practices.

Chiropractic

This is a system of healing based on the premise that poor spinal health (subluxations) leads to improper nerve flow and disease. Through specific adjustments of the spine and the extremities, one can restore spinal health and normal body function. Doctors of chiropractic are trained as primary health-care physicians.

Craniosacral Therapy

Craniosacral therapy is regarded as a gentle, noninvasive type of bodywork. The craniosacral system consists of the membranes and the fluid that surround and support the brain and the spinal cord. The craniosacral system extends from the bones of the head (cranium) down to the bones at the base of the spine (sacrum). The fluid within the membranes is continuously draining and refilling. The filling and draining create gentle, rhythmic, expanding and contracting movements that can be felt and monitored by a craniosacral therapist. The therapist then applies gentle manipulations to correct imbalances and reestablish proper fluid movement. Specific training is required to become a craniosacral therapist.

Hydrotherapy

Hydrotherapy is a type of bodywork that uses water as a healing agent to stimulate healing. It can involve water in the form of a liquid (such as a bath), a solid (ice), or a vapor (steam sauna). Various practitioners are trained in many forms of hydrotherapy.

Magnet Therapy

Magnets are used on or near the skin to positively influence the magnetic field of the body to stimulate healing. They have been shown to reduce pain and inflammation.

Massage

Massage is the therapeutic use of external pressure applied to the skin and the muscles of the body. Many different types of techniques are used by massage therapists.

Osteopathic Medicine

Osteopathy or osteopathic medicine is a system of medicine based on the premise that the bone structure (the spine and the extremities) is related to the internal health of the body. Osteopathic doctors may use spinal manipulation (osteopathic manipulative treatment) to help patients with musculoskeletal and systemic disorders. They are also trained in drugs and surgery, and they practice as primary-care doctors.

Physiotherapy

Physiotherapy is the use of external therapies to prevent and treat health conditions. It may involve the use of heat, cold, light, and physical and mechanical means to enhance healing within the body. Physiotherapists are health-care specialists trained in the use of physiotherapy. Many holistic doctors incorporate physiotherapy techniques and methods into their practices.

Reflexology

Reflexology involves the use of therapeutic pressure on the reflex points of the foot to enhance the innate healing mechanisms of the body. It is based on the premise that internal organs can be positively influenced by the proper application of pressure applied to specific reflex points on the hands and the feet. Many massage therapists are trained in reflexology.

Sinus (tips of toes)

Lymphs
(between toes, marked *)

Sinus (tips of toes)

Eyes

Ears

Chronic
Eyes/Ears

Liver

Gallbladder

Duodenum

Transverse
Colon

Ascending
Colon

Pituitary-Pineal

Thyroid-Parathyroid

Lungs

Spine

Solar Plexus

Adrenals

Kidneys

Waist

Hips

Small Intestine

Bladder

Spine

Sciatic Nerve

Tailbone

Eyes

Ears

Chronic
Eyes/Ears

Heart

Stomach

Pancreas

Transverse
Colon

Descending
Colon

Rectum

Sigmoid
Colon

Reflexology points

Exercise and Stress Reduction

You have heard the expression "Stress kills." There is some truth to this statement, although the way you perceive and respond to stress is more important. One crucial thing we can do as doctors and educators is to help people realize how stress is affecting their health and then recommend stress-reduction techniques to help people better handle their stress. In many instances, we have found that how patients handle stress makes all the difference between their healing or remaining ill.

Many people fail to see the connection between their health problems and how they handle their stress. Unfortunately, many doctors fail to see the connection as well. Research continues to show that how one handles stress is paramount to one's physical, mental, and emotional health.

The body responds to stress by releasing adrenal hormones, such as cortisol, DHEA, and other hormonal and neural chemicals, into the bloodstream. These "stress hormones" are powerful chemicals. When they are heightened or depressed for too long of a period of time, as a result of stress, a person becomes susceptible to disease. For example, high levels of cortisol are associated with an increased risk of Alzheimer's disease, diabetes, heart disease, certain cancers, and other serious illnesses.

The stress-reduction techniques in this chapter will help you to lessen the effects of stress on your body. Keep in mind that everyone is different, so you should choose the technique(s) that interest you most. As with anything, the more you practice them, the more helpful they will be in preventing and treating health problems. Many professionals in these areas can be of assistance.

You can use the following techniques to reduce the effects of stress and improve your health.

Deep Breathing

Proper breathing is key in reducing the effects of stress and improving your energy and concentration levels. Every time you breathe in, cells are replenished with oxygen that sustains life. When you breathe out, carbon dioxide and other toxins are released from the lungs. Numerous studies have shown that deep breathing relaxes the mind, calms the nervous system, improves mental focus, and improves energy.

When you look at a young child, you can observe the proper way to breathe. Children breathe from the belly, not the chest. This allows for maximal oxygen intake and carbon dioxide release, because the diaphragm comes into play. During deep breathing, this muscular covering over the top of the abdominal cavity has a massaging effect on the internal organs.

To deep breathe properly, you should first find a quiet, comfortable place. Stand or sit up straight, with your belly and chest relaxed. Breathe in through your nose slowly for a count of five, hold for two seconds, and then exhale through your mouth. Please note that when you inhale, your stomach, not your chest, should expand outward. This is how to assess whether you are breathing deeply and using your diaphragm. As you breathe out, your stomach should flatten.

Exercise

Exercise is one of the simplest and most underrated ways to reduce the effects of stress on the body. Few people would argue that exercise calms the mind, improves energy, and makes one more resilient to stress. Exercise has been shown in numerous studies to be very effective in reducing anxiety and depression, two conditions that millions of Americans deal with. Exercise also offers an opportunity to enjoy more social contact, which is healthful for the mind and the spirit.

One key we have found to long-term exercise commitment is choosing exercise(s) that you truly enjoy. Too many people join a local gym or begin an exercise regimen with a friend, but it is short lived since they really don't enjoy it. Think of a type of exercise that makes you excited enough to get out and do it. It may be something as simple as walking or biking, or it may be more involved, such as joining a gym or a sports team.

Before you begin a new exercise, get evaluated by your doctor. With all forms of exercise, start with a warm-up period, in which you loosen up and perform mild stretches. Then, after the activity, spend even more time stretching and cooling down to prevent injury and soreness. You should try to exercise a minimum of three times a week for twenty minutes. If you have not been physically active for a while, start with a lesser amount of time and gradually increase it every week. As long as you can recover from your exercise and do not remain stiff and sore for more than a day or two, you are on the right track.

Optimally, it is most beneficial to choose exercises that target the cardiovascular system (such as walking, biking, jogging, swimming, hiking, dancing, etc.), along with those that build lean muscle and bone density (weightlifting).

Laughter

A good laugh can go a long way toward reducing the effects of stress. Research shows that laughter prevents inflammatory triggers that lead to heart and artery damage, and it reduces the effects of stress. Research done at the University of Maryland School of Medicine found that laugher and a good sense of humor resulted in protection against heart disease. In this study, researchers evaluated the responses of three hundred people to potentially humorous situations. For example, one questionnaire asked how they would respond to a specific scenario that could cause a stress response, such as having a drink accidentally spilled on them by a waiter while dining with friends, or arriving at a party dressed in clothing identical to one of the other guests. People with the highest "humor scores" had a 48 percent lower risk of heart disease, independent of their age or sex. However, those with heart disease were much less likely to use humor as an adaptive mechanism.

Music Therapy

The human brain has been programmed to be responsive to music. Examine any culture throughout the world, and you are sure to find music being used as a way to relax and combat the effect of stress. Certain types of music induce a relaxation state. This, of course, depends on each individual's music interests. On the other hand, some types of music are stimulating and should be avoided when you are trying to achieve a relaxation response.

Prayer

The most powerful mind-body relaxation technique, in our opinion, is prayer. It offers an opportunity to communicate with the Creator and cast your doubts and cares upon Him. This is the time to "Be still" and hear from God. Make prayer a daily habit, and it will help you relax and achieve a more healthful life.

Progressive Muscle Relaxation

A popular technique to help people relax is to tighten and relax muscles throughout the body. People do not realize how tight their muscles are until they consciously tighten and relax them.

Starting by curling your toes and holding them tightened for three seconds, then relax them. Work your way up the body, focusing on how each muscle group feels as you tighten and relax it. This is a great technique for unwinding at the end of the day or reducing anxiety that is troubling you.

Tai Chi and Qigong

Tai Chi and Qigong are two aspects of Traditional Chinese Medicine that have become popular in the West as forms of exercise and stress reduction. They involve specific body movements and deep breathing. Videos and public classes are readily available to help you learn these two systems of movement and relaxation.

Visualization

The use of positive imagery is a potent tool in the war against stress. The visualization of positive images invokes a relaxation response. Find a quiet, comfortable place and visualize images that make you feel relaxed and content. You can also visualize yourself feeling relaxed and healthy.

Yoga

Yoga has become a popular way to relax the body. It involves deep breathing, stretches, and meditation. Take classes from a yoga instructor whom you are comfortable with. There are many different types of yoga, so research the styles to see what you prefer.

References: Stress Reduction and Exercise

Clark, A., A. Seidler, and M. Miller. 2000. Coronary disease and reduced situational humor-response: Is laughter cardioprotective? [Abstract] Presented at the 73rd Scientific Session of the American Heart Association, November 15th, New Orleans.

PART THREE

Appendix

A Natural Health-Care Modalities and Resource Guide

Acupuncture/Acupressure

These therapies are based on the ancient Chinese medicine concept that the body contains twelve main channels of acupuncture/acupressure points. Through these channels run the life-giving energy referred to as qi (pronounced *chee*, also written as "chi"). Disease arises when one or more of these channels (meridians) are blocked. Using needles (acupuncture) or pressing on specific points (acupressure) will reestablish energy flow and balance in the body. There are hundreds of acupuncture/acupressure points. Each point has one or more indications. Practitioners of Oriental medicine use acupuncture and acupressure in their practices.

American Oriental Bodywork Therapy Association
1010 Haddonfield-Berlin Road, Suite 408
Voorhees, NJ 08043
(856) 782-1616

American Association of Oriental Medicine
433 Front Street
Catasauqua, PA 18032
(610) 266-1433
www.aaom.org

Aromatherapy

The use of essential oils made from plants, leaves, bark, roots, seeds, and flowers can treat a wide range of conditions. Aromatherapists use essential oils that have specific properties to prevent or alleviate symptoms or conditions. The scents from these essential oils stimulate the healing mechanisms of the body.

The National Association for Holistic Aromatherapy
4509 Interlake Ave N., #233
Seattle, WA 98103-6773
888-ASK-NAHA
http://www.naha.org

Ayurvedic Medicine

Ayurveda is a Sanskrit word that is translated as "science of life" or "knowledge of how to live." Ayurveda is an ancient East Indian system of healing that seeks to promote balance through a healthful lifestyle and various natural healing methods. Ayurveda practitioners tailor treatments to each person's unique condition.

American Academy of Ayurvedic Medicine
100 Jersey Avenue
Building B, Suite 300
New Brunswick, NJ 08901
(732) 247-3301
www.ayurvedicacademy.com

Biofeedback

Biofeedback consists of information supplied instantaneously about an individual's own physiological processes. Data concerning cardiovascular activity (blood pressure and heart rate), temperature, brain waves, or muscle tension are monitored electronically and returned, or "fed back," to each person via a gauge on a meter, a light, or a sound. It has been shown that an individual can be taught to use biofeedback to voluntarily control the body's reactions to stress or "outside-the-skin" events. An individual learns through biofeedback training to detect his or her physical reactions (inside-the-skin events) and establish control over them. An example would be a child with anxiety who learns to calm his or her nervous system by using biofeedback. Clinical psychologists, counselors, and some health practitioners use biofeedback in their practices.

Biofeedback Certification Institute of America
10200 West 44th Avenue, Suite 310
Wheat Ridge, CO 80033
(303) 420-2902
http://www.bcia.org

Chelation Therapy

Chelation therapy is the use of certain agents or nutrients to help pull toxic substances out of the body (e.g., heavy metals such as lead). This can be done intravenously, with chelating agents, such as ethylenediaminetetraacetic acid (EDTA), or with oral agents (e.g., DMSA, or certain vitamins and minerals).

American College for Advancement in Medicine
23121 Verdugo Drive, Suite 204
Laguna Hills, CA 92653
http://www.acam.org

The American Association of Naturopathic
    Physicians
3201 New Mexico Avenue, NW Suite 350
Washington, DC 20016
Toll free: 1-866-538-2267
http://www.naturopathic.org

Chiropractic

This is a system of healing based on the premise that poor spinal health (subluxations) leads to improper nerve flow and disease. Through specific adjustments of the spine and the extremities, one can restore spinal health and normal body function. Doctors of Chiropractic are trained as primary health-care physicians.

American Chiropractic Association
1701 Clarendon Boulevard
Arlington, VA 22209
(703) 276-8800
www.amerchiro.org

Craniosacral Therapy

Craniosacral therapy is regarded as a gentle, noninvasive type of bodywork. The craniosacral system consists of the membranes and the fluid that surround and support the brain and the spinal cord. The craniosacral system extends from the bones of the head (cranium) down to the bones at the base of the spine (sacrum). The fluid within the membranes is continuously draining and refilling. The filling and draining create gentle, rhythmic, expanding and contracting movements that can be felt and monitored by a craniosacral therapist. The therapist then applies gentle manipulations to correct imbalances and reestablish proper fluid movement. Specific training is required to become a craniosacral therapist.

The Upledger Institute, Inc.
1211 Prosperity Farms Road, Suite D-325
Palm Beach Gardens, FL 33410
800-233-5880
www.upledger.com

Guided Imagery

This is the use of imaging techniques in one's mind to enhance health and well-being. Studies have shown a benefit to the immune system from guided imagery. For example, many people with cancer are taught to visualize their immune cells becoming active and fighting cancer cells. Clinical psychologists, counselors, naturopathic and medical doctors, and various health practitioners recommend guided imagery.

The Academy for Guided Imagery
30765 Pacific Coast Highway #369
Malibu, CA 90265
800-726-2070
www.healthy.net/agi

Herbal Medicine

Herbal medicine is the therapeutic use of plant extracts for the prevention and the treatment of illness. Herbalists and naturopathic doctors are trained extensively in the therapeutic uses of herbs as medicine.

American Botanical Council
P.O. Box 144345
Austin, TX 78714-4345
(512) 926-4900
http://www.herbalgram.org

Herb Research Foundation
1007 Pearl Street, Suite 200
Boulder, CO 80302
(303) 449-2265
www.herbs.org

Holistic Dentistry

Holistic dentistry refers to dentists who view the body as a whole. They utilize nontoxic materials whenever possible—for example, by avoiding the use of amalgam fillings.

Holistic Dental Association
P.O. Box 5007
Durango, CO 81301
http://www.holisticdental.org

Homeopathy

Homeopathy is a system of natural healing based on the premise that "like cures like." Homeopathic remedies are highly diluted medicines that stimulate the healing response of the body. Homeopaths, homeopathic doctors, and naturopathic doctors have had extensive training in this field.

National Center for Homeopathy
801 N. Fairfax St., Suite 306
Alexandria, VA 22314
(703) 548-7790
www.homeopathic.org

Homeopathic Academy of Naturopathic Physicians
12132 SE Foster Place
Portland, OR 97266
(503) 761-3298
http://www.naturopathic.org

Hydrotherapy

Hydrotherapy is a type of bodywork that uses water as a healing agent to stimulate healing. It can involve water in the form of a liquid (such as a bath), a solid (ice), or a vapor (steam sauna). Various practitioners are trained in many forms of hydrotherapy.

The American Association of Naturopathic Physicians
3201 New Mexico Avenue, NW Suite 350
Washington, DC 20016
Toll free: 1-866-538-2267
http://www.naturopathic.org

Massage

Massage is the therapeutic use of external pressure applied to the skin and the muscles of the body.

American Massage Therapy Association
820 Davis St., Suite 100
Evanston, IL 60201-4444
(847) 864-0123
http://www.amtamassage.org

Naturopathic Medicine

Naturopathic medicine is a system of natural medicine that focuses on working with the healing systems of the body. Naturopathic doctors are trained as primary health-care providers. As general practitioners, they work to restore health by using clinical nutrition, herbal medicine, homeopathy, physical medicine, counseling, nutritional supplementation, natural hormones, hydrotherapy, and other forms of natural healing. They are also trained in the use of pharmaceutical medicines and minor surgery.

The American Association of Naturopathic
    Physicians
3201 New Mexico Avenue, NW Suite 350
Washington, DC 20016
Toll free: 1-866-538-2267
http://www.naturopathic.org

Canadian Naturopathic Association
4174 Dundas St. W, Ste. 303
Etobicoke, Ontario
M8X 1X3 Canada
(416) 233-2924

Nutrition

The use of clinical nutrition means the therapeutic use of foods as medicine. Many practitioners of holistic and natural medicine use nutrition as the basis for their treatment.

Osteopathic Medicine

Osteopathy or osteopathic medicine is a system of medicine based on the premise that the bone structure (the spine and the extremities) is related to the internal health of the body. Osteopathic doctors may use spinal manipulation (osteopathic manipulative treatment) to help patients with musculoskeletal and systemic disorders. They are also trained in drugs and surgery, and they practice as primary-care doctors.

American Osteopathic Association
142 East Ontario Street
Chicago, IL 60611
(800) 621-1773 | (312) 202-8000
http://www.aoa-net.org

Physiotherapy

Physiotherapy is the use of external therapies to prevent and treat health conditions. Physiotherapy uses heat, cold, light, and physical and mechanical means to enhance healing within the body. Physiotherapists are health-care specialists trained in the use of physiotherapy. Many holistic doctors incorporate physiotherapy techniques and methods into their practices.

Reflexology

Reflexology involves the use of therapeutic pressure on the reflex points of the foot to enhance the innate healing mechanisms of the body. It is based on the premise that internal organs can be positively influenced by the proper application of pressure applied to specific reflex points on the hands and the feet. Many massage therapists are trained in reflexology.

Reflexology Association of America
4012 Rainbow Suite K-PMB #585
Las Vegas, NV 89103-2059
http://www.reflexology-usa.org

Yoga

The word *yoga* means "to join or yoke together," and this discipline is said to bring the body and the mind together. Yoga involves exercise, breathing, and meditation. There are many different types of yoga.

American Yoga Association
P.O. Box 19986
Sarasota, FL 34276
(941) 927-4977
http://www.americanyogaassociation.org

Glossary

absorption The process of assimilation, whereby nutrients are absorbed through the digestive tract and into the bloodstream, then into the body's cells.

acetylcholine A neurotransmitter that's involved in nerve-muscle activity and memory.

acidophilus A species of healthful or friendly bacteria found throughout the body, especially in the digestive tract.

acupressure The use of pressure and massage techniques along the meridians and at acupressure points to promote balance and good health.

acupuncture The use of needles inserted in specific spots along the body's meridians to relieve pain or create balance in the body.

acute illness An illness that may cause relatively severe symptoms but is of limited duration; a type of disease or disorder having a sudden onset, with severe symptoms, and generally a short or self-limited duration (such as a head cold or a sprain). The opposite of chronic.

adaptogen An agent, such as an herb, that helps the body adapt to various stressors, whether they be physical, mental, or emotional. Often referred to as a "tonic." Many adaptogen herbs work, in part, by supporting adrenal gland function. Ginseng is a classic example.

additive A substance added to food as a preservative to extend the shelf life or the nutritional value. They can be made from natural sources or synthetically.

adrenal glands A pair of glands situated above the kidneys that secrete the stress hormones epinephrine (adrenaline) and cortisol, as well as the sex steroids DHEA and pregnenolone.

aggravation When symptoms worsen for a short time after a patient begins a homeopathic or natural treatment. Also known as a healing crisis.

allergen A substance that provokes an allergic response.

allergy Hypersensitivity caused by a foreign substance, small doses of which produce a bodily reaction; an immune system response to a normally harmless substance, which can affect any of the tissues in the body.

alopecia Baldness, loss of hair.

alternative medicine Health care existing outside the established medical system—for example, herbalism, nutrition, chiropractic, naturopathic medicine, and so on.

amino acids The individual building blocks of protein. There are approximately twenty different amino acids. Ten of the amino acids are known as "essential amino acids," which means that our bodies cannot manufacture them, so it is essential that we consume them in our diets. The remaining ten nonessential amino acids can be manufactured in the body.

analgesic A substance that reduces or relieves pain.

anemia A blood condition in which there are too few red blood cells or the red blood cells are deficient in hemoglobin. The most common form of anemia is caused by iron deficiency, although B12 and folic acid anemias commonly occur as well.

aneurysm An enlarged dilated artery that results from a weakened artery wall.

antibiotics A substance (natural or synthetic) that destroys or reduces the growth of bacteria or fungi.

antibody A protein molecule made by the immune system that intercepts and neutralizes a specific invading organism or other foreign substance.

anticoagulant A substance that thins the blood. Used to avoid blood clots.

antigen A substance that can cause the formation of an antibody when introduced into the body.

antihistamine A substance that reduces or blocks the histamine response.

anti-inflammatory A substance that is used to relieve inflammation.

antimicrobial A substance or a treatment that destroys or neutralizes microorganisms (bacteria, virus, fungus, etc.).

antioxidants This refers to substances that neutralize or reduce the effects of cell-damaging free radicals. Common examples include vitamins A, C, and E and selenium.

antiparasitic A substance (natural or synthetic) that kills or reduces the growth of parasites.

antispasmodic Protects against muscle spasms.

aromatherapy The use of essential oils and other pure plant extracts to treat a variety of conditions through inhalation and/or absorption through the skin.

arrhythmias An abnormal or irregular heart rhythm.

atherosclerosis The most common type of arteriosclerosis, where fatty deposits accumulate within the blood vessel walls of medium and large arteries.

arteriosclerosis Hardening of the arteries created when plaque and calcium attach to the interiors of the arterial walls. This causes a loss in elasticity and flexibility of the artery, resulting in reduced circulation.

artery   A blood vessel through which blood is pumped from the heart to all the organs, glands, and other tissues of the body.

ascorbic acid   Refers to vitamin C.

aspartame   An artificial sweetener that is used as a sugar substitute.

autoimmune disease   One of several conditions where the immune system attacks and damages its own tissues. A common example is rheumatoid arthritis.

bacteria   Single-celled microorganisms. Some bacteria can cause disease; other ("friendly") bacteria are normally present in the body and perform such useful functions as aiding digestion and protecting the body from harmful invading organisms.

benign   Literally means "harmless"; it refers to cells, especially cells growing in inappropriate locations, that are not malignant (noncancerous).

bile   A greenish-yellow substance that the liver releases into the intestines; it assists in the digestion of fats, the elimination of toxins, and the absorption of fat-soluble vitamins.

biofeedback   Information supplied instantaneously about an individual's own physiological processes. Data concerning a person's physiological processes (blood pressure, heart rate, temperature, brain waves, muscle tension) are monitored electronically and returned to that person by a gauge on a meter, a light, or a sound. This information is used to help a person learn how to voluntarily control body reactions to stress or related events.

bioflavonoid   Biologically active flavonoids that act synergistically with vitamin C; they are not technically vitamins but are often referred to as vitamin P.

bitters   An herbal term for a substance that tastes bitter and stimulates stomach and digestive activity.

bronchi   The two branches of the trachea (windpipe) that transport oxygen to and carbon dioxide from the lungs.

bronchodilator   A substance that relaxes and dilates the airway passages.

candida   A fungus that normally inhabits the human body. Overgrowth of this organism can lead to a systemic infection, including immune system suppression, fatigue, and a multitude of other potential symptoms. Woman experience vaginal infections caused by candida.

Candida albicans   A type of fungus that normally inhabits the digestive tract and the body and results in systemic disease when it overwhelms the body's immune system.

capillaries   The smallest vessel that connects small arteries with small veins for the exchange of nutrients and waste products.

carbohydrate   A term that refers to a food compound that contains carbon and water molecules, which provides an energy source for the body.

carcinogen   A substance or an agent that is known to cause cancerous changes in the body.

cardiac   Refers to the heart.

carotenoids   A group of fat-soluble pigments (i.e., colors) found in plants or nutritional supplements that are known to have antioxidant properties.

cardiovascular disease   Disease of the heart and the blood vessels.

carrier oil   A pure plant oil, such as sweet almond oil, used to dilute essential oils for aromatherapy. Cold-pressed, unrefined oils are preferred.

cell   The smallest independently functioning unit in the structure of an organism.

cellulose   The indigestible portion of a carbohydrate (plant food).

cerebral   Refers to the brain.

cervical   Refers to the neck.

cervix   Refers to the portion of the vagina that connects to the uterus.

chelation therapy   The use of certain agents or nutrients to pull toxic substances out of the body; commonly used for toxic metals (e.g., lead, mercury, etc.).

chemotherapy   The use of chemical agents to treat disease—most commonly, cancer.

chiropractic   A system of healing based on the premise that poor spinal health (subluxations) leads to improper nerve flow and disease. Through specific adjustments of the spine and the extremities, one can restore normal health.

chlorophyll   A green plant pigment that's responsible for capturing the light energy needed for photosynthesis. It is used in natural medicine for detoxification, red blood cell support, and antioxidant properties.

cholesterol   A yellow, waxy substance that is necessary for life; an important component of cell walls. It is used to manufacture hormones and other life-giving substances.

chronic illness   When a patient experiences gradually eroding health associated with a long-term illness.

coenzyme   A substance that works with enzymes to activate a specific reaction in the body. For example, coenzyme Q10 is required for energy production within cells.

collagen   A protein matrix that holds connective tissue and skin together.

contagious   A disease or condition that is spread from one person or animal to another person.

craniosacral therapy   The use of gentle manual techniques to correct or balance the flow of fluid through the craniosacral system and relieve undue pressure on the brain and the spinal cord, resulting in a healthier nervous system.

CT scan (computerized axial tomography) A diagnostic image involving X-rays and a computer that allows for a three-dimensional picture inside of the body.

decoction The heating of herbs to make a tea.

dementia Refers to the deterioration or the impairment of mental functioning.

detoxification The process of eliminating toxins and waste products in the body.

diffusor A device used to spread essential oil molecules through the air. It may operate on electricity or with a heat source, such as a candle or a lightbulb.

digestion The chemical and physical process of breaking down and assimilating food.

digestive enzyme A supplement that acts as a catalyst in the breakdown of food.

diuretic A substance or a drug that increases the amount of urine flow.

DNA (deoxyribonucleic acid) A nucleic acid molecule that contains the "genetic blueprint" for protein synthesis and cell reproduction and is responsible for passing along hereditary characteristics from one generation to the next.

dysmenorrhea Refers to menstrual cramps or pain around the time of menses.

dyspepsia Indigestion.

dyspnea Shortness of breath.

edema A build-up of fluid in the tissues that results in swelling.

electrolytes Minerals that are required for body functioning, especially sodium, potassium, calcium, magnesium, and chloride. Electrolytes help to control fluid levels in the body, maintain normal pH levels, and ensure the transmission of nerve signals.

endorphin A substance produced in the brain that reduces pain.

enema The use of an aid to move the bowels and eliminate waste material. It involves the administration of water or a solution into the rectum.

enteric-coated Refers to a supplement that has a special coating on the exterior so that it does not become inactivated by stomach acid and can then be absorbed in the small intestines.

enzyme A protein produced by cells or taken in supplement form that acts as a catalyst for a specific biochemical reaction, such as digestion or energy production.

essential amino acids Amino acids are the individual building blocks of protein. There are approximately twenty different amino acids. Ten of the amino acids are known as "essential amino acids," which means that our body cannot manufacture them, so it is essential that we consume them in our diets.

essential fatty acids Fats that the body cannot manufacture and that are required by every cell in the body. The two essential fatty acids are alpha linolenic acid (ALA), of the omega-3 family, and linoleic acid (LA), from the omega-6 family.

essential oils A material that is present in plant cells and that is extracted by various physical processes and used in aromatherapy.

fat soluble Refers to something that dissolves in fats and oils. Fat-soluble vitamins require a source of fat for optimal absorption.

fermented food A biochemical process in which a microorganism breaks down a substance into a simpler one, using enzymes from bacteria, yeast, or molds. Examples of fermented foods include cheese and yogurt.

fiber The indigestible portion of plant food. It helps us to eliminate waste from the body.

free radicals Unstable, negatively charged molecules that are potentially damaging to the organs and the tissues of the body. They are formed by the normal process of energy production within cells, as well as from pollution, toxins, and radiation. Antioxidant enzyme systems within the body, as well as antioxidants from foods or supplements, protect against free radicals. Free radicals can also have beneficial properties, as part of the immune response to destroying microbes.

fungus A single-celled or multicellular organism that reproduces by spores and lives by absorbing nutrients from organic matter. Examples include mildews, molds, mushrooms, and yeasts.

gastrointestinal tract Refers to the stomach, the small intestine, and the large intestine.

genetic Refers to one's genes or inherited traits.

gland An organ or a group of cells that secretes substances such as hormones. Endocrine glands such as the thyroid are ductless and secrete directly into the bloodstream, while exocrine glands—for example, the salivary glands—secrete via ducts to a surface.

glucose A simple sugar that is the body's preferred fuel source.

gluten A protein combination found in many grains, such as wheat, spelt, barley, rye, and oats.

glyconutrients Food and supplements that contain some or all of the eight essential saccharides.

guided imagery The use of imaging techniques in one's mind to enhance health and well-being.

hair analysis A laboratory technique used to identify mineral balance and heavy metal toxicity from a person's hair.

heavy metal A metal with high relative density (relative density of 5.0 or higher) that is often toxic to humans. Examples include lead, mercury, copper, and cadmium. Also referred to as toxic metals.

hemoglobin The iron-containing portion of red blood cells that transports oxygen to cells.

hemorrhage Excessive or uncontrollable bleeding.

hepatic   Refers to the liver.

herbicide   A class of chemicals used to kill weeds.

histamine   A chemical released by the immune system (from mast cells) in response to an allergen, resulting in allergy symptoms (runny nose, watery eyes, sneezing, skin rash, etc.).

holistic   From the Greek term *holos,* for "whole." Pertaining to the "whole" person in mind, body, and spirit. Often used in the term *holistic medicine.*

hormone   A substance produced by an endocrine gland that regulates the function of cells and organs.

hydrogenation   A chemical process that uses hydrogen to turn liquid oils into solids. This results in trans-fatty acids that are harmful to the human body. Examples include margarine and shortenings.

hydrotherapy   A type of bodywork that uses water as a healing agent. It can involve water in the form of a liquid, a solid, or a vapor.

hypoallergenic   A substance that is unlikely to cause an allergic reaction.

hypoglycemia   Refers to low blood-sugar levels.

hypothalamus gland   Located in the brain and involved with the regulation of body temperature and other metabolic processes.

immune system   The body's complex defense system, which recognizes and protects against disease. It is also involved in the healing of damaged tissues. It's composed of a variety of white blood cells, the lymphatic system, and other specialized substances.

infection   The invasion and the proliferation of microorganisms within the body.

inflammation   The immune system's reaction to an illness, an irritation, or an injury that results in heat, pain, redness, and/or swelling.

infusion   The use of hot water to make an herbal tea.

insulin   A hormone that is secreted by the pancreas for the function of regulating blood-sugar levels by transporting glucose into the cells.

International Unit (IU)   A unit of potency for certain vitamins, such as A and E.

intolerance   An adverse but not life-threatening reaction to a food, a chemical, or another substance.

intravenous   Refers to the administration of drugs, nutrients, fluids, or other substances directly into a vein.

IU   See International Unit.

Lactobacillus acidophilus   Refers to "friendly bacteria" found throughout the digestive tract and other mucous membrane areas of the body. The bacteria are involved with digestion, vitamin synthesis, and immunity.

laxative   A substance that promotes bowel movements.

lesion   Abnormal tissue due to an injury, an infection, or a cancerous growth.

ligament   The connective tissue that connects bones to each other.

lignans   Plant substances that have hormone-balancing, cholesterol-lowering, and immune-enhancing properties. The lignans found in flaxseeds are a common example.

lipid   A group of compounds consisting of fats or oils; also used to describe cholesterol and triglycerides in medical terms.

liver   The primary filter for cleansing the blood. It metabolizes hormones, toxins, and other substances that enter the bloodstream and also stores carbohydrates, vitamins, and minerals.

lumbar   Refers to the lower back area.

lymph   Part of the lymphatic system, which carries lymphocytes and nutrients to cells and expels toxins.

lymph node   A small structure located in lymphatic vessels that produces white blood cells, known as lymphocytes, that fight infection and remove toxic debris.

magnetic resonance imaging (MRI)   A diagnostic image that uses electromagnetic radiation to obtain images of the body's soft tissues—for example, the brain and the spinal cord.

malignant   A medical term that refers to cancerous cells.

melatonin   A natural hormone produced by the body at night to promote sleep. It's also available in supplement form.

meridian   In Chinese medicine, a conduit that can be compared to an imaginary line (or a channel) linking points on the body's surface with internal organs, in which qi (chi) flows. Traditional Chinese medicine defines twelve main meridians and several supporting meridians. The surface points are used in acupuncture.

metabolism   The chemical and physical interactions taking place in the body that provide the energy and the nutrients needed to sustain life.

metabolite   A substance that is a by-product of metabolism.

mg   See milligram.

microgram (mcg)   A measure of weight equivalent to 1/1000 mg or one millionth part of a gram.

micronutrient   A substance, such as a mineral, that is required in minute amounts by the body.

microorganism   An organism that is not visible to the naked eye, such as a bacteria, a virus, a fungus, or a parasite.

milligram   A measurement of weight that is 1/1000 of a gram.

minerals   Inorganic substances that are important components of tissues and fluids. They are necessary for the proper functioning of vitamins, enzymes, hormones, and other metabolic activities in the body.

monosodium glutamate (MSG)   An additive commonly used to increase the flavor of foods. It is known to cause allergic reactions, such as headaches, in some sensitive individuals.

MRI   See magnetic resonance imaging.

MSG   See monosodium glutamate.

naturopathic medicine   A system of natural medicine that focuses on working with the healing systems of the body. Naturopathic doctors are trained as primary health-care providers. As general practitioners, they work to restore health by using clinical nutrition, herbal medicine, homeopathy, physical medicine, counseling, nutritional supplementation, natural hormones, hydrotherapy, and other forms of natural healing. They are also trained in the use of pharmaceutical medicines and minor surgery.

nerves   The body's complex wiring, which carries messages to and from the brain.

neural   Refers to the nerves.

neuralgia   Pain along a nerve.

neuropathy   A disease or a disorder that affects the nerves.

neurotransmitter   A chemical that carries messages between nerve cells of the brain and the nervous system.

nonsteroidal anti-inflammatory drugs (NSAID)   A class of drugs used to reduce pain and inflammation.

NSAID   See nonsteroidal anti-inflammatory drugs.

nucleus   The central part of the cell containing the DNA and the RNA (genetic information), which are necessary to control cell growth and reproduction.

nutraceutical   A natural substance that is usually of plant origin, which is taken as a dietary supplement for therapeutic use.

nutrition-oriented doctors   Doctors who place an emphasis on the role of nutrition with patients.

organic   A term used to describe foods grown without the use of artificial chemicals, such as pesticides, herbicides, or hormones.

oxidation   A chemical reaction between oxygen and another substance.

parasite   An organism that requires a host to receive nourishment. Certain parasites cause diseases in humans and animals.

parotid gland   A salivary gland located below each ear.

pathogen   Something that causes disease.

peristalsis   A series of wavelike muscle contractions that moves food and waste material through the digestive tract.

pH   A scale of measurement of the acidity or the alkalinity of a substance. The scale runs from zero to fourteen. A pH of seven is considered neutral, anything below seven is acidic, and values above seven are considered alkaline.

pharmacognosy   A study of the biochemistry and the pharmacology of plant drugs, herbs, and spices.

pharyngitis   Refers to a sore throat.

phytochemicals   See phytonutrients.

phytonutrients   These naturally occurring substances give plants their characteristic flavor, color, aroma, and resistance to disease. Thousands of phytonutrients have been identified in fruits, vegetables, grains, seeds, algae, and nuts. They have tremendous benefits for people because they help prevent and treat disease. They are also referred to as phytochemicals.

pituitary gland   An endocrine gland located at the base of the brain that controls growth, metabolism, and other glands in the body. The "Master Endocrine Gland."

placebo   A "sugar pill" or another inactive substance that helps researchers determine the effects of a drug or substance being tested.

platelets   Blood cells that are responsible for clotting.

prebiotic   A substance that assists in the formation of a probiotic. For example, fructooligosaccharides are a type of sugar that promotes the growth of the friendly bacteria *Lactobacillus acidophilus* and *Bifidobacterium*.

precursor   A substance required for another substance to be formed or utilized. For example, beta-carotene is a precursor for vitamin A, and DHEA is a precursor hormone that the body converts into testosterone.

preservative   Refers to an additive that extends shelf life or preserves color.

probiotic   A substance that contains friendly flora such as *Lactobacillus acidophilus* and *Bifidobacterium*.

proteolytic enzymes   Enzymes that break down protein when taken with food. They also have an anti-inflammatory effect when taken between meals.

protein   A nitrogen-containing compound found in plant and animal foods. The body uses protein as a fuel source and to form or repair tissues, organs, and muscles. Protein comprises enzymes and hormones and is found in every cell in the body. Amino acids are the individual building blocks of protein. There are approximately twenty different amino acids.

pustule   A small, raised lesion that usually contains white or yellow pus.

qi (chi)   In Chinese medicine, it is a reference to the body's vital energy.

radiation therapy   The use of radiation to treat certain types of cancers; also known as radiotherapy.

RDA   See Recommended Daily Allowance.

Recommended Daily Allowance (RDA)   The average daily dietary intake level that is sufficient to meet the nutrient requirement of nearly all (97 to 98 percent) healthy individuals in a group. In other words, the RDA is the amount of vitamins and minerals that a healthy person requires to stay healthy. This standard is regarded as woefully inadequate for optimal health by most nutrition-oriented doctors.

saturated fat   Refers to a fat that is full or "saturated" with hydrogen molecules. Saturated fats are semisolid to solid at room temperature. Examples include butter and lard. Dairy products and red meat products contain higher percentages of saturated fats than most foods. Too much saturated fat in the diet is associated with various diseases, such as arthritis and cancer.

sebaceous glands   Glands located in the skin that secrete sebum.

sebum   An oily lubricant secreted by the sebaceous glands of the skin. This lubricant is necessary for protecting the skin from the elements and for keeping it moist.

secondary infection   An infection that occurs after an initial infection. For example, a cold that turns into bronchitis.

sedative   Promoting sleep or a deep sense of relaxation.

sensitivity   An adverse but not life-threatening reaction to a food, a chemical, or another substance.

serotonin   A neurotransmitter that influences mood and sleep, as well as other mechanisms in the body.

simple carbohydrate   Refers to a carbohydrate that is broken down and absorbed quickly in the body. Examples include table sugar, honey, and fruit sugars.

steam inhalation   An aromatherapy technique that uses steamy water to carry essential oil molecules into the nose, the mouth, and the sinuses and into the body to heal. It's especially useful for respiratory ailments.

sublingual   A supplement that dissolves beneath the tongue, directly into the bloodstream.

systemic   Referring to the entire body.

tendon   Connective tissue that joins bones and muscles together.

thrombus   A blood clot.

tincture   A tincture, or liquid extract, is the preservation of herbs in water and alcohol.

tonic   A substance, such as an herb, that renews and supports the body as the body rebuilds its strength.

tonify   Strengthen and restore.

toxins   Any impure, poisonous substances that impair the body's functions.

trace element   A substance, such as a mineral, that the body requires in minute amounts. An example would be chromium.

trans-fatty acids   Harmful fatty acids that are formed during a chemical process that uses hydrogen to turn liquid oils into a solid.

triglyceride   A chemical compound formed from a molecule of the alcohol glycerol and three molecules of fatty acids. Triglycerides constitute many of the fats and the oils in the diet.

tumor   An uncontrolled growth of cells or tissues. Benign tumors are generally harmless, while malignant tumors can interfere with body functions or, in more advanced cases, cause death.

unsaturated fat   Fat that is liquid at room temperature. These fats come from vegetable oils. An example is olive oil.

urticaria   The medical term for hives.

uric acid   The by-product of protein metabolism. High levels are associated with gout and kidney stones.

vaccine   The administration of a substance to stimulate immunity to a particular disease.

vasoconstriction   The constriction of blood vessels, resulting in less blood flow.

vasodilation   The relaxation of blood vessel walls, resulting in increased blood flow.

venous return   Blood flow from the extremities through the veins back to the heart.

virus   A large class of parasitic structures, each of which consists of a nucleic acid core and a protein covering. A virus requires a host to replicate itself.

vitamin   A vitamin is an organic substance that is essential ("vital") for life. Most vitamins cannot be synthesized in the body and so must be attained through the diet or from supplements. Vitamins fall into two main groups. Fat-soluble vitamins require some amount of fat to be absorbed. They are also stored longer in the body. Common examples of fat-soluble vitamins include vitamins A, D, K, and E. The second major group of vitamins is termed water-soluble. These vitamins do not need fat to be absorbed and are excreted out of the body much more readily than fat-soluble vitamins are. Vitamin C and the B vitamins are water-soluble.

volatile oil   An easily evaporated oil. Essential oils are volatile oils. They evaporate and leave no oily residue.

water-soluble   A substance that dissolves easily in water.

white blood cells   Immune cells that prevent and fight against infection and tissue damage.

withdrawal   A period during which someone who is addicted to a drug or another addictive substance stops taking it, which results in uncomfortable symptoms.

yeast   A single-celled organism that can cause infection in the body.

Index

About the Authors

JAMES BALCH, M.D.

Dr. Balch has been a physician and a surgeon for over thirty-five years. A Certified Nutritional Consultant, a member of the American Medical Association, a Fellow in the American College of Surgeons, and a leading authority on integrative medicine and nutritional healing, Dr. Balch visits clinics worldwide, sharing his ideas with doctors of various health-care disciplines. He has written several books and has coauthored two best-selling books, including the well-known *Prescription for Nutritional Healing,* which has sold over 8 million copies. Dr. Balch also writes a monthly newsletter, *Prescription for Healthy Living.* He has appeared on ABC, Fox, and CBS, and has been interviewed on various national radio talk shows. He is the host of *Prescriptions for Healthy Living* radio show. Dr. Balch continues to produce publications that address a broad range of health and nutrition topics. He has lectured extensively across the United States, Canada, and overseas, encouraging patients to seek wise counsel in order to maintain good health and prevent disease, which he believes is wisdom in action.

MARK STENGLER, N.D.

Mark Stengler, N.D., is a licensed naturopathic doctor, an author, and a lecturer with expertise in nutrition, herbal therapy, vitamin therapy, homeopathy, natural hormones, and integrated medicine. He has served on a medical advisory committee for the Yale University Complementary Medicine Outcomes Research Project. Dr. Stengler received his doctorate from the National College of Naturopathic Medicine. He has also been an associate clinical professor at the National College of Naturopathic Medicine and at Bastyr University. Dr. Stengler is a member of the American Association of Naturopathic Physicians and the California Association of Naturopathic Physicians. He is the author of fifteen books, including the best-selling *Natural Physician's Healing Therapies.* Dr. Stengler is a contributing author for several health magazines and is the co-host of two weekly radio shows. Dr. Mark has been interviewed on dozens of television shows on Fox, CBS, and NBC, as well as for two PBS documentaries. He is the owner and the director of the La Jolla Whole Health Clinic in La Jolla, California. Visit Dr. Stengler's Web site, www.lajollawholehealth.com.